Anticoagulation, Hemostasis, and Blood Preservation in Cardiovascular Surgery

ROQUE PIFARRÉ, MD
Professor and Chairman
Department of Thoracic and Cardiovascular Surgery
Loyola University of Chicago Stritch School of Medicine
Maywood, Illinois

HANLEY & BELFUS, INC./Philadelphia
MOSBY/St. Louis • Baltimore • Boston • Chicago
London • Philadelphia • Sydney • Toronto

Publisher: HANLEY & BELFUS, INC.
Medical Publishers
210 South 13th Street
Philadelphia, PA 19107
(215) 546-7293
Fax (215) 790-9330

North American and worldwide sales and distribution:

MOSBY
11830 Westline Industrial Drive
St. Louis, MO 63146

In Canada: Times Mirror Professional Publishing Ltd.
130 Flaska Drive
Markham, Ontario L6G 1B8
Canada

**Anticoagulation, Hemostasis, and
Blood Preservation in Cardiovascular Surgery**   ISBN 1-56053-098-7

© 1993 by Hanley & Belfus, Inc. All rights reserved. No part of this book may be reproduced, reused, republished, or transmitted in any form or by any means without written permission of the publisher.

Library of Congress catalog card number 93-77761

Last digit is the print number: 9 8 7 6 5 4 3 2 1

To my wife Teresa
and
in memory of my teachers Charles A. Hufnagel
and Arthur M. Vineberg

CONTRIBUTORS

CHRISTOPHER P. CANNON, M.D.
Instructor in Medicine, Cardiovascular Division, Harvard Medical School; Associate Physician, Brigham and Women's Hospital, Boston, Massachusetts

JOSEPH A. CAPRINI, M.D.
Clinical Professor of Surgery, Northwestern University Medical School, Chicago, Illinois

JOY V. CUNNINGHAM, JD
Associate General Counsel, Office of the General Counsel, Loyola University of Chicago, Chicago, Illinois

SERAFIN Y. DeLEON, M.D.
Professor and Chief of Pediatric Cardiac Surgery, Department of Thoracic and Cardiovascular Surgery, Loyola University of Chicago Stritch School of Medicine, Maywood, Illinois

JAWED FAREED, Ph.D.
Professor of Pathology and Pharmacology, Loyola University of Chicago Stritch School of Medicine, Maywood, Illinois

JENNY E. FREEMAN, M.D.
Assistant Professor, Department of Thoracic and Cardiovascular Surgery/Pediatric Cardiac Surgery, Loyola University of Chicago Stritch School of Medicine, Maywood, Illinois

VALENTIN FUSTER, M.D., Ph.D.
Mallinkrodt Professor of Medicine, and Chief, Cardiac Unit, Harvard Medical School, Boston, Massachusetts

JOHN E. GODWIN, M.D.
Assistant Professor of Medicine, Division of Hematology/Oncology, Loyola University of Chicago Stritch School of Medicine, Maywood, Illinois

ROLF M. GUNNAR, M.D., FACP
Director of Medical Affairs, MacNeal Hospital, Berwyn, Illinois; Emeritus Professor of Medicine, Loyola University of Chicago Stritch School of Medicine, Maywood, Illinois

ALAN W. HELDMAN, M.D.
Fellow in Cardiology, Department of Medicine, The Johns Hopkins University School of Medicine, Baltimore, Maryland

DEBRA HOPPENSTEADT, M.S.
Department of Pathology, Loyola University of Chicago Stritch School of Medicine, Maywood, Illinois

LI-CHIEN HSU, Ph.D.
Baxter Scientist, Bentley Laboratories Division, Baxter Healthcare Corporation, Irvine, California

MAHER ISTANBOULI, CCP
Director, Loyola University School of Perfusion, Department of Thoracic and and Cardiovascular Surgery, Loyola University of Chicago Stritch School of Medicine, Maywood, Illinois

IK-KYUNG JANG, M.D., Ph.D.
Assistant Professor of Medicine, Harvard Medical School, Boston, Massachusetts

CONTRIBUTORS

PAOLO ARCIERI, M.D.

Department of Human Biopathology, Section of Hematology, Thrombosis Research Center, University of Rome "La Sapienza," Rome, Italy

WILLIAM R. BELL, JR., M.D., FACP

Edythe Harris Lucas-Clara Lucas Lynn Professor in Hematology, Professor of Medicine, Radiology, and Nuclear Medicine, Department Medicine, Division of Hematology, The Johns Hopkins University School of Medicine, Baltimore; Director, Special Coagulation Laboratory, The Johns Hopkins University Hospital, Baltimore, Maryland

RODGER L. BICK, M.D., FACP

Clinical Professor of Medicine, UCLA; Medical Director of Oncology and Hematology, Presbyterian Comprehensive Cancer Center, Presbyterian Hospital of Dallas, Dallas, Texas

BRADFORD P. BLAKEMAN, M.D.

Associate Professor, Department of Thoracic and Cardiovascular Surgery, Loyola University of Chicago Stritch School of Medicine, Maywood, Illinois

BARBARA BOCZKOWSKA-RADZIWON, M.D.

Department of Angiology, Center of Internal Medicine, J.W. Goethe University, Frankfurt, Germany

HANS KLAUS BREDDIN, M.D.

Professor of Medicine, Department of Angiology, Center of Internal Medicine, J.W. Goethe University, Frankfurt, Germany

JULIAN BREILLATT, PH.D.

Research Director, Applied Sciences, Baxter Healthcare Corporation, Round Lake, Illinois

BRIAN S. BULL, M.D.

Professor and Chairman, Department of Pathology and Laboratory Medicine, Loma Linda University School of Medicine, Loma Linda, California

MAUREEN H. BULL, M.D.

Associate Professor of Anesthesiology, Loma Linda University School of Medicine, Loma Linda, California

CHRISTIAN CABROL, M.D.

Consultant (Former Chief), Department of Cardiovascular Surgery, La Pitié Hospital, Paris, France

DAVID B. CALANDRA, M.D.

Assistant Professor, Department of Thoracic and Cardiovascular Surgery, Loyola University of Chicago Stritch School of Medicine, Maywood, Illinois

Chapter 22
Perioperative Antiplatelet Therapy and Management in Cardiovascular Surgery: Assessment of Bleeding Risk 317
*Thomas P. Lecompte, M.D., Pierre L. Julia, M.D.,
Simone Massonnet-Castel, M.D., and Michel Meyer Samama, M.D.*

Chapter 23
Anticoagulants for Peripheral Vascular Disease 327
*Hans Klaus Breddin, M.D., Piotr Radziwon, M.D.,
and Barbara Boczkowska-Radziwon, M.D.*

Chapter 24
Potential Use of New Thrombin Inhibitors and Low-Molecular-Weight Heparins as Anticoagulants in Cardiopulmonary Bypass Surgery 343
*Jeanine M. Walenga, Ph.D., Michael J. Koza, B.S., MT(ASCP),
and Roque Pifarré, M.D.*

Chapter 25
Antithrombotic Biomaterials for Cardiovascular Surgery 353
Julian Breillatt, Ph.D., and Li-Chien Hsu, Ph.D.

Chapter 26
Medicolegal Aspects of Blood Transfusions 363
Joy V. Cunningham, J.D., and Jill M. Rappis, J.D.

Index 381

Chapter 11
The Use of Desmopressin in Cardiopulmonary Bypass Surgery 167
G. Mariani, M.D., P. Arcieri, M.D., and F. Pizzo, M.D.

Chapter 12
Management of Patients with Acute Myocardial Infarction Who Require Cardiac Surgery after Failed Thrombolysis 177
Alan W. Heldman, M.D., and William R. Bell, Jr., M.D.

Chapter 13
Heparin-Induced Thrombocytopenia and Platelet Activation in Cardiovascular Surgery 185
Harry L. Messmore, M.D., Sucha Nand, M.D., and John Godwin, M.D.

Chapter 14
Monitoring of Platelet Function in the Cardiovascular Surgery Patient 201
Ricardo Manrique, M.D.

Chapter 15
Blood Utilization and the Role of the Transfusion Medicine Specialist in Cardiac Surgery 215
David B. Calandra, M.D., and Roland E. Lonser, M.D.

Chapter 16
The Use of Apheresis in Cardiac Surgery 225
John A. Robinson, M.D.

Chapter 17
Control and Treatment of Hemostasis in Patients with a Total Artificial Heart: The Experience of La Pitié 237
Jacques Szefner, M.D., and Christian Cabrol, M.D.

Chapter 18
Anticoagulation for Ventricular Assist Devices 265
A. Montoya, M.D., V.A. Lonchyna, M.D., and N. Moreno, M.D.

Chapter 19
Surgical Considerations for Postoperative Bleeding 271
Bradford P. Blakeman, M.D., and Henry J. Sullivan, M.D.

Chapter 20
Cardiopulmonary Bypass in Children: Current Strategies in Anticoagulation and Hemostasis 287
Serafin Y. DeLeon, M.D., Jenny E. Freeman, M.D., Kalavathi P. Shenoy, M.D., and Carlos R. Suarez, M.D.

Chapter 21
Antithrombotic Therapy in Patients with Substitute Heart Valves 301
Sheldon M. Kahn, M.D., FACP, and Rolf M. Gunnar, M.D., FACP, FRCP(E)

CONTENTS

Chapter 1
The Pharmacology of Anticoagulation 1
Christopher P. Cannon, M.D.

Chapter 2
Physiology and Pathology of Hemostasis During Cardiac Surgery 23
Rodger L. Bick, M.D., FACP

Chapter 3
Protocol for Anticoagulation During Cardiopulmonary Bypass 57
Roque Pifarré, M.D., Maher Istanbouli, C.C.P., and Jamal Sinno, C.C.P.

Chapter 4
Monitoring Systemic Anticoagulation in Cardiovascular Surgery 65
Clara I. Traverso, M.D., Ph.D., and Joseph A. Caprini, M.D., FACS

Chapter 5
**Blood Preservation in Cardiac Surgery
at Loyola University Medical Center** 77
Jeanine M. Walenga, Ph.D., and Roque Pifarré, M.D.

Chapter 6
Cardiopulmonary Bypass and the Salvaged Blood Syndrome 85
Brian S. Bull, M.D., and Maureen H. Bull, M.D.

Chapter 7
Antithrombotic Therapy in Cardiology and Cardiovascular Surgery 95
Ik-Kyung Jang, M.D., Ph.D., and Valentin Fuster, M.D., Ph.D.

Chapter 8
An Overview of Current Anticoagulant and Antithrombotic Drugs 111
*Jawed Fareed, Ph.D., Debra Hoppensteadt, M.S., MT (ASCP),
Jeanine M. Walenga, Ph.D., and Roque Pifarré, M.D.*

Chapter 9
**Effect of Aprotinin on Blood Loss and
Blood Use after Cardiopulmonary Bypass** 129
Kenneth M. Taylor, M.D., FRCS (Eng), FRCS (Glasg), FSA

Chapter 10
Controversies in the Practical Use of Aprotinin 147
David Royston, FFARCS

PIERRE L. JULIA, M.D.
Chief Resident, Cardiovascular Surgery, Broussais Hospital, Paris, France

SHELDON M. KAHN, M.D., FACP
Clinical Professor of Medicine, University of Illinois College of Medicine, Chicago; Attending Physician, Department of Medicine, MacNeal Hospital, Berwyn, Illinois

MICHAEL J. KOZA, B.S., MT(ASCP)
Department of Thoracic and Cardiovascular Surgery, Loyola University of Chicago Stritch School of Medicine, Maywood, Illinois

THOMAS P. LECOMPTE, M.D.
Maître de Conference des Universités, Department of Hematology, Hôtel Dieu University Hospital, Paris, France

VASSYL A. LONCHYNA, M.D.
Assistant Professor, Department of Thoracic and Cardiovascular Surgery, Loyola University of Chicago Stritch School of Medicine, Maywood, Illinois

ROLAND E. LONSER, M.D.
Director of Transfusion Medicine, and Chairman and Medical Director, Department of Pathology and Laboratory Medicine, Hinsdale Hospital, Hinsdale, Illinois

RICARDO MANRIQUE, M.D., PH.D.
Instituto Dante Pazzanese de Cardiologia, Hospital de Coracao, São Paulo, Brazil

GUGLIELMO MARIANI, M.D.
Professor of Hematology, Department of Human Biopathology, Section of Hematology, Thrombosis Research Center, University of Rome "La Sapienza," Rome, Italy

SIMONE MASSONNET-CASTEL, M.D.
Practicien Hospitalier, Hémobiologie, Broussais Hotel Dieu, Paris, France

HARRY L. MESSMORE, M.D.
Professor of Medicine and Pathology, Loyola University of Chicago Stritch School of Medicine, Maywood, Illinois

MICHEL MEYER SAMAMA, M.D.
Professor of Hematology, Hotel Dieu University Hospital, Paris, France

ALVARO MONTOYA, M.D.
Professor, Department of Thoracic and Cardiovascular Surgery, Loyola University of Chicago Stritch School of Medicine, Maywood, Illinois

NIBERTO MORENO, M.D.
Department of Thoracic and Cardiovascular Surgery, Loyola University of Chicago Stritch School of Medicine, Maywood, Illinois

SUCHA NAND, M.D.
Associate Professor of Medicine, Division of Hematology/Oncology, Loyola University of Chicago Stritch School of Medicine, Maywood, Illinois

ROQUE PIFARRÉ, M.D.
Professor and Chairman, Department of Thoracic and Cardiovascular Surgery, Loyola University of Chicago Stritch School of Medicine, Maywood, Illinois

FRANCESCO PIZZO, M.D.
Department of Human Biopathology, Section of Hematology, Thrombosis Research Center, University of Rome "La Sapienza," Rome, Italy

PIOTR RADZIWON, M.D.
Department of Angiology, Center of Internal Medicine, J.W. Goethe University, Frankfurt, Germany

JILL M. RAPPIS, J.D.
Assistant General Counsel, Office of the General Counsel, Loyola University of Chicago, Chicago, Illinois

JOHN A. ROBINSON, M.D.
Professor of Medicine/Microbiology and Associate Dean for Research, Loyola University of Chicago Stritch School of Medicine, Maywood, Illinois

DAVID ROYSTON, M.D., FFARCS
Consultant in Cardiothoracic Anaesthesia, Harefield Hospital, Harefield, Middlesex, United Kingdom

KALAVATHI P. SHENOY, M.D.
Assistant Professor, Department of Anesthesiology, Loyola University of Chicago Stritch School of Medicine, Maywood, Illinois

JAMAL SINNO, CCP
Co-Director, Loyola University School of Perfusion, Department of Thoracic and Cardiovascular Surgery, Loyola University of Chicago Stritch School of Medicine, Maywood, Illinois

CARLOS R. SUAREZ, M.D.
Associate Professor and Director, Section of Hematology/Oncology, Department of Pediatrics, Loyola University of Chicago Stritch School of Medicine, Maywood, Illinois

HENRY J. SULLIVAN, M.D.
Professor and Vice-Chairman, Department of Thoracic and Cardiovascular Surgery, Loyola University of Chicago Stritch School of Medicine, Maywood, Illinois

JACQUES SZEFNER, M.D.
Chief, Laboratory of Hemostasis, Cardiovascular Surgery Department, La Pitié Hospital, Paris, France

KENNETH M. TAYLOR, M.D., FRCS, FRCSE, FSA
British Heart Foundation Professor of Cardiac Surgery, Royal Postgraduate Medical School, and Head of Cardiothoracic Surgery, Hammersmith Hospital, London, England

CLARA I. TRAVERSO, M.D., PH.D.
Assistant Professor, Department of Surgery and Related Specialties, University of Granada School of Medicine, Granada, Spain

JEANINE W. WALENGA, PH.D.
Assistant Professor, Department of Thoracic and Cardiovascular Surgery and Pathology, Loyola University of Chicago Stritch School of Medicine, Maywood, Illinois

FOREWORD

Our current approach to the diagnosis and treatment of the hemostatic systems in cardiac surgery and mechanical circulatory support systems has profound effects on the morbidity and mortality associated with our operations and mechanical circulatory support systems. I do not doubt that if aprotinin were available in the United States, as it is in Europe in early 1993, thousands of liters of blood would be saved each week; the risk of blood-mediated infection would be considerably reduced; and surgeons would be more willing to offer operations associated with high risk for bleeding. I am equally convinced that if we used multisystem diagnosis and treatment, focused at the fibrinolytic, procoagulant, and platelet systems, we could better control the complications of devices placed in the bloodstream. Finally, having seen the great variability from patient to patient in the effects of "state of the art" therapy with aspirin and with warfarin, I am skeptical of these therapies unless they are closely controlled.

As a cardiac surgeon, I have "grown up" in an environment that is probably typical of many of my colleagues. There were, and are, only three clotting tests (PT, PTT, and platelet count) and two anticoagulants (heparin and warfarin). Aspirin has recently become recognized for its antiplatelet effects in many settings. We occasionally test for platelet function with the bleeding time or even more rarely with platelet aggregation studies. Armed with this small amount of information, we have done the full spectrum of open-heart procedures, implanting patches, grafts, valves, conduits, and devices. We have generally been self-sufficient. Few real experts in hemostasis are available and only a rare one has serious interest in cardiac surgery.

Perhaps my own naiveté is showing, but my impression is that we, along with our more learned consultants, understand only a small part of the hemostatic phenomena that we witness daily in the operating room and clinic. I think that we are just beginning to appreciate the complexity of the various homeostatic systems that are delicately balanced, preventing bleeding and thrombosis. As we learn more, perhaps we will be better at assessing and controlling the imbalances created by our therapies. Until then, we are obliged to spend many hours stopping the bleeding we have created, replacing units of blood, witnessing the tragedy of thromboembolism, and regretting the morbidity and mortality from each of these.

I congratulate Dr. Pifarre and the other authors of this book for bringing together a text that is useful, documenting what we know. It also stimulates us with new ideas and techniques. This book is a step toward better understanding and control of the hemostatic systems in cardiac surgery.

Jack G. Copeland, M.D.
Michael Drummond Distinguished Professor
of Cardiothoracic Surgery
University of Arizona College of Medicine
Tucson, Arizona

PREFACE

The discovery and clinical use of heparin made possible the initiation of extracorporeal circulation. The protamine neutralization of the effects of heparin, returning coagulation to normal, made possible the clinical application of cardiopulmonary bypass. With the advent of anticoagulation, extraordinary progress has been made in the past forty years in cardiovascular surgery and the surgical treatment of congenital defects, valvular lesions, and coronary artery disease and its complications.

The large surface of the extracorporeal circulation apparatus results in a massive thrombotic stimulus. The early reactions that lead to activation of the contact system of plasma proteins, white cells, fibrinolysis, platelets, and complement are not inhibited because heparin acts near the end of the coagulation cascade. The consequences of these early reactions are: potential bleeding, thrombotic complications, and inflammatory reactions associated with cardiopulmonary bypass. It is of paramount importance that cardiovascular surgeons have a clear understanding of the use of anticoagulant, hemostatic, and adjunct drugs with respect to their safety and efficacy in cardiovascular surgical procedures. Accordingly, the need for a text that provides current information on the subject was evident. The purpose of this book is to provide an updated review of the most important developments in blood anticoagulation and blood preservation and their application in cardiovascular surgery.

The AIDS crisis has made the public aware of the problem of transfusion-borne disease. Patients are afraid to receive banked blood. The use of autologous transfusion and cell-saver devices has become routine. All cardiovascular surgical teams are aware of the need for blood preservation, and new protocols (for blood preservation) are being implemented. Litigation over blood-related complications is not uncommon.

To my knowledge, this is the first time that a variety of specialists such as cardiovascular surgeons, cardiologists, hematologists, pharmacologists, anesthesiologists, pathologists, and attorneys have collaborated to present their expertise on this complex and very important topic. I would like to express my gratitude to the authors for their efforts and cooperation.

Roque Pifarré, M.D.
Editor

Chapter 1

The Pharmacology of Anticoagulation

Christopher P. Cannon, M.D.

Anticoagulation has become crucially important to the field of cardiac disease. Currently, anticoagulants and antiplatelet drugs are central to the treatment as well as the primary and secondary prevention of coronary artery disease.[33,44,52,53,58,68] In patients undergoing cardiac surgery, antiplatelet drugs improve coronary bypass graft patency,[55] and anticoagulants are of obvious importance in valve surgery.

Clinical pharmacology encompasses the major aspects of therapeutic actions of medicines: mechanisms of action, relationship between administration of a drug and its blood level, and ultimately the therapeutic (and untoward) effects.[3] These aspects are especially important in anticoagulation because the drugs have intricate interactions with several components of the clotting cascade rather than a single receptor. Each of the four basic areas of pharmacology—pharmacokinetics, pharmacodynamics, pharmacotherapeutics, and toxicology—has several determinants[4] (Table 1). Pharmacokinetics has been defined as what the body does to the drug and pharmacodynamics as what the drug does to the body.[3] The actual pharmacotherapeutic effect of the drug in prevention and treatment of disease is found in clinical practice. These effects must be balanced, however, by the toxicology of the drug. In combination, these factors establish the therapeutic window of a drug and its benefit/risk ratio in clinical practice.

This chapter reviews the clinical pharmacology of anticoagulants as they interact with components of the clotting cascade. General principles of pharmacokinetics and pharmacodynamics are discussed, followed by specifics for the major anticoagulants in current clinical use. The pharmacotherapeutic effects of anticoagulants are the focus of other chapters in this volume.

NORMAL HEMOSTASIS

Hemostasis consists of two interrelated stages, primary hemostasis and secondary hemostasis.[14,21] The first stage is initiated by platelets as they adhere to damaged vessels and form a platelet plug. The second phase involves

TABLE 1. Aspects of Clinical Pharmacology

Pharmacokinetics	Pharmacodynamics
Absorption	Mechanism of action
Route of administration	Physiologic effects
Bioavailability	Physiologic half-life
Distribution	Toxicology
Biotransformation	Side effects at therapeutic doses
Excretion	Effects at high doses
Half-life	Pharmacotherapeutics
Drug interactions	Effect of drug in preventing and treating disease
Inhibitors	Benefit/risk ratio

activation of the coagulation system: a series of inactive proteins (zymogens) are activated by proteolytic cleavage into active enzymes that ultimately cleave fibrinogen into fibrin to form a hemostatic clot.[62]

Primary Hemostasis

In normal blood vessels lined with endothelium, platelets circulate in the blood and do not interact with the vessel wall. In the presence of a damaged vascular site, platelets play the initial role in hemostasis by forming the platelet plug, a process that has three components: platelet adhesion, granule secretion, and aggregation.[21] Platelets adhere to the subendothelium principally by means of the glycoprotein (GP) Ib[21,22] (Fig. 1). The binding of platelets by GPIb is mediated by von Willebrand's factor (vWF), which is made by endothelial cells, circulates in the plasma, and binds to exposed collagen in the subendothelium.[22] It also plays a role in facilitating platelet–platelet cohesion and aggregation and stabilizes the attachment of platelets to the vessel wall under conditions of high shear stress.[29] Collagen (via platelet GPIa) and the adhesive proteins fibronectin, vitronectin, and thrombospondin also participate in the adhesion of platelets to subendothelium.[22]

Once platelets adhere to the wall, platelet activation and degranulation follow (Fig. 2). Platelet adhesion induces (1) the release of dense and α-granule constituents, including adenosine diphosphate (ADP), fibrinogen, vWF, fibronectin, vitronectin, thrombospondin, platelet factor 4, and others, and (2) the activation of platelet membrane phospholipase complex and generation of thromboxane A_2 (TxA_2), a potent vasoconstrictor and platelet agonist.[21,60] Under the influence of mediators such as ADP and TxA_2, additional circulating platelets are recruited to bind to the adherent monolayer, thus forming a platelet aggregate.[21,22]

Platelet Aggregation

The binding of ADP to the platelet receptor induces a change in the shape of the platelet and in the conformation of the GPIIb/IIIa receptor, which in turn binds fibrinogen.[21] Fibrinogen is an essential cofactor for platelet aggregation because it forms the bridge between platelets in the platelet plug[5] (Fig. 1). In the arterial system, where sheer stress is high, the platelet plug is central to the formation of a hemostatic clot.

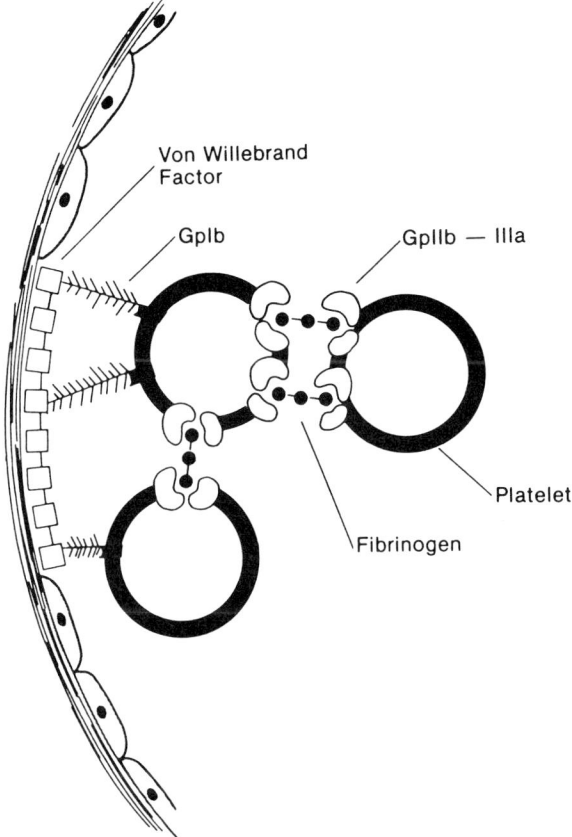

FIGURE 1. Mechanisms of platelet adhesion and aggregation. Von Willebrand's factor binds to exposed collagen of the vascular subendothelium, and platelets then adhere via glycoprotein Ib. This interaction stabilizes platelets so that they remain attached to the vessel wall despite the high sheer forces of arterial blood flow. Platelet–platelet aggregation takes place via the glycoprotein IIb/IIIa. Fibrinogen molecules link platelets together to form the hemostatic plug. (From Handin RI, Loscalzo J: Hemostasis, thrombosis, fibrinolysis, and cardiovascular disease. In Braunwald E (ed): Heart Disease, 4th ed. Philadelphia, W.B. Saunders, 1992, p 1768, with permission.)

Secondary Hemostasis

Simultaneously with formation of the platelet plug, the plasma coagulation system is activated: a series of plasma proteins become activated into catalytic enzymes that convert a second zymogen protein by proteolytic cleavage into an active enzyme. This process is frequently described as the fluid phase of coagulation; however, the majority of the reactions proceed on vascular subendothelium or on negatively charged, phospholipid-rich surfaces such as activated platelets or endothelial cells.[21]

Traditionally, the coagulation cascade has been divided into two pathways; the "extrinsic" or contact system and the "intrinsic" system. Recent evidence, however, has revised the understanding of coagulation into a single interrelated system.[6,43] The extrinsic pathway, initiated by release of tissue factor, is now

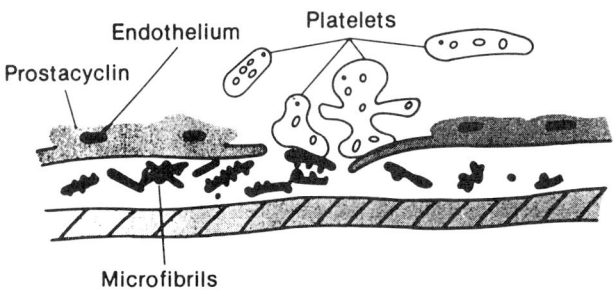

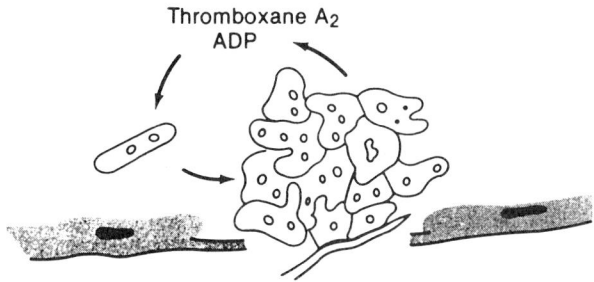

FIGURE 2. Primary hemostasis. The first event is platelet adhesion to vascular subendothelium. Platelets become stimulated to release their granule contents, including ADP, and to generate thromboxane A_2, which both recruit other platelets to form a platelet plug. (From Handin RI, Loscalzo J: Hemostasis, thrombosis, fibrinolysis, and cardiovascular disease. In Braunwald E (ed): Heart Disease, 4th ed. Philadelphia, W.B. Saunders, 1992, p 1770, with permission.)

believed to be the predominant mechanism for initiating hemostasis.[6,18] This view is consistent with the longstanding clinical observation that patients deficient in one of the contact factors that initiate the intrinsic pathway—factor XII (Hageman factor), high-molecular-weight kininogen (HMWK), or prekallikrein (PK)—do not bleed excessively. Ultimately, factor X is activated and leads to formation of thrombin, which in turn cleaves fibrinogen to fibrin.

Blood clotting is an autocatalytic process but also a self-limiting one.[62] One factor that controls clotting is localization of coagulation to the site of injury. Clotting interactions take place mainly on negatively charged surfaces, such as activated platelet membranes, activated endothelial cells, or other phospholipid surfaces.[21,62] Because the overall concentration of circulating coagulant factors in the bloodstream is relatively low, the binding or adsorption of clotting factors at the sites of injury increases the local concentration of clotting factors and helps to localize the process. One mechanism of localization is that six coagulation factors (factor VII, IX, X thrombin, and proteins C and S) contain residues of vitamin K-dependent γ-carboxylated glutamic acid, by which they can become fixed through calcium (Ca^{++})-bridges to negatively charged phospholipid membranes.[62] A second method of regulation of coagulation depends on a complex interaction of positive and negative feedback loops (Fig. 3). In addition, there are several inhibitors of the coagulation cascade, or natural anticoagulants.

Extrinsic Pathway. Under the current hypothesis, blood coagulation is principally initiated by tissue factor, an integral membrane protein made by tissue cells beneath the endothelial surface (e.g., fibroblasts and smooth muscle cells.)[6,18,39] When vascular cells are injured, tissue factor (also called tissue thromboplastin) is exposed and binds to factor VII, a glycoprotein synthesized by the liver that circulates in both its native and activated form.[6] The binding of tissue factor and factor VIIa forms a complex that activates factor X to Xa in the presence of phospholipid (activated platelets or endothelial cells) and calcium.[6] The extrinsic pathway can also be activated by tissue factor released from monocytes when they are stimulated by agents such as endotoxin, antigen-antibody complexes, or products of the complement system. This may be the mechanism of disseminated intravascular coagulation in sepsis and similar pathologic conditions.[21,38]

Clotting on Foreign Surfaces. The placement of foreign surfaces in contact with blood is a stimulus for thrombosis, but not by the pathway described, because neither tissue factor nor subendothelium is present in the metallic or synthetic materials used in cardiac surgery. Because they are negatively charged, however, these synthetic surfaces are ideal for initiation of the intrinsic or contact pathway.[62] Thus, although the extrinsic pathway appears to be the principal means by which coagulation is initiated in vivo at sites of damaged vessels, the intrinsic pathway is important in cardiac surgery because prosthetic materials are used either during perfusion on cardiac bypass or as valves or grafts in the patient.

Intrinsic Pathway. The intrinsic pathway is initiated by exposure of the vascular subendothelium or a foreign surface, which adsorb several clotting factors.[21,62] In plasma, HMWK and PK readily associate to form a noncovalent complex (Fig. 3). When the complex is adsorbed to a suitable surface, factor XII binds to the complex and is activated to factor XIIa. This complex in turn releases kallikrein and bradykinin, which accelerate the activation of factor XII.[21] Factor XI is then activated by surface bound factor XIIa. Factor XIa then activates factor IX to IXa, which feeds into the common pathway.[62]

Both the extrinsic and intrinsic pathways can activate factor X: the complex of tissue factor and factor VIIa can generate factor Xa, as can factor IXa in conjunction with factor VIII, Ca^{++}, and phospholipid (i.e., activated platelets or endothelial cells) (Fig. 3).[6,18,45] Factor VIII is not a proteolytic enzyme and has minimal activity until activation by trace amounts of thrombin.[21]

Connections Between the Two Pathways. Factor IXa can be generated from two sources: the intrinsic pathway, as discussed above, or the tissue factor-VIIa complex, which marks one of the several recently understood connections between the extrinsic and intrinsic pathways. Indeed, when the initial stimulus is the extrinsic pathway, two sources of factor IX activation must be present for normal hemostasis to occur.[6,18] Upon initial generation of factor Xa by the extrinsic pathway, an inhibitor of the tissue factor-VIIa complex (called the tissue factor pathway inhibitor [TFPI]) is stimulated immediately to inhibit the Xa-tissue factor-VIIa complex as it is formed, thereby preventing further generation of Xa (Fig. 3). Additional factor Xa must be produced by the generation of factor IXa via the TF-VIIa complex.[6]

Common Pathway. Once a sufficient amount is generated, factor Xa associates with factor Va, a nonenzymatic cofactor, again in association with Ca^{++} and phospholipids, to convert prothrombin to thrombin. This enzymatic cleavage releases prothrombin fragment 1.2, the measurement of which is a direct measurement in vivo of the generation of thrombin.[56]

Thrombin plays the central roles in coagulation.[22,23,62] The most important is cleavage of pairs of fibrinopeptides A and B from fibrinogen to form fibrin monomers, which then polymerize by weak hydrophobic and/or salt bridges into large fibrillar polymers (Fig. 3). The generation of thrombin leads to several positive feedback loops. First, thrombin activates factors V and VIII;[21] their generation leads to increased rates of activation of factor Xa. In addition, thrombin has been shown to activate factor XI, which feeds back into the extrinsic pathway.[6,42] In the final step of coagulation, thrombin activates factor XIII, which forms covalent bonds between the fibrin polymers (Fig. 3). These covalent bonds strengthen and stabilize the clot. Thus, the process of blood coagulation, with its many interrelated and positive feedback reactions, provides a rapid response to vessel injury and restores vascular integrity.

Natural Anticoagulants

Tight regulation of the coagulation cascade is needed, however, because the inactive clotting factors present in a single milliliter of blood are sufficient to clot the entire volume of blood within 15 seconds if no regulation existed.[21] The requirement for many of the clotting reactions to occur on suitable surfaces, such as subendothelium or activated platelets, limits reaction to the local area of vascular injury.[62] The natural anticoagulants, however, provide direct regulation of the activated clotting factors and thereby prevent the local clotting from becoming systemic.[21] The major natural anticoagulants are antithrombin III, protein C, protein S, and TFPI.

Antithrombin III. Antithrombin III is a serine protease inhibitor protein synthesized in the liver. Its major action is to bind to thrombin at its active site, thereby inhibiting its action. Under normal circumstances this binding occurs at a very slow rate; in the presence of heparin, the rate is enhanced 1000-fold.[46] Thrombin and antithrombin III bind tightly in a 1:1 stoichiometric complex: the active center of thrombin (serine) reacts with the reactive arginine center of antithrombin III[46,62] (Fig. 4). Heparin binds to a separate site on antithrombin III and thus acts as an allosteric catalyst for the interaction of thrombin and

---

FIGURE 3 *(facing page).* The clotting cascade, including recent findings of interactions between the two pathways of coagulation initiation. Blood coagulation is believed to be predominantly initiated by the extrinsic pathway by release of tissue factor, which binds to factor VII. The tissue factor/VIIa complex can activate factor X directly or activate factor IX, which then activates factor Xa. Clotting can also be initiated by the intrinsic or contact pathway, which is the major mechanism of clotting on foreign surfaces. Contact factors prekallikrein (PK) and high-molecular-weight kininogen (HMWK), when bound to a negatively charged surface, activate factor XII, which in turn activates factor XI, IX, and then X, thereby feeding into the common pathway. In the common pathway, factor Xa, in conjunction with factor Va, calcium, and phospholipid (activated platelet membranes or endothelial cells) cleaves prothrombin to thrombin. Thrombin is central to coagulation: its principle action is to cleave fibrinogen to fibrin, which then polymerizes to form a hemostatic clot. Thrombin also stimulates factor XIII, which acts to strengthen and stabilize the clot, and activates factors V and VII, thereby generating an autocatalytic reaction that generates more thrombin. (From Roberts HR, Lozier JN: New perspectives on the coagulation cascade. Hospital Pract Jan 15, 1992, p 74, with permission.)

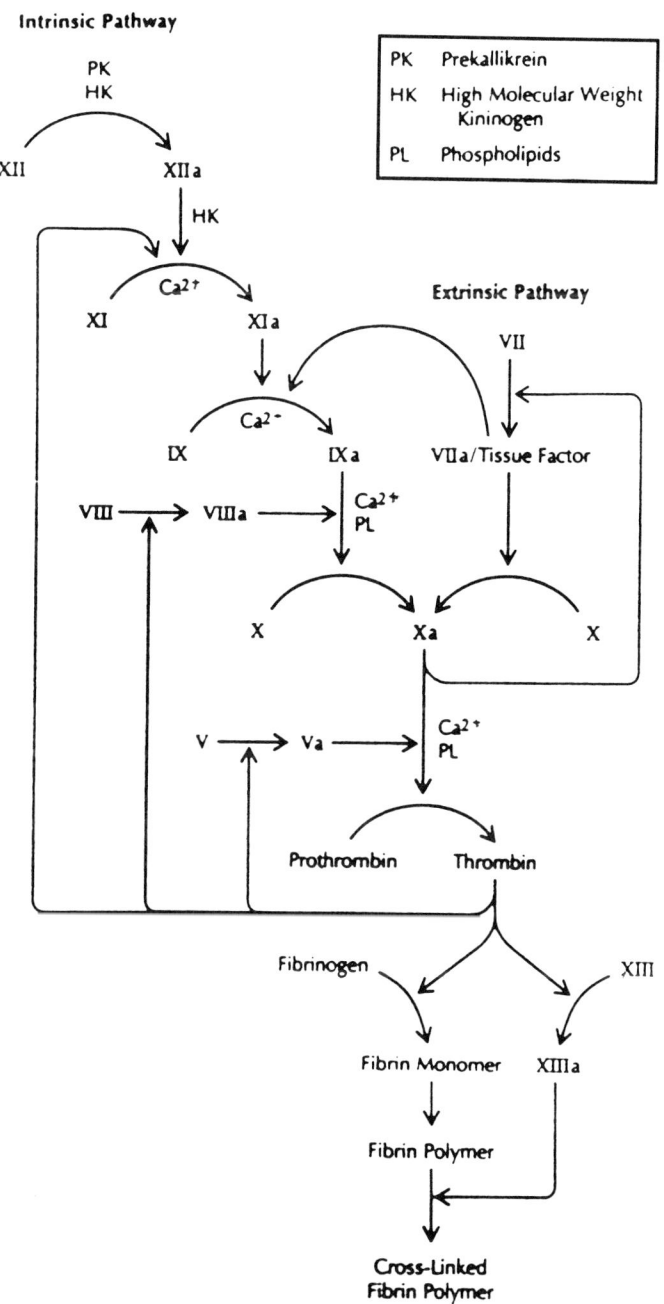

FIGURE 3.

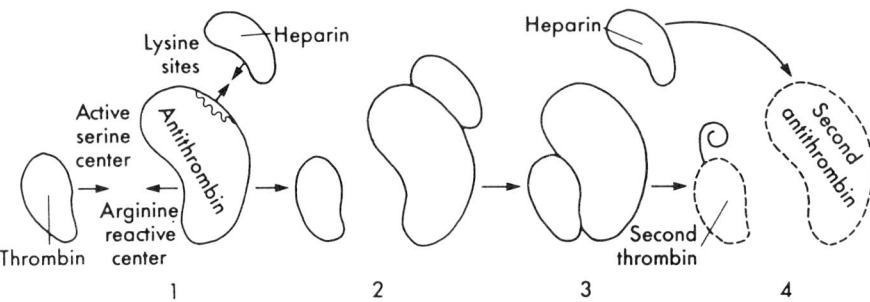

FIGURE 4. The mechanism of action of antithrombin III and its interaction with heparin. The arginine reactive center of antithrombin III binds to the serine at the active site of thrombin to form a permanent bond. Heparin acts as a catalyst for this reaction by binding to the lysine sites of antithrombin III, thus inducing a conformational change in the antithrombin III molecule and enhancing its inhibition of thrombin 1000-fold. Once the thrombin-antithrombin III complex is formed, heparin dissociates and is free to bind to a second antithrombin III molecule. (From Rosenberg RD: The heparin-antithrombin system: A natural anticoagulant mechanism. In Colman RW, Marder VJ, Salzman EW, Hirsh J (eds): Hemostasis and Thrombosis: Basic Principles and Clinical Practice. Philadelphia, J.B. Lippincott, 1987, p 1375, with permission.)

antithrombin III. Once the thrombin-antithrombin III complex is formed, heparin dissociates and can bind to additional molecules of antithrombin III, whereas the thrombin-antithrombin III complex is cleared by the reticuloendothelial system.

In normal hemostasis, antithrombin III is activated by binding to heparan sulfates, and glycosaminoglycans, which resemble heparin and line the surface of endothelial cells (Fig. 5).[21] Although the inhibition of thrombin is the most significant in the clinical setting, antithrombin III also inhibits several other coagulation factors (all serine proteases): factors XIIa, XIa, IXa, Xa, plasmin, and kallikrein.[25,26] Low-molecular-weight heparin's effect is based on inhibition of factor Xa by antithrombin III (see below).

Proteins C and S. A secondary regulatory system involves both proteins C and S, which are vitamin K-dependent proteins made in the liver. The intact endothelium contains a membrane protein thrombomodulin (Fig. 5). When thrombin binds to thrombomodulin, it activates protein C and simultaneously loses its affinity for fibrinogen. Activated protein C then inactivates factors Va and VIIIa, thereby slowing coagulation.[13] Protein S acts as a cofactor by increasing the rate of inhibition of Va and VIIIa by protein C.[65]

Tissue Factor Pathway Inhibitor. The recent rediscovery of TFPI, the third major inhibitor, has helped to revise the understanding of the clotting cascade. TFPI has also been termed the lipoprotein-associated coagulation inhibitor (LACI) or the extrinsic pathway inhibitor (EPI).[7,43] TFPI, a protein that circulates bound to lipoproteins LDL and HDL,[30] is known to inhibit both the VIIa/tissue factor complex and factor Xa. It can either form a quaternary complex with the VIIa/tissue factor/factor Xa complex or bind directly with factor Xa alone.[6] In the clotting cascade, TFPI inhibits the production of factor Xa generated by the extrinsic pathway, thus inhibiting coagulation more proximally than antithrombin III and protein C.[6]

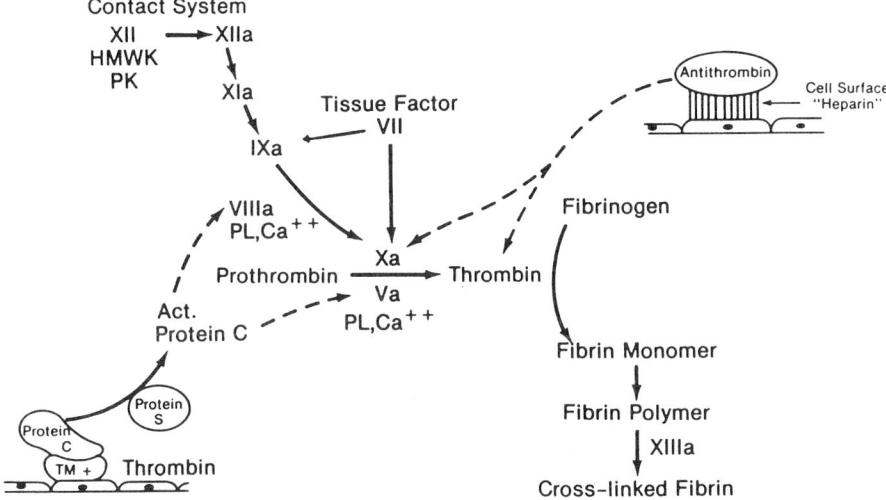

FIGURE 5. The clotting cascade, including several of the natural anticoagulants. Heparan sulfates are glycoproteins found on the endothelial cell surfaces and act as "cell surface heparin" to stimulate antithrombin III to inhibit thrombin and factor Xa. Protein C is activated when thrombin binds to thrombomodulin (TM). Activated protein C inhibits activated factors Va and VIIIa, a reaction which is speeded by protein S. Not shown: tissue factor pathway inhibitor (TFPI) can bind to either the tissue factor-VIIa-Xa complex or to factor Xa alone, thereby inhibiting the generation of thrombin. (From Handin RI: Bleeding and thrombosis. In Wilson J, et al (eds): Harrison's Principles of Internal Medicine, 12th ed. New York, McGraw-Hill, 1991, p 350, with permission.)

CLINICAL PHARMACOLOGY: GENERAL PRINCIPLES

All medications must be delivered to their target at a concentration that yields therapeutic efficacy within a range that does not generate toxicity or excessive effect. The desired range of an anticoagulant prevents thrombosis but does not result in uncontrolled bleeding.

Pharmacokinetics

Pharmacokinetics describes the interaction of the absorption of a drug, its distribution in body tissues, its biotransformation, and its excretion[4] (Fig. 6). In addition, inhibitors of the drug, as well as drug–drug interactions, are important in determining the overall effect. Finally, available antidotes to reverse the drug's effects, if needed, must be understood.

Absorption of a drug can be immediate, as with intravenous administration, or of longer duration, as with subcutaneous injection, whereby drug is slowly released from the subcutaneous tissues and reaches the bloodstream over a period of hours[64] (Fig. 7). With oral administration, bioavailability of the preparation indicates what percentage of the drug actually reaches the bloodstream. Bioavailability, which can vary greatly among preparations, is a potential hazard in changing from one brand of medication to another.

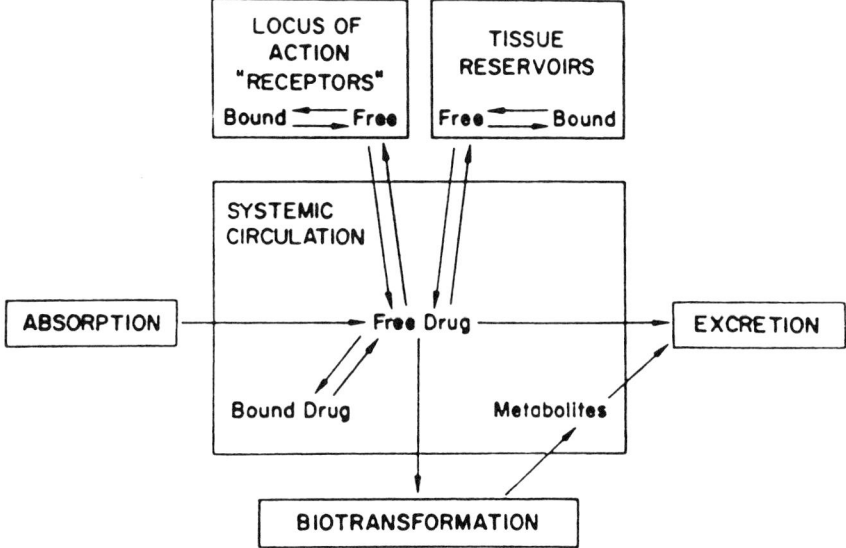

FIGURE 6. The many pathways a drug takes between absorption and excretion. (From Benet LZ, Mitchell JR, Sheiner LB: Pharmacokinetics: The dynamics of drug absorption, distribution, and elimination. In Gilman AG, Rall TW, Nies AS, Taylor P (eds): The Pharmacological Basis of Therapeutics. New York, Pergamon Press, 1990, p 3, with permission of McGraw-Hill.)

Once a drug has reached the bloodstream, it is distributed throughout the body and delivered to various organs[4] (Fig. 6). Relatively lipid-soluble drugs distribute extensively into fat stores, thus forming a reservoir in the body. Conversely, if a drug is highly bound to plasma proteins, it is maintained in the circulation. Some drugs can cross the placenta (e.g, warfarin), thus creating potential hazards to the fetus. Biotransformation is one mechanism by which the body processes drugs for excretion. A whole series of possible modifications are possible, including oxidation, hydrolysis, reduction, or conjugations, many of which are performed in the liver.[4] The drug metabolites are then eliminated, usually in the urine. Some medications are excreted unchanged in the urine (e.g., penicillin).

The ultimate goal of understanding these parameters is to determine a dosing schedule that delivers the appropriate amount of drug in a timely fashion and at a steady rate. The route of administration as well as loading and maintenance dosing can be determined for each medication, but frequently they differ with the clinical situation. To gauge the overall rate of elimination, the plasma half-life is frequently used in clinical medicine. The half-life is the time that it takes for plasma concentration of the drug to be reduced by 50% ($t_{1/2}$):

$$t_{1/2} = 0.693 \times Vd/Cl,$$

where Vd = volume of distribution and Cl = rate of clearance (Cl).[4] The faster the rate of elimination, the shorter the half-life. For drugs that distribute into the fatty tissues and thus have a large volume of distribution, the half-life is longer.

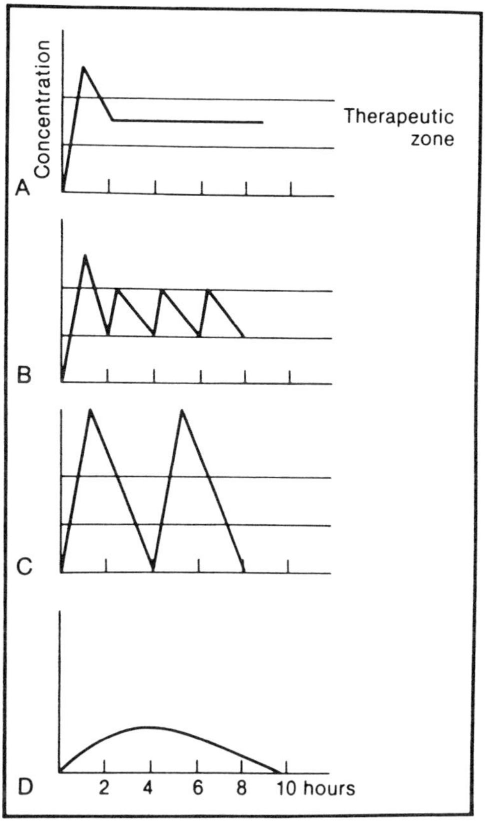

FIGURE 7. The pharmacokinetics of heparin after various routes of administration. The concentration of heparin in blood is shown after intravenous administration, a bolus followed by a constant infusion (*A*), after intermittent intravenous boluses (*B,C*), and after subcutaneous injection (*D*). (From Verstraete M, Vermylen J: Thrombosis. London, Pergamon Press, 1984, p 85, with permission).

Pharmacodynamics

Pharmacodynamics encompasses the mechanism of action of the drug and its physiologic effects (Table 1). For anticoagulants, the physiologic effects include both the desired therapeutic effects (resolution or prevention of thrombus formation), parallel effects that help monitor the medication (prolongation of activated partial thromboplastin time [APTT] or prothrombin time [PT]), as well as the undesired side effects, such as bleeding. Ultimately, based on clinical testing, the effect of the drug in preventing or treating disease is assessed with an overall benefit/risk ratio.

PHARMACOLOGY OF CURRENT ANTICOAGULANTS

Heparin

At present, heparin is the most widely used anticoagulant for cardiac surgery, venous thromboembolism, and coronary ischemic syndromes such as acute myocardial infarction and unstable angina. Heparin is an indirect anticoagulant: it achieves the majority of its effect by stimulating the natural anticoagulant antithrombin III to inhibit thrombin.[21]

Structure. Heparin is not a single molecule; it consists of a heterogeneous mixture of long polysaccharide chains, with repeating units of glucosamine and glucuronic acid.[26,61] These polysaccharide chains undergo a series of modifications, including sulfation and N-deacetylation, but these reactions are incomplete, leading to a wide variety of different molecules.[39,59,61] The anticoagulant activity of heparin is contained in a specific pentasaccharide sequence with several sulfate groups that bind to lysine sites on antithrombin III[12,47,48] (Fig. 4). Commercial preparations of heparin are heterogeneous mixtures of these mucopolysaccharides, with the molecular weights ranging from 3,000–30,000 (mean: 15,000).[26] Only one-third of the heparin is able to bind to antithrombin III; the remaining two-thirds have no significant anticoagulant activity at clinical concentrations.[26]

Mechanism of Action. The majority of heparin's anticoagulant activity is derived from its interaction with antithrombin III,[46] a circulating protein with an arginine center that binds to the active center serine of thrombin (and other coagulation factors) to form a covalent bond[19,59] (Fig. 4). Normally this reaction proceeds very slowly; however, heparin binds to lysine sites on antithrombin III and induces a conformational change at the arginine center of antithrombin III, thereby leading to 1000-fold acceleration of the enzyme-inhibitor complex formation.[46,61]

Heparin also acts as a template that helps bring thrombin in close proximity to antithrombin III[26,59] (Fig. 8). Thrombin then cleaves the reactive site bond of antithrombin III, to which it becomes covalently bound and thus is irreversibly inhibited.[59] The heparin-antithrombin III complex can also inhibit activated factors Xa, XIIa, XIa and IXa, although factor Xa, the next most susceptible to inhibition, is an order of magnitude less sensitive to inhibition than thrombin.[26,46,61] Heparin does not act as a template for the interaction of antithrombin III and factor Xa.[10] Thus smaller heparin molecules, such as low-molecular-weight heparin, are able to inhibit factor Xa but cannot inhibit thrombin.[61]

Pharmacokinetics. Heparin is not absorbed by the gastrointestinal tract and thus must be given parenterally.[39] Because there is no suitable chemical assay to measure drug level, investigation of the pharmacokinetics of heparin depends on measuring its pharmacodynamic effects on anticoagulation.[26] Although its onset of action is immediate with intravenous administration, the bioavailability and anticoagulant response with subcutaneous administration are quite variable.[35,39,59] The onset of action usually occurs between 20 and 60 minutes, but the peak level is not reached until 4–6 hours later[21,59] (Fig. 7). Its distribution in the body is largely intravascular, although, in the setting of open heart surgery, heparin appears to be liberated from fat stores upon rewarming of the patient.[1]

The elimination of heparin can be described by first-order kinetics, although the half-life appears to be dose-related.[26,41,59] In clinical doses, the half-life is between 60 and 90 minutes.[26,39,41,59] Heparin appears to be cleared and degraded primarily by the reticuloendothelial system, with small amounts excreted unchanged in the urine.[39,59] The half-life of heparin is shortened in acute pulmonary embolism[28] and prolonged in hepatic cirrhosis and endstage renal disease.[39,59] Because heparin does not cross the placenta, it is the drug of choice for anticoagulation during pregnancy.[26,59]

Many substances can inhibit heparin and may contribute to the variability in anticoagulant response seen in many patients, especially those with acute coronary thrombosis.[26,40] In vivo, many proteins can neutralize heparin,

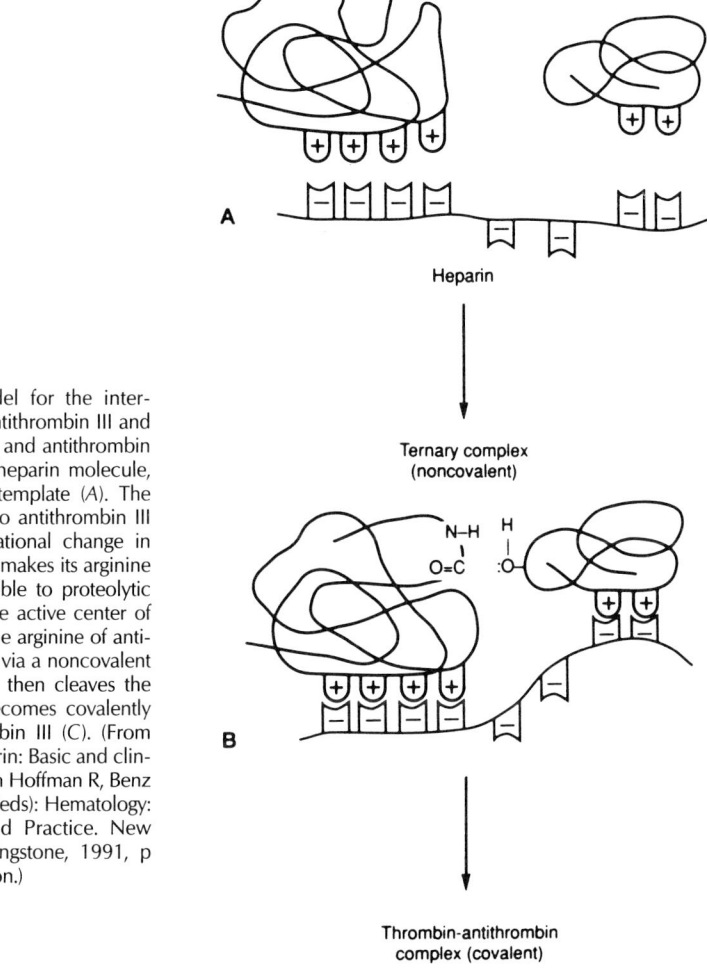

FIGURE 8. Model for the interaction of heparin, antithrombin III and thrombin. Thrombin and antithrombin III bind to a single heparin molecule, which serves as a template (A). The binding of heparin to antithrombin III induces a conformational change in antithrombin III and makes its arginine center more accessible to proteolytic attack (B). The serine active center of thrombin binds to the arginine of antithrombin III, initially via a noncovalent bond, but thrombin then cleaves the reactive site and becomes covalently bound to antithrombin III (C). (From Tollefsen DM: Heparin: Basic and clinical pharmacology. In Hoffman R, Benz EJ Jr, Shattil SJ, et al (eds): Hematology: Basic Principles and Practice. New York, Churchill Livingstone, 1991, p 1439, with permission.)

including platelet factor 4 (secreted by activated platelets), histidine-rich glycoprotein, and vitronectin.[26]

Antagonists. Protamine sulfate, a mixture of basic polypeptides isolated from fish sperm, is an effective antidote for heparin. It can be given intravenously and immediately binds to and neutralizes heparin.[59] Protamine also interacts with platelets, fibrinogen and other plasma proteins, so the dose given must approximate the amount of heparin in the patient at a ratio of 1 mg of protamine to every 100 U heparin.[39] Recombinant platelet factor 4 also can reverse heparin anticoagulation.[15] Drug-drug interactions with heparin are few; intravenous nitroglycerin, when given at high doses, has been reported to increase the requirement for heparin,[26] an effect which may be due to an alteration of the antithrombin III molecule.[2]

Toxicity. The most common side effect of heparin is bleeding. The risk of bleeding ranges from 1-33% of patients.[36] The risk increases with increasing total dose of heparin and with the degree of clotting parameter prolongation.[36] Use of aspirin has been reported to increase bleeding, notably postoperative bleeding in patients undergoing open-heart surgery.[51] Heparin and aspirin are widely used together, however, in the setting of percutaneous transluminal coronary angioplasty (PTCA) and the medical treatment of patients with acute coronary syndromes with acceptable rates of bleeding.[26,54,58]

Thrombocytopenia is a well-recognized side effect that presents in two forms.[59] In up to 25% of patients, mild thrombocytopenia occurs with 1-2 weeks of therapy, apparently due to platelet aggregation.[49,59] In these patients heparin can be continued without undue risk of bleeding.[59] In a small percentage of patients, severe thrombocytopenia occurs, with platelet counts falling below 50,000/dl, a process that appears to be mediated by immune mechanisms.[34,66] The platelet count usually returns to normal 4 days after discontinuation of heparin.[26,59,66] Acute arterial thrombosis has occurred in rare cases of heparin-induced thrombocytopenia.[66] Long-term administration of heparin has been associated with osteoporosis.[39]

Low-molecular-weight Heparin

Low-molecular-weight heparin refers to preparations that have been fractionated to contain molecules of heparin with a molecular weight <9000 daltons (mean: 4000-5000).[61] Many preparations exist, including Fragmin, Enoxaparin, Fraxiparine, CY 222, and ORG 10172.[61] All share the same basic principle: the heparin molecules with small molecular weights bind to antithrombin III but do not act as a template for thrombin; thus, their anticoagulant activity is based on inhibition of factor Xa.[10,61] However, only free factor Xa in the plasma is susceptible to inhibition by low-molecular-weight heparin; factor Xa that is bound to the platelet surface is not inhibited.[57] Because thrombin is not inhibited, the APTT is minimally prolonged.[32,61]

Low-molecular-weight heparin is eliminated more slowly than unfractionated heparin; its biological half-life is approximately twice as long as that of unfractionated heparin.[39,61] Low-molecular-weight heparin appears to interfere less with platelet function and may be associated with less bleeding than unfractionated heparin.[32,37]

Oral Anticoagulants

The vitamin K antagonists were discovered as a result of investigation of a hemorrhagic disease of cattle in the 1920s.[50] Of the currently available vitamin K antagonists, warfarin is the most widely used in North America[17,27] (Fig. 9). Warfarin is a racemic mixture of two active isomers, the R and S forms, which are present in roughly equal amounts.[27]

Mechanism of Action. Warfarin achieves anticoagulation by inhibiting the synthesis of vitamin K-dependent coagulation factors, including prothrombin, factors VII, IX, X, and proteins C and S.[17,27] These coagulation factors require vitamin K-dependent γ-carboxylation of their glutamic acid residues in order to retain functional activity.[17,27] Warfarin interferes with the cyclic conversion of vitamin K to its active epoxide, thereby reducing the amount of

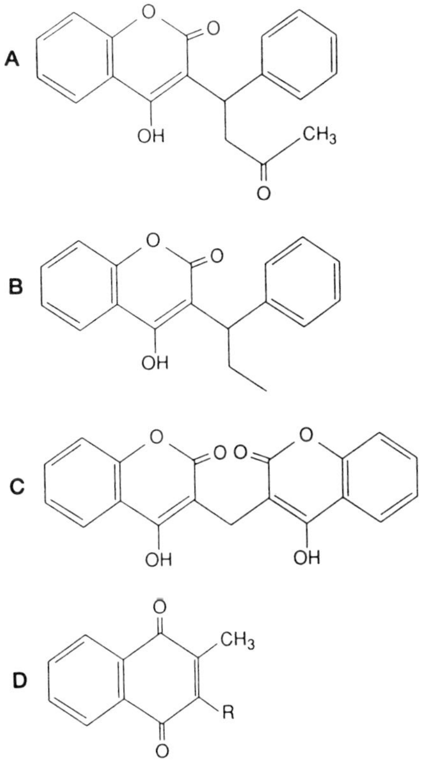

FIGURE 9. The structure of oral anticoagulants and their relationship to vitamin K. Warfarin (A), phenprocoumon (B), and dicoumarol (C) all share a similar ring structure to vitamin K (D). (From Furie B: Oral anticoagulant therapy. In Hoffman R, Benz EJ Jr, Shattil SJ, et al (eds): Hematology: Basic Principles and Practice. New York, Churchill Livingstone, 1991, p 1431, with permission.)

active vitamin K available to serve as a cofactor of γ-carboxylation.[17,21] Normal vitamin K-dependent coagulation factors normally contain 10–13 residues of γ-carboxylated glutamic acid; oral anticoagulants induce hepatic production of partially carboxylated factors.[27] Reducing the concentration of functional clotting factors in the bloodstream impairs coagulation.[21]

Pharmacokinetics. Warfarin is almost always used as an oral anticoagulant since perenteral administration does not alter the speed of its anticoagulant effect.[27,39] It is absorbed almost completely, with peak blood levels achieved after approximately 90 minutes.[27] Over 97% of warfarin circulates bound to albumin; only the free drug is biologically active. Warfarin is metabolized in the liver and kidneys into inactive metabolites excreted in the urine.[17,39] The plasma half-life of warfarin is between 36–42 hours.[17,27]

Pharmacodynamics. The pharmacodynamic anticoagulant effects of warfarin lag far behind, because warfarin inhibits the formation of new clotting factors and does not affect the plasma half-life of previously synthesized factors.[17] The disappearance of these clotting factors thus determines the onset of the anticoagulant effect. Factor VII disappears most rapidly, with a half-life of about 6 hours. Protein C has a half-life of 8 hours; factors IX and X, approximately 24 hours; and prothrombin, approximately 72 hours (Fig. 10).[17,39] Effective antithrombotic effects are not achieved until all the factors (VII, IX, X, and prothrombin) are reduced in concentration, which usually occurs 3–5 days after initiating therapy.[17,21]

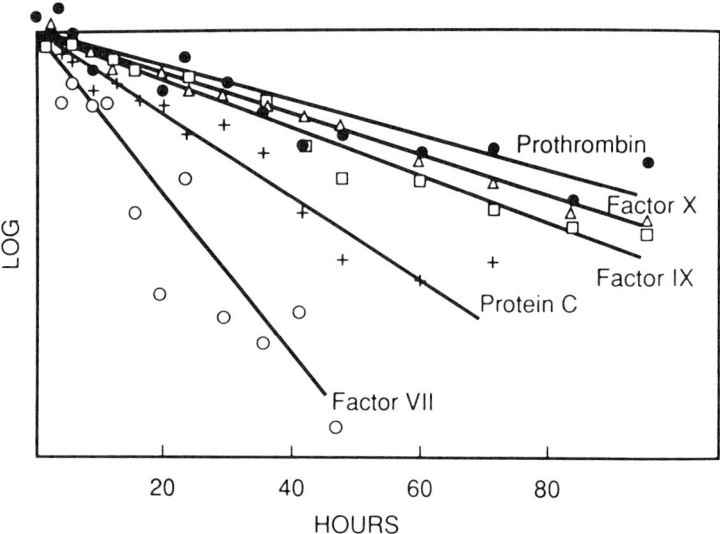

FIGURE 10. The decrease in activity of the vitamin K-dependent coagulation factors plotted on a log scale. Factor VII is the most sensitive to inhibition by vitamin K antagonists, disappearing with a half-life of approximately 6 hours, whereas factors IX, X and prothrombin activity disappear more slowly. Because the prothrombin time is so sensitive to the factor VII concentration, after initiation of warfarin therapy the prothrombin time can be disproportionately prolonged before the levels of factors IX, X, and prothrombin are reduced sufficiently to produce an antithrombotic effect. (From Furie B: Oral anticoagulant therapy. In Hoffman R, Benz EJ Jr, Shattil SJ, et al (eds): Hematology: Basic Principles and Practice. New York, Churchill Livingstone, 1991, p 1432, with permission).

TABLE 2. Drugs That Alter Prothrombin Time by Interacting with Warfarin, According to Type of Interaction

Pharmacokinetic (Drugs That Change Warfarin Levels)	Pharmacodynamic (Drugs That Do Not Change Warfarin Levels)	Mechanism Unknown (Drugs Whose Effect on Warfarin Levels Is Unknown)
Prolongs prothrombin time	**Prolongs prothrombin time**	**Prolongs prothrombin time**
Stereoselective inhibition of clearance of S isomer	Inhibits cyclic interconversion of vitamin K	Evidence for interaction convincing
Phenylbutazone	2nd- and 3rd-generation cephalosporins	Erythromycin
Metronidazole		Anabolic steroids
Sulfinpyrazone	Other mechanisms	Evidence for interaction less convincing
Trimethoprim–sulfamethoxazole	Clofibrate	
Disulfiram	Inhibits blood coagulation	Ketoconazole
Stereoselective inhibition of clearance of R isomer	Heparin	Fluconazole
	Increases metabolism of coagulation factors	Isoniazid
Cimetidine*		Piroxicam
Omeprazole*	Thyroxine	Tamoxifen
Nonstereoselective inhibitions of clearance of R and S isomers		Quinidine
		Vitamin E (megadose)
Amiodarone		Phenytoin
Reduces prothrombin time	**Inhibits platelet function**	**Reduces prothrombin time**
Reduces absorption	Aspirin	Penicillins
Cholestyramine	Other nonsteroidal anti-inflammatory drugs	Griseofulvin†
Increases metabolic clearance		
Barbiturates	Ticlopidine	
Rifampin	Moxalactam	
Griseofulvin	Carbenicillin and high doses of other penicillins	
Carbamazepine		

From Hirsh J: Heparin. N Engl J Med 324:1565–1574, 1991, with permission.
* Causes minimal prolongation of the prothrombin time.
† Has been proposed to cause increased metabolic clearance.

Variation in the anticoagulant response to a fixed dose of warfarin may be due to changes in dietary vitamin K, patient compliance, absorption from the GI tract (i.e., diarrhea), or various other factors. Alternatively, changes in laboratory reagents may alter the reported PT.[21,27] Recent improvements in the monitoring of warfarin therapy are covered in a subsequent chapter.

Drug Interactions. Many drugs interact with warfarin to alter its anticoagulant response (Table 2).[27] Drugs can either have a pharmacokinetic effect by affecting warfarin levels or alter the anticoagulant response by affecting other components of the clotting cascade.[27] Particular attention has been paid to the combination of aspirin and warfarin. Increased bleeding has previously been noted in trials when large doses of aspirin (1 g/day) are used in conjunction with high-intensity warfarin therapy.[11,16] Whether lower doses of aspirin can be used safely with warfarin is at present unproved but under investigation.

Antagonists. The effects of warfarin can be reversed by administration of vitamin K. However, the depleted clotting proteins need to be synthesized by the liver, leading to a delay of 12–24 hours before clotting parameters return toward normal.[17] More rapid reversal can be achieved by repletion of vitamin K-dependent clotting factors with fresh frozen plasma.[17]

Toxicity. Bleeding is the major complication of warfarin therapy. The reported incidence of bleeding ranges from 1–5% of patients/year.[21,27,52] The risk of bleeding is related to the intensity of anticoagulant therapy.[27] In addition, various risk factors for bleeding have been reported: age >65 years, history of stroke or gastrointestinal bleeding, atrial fibrillation, and other serious conditions, such as renal disease.[27] Reduction of the risk of bleeding has been noted with less aggressive regimens of anticoagulation, without reduction in antithrombotic effects.[27,31]

Warfarin-induced skin necrosis is a rare complication most commonly seen in patients with congenital deficiencies of protein C or S.[17] In such patients heparin should be administered for 4-5 days before warfarin.[17] Oral anticoagulants cross the placenta and have been associated with embryopathies, central nervous system abnormalities, or fetal bleeding in approximately one-third of patients.[20] For this reason, warfarin is avoided during pregnancy, and heparin is substituted.[27]

Anticoagulants of the Future

Numerous new anticoagulants are currently under laboratory and clinical investigation, some of which may soon be available.[63] Selective thrombin inhibitors, such as hirudin and hirulog, are more effective than heparin in inactivating clot-bound thrombin[67] and have shown promise in experimental models of thrombosis.[24] Preliminary results in patients have been favorable.[8,9] A review of the pharmacology of anticoagulation five years from now will likely include many new agents.

REFERENCES

1. Antman EM: Medical management of the patient undergoing cardiac surgery. In Braunwald E (ed): Heart Disease: A Textbook of Cardiovascular Medicine, 4th ed. Philadelphia, W.B. Saunders, 1992, pp 1670-1693.
2. Becker RC, Corrao JM, Bovill EG, et al: Intravenous nitroglycerin-induced heparin resistance: A qualitative antithrombin III abnormality. Am Heart J 119:1254-1261, 1990.
3. Benet LZ, Mitchell JR, Sheiner LB: Introduction. In Gilman AG, Rall TW, Nies AS, Taylor P (eds): The Pharmacological Basis of Therapeutics, 8th ed. New York, Pergamon Press, 1990, pp 1-2.
4. Benet LZ, Mitchell JR, Sheiner LB: Pharmacokinetics: The dynamics of drug absorption, distribution, and elimination. In Gilman AG, Rall TW, Nies AS, Taylor P (eds): The Pharmacological Basis of Therapeutics, 8th ed. New York, Pergamon Press, 1990, pp 3-32.
5. Bennett JS, Vilaire G, Cines DB: Identification of the fibrinogen receptor on human platelets by photoaffinity labeling. J Biol Chem 257:8049-8054, 1982.
6. Broze GJ Jr: The role of tissue factor pathway inhibitor in a revised coagulation cascade. Semin Hematol 29:159-169, 1992.
7. Broze GJ Jr, Warren LA, Novotny WF, et al: The lipoprotein-associated coagulation inhibitor that inhibits the factor VII-tissue factor complex also inhibits factor Xa: Insight into the possible mechanism of action. Blood 71:335-343, 1988.
8. Cannon CP, Maraganore JM, Loscalzo J, et al: Anticoagulant effects of Hirulog, a novel thrombin inhibitor, in patients with coronary artery disease. Am J Cardiol 71(in press), 1993.
9. Cannon CP, McCabe CH, Henry TD, et al, for the TIMI 5 Investigators: Hirudin reduces reocclusion compared to heparin following thrombolysis in acute myocardial infarction: Results of the TIMI 5 Trial. J Am Coll Cardiol 21(Suppl A):136A, 1993.
10. Casu B, Oreste P, Torri G, et al: The structure of heparin oligosaccharide fragments with high anti-(factor Xa) activity containing the minimal antithrombin III-binding sequence. Biochem J 197:599-609, 1981.
11. Chesebro JH, Fuster V, Elveback LR, et al: Trial of combined warfarin plus dipyridamole or aspirin therapy in prosthetic heart valve replacement: Danger of aspirin compared with dipyridamole. Am J Cardiol 51:1537-1541, 1983.

12. Choay J, Lormeau JC, Petitou M, et al: Structural studies on a biologically active hexasaccharide obtained from heparin. Ann NY Acad Sci 370:644-649, 1981.
13. Clouse LH, Comp P: The regulation of hemostasis: The protein C system. N Engl J Med 314:1298-1304, 1986.
14. Colman RW, Marder VJ, Salzman EW, Hirsh J: Overview of hemostasis. In Colman RW, Marder VJ, Salzman EW, Hirsh J (eds): Hemostasis and Thrombosis: Basic Principles and Clinical Practice, 2nd ed. Philadelphia, J.B. Lippincott, 1987, pp 3-17.
15. Cook JJ, Niewiarowski S, Yan Z, et al: Platelet factor 4 efficiently reverses heparin anticoagulation in the rat without adverse effects of heparin-protamine complexes. Circulation 85:1102-1109, 1992.
16. Dale J, Myhre E, Loew D: Bleeding during acetylsalicylic acid and anticoagulant therapy in patients with reduced platelet reactivity after aortic valve replacement. Am Heart J 99:746-752, 1980.
17. Furie B: Oral anticoagulant therapy. In Hoffman R, Benz EJ Jr, Shattil SJ, et al (eds): Hematology: Basic Principles and Practice. New York, Churchill Livingstone, 1991, pp 1431-1435.
18. Furie B, Furie BC: Molecular and cellular biology of blood coagulation. N Engl J Med 326:800-806, 1992.
19. Griffith MJ: Heparin-catalyzed inhibitor/protease reactions: Kinetic evidence of for a common mechanism of action of heparin. Proc Natl Acad Sci USA 80:5460-5464, 1983.
20. Hall JG, Pauli RM, Wilson KM: Maternal and fetal sequelae of anticoagulation during pregnancy. Am J Med 68:122-141, 1980.
21. Handin RI, Loscalzo J: Hemostasis, thrombosis, fibrinolysis, and cardiovascular disease. In Braunwald E (ed): Heart Disease: A Textbook of Cardiovascular Medicine, 4th ed. Philadelphia, W.B. Saunders, 1992, pp 1767-1789.
22. Harker LA: Pathogenesis of thrombosis. In Williams WJ, Beutler E, Erslev AJ, Lichtman MA (eds): Hematology, 4th ed. New York, McGraw-Hill, 1990, pp 1559-1569.
23. Heras M, Chesebro JH, Penny WJ, et al: Effects of thrombin inhibition on the development of acute platelet-thrombus disposition during angioplasty in pigs. Heparin versus recombinant hirudin, a specific thrombin inhibitor. Circulation 79:657-665, 1989.
24. Heras M, Chesebro JH, Webster MWI, et al: Hirudin, heparin and placebo during deep arterial injury in the pig: The in vivo role of thrombin in platelet-mediated thrombosis. Circulation 82:1476-1484, 1990.
25. Hirsh J: Mechanism of action and monitoring of anticoagulants. Semin Thromb Hemost 12:1-11, 1986.
26. Hirsh J: Heparin. N Engl J Med 324:1565-1574, 1991.
27. Hirsh J: Oral anticoagulant drugs. N Engl J Med 324:1865-1875, 1991.
28. Hirsh J, van Aken WG, Gallus AS, et al: Heparin kinetics in venous thrombosis and pulmonary embolism. Circulation 53:691-695, 1976.
29. Houdjik WPM, Sakariassen KS, Nievelstein PFEM, Sixma JJ: Role of factor VIII-von Willebrand factor and fibronectin in the interaction of platelets in flowing blood with monomeric and fibrillar human collagen types I and III. J Clin Invest 75:531-540, 1985.
30. Hubbard AR, Jennings CA: Inhibition of the tissue factor-factor VII complex: Involvement of factor Xa and lipoproteins. Thromb Res 46:527-537, 1987.
31. Hull R, Hirsh J, Jay R, et al: Different intensities of oral anticoagulant therapy in the treatment of proximal-vein thrombosis. N Engl J Med 307:1676-1681, 1982.
32. Hull RD, Raskob GE, Pineo GF, et al: Subcutaneous low-molecular-weight heparin compared with continuous intravenous heparin in the treatment of proximal-vein thrombosis. N Engl J Med 326:975-982, 1992.
33. ISIS-2 (Second International Study of Infarct Survival) Collaborative Group: Randomized trial of intravenous streptokinase, oral aspirin, both, or neither among 17,187 cases of suspected acute myocardial infarction: ISIS-2. Lancet 349-360, 1988.
34. King DJ, Jelton JG: Heparin-associated thrombocytopenia. Ann Intern Med 100:535-540, 1984.
35. Kroon C, ten Hove WR, de Boer A, et al: Highly variable anticoagulant response after subcutaneous administration of high-dose (12,500 IU) heparin in patients with myocardial infarction and healthy volunteers. Circulation 86:1370-1375, 1992.
36. Levine M, Hirsh J: Hemorrhagic complications of anticoagulant therapy. Semin Thromb Hemost 12:39-57, 1992.
37. Levine M, Hirsh J, Gent G, et al: Prevention of deep vein thrombosis after elective hip surgery. A randomized trial comparing low molecular weight heparin with standard unfractionated heparin. Ann Intern Med 114:545-551, 1991.

38. Lyberg T, Galdal KS, Evensen SA, Prydz H: Cellular cooperation in endothelial cell thromboplastin synthesis. Br J Haematol 53:89-95, 1983.
39. Majerus PW, Broze GJ, Miletich JP, Tollefsen DM: Anticoagulant, thrombolytic, and antiplatelet drugs. In Gilman AG, Rall TW, Nies AS, Taylor P (eds): The Pharmacological Basis of Therapeutics, 8th ed. New York, Pergamon Press, 1990, pp 1-2.
40. Maraganore JM, Bourdan P, Adelman B, et al: Heparin variability and resistance: Comparisons with a direct thrombin inhibitor. Circulation 86(Suppl I):I-386, 1992 [abstract].
41. McAvoy TJ: Pharmacokinetic modeling of heparin and its clinical implications. J Pharm Biopharm 7:331-354, 1979.
42. Naito K, Fujikawa K: Activation of human blood coagulation factor XI independent of factor XII: Factor XI is activated by thrombin and factor XIa in the presence of negatively charged surfaces. J Biol Chem 266:7353-7358, 1991.
43. Osterud B, Rapaport S: Activation of factor IX of the reaction product of tissue factor and factor VII. Additional pathway for initiating blood coagulation. Proc Natl Acad Sci USA 74:5260-5264, 1977.
44. Ridker PM, Manson JE, Gaziano JM, et al: Low-dose aspirin therapy for chronic stable angina. A randomized, placebo-controlled clinical trial. Ann Intern Med 114:835-839, 1991.
45. Roberts HR, Lozier JN: New perspectives in the coagulation cascade. Hosp Prac January 15:73-88, 1992.
46. Rosenberg RD: The heparin-antithrombin system: A natural anticoagulant mechanism. In Colman RW, Marder VJ, Salzman EW, Hirsh J (eds): Hemostasis and Thrombosis: Basic Principles and Clinical Practice, 2nd ed. Philadelphia, J.B. Lippincott, 1987, pp 1373-1392.
47. Rosenberg RD, Armand H, Lam L: Structure-function relationship of heparin species. Proc Natl Acad Sci USA 75:3065-3069, 1978.
48. Rosenberg RD, Lam LH: Correlation between structure and function of heparin. Proc Natl Acad Sci USA 75:1218-1222, 1979.
49. Salzman EW, Rosenberg RD, Smith MH, et al: Effect of heparin and heparin fractions on platelet aggregation. J Clin Invest 65:64-73, 1980.
50. Schofield FW: A brief account of a disease in cattle simulating hemorrhagic septicemia due to feeding sweet clover. Can Vet Rec 3:74, 1922.
51. Sethi HK, Copeland JG, Goldman S, et al: Implications of preoperative administration of aspirin in patients undergoing coronary artery bypass grafting. J Am Coll Cardiol 15:15-20, 1990.
52. Smith P, Arnesen H, Holme I: The effect of warfarin on mortality and reinfarction after myocardial infarction. N Engl J Med 323:147-152, 1990.
53. Steering Committee of the Physicians' Health Study Research Group: Final report on the aspirin component of the ongoing Physicians' Health Study. N Engl J Med 321:129-135, 1989.
54. Stein B, Fuster V, Halperin JL, Chesebro JH: Antithrombotic therapy in cardiac disease. An emerging approach based on pathogenesis and risk. Circulation 80:1501-1513, 1989.
55. Stein B, Fuster V, Israel DH, et al: Platelet inhibitor agents in cardiovascular disease: An update. J Am Coll Cardiol 14:813-836, 1989.
56. Teitel JM, Bauer KA, Lau HK, Rosenberg RD: Studies of the prothrombin activation pathway utilizing radioimmunoassays for the F2/F1+2 fragment and thrombin-antithrombin complex. Blood 59:1086-1097, 1982.
57. Teitel JM, Rosenberg RD: Protection of factor Xa from neutralization by the heparin antithrombin III complex. J Clin Invest 71:1383-1391, 1983.
58. Theroux P, Ouimet H, McCans J, et al: Aspirin, heparin or both to treat unstable angina. N Engl J Med 319:1105-1111, 1988.
59. Tollefsen DM: Heparin: Basic and clinical pharmacology. In Hoffman R, Benz EJ Jr, Shattil SJ, et al (eds): Hematology: Basic Principles and Practice. New York, Churchill Livingstone, 1991, pp 1436-1445.
60. Vermylen J, Badenhorst PN, Deckmyn H, Arnout J: Normal mechanisms of platelet function. In Harker LA, Zimmerman TS (eds): Clinics in Hematology. London, Saunders, 1983, pp 107-151.
61. Verstraete M: Heparin. In Messerli FH (ed) Cardiovascular Drug Therapy. Philadelphia, W.B. Saunders, 1990, pp 1457-1469.
62. Verstraete M: Biology and chemistry of thrombosis. In Haber E, Braunwald E (eds): Thrombolysis. Basic Contributions and Clinical Progress. St. Louis, Mosby-Year Book, 1991, pp 3-16.

63. Verstraete M: Novelties in antithrombotic and thrombolytic therapy: A latest update. In Fuster V, Verstraete M (eds): Thrombosis in Cardiovascular Disorders. Philadelphia, W.B. Saunders, 1992, pp 529-543.
64. Verstraete M, Vermylen J: Thrombosis. London, Pergamon Press, 1984.
65. Walker FJ: Regulation of activated protein C by a new protein: A possible function for protein S. J Biol Chem 255:5521-5524, 1980.
66. Warkentin TE: Heparin-induced thrombocytopenia. Annu Rev Med 40:31-44, 1989.
67. Weitz JI, Hudoba M, Massel D, et al: Clot-bound thrombin is protected from inhibition by heparin-antithrombin III but is susceptible to inactivation by antithrombin III-independent inhibitors. J Clin Invest 86:385-391, 1990.
68. Willard JE, Lange RA, Hillis LD: The use of aspirin in ischemic heart disease. N Engl J Med 327:175-181, 1992.

Chapter 2

Physiology and Pathology of Hemostasis During Cardiac Surgery

Rodger L. Bick, M.D., FACP

PHYSIOLOGY OF HEMOSTASIS

Mastering the basic physiology of hemostasis is important for many reasons, including interpretation of new testing modalities, appreciation of the enormously complex nature of hemostasis, and understanding of the novel and specific pharmacologic interventions now being used or explored for treating disorders of hemostasis and thrombosis.

The three hemostasis compartments (Fig. 1) are equally important[1,2]: (1) the platelets, which must be normal in both number and function; (2) the blood proteins, which include procoagulants, anticoagulants, and fibrinolytic proteins; and (3) the vasculature, which remains the last frontier and least understood of the three. These three compartments are intricately interrelated, and disturbances of delicately balanced interrelationships may lead to serious clinical consequences.[2]

Vascular Function

Normal vascular morphology consists of three discrete layers: the intima, media, and adventitia.[3-5] The intima has a monolayer of nonthrombogenic endothelial cells and an internal elastic membrane. The media has smooth muscle cells; its size varies with the type (arterial/venous) and size of the vasculature. The adventitia consists of an external elastic lamina or membrane and supportive connective tissue.

When endothelial sloughing occurs with the subsequent exposure of subendothelial collagen and basement membrane, platelets are immediately recruited to fill the gap.[2,6,7] Both subendothelial collagen and subendothelial basement membrane recruit platelets to form a primary hemostatic plug, thereby stopping blood from leaving the vascular compartment. As the primary hemostatic plug is formed, subsequent reparative events ensue. If

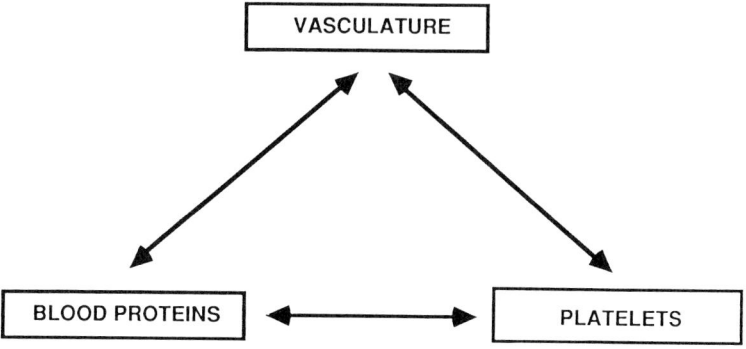

FIGURE 1. The three compartments of hemostasis.

endothelial damage occurs repeatedly in the same area over a protracted period of time, then as smooth muscle or other cells dedifferentiate and migrate into the intima of the vessel, compounds are released to attract macrophages, which ingest cholesterol and other materials. An atherosclerotic plaque eventually develops.[2,8]

Permeability, fragility, and vasoconstriction are properties of the vasculature.[2] Increased vascular permeability results in exit of blood from the vessel and manifests as petechiae and purpura or occasionally as large ecchymoses. If fragility increases, the vasculature may rupture, resulting in petechiae and purpura, especially in the integument and mucous membranes; large ecchymoses; and potential serious deep-tissue hemorrhage. If vasoconstriction is inappropriately intense, thrombus may form. Vasoconstriction is under local, neural, and humoral control. Also of importance are cellular interactions between the endothelium and other cells, including neutrophils and cells of the monocyte-macrophage system; these interactions are important not only in hemostasis, but also in mediation of inflammatory and immune responses.[9-11]

Platelet Function

The platelet consists of three primary zones: (1) a peripheral zone, (2) a sol-gel zone, and (3) an organelle zone.[12] The peripheral zone is an extramembranous glycocalyx that contains a plasma membrane, similar to any other trilamellar cellular plasma membrane. Under the plasma membrane is an open canalicular system. The sol-gel zone contains microtubules and microfilaments as well as a dense tubular system that transports adenine nucleotides and calcium. In the sol-gel zone is found the contractile platelet protein, thrombosthenin, which is similar to actomyosin. The organelle zone consists of dense bodies, alpha granules, mitochondria, and many other organelles found in other cellular systems, including lysosomes and endoplasmic reticulum. Alpha granules contain fibrinogen and lysosome enzymes, whereas dense bodies contain and release adenine nucleotides, serotonin, catecholamines, and platelet factor 4.[13-16] Table 1 summarizes factors necessary for normal platelet function.

Many stimuli will induce a platelet release reaction,[17-20] including subendothelial collagen and basement membrane. Other potent inducers are

TABLE 1. Factors Necessary for Normal Platelet Function

Adequate number of platelets (>100,000 mm^3)	Adequate cationic proteins
Adequate energy metabolism	Adequate membrane receptors and responsiveness
Adequate number and contents of storage granules	Adequate divalent cations (Mg^{++} and Ca^{++})
	Adequate physical conditions (pH, temperature)
Adequate storage granule release	

thrombin, soluble fibrin monomer, fibrinogen degradation products (especially fragment X), endotoxin, circulating antigen-antibody complex, gammaglobulin-coated surfaces, various viruses, adenosine diphosphate (ADP), catecholamines, and free fatty acids.[21-24]

As platelets become activated, they contract and form pseudopods. During contraction the many intraplatelet compounds and granules are concentrated at the center of the platelet. At the same time the platelet organelles, including alpha granules and dense bodies, are concentrated at the center of the platelet, where organelle membranes disrupt. Their contents are released and transported outside the platelet via the open canalicular system. These compounds then interact with platelet membrane receptors of adjacent platelets, causing further platelet activation in a type of amplifying process by which numerous platelets become activated.[2] In addition, many of these compounds may interact with adjacent endothelium. Pseudopod formation enhances platelet-surface interactions (adhesion) and platelet-platelet interaction (cohesion).[2]

Figure 2 presents a summary of platelet function. The first process that occurs during platelet activation is platelet adhesion,[2] which refers to a platelet's adhering to something other than another platelet; for example, a glass bead, other artificial surface, or collagen/basement membrane. Early release of intraplatelet ADP follows platelet adhesion. This reversible process, called primary (reversible) aggregation, accounts for the primary wave on an aggregation pattern. As the concentration of ADP increases, platelet cohesion occurs. Platelet cohesion refers to platelets adhering to other platelets. As this occurs, more and more ADP, as well as other compounds (including serotonin), are released. These compounds not only activate adjacent platelets but also induce vascular constriction to prepare for an effective primary hemostatic plug or primary platelet/fibrin clot. During this increased reaction, when the ADP concentration reaches a critical point, an irreversible conformational change in the platelet membrane takes place, making available platelet factor 3 (platelet membrane phospholipid-type activity). This material serves as a primary surface in mediating the formation of complexes in the coagulation protein sequence. The sequence of platelet cohesion, increased release reaction, and conformational changes leading to the availability of platelet factor 3 is an irreversible process and accounts for the secondary wave seen on a platelet aggregation pattern.[2] In vivo, the final result is the formation of a platelet/fibrin plug, or primary hemostatic plug, the function of which is rendered most efficient by vasoconstriction induced by compounds released from platelets.

Platelet and endothelial cell membrane phospholipids are converted into arachidonic acid by the enzyme, phospholipase A$_2$,[25-27] which is activated by both thrombin and collagen and inhibited by dipyridamole. Arachidonic acid is converted into prostaglandin intermediates, prostaglandin G$_2$ (PGG$_2$), and

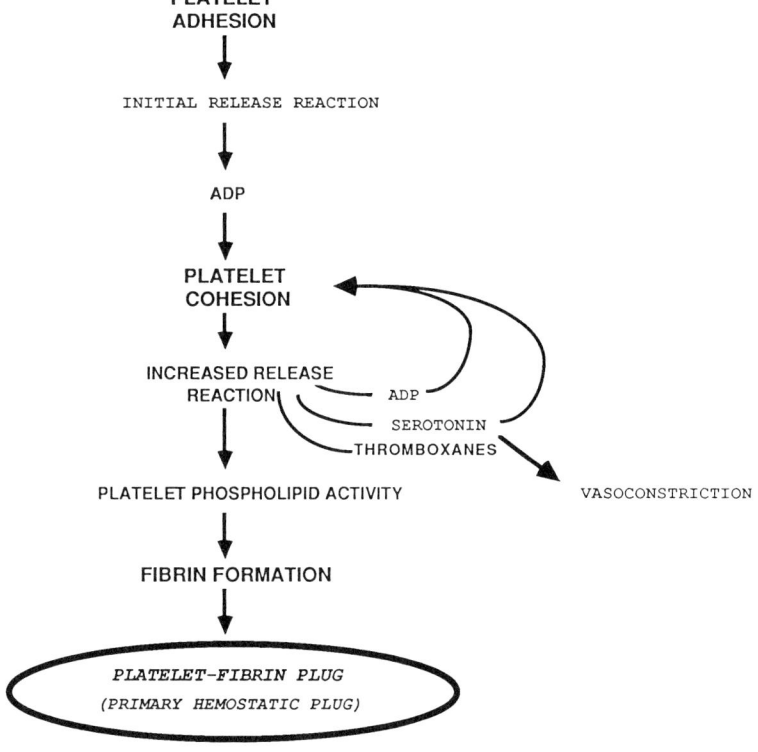

FIGURE 2. Simplified platelet function.

prostaglandin H_2 (PGH_2) by the enzyme cyclooxygenase. In the platelet membrane thromboxane synthetase converts PGH_2 into thromboxane A_2, one of the most potent aggregating agents described.[2] Thromboxane A_2 also has potent vasoconstricting activity. In the endothelial cell, and in some subendothelial muscle cells, prostacyclin synthetase converts PGH_2 into prostacyclin, a potent inhibitor of aggregation as well as a potent vasodilator.[28-30] Prostacyclin is being assessed in clinical trials for thromboembolic and vasoocclusive disease.[31,32] Cyclooxygenase is inhibited by aspirin and sulfinpyrazone, two popular antiplatelet agents.[2,33] Thromboxane A_2 is a potent inhibitor of adenylate cyclase, and prostacyclin is a potent stimulator of adenylate cyclase. Therefore, the presence of bleeding or thrombosis may depend on the relative concentrations of these two compounds.

Platelet interactions with the vasculature (adhesion) and with other platelets (cohesion), as well as plasma protein reactions, occur at the platelet membrane surface; these many interactions are mediated by various platelet membrane glycoproteins (PMGPs).[34]

Plasma Protein Function

Plasma protein function in hemostasis involves numerous systems, the five most important of which are depicted in Table 2: (1) the coagulation protein system, (2) the fibrino(geno)lytic system, (3) the kinin system, (4) the

TABLE 2. Blood Protein Function: The Five Interactive Systems

Coagulation protein system	Kinin system
Fibrinolytic enzyme system	Inhibitors of the first four systems
Complement system	

complement system, and (5) the inhibitors for the first four systems.[2] Kinin generation and complement generation (activation) are often not appreciated as important participants in thrombohemorrhagic disorders. These systems assume extreme pathophysiologic importance, especially in disorders such as disseminated intravascular coagulation (DIC).[35]

Coagulation Proteins

Coagulation proteins and their synonyms are summarized in Table 3. The Roman numeral system is most widely used, although in some instances no Roman numerals have been assigned. Fletcher factor is synonymous with prekallikrein; Fitzgerald factor, also called Williams factor, Flaujac factor, Reid factor, and Fujiwara factor, is high-molecular-weight kininogen.[36-38] The chromosome location containing genetic information for synthesis of almost all the coagulation factors is known[39,40] (Table 4).

The formation of a fibrin clot is best viewed as consisting of four key reactions: (1) contact activation, (2) formation of factor Xa, (3) formation of thrombin, and (4) formation of fibrin (Table 5). Appreciating these four key reactions is of help in remembering the entire blood coagulation system as well as the order and interplay of reactions.

The contact activation phase of coagulation begins with the activation of Hageman factor or factor XII. Factor XII can be activated by many potential mechanisms, including phospholipids, collagen, subendothelial collagen, and kallikrein (activated Fletcher factor).[41-44] Active Hageman factor, also a serine protease, then converts factor XI into factor XIa. This reaction occurs quickly in the presence of Fitzgerald factor (high-molecular-weight kininogen) and slowly in its absence.[45,46] The role of factor XIa is to convert factor IX into

TABLE 3. Coagulation Factors and Synonyms

Factor	Synonym
I	Fibrinogen
II	Prothrombin
V	AC-globulin
VII	Prothrombin conversion accelerator
VIII:C	Antihemophilic factor
IX	Christmas factor (PTC)
X	Stuart-Prower factor
XI	Thromboplastin antecedent (TPA)
XII	Hageman (contact) factor
XIII	Profibrinoligase
Fletcher factor	Prekallikrein
Fitzgerald factor	High-molecular-weight kininogen
Protein C	Xa inhibitor
Protein S	None

TABLE 4. Chromosomal Location Containing Coagulation Factor Information

Factor	Inheritance	Chromosome	Region
I	AD	4	q26-31
II	AD	11	p11-q12
V	AR	1	q21-25
VII	AR	13	q34
VIII:C	SLR	X	q28
von Willebrand's factor	AD	12	p12-13
IX	SLR	X	q27
X	AR	13	q34
XI	AR	4	q35
XII	AR	5	q33
XIII	AD	6	p24-25
Antithrombin III	AD	1	p23
Protein C	AD	2	q13-14
Protein S	AD	3	p21
Plasminogen	AD	6	q26-27
Thromboplastin antecedent (TPA)	AD	8	p12
TPA-1-1	AD	7	q21-22
TPA-1-2	AD	18	q21-22
Antiplasmin	AR	18	?
Fletcher factor	AR	?	?
Fitzgerald factor	AR	?	?
Heparin cofactor II	AD	22	?

Inheritance = usual mode of inheritance; AD = autosomal dominant; AR = autosomal recessive; SLR = sex-linked recessive.

factor IXa. Factor IXa is the enzyme responsible for the second key reaction, the generation of factor Xa.[2]

The formation of factor Xa requires five components: (1) a substrate (factor X), (2) an enzyme (factor IXa), (3) a determiner or cofactor (factor VIII:C), (4) a surface (platelet factor 3), and (5) calcium ions.[47,48] The third key reaction is the formation of thrombin, which also requires five components: (1) a substrate (factor II), (2) an enzyme (factor Xa), (3) a determiner/cofactor (factor V), (4) platelet factor 3 or platelet membrane phospholipoprotein, which acts as a surface, and (5) calcium ions.[49-51] Figure 3 summarizes the second two key reactions, emphasizing that both require five similar components.

The two previous reactions, generation of factor Xa and factor IIa (thrombin), depend on many vitamin K-dependent factors, including factors II, VII, IX, and X and proteins C and S. Prothrombin and the other prothrombin complex factors, VII, IX, and X and proteins C and S, can be synthesized in a normal form or in a so-called plasma abnormal form.[52-54] The role of vitamin K in synthesizing these factors is postribosomal attachment of a calcium-binding prosthetic site to each protein.[2] In the absence of vitamin K—for

TABLE 5. The Four Key Procoagulant Reactions

Contact activation (generation of IXa)	Generation of thrombin (IIa)
Generation of factor Xa	Generation of fibrin

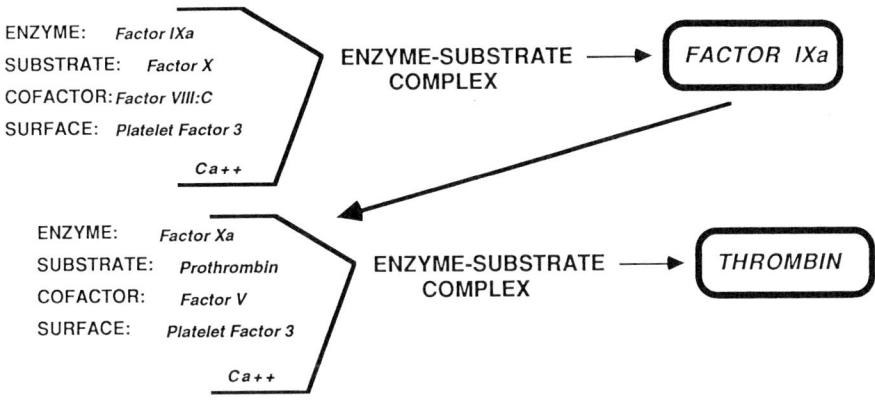

FIGURE 3. The formation of Xa and thrombin.

example, in a patient on warfarin therapy—calcium-binding sites are not attached, although a complete protein is synthesized. Thus, either plasma abnormal prothrombin complex factors or normal plasma prothrombin complex factors can be synthesized, depending on the absence or presence of vitamin K. These abnormal vitamin K-dependent factors are called proteins induced by vitamin K absence (or antagonists) (PIVKAs).[55]

The fourth key reaction is the formation of fibrin. The third key reaction, discussed earlier, generates thrombin, the primary role of which is to remove two small peptides, fibrinopeptide A and fibrinopeptide B, from fibrinogen, thus leaving fibrin monomer.[2,56,57] Fibrin monomer, void of fibrinopeptides A and B, begins to aggregate end-to-end and side-to-side; these aggregates are held together by hydrophobic bonds.[4] Another important role of thrombin is to activate factor XIII (profibrinoligase) to factor XIIIa (fibrinoligase), which replaces hydrophobic bonds with peptide bonds, resulting in an insoluble, stable fibrin clot.[58,59]

Fibrinolytic System

The fibrinolytic system (the second plasma protein system) is responsible for the destruction of a fibrin clot. In theory, small amounts of fibrin are constantly and probably systemically deposited, with subsequent lysis of the deposits.[2,60,61] Thus the presence or absence of hemorrhage or thrombosis depends on a delicate balance between the procoagulant system and the fibrinolytic system.[2,62] The fibrinolytic system consists of a proenzyme (plasminogen), which is converted via many mechanisms into the active enzyme, plasmin.[63] Plasmin, a serine protease, is not specific and has equal affinity for fibrinogen and fibrin, degrading both into fibrin(ogen) degradation products (FDPs).[64] In addition, plasmin may biodegrade factors V, VIII, IX, and XI as well as adrenocorticotropic hormone (ACTH), growth hormone, insulin, and probably many other plasma proteins.[2,62,65-68] There are two primary physiologic (and pathologic) activation pathways for the fibrinolytic system: (1) endothelial plasminogen activator activity[69] and (2) Hageman factor activation.[70] Moreover, pharmacologic activators are currently used, including streptokinase, urokinase, tissue plasminogen activator (TPA), and acyl-plasminogen-streptokinase activator complex (APSAC), used for therapeutic thrombolysis.[71] Urokinase directly activates plasminogen into plasmin; however, streptokinase forms a streptokinase-plasminogen complex that converts plasminogen into plasmin.[2,72]

The two pharmacologic inhibitors of the fibrinolytic system are aminocaproic acid and tranexamic acid, but there are several physiologic inhibitors as well. Alpha-2-antiplasmin is a rapid inhibitor of plasmin activity, whereas alpha-2-macroglobulin is effective but slow.[61,73] There are two known inhibitors of TPA: plasminogen activator inhibitors types 1 and 2 (PAI-1 and PAI-2).[74,75] PAI-1 is found in endothelial cells, platelets, smooth muscle cells, and hepatocytes.[76-80] PAI-2, first isolated from placental tissue, is also found in granulocytes and monocyte-macrophage cells.[81,82]

Complement Activation and Hemostasis

The next plasma protein system is complement and its interrelationships with coagulation. Complement activation is often not considered important in hemostasis, but complement interactions with hemostatic components are of major importance in many thrombohemorrhagic disorders. The complement system is capable of increasing vascular permeability and thus leading to hypotension and shock, common occurrences in disseminated intravascular coagulation and other thrombohemorrhagic disorders.[2,83,84] Complement activation to the C 8-9 (attack) phase leads to osmotic lysis of red cells and platelets.[85,86] The lysis and disruption of red cells and/or platelets lead to release of procoagulant material that usually accelerates a procoagulant process.[2] Plasmin is capable of directly activating C1 or C3, providing two independent pathways for plasmin activation of complement. Plasmin-induced activation of the complement system leads to serious clinical consequences in many instances of thrombohemorrhagic disease.[2,35,66,87]

Kinins and Coagulation

The next plasma protein system is the kinin system. Only recently has the importance of kinin generation during pathologic thrombohemorrhagic phenomena been appreciated.[2] Kinins are capable of vascular dilatation that leads to hypotension, shock, and other potential end-organ damage.[2,88-90] Kinins also increase vascular permeability, with ensuing hypotension and shock. Like complement activation, activation of kinins centers on activation of Hageman factor. Factor XIIa converts prekallikrein (Fletcher factor) into kallikrein; kallikrein converts kininogens into kinins.

Inhibitor Systems

The most important inhibitors of the procoagulant system are antithrombin III (AT III), protein S, and protein C.[2,91,92] Most of these inhibitory mechanisms are important physiologically, and some assume major importance in pathophysiology. Factors V and VIII:C are activated by thrombin and inactivated by protein C (protein Ca) and protein S.[93,94] The serine proteases, thrombin, factors Xa, IXa, XIa, and XIIa, and kallikrein are inhibited to a major degree by AT III.[95-98] The inhibitory activity of AT III is markedly enhanced by heparin.[99-101]

PATHOLOGY OF HEMOSTASIS DURING CARDIAC SURGERY

Cardiopulmonary bypass (CPB) surgery, which has become routine in clinical medicine, may result in severe defects in hemostasis that dramatically increase morbidity or mortality.

Prevention of Cardiac Surgical Bleeding

Hemorrhage associated with cardiac surgery may be devastating and life-threatening; great caution regarding prevention, differential diagnosis, and rapid effective therapy is essential. Attention must be given to preventing surgical hemorrhage by uncovering hereditary, acquired, or drug-induced bleeding tendencies before CPB. A preexisting bleeding diathesis, although mild, may lead to calamitous results when coupled with the changes of hemostasis induced by cardiac surgery.[102]

Laboratory Screening

Any preoperative laboratory and hemostasis screen should generally be simple and involve minimal expense to the patient while providing adequate information; however, presurgical or precardiac bypass hemostasis screens are often insufficient.[103-105] When a surgical procedure is planned, screening for defects in hemostasis requires as much knowledge as an adequate history or physical examination. When preexisting hemostatic defects are combined with the defects created by CPB, the resultant hemorrhage is often catastrophic, but frequently it can be averted by wise screening of patients. The usually ordered SMA 12/60 biochemical screening survey, electrolytes, and complete blood and platelet count detect the commonly acquired disorders often associated with a bleeding tendency, such as chronic liver disease, renal disease, and hypersplenism or bone-marrow failure. Most commonly, a presurgical screen consists only of a prothrombin time (PT), activated partial thromboplastin time (APTT), and a platelet count. Although these simple tests detect most coagulation protein problems and thrombocytopenia, they provide absolutely no information about vascular or platelet function and disregard the possibility of pathologic fibrinolysis.

Nontechnical hemorrhage associated with cardiac surgery is caused most commonly by platelet function defects, less commonly by coagulation protein or vascular defects. Therefore, one simple procedure is added to the routine preoperative surgical screen: the standardized template bleeding time, as described by Mielke and coworkers,[106] which provides a reasonable screen for adequate vascular and platelet function.[107] The template bleeding time should not be assessed until adequate platelet numbers ($>100,000/mm^3$) are documented by count or smear evaluation. For CPB surgery, a thrombin time is added to the preoperative screen.[108,109] In addition, the resultant clot should be observed for 5 minutes after the test is done. A normal thrombin time assures the absence of significant hypofibrinogenemia, dysfibrinogenemia, fibrinolysis, or elevated FDPs. The addition of these tests to the presurgical screen adds minimal cost and laboratory time while providing valuable information not given by a simple PT, APPT, or platelet count. If hypothermic perfusion is to be performed, cryoglobulins and cold agglutinins should also be assessed before

TABLE 6. Presurgical Hemostasis Screen (Minimal Requirements)

Complete blood and platelet count (CBC)	Thrombin time (cardiopulmonary bypass surgery)
Prothrombin time	(Observe clot for 5 minutes)
Partial thromboplastin time	Cryoglobulins and cold agglutinins
Template bleeding time (duplicate)	(Hypothermic cardiopulmonary bypass)

bypass.[110-115] The preoperative surgical and bypass hemostasis screen is summarized in Table 6.[106,116-119]

Hemostasis in Cardiac Surgery

Hemorrhage during or after bypass is of more than fleeting significance because it may lead to substantial morbidity and mortality from an elective procedure, places formidable demands on blood bank facilities, and can lead to prolonged, expensive hospitalizations.[109,120-123] The actual incidence of life-threatening hemorrhage associated with CPB varies from 5-25%.[109,120,123-126]

Until recently, the pathophysiology of altered hemostasis created by CPB was poorly understood. Various investigators attributed the hemorrhagic syndrome of CPB surgery to an assorted spectrum of defects; each investigator, moreover, assigned diverse degrees of importance to each defect, depending on which particular hemostatic parameters were monitored. In the past, the abnormalities most frequently cited to account for CPB hemorrhage included (1) inadequate heparin neutralization, (2) protamine excess, (3) heparin rebound, (4) thrombocytopenia, (5) hypofibrinogenemia, (6) primary fibrinolysis, (7) DIC, (8) isolated coagulation factor deficiencies, (9) transfusion reactions, and (10) hypocalcemia. The suggestion that all these defects may contribute to CPB hemorrhage clearly shows that despite the finding of multiple defects in hemostasis, the basic pathophysiology of altered hemostasis during CPB is bewildering to many. Basic mechanisms of altered hemostasis associated with CPB must be completely understood and appreciated before an appropriate approach to rapid diagnosis and effective therapy can be rationally designed.

Thrombocytopenia

Early studies of hemostasis during CPB noted significant thrombocytopenia (about 50,000/mm³); many authors attributed bypass hemorrhage to this factor. In addition, Kevy noted that thrombocytopenia was related to time on bypass and was more pronounced with perfusions lasting > 60 minutes.[127] A relationship between thrombocytopenia and time on bypass was also reported by Signore.[128] Later studies noted similar findings.[129,130] Porter and Silver observed that in most patients undergoing CPB, the platelet count fell to one-third of the preoperative level; in addition, thrombocytopenia did not abate until several days after CPB.[49] Earlier studies by Wright[131] and von Kaulla and Swan[132] also recognized thrombocytopenia in association with CPB, but these investigators concluded that thrombocytopenia bore little, if any, relationship to actual bypass hemorrhage. Some studies concluded that thrombocytopenia during CPB was associated with DIC.[133-136] Bick[105,109,121,137-140] and others[141-143] have failed to find significant thrombocytopenia during CPB. This wide variability in experience probably reflect differences in surgical and pumping techniques,

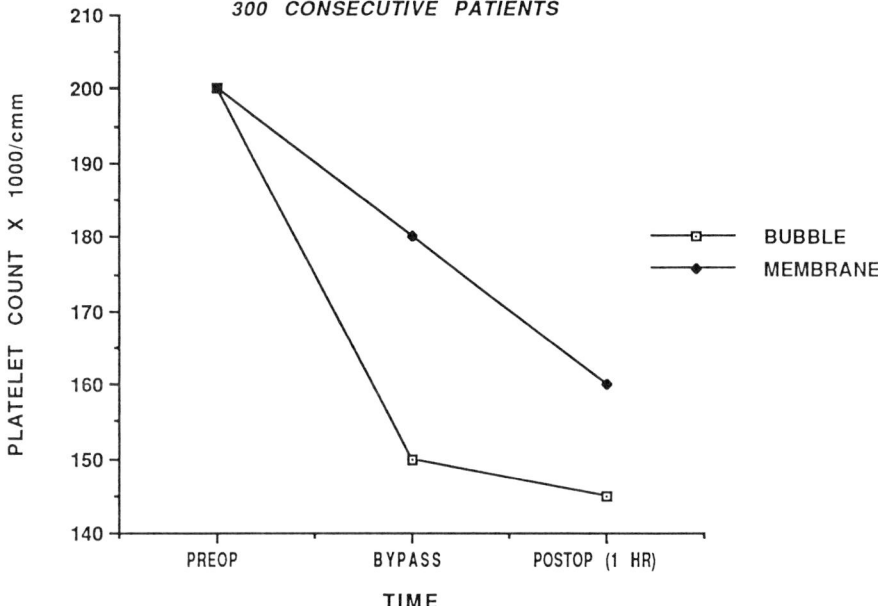

FIGURE 4. Platelet count during cardiopulmonary bypass. Membrane versus bubble oxygenation. (300 consecutive patients).

such as flow rates, normothermic or hypothermic perfusion, oxygenation system, time on bypass, and priming solution.

Figure 4 shows changes in platelet number during CPB for 300 consecutive patients. The dotted line represents the mean platelet counts in patients pumped with membrane oxygenation, and the solid line represents patients with bubble oxygenation.[105,121,144] In our experience, the type of oxygenation mechanism appears to play a minor role, if any, in causing clinically significant thrombocytopenia.[105,121,144] Thrombocytopenia with bubble oxygenators is slightly greater than that with membrane oxygenators, but the difference does not often reach clinical significance. The most commonly cited mechanisms for the development of CPB thrombocytopenia are (1) hemodilution, (2) formation of intravascular platelet thrombi, (3) platelet use in the pump or oxygenation system, and (4) peripheral use because of DIC. Our failure to find a correlation between CPB hematocrit and platelet count suggests that hemodilution is not a major factor.[104,140,145] The role, if any, of these mechanisms in producing CPB thrombocytopenia is unclear.

Platelet Function Defects

In contrast with the prolific investigations regarding platelet number during CPB, the lack of interest in assessing platelet function is surprising. Early investigators suspected that abnormalities of platelet function might occur, because faulty clot retraction was noted.[128] These results were of unclear significance, however, because other changes known to affect clot retraction, such as hypofibrinogenemia and thrombocytopenia, were also present. Another early study assessed platelet function before placing patients on CPB but did not evaluate platelet function during or after bypass.[146] In this study, abnormal preoperative platelet adhesion in glass bead columns was associated with increased postoperative bleeding. Salzman[147] studied platelet adhesion before, during, and after bypass and noted decreased adhesion to glass bead columns during bypass; however, the significance of this defect was difficult to evaluate because all patients had marked thrombocytopenia, which is definitely known to alter adhesion studies.[148-150] In addition, adhesion studies are now generally thought to have no particular clinical significance.[107,151,152] This study also indicated that heparin, in doses used during CPB, did not alter platelet adhesion. Salzman concluded that a circulating anticoagulant might be responsible for the platelet function defect noted, because plasma from CPB patients altered adhesion when added to normal platelets. This circulating anticoagulant probably represented FDPs.[109] Salzman also noted that perfusion temperature and the type of priming solution did not correlate with development of abnormal platelet function.

Platelet adhesion studies have also been performed in patients undergoing CPB without significant thrombocytopenia.[137,139,140,145] In these studies platelet function, as measured by adhesion, decreased profoundly in all patients at the initiation of bypass; in most patients adhesion decreased to 17% of preoperative levels. In one study little correlation was noted between hematocrit, fibrinogen level, or FDP titer and abnormal adhesion.[139] In addition, poor correlation was noted between chest-tube blood loss and abnormal platelet function, as assessed by adhesion. It must again be stressed that recent studies have questioned the clinical significance of platelet adhesion by the glass-bead column technique.[107,151,152] However, this degree of abnormal platelet function would surely be expected to result in severe compromise of hemostasis. The platelet function defect is slightly more severe and tends to correct more slowly when a membrane oxygenator is used compared with a bubble oxygenator. Platelet function, as assessed by template bleeding times, platelet aggregation, or lumiaggregation, is abnormal in patients with platelet function defects,[107,150] von Willebrand's syndrome (ristocetin aggregation only),[149] or myeloproliferative disorders.[153]

Many factors, some possibly altered by CPB, may affect platelet function, including (1) pH, (2) absolute platelet count, (3) hematocrit, (4) drugs, (5) the presence of FDPs, (6) the type of pump prime, and (7) the type of oxygenation system.[109,154-160] Although most studies do not clearly define the reasons for abnormal platelet function during CPB, they do suggest that several of the above mechanisms are probably not involved. The finding of platelet counts >100,000/mm^3 and hematocrits >30% in most patients with marked platelet dysfunction 1 hour after CPB suggests that absolute platelet count and hematocrit do not account for altered platelet function. Moreover, because most patients have a normal or near normal pH 1 hour after CPB surgery, a change in pH is unlikely to account for abnormal platelet function. Heparin, at levels higher than those attained in patients undergoing CPB, has been shown not to alter platelet function.[120,147,150] Circulating FDPs, which are known to interfere with platelet function, are present in about 85% of patients undergoing CPB.[109,155,159] However, the correlation between levels of circulating FDPs and abnormal platelet function during bypass surgery is poor.[139,145] In addition, because defective platelet function occurs in 100% of patients undergoing CPB, circulating FDPs cannot be the cause in many instances.[104,109,121,139,145]

Other possible mechanisms of altered platelet function during CPB include platelet membrane damage by shearing force or contact with foreign material, which may result in partial release of platelet contents, coating of platelet membrane with nonspecific proteins or protein degradation products, incomplete release reaction, or nonspecific platelet damage induced by flow rates. More recent studies have shown that selective platelet degranulation occurs during bypass surgery.[161] However, no studies yet reported allow conclusions to be drawn about the contribution of any of these mechanisms to altered platelet function during CPB. One preliminary study has reported platelet aggregation studies during CPR in a series of 29 patients. Only 20% developed aggregation abnormalities during CPB; however, after heparin reversal with protamine sulfate, 90% of patients developed aggregation abnormalities. The authors attributed this finding to a protamine/platelet interaction rather than to CPB itself.[162] We have evaluated platelets by lumiaggregation in patients undergoing CPB surgery, and platelet aggregation and platelet release were markedly altered in 100%.[120,121,163] Typical midbypass and postbypass lumiaggregation patterns seen in cardiac surgery patients are depicted in Figures 5 and 6. In addition, in all patients assessed, the aggregation and release reaction defect occurred within 10–15 minutes of initiating bypass. We

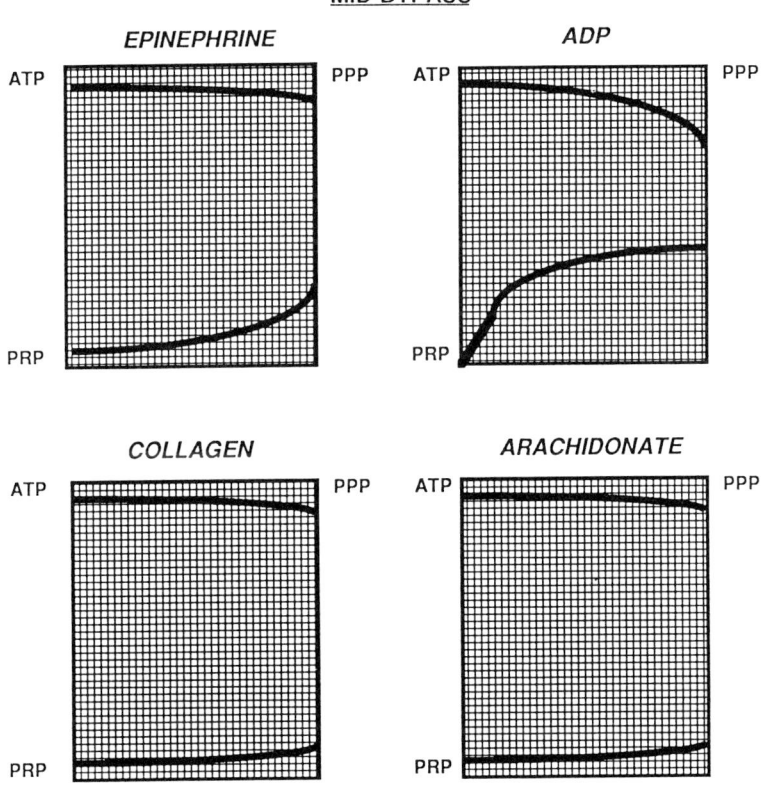

FIGURE 5. Cardiopulmonary bypass surgery platelet lumiaggregation patterns. PRP = platelet-rich plasma; PPP = platelet-poor plasma; ATP = ATP release.

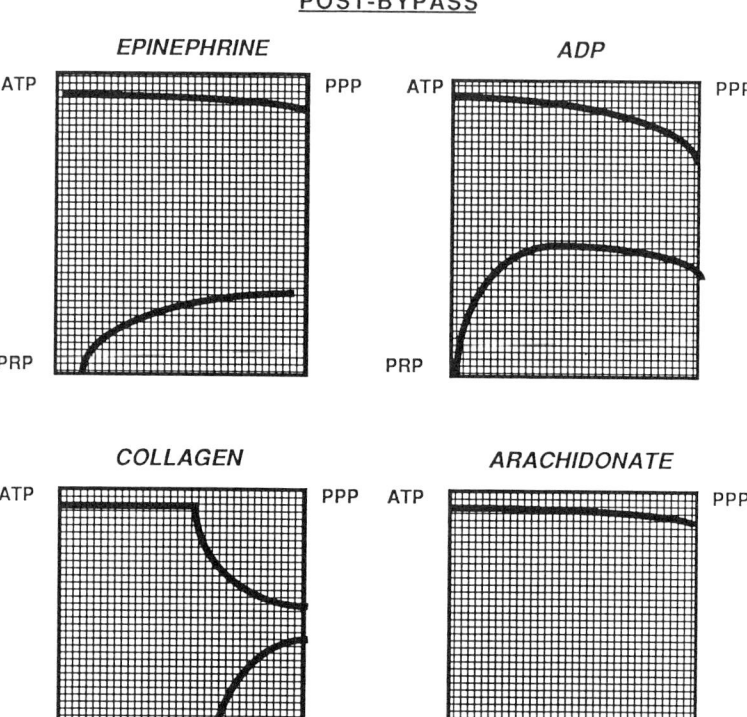

FIGURE 6. Cardiopulmonary bypass surgery platelet lumiaggregation patterns. PRP = platelet-rich plasma; PPP = platelet-poor plasma; ATP = ATP release.

have also noted that in all patients levels of platelet factor 4 rise rapidly with initiation of bypass. The aggregation defects appear to be similar with both membrane and bubble oxygenators; however, the type of priming solution (albumin vs. hydroxyethyl starch) seems to change the type of defects.[163]

Despite the mechanism(s) involved, studies to date clearly disclose a significant defect in platelet function among all patients undergoing CPB surgery. The magnitude of this defect certainly would be expected to have potential serious consequences for hemostasis during and after bypass. In addition, patients who have ingested drugs known to interfere with platelet function would be expected to lose more blood than other patients because the drugs are likely to compound the defects already induced by CPB and to potentiate the chance for hemorrhage. One small study has provided evidence for this conclusion.[158]

Although diagnosis and management of hemorrhage associated with CPB are discussed later, the defect in platelet function is obviously of major significance in post-CPB hemorrhage. Usually platelet concentrates in the face of a normal platelet count promptly correct or significantly reduce most episodes of CPB or post-CPB hemorrhage. Desmopressin acetate (DDAVP) was initially thought to decrease bleeding after open-heart surgery; thus many surgeons began the empirical and sometimes irrational use of DDAVP during and after open-heart surgery. However, more recent blinded, randomized trials have failed to show any significant differences in post-CPB blood loss between DDAVP and placebo.[164-166] Furthermore, DDAVP releases TPA, potentially activating the fibrinolytic system and enhancing or inducing hemorrhage; thus many investigators using this agent recommend the concomitant use of aminocaproic acid to abort any possible hemorrhage.[167-170] Current evidence suggests little, if any, rationale for the empirical use of DDAVP during CPB; those using the agent should be aware of the potential for enhancing hemorrhage and increasing risk of coronary artery and cerebrovascular thrombosis.

Isolated Coagulation Factor Defects

Many studies have examined and reported coagulation factor deficiencies during CPB. The wide variety of findings, like the finding of thrombocytopenia, may reflect only differences in surgical or pumping techniques, such as flow rate and priming solution. Most studies have noted significant hypofibrinogenemia that does not seem to be correlated with perfusion time.[124,129-131,139,140] We[139,140,155] and others[124,130] have found fibrinogen levels to be closely correlated with CPB fibrinolysis; however, other investigators report little correlation between hypofibrinogenemia and degree of CPB fibrinolysis.[127,171] Figure 7

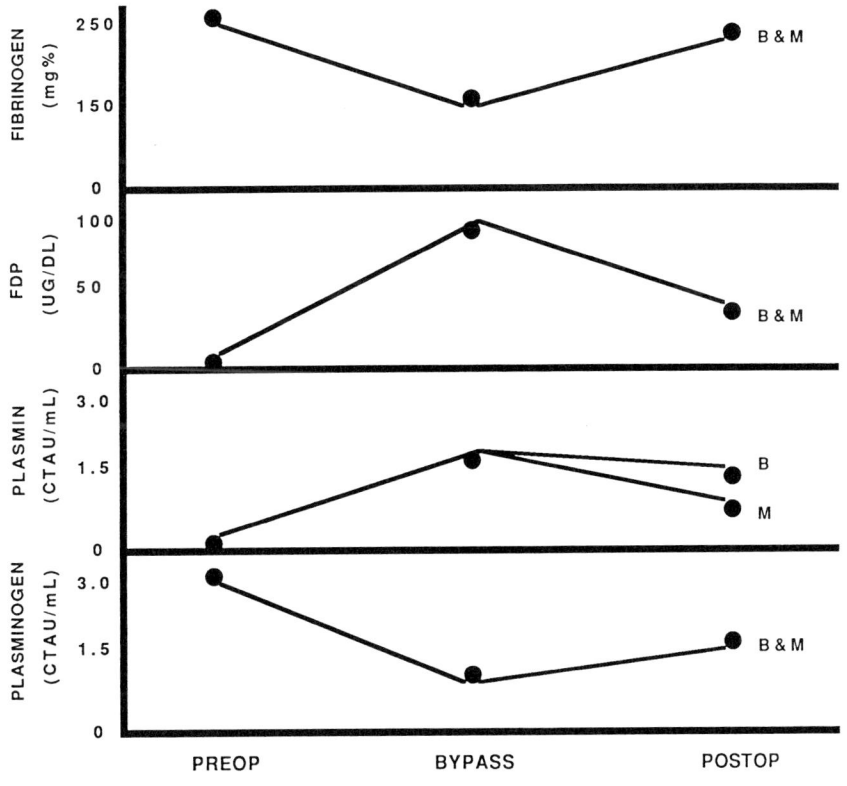

FIGURE 7. Fibrinolytic activity during cardiopulmonary bypass.

depicts correlations noted between fibrinogen, plasminogen, circulating plasmin, and FDPs during CPB. The dashed lines represent membrane-pumped patients and the solid lines represent bubble oxygenator-pumped patients.[104,121,144] Some studies have concluded that hypofibrinogenemia occurs primarily because of DIC during pump surgery;[133,135,136] however, others have failed to find hypofibrinogenemia during CPB.[172,173] It seems reasonable to conclude that hypofibrinogenemia secondary to hyperfibrinolysis may be a frequent occurrence during CPB. Fibrinolysis occurs in about 85% of patients undergoing bypass surgery. Most studies have also noted other coagulation deficiencies in association with CPB, most commonly decreases in factors II, V, and VIII:C.[124,127,130,131,133,136] Some patients undergoing CPB for valvular heart disease have low counts of factor VIII:vW high-molecular-weight monomers; these monomers may also increase during CPB.[165] Some conclude that the changes are secondary to DIC,[133,143] whereas others attribute them to a primary fibrinolytic syndrome and plasmin-induced degradation of coagulation proteins.[104,109,124,139,140,155] Still others have failed to find a significant decrease in most coagulation factors during bypass surgery,[127,172,173] and two authors have reported increased levels of factor VIII:C during perfusion.[172,174]

Disseminated Intravascular Coagulation

The question of whether DIC develops during bypass surgery has caused much confusion regarding altered hemostasis, both during and after bypass. Many early studies of hemostasis during CPB concluded that DIC occurred.[133,135,136,175,176] However, many such studies monitored only isolated coagulation factors; the measured decreases were empirically ascribed to presumed DIC because no other explanation was evident. Specifically, the findings of isolated deficiencies in fibrinogen, factor VIII:C,[131,135] or prothrombin complex factor[142] were often assumed, usually erroneously, to be secondary to DIC, without proper confirmatory testing. In addition, two more recent reports have concluded that DIC accounts for altered hemostasis during CPB.[143,177] These reports of 9 patients concluded that DIC was present after noting that several parameters of hemostasis worsened following reversal of heparin with protamine. Specifically, FDP elevation, hypofibrinogenemia, and hypoplasminogenemia appeared to be accentuated after the infusion of protamine. However, our experience[104,105,109,120,139,140] and that of others[124,128,129,132,173,178] have been the opposite; hypofibrinogenemia, hypoplasminogenemia, and FDP elevation usually correct rapidly and uniformly after the administration of protamine sulfate.

These findings suggest that DIC is not generally associated with CPB surgery. DIC during cardiac surgery also seems unlikely in view of the many reports of massive heparinization and absence of significant or uniform thrombocytopenia despite markedly abnormal hemostasis. Another finding that surely argues against DIC is the presence of normal or near-normal levels of AT III during CPB;[104,120,124,145] evidence suggests that decreased levels of AT III are a good indicator of the development of acute or chronic DIC.[179,180-182] Only one study has shown decreased AT III during CPB;[143] however, all of the 9 patients had low levels of AT III before bypass was started. In addition, because the method used was quite old and possibly influenced by the presence of FDPs or heparin, interpretation of these results is unclear.

Another consideration negating the probability of DIC is that if it were present in patients undergoing CPB, the infusion of intravenous protamine sulfate would be expected to cause a massive precipitation of soluble fibrin monomer, with resultant extensive micro- or macrovascular occlusion. In this author's experience, only 2 out of several thousand patients have had true DIC in association with CPB.[104,109,121] Both patients developed DIC before CPB, one from cardiac arrest and the other from septicemia. In these two patients bypass surgery was accomplished without incident; however, when protamine sulfate was infused, massive vascular occlusion, including carotid and renal artery thrombosis, occurred.

Although most early and several recent studies have detected primary fibrinolysis in association with CPB, only a few have concluded that DIC might occur. This conclusion probably results from the marked superficial similarities between primary or secondary fibrinolysis and DIC and from the difficulty in making a clearcut differential diagnosis between these two states without sophisticated and complete coagulation studies.

Primary Fibrinolysis

Fibrinolytic activity is generally decreased or inhibited during and after most general surgical procedures.[183-186] However, most studies using a variety of laboratory modalities have found increased fibrinolysis during and after CPB surgery.[104,109,121,124,139-141,155-157,163,171,173,178,187] Many earlier studies of hemostasis during CPB assessed fibrinolysis with the euglobulin lysis time; the finding of fibrinolysis was of unclear significance for a long time.[188,189] More recent studies of CPB hemostasis,[104,120,121,129,139,140,145] which have used more specific methods for assessing fibrinolysis—primarily synthetic substrate assays[181,190,191-194]—have confirmed earlier reports of a primary fibrino(geno)lytic syndrome in most patients undergoing CPB surgery (Fig. 7). Because of early reports detecting primary fibrinolysis during CPB, the empirical use of antifibrinolytics, usually epsilon aminocaproic acid (EACA), has become commonplace. Many cardiovascular surgeons have frequently used this drug despite its attendant hazards, which include hypokalemia, hypotension, ventricular arrhythmias, local or disseminated thromboses, and DIC syndromes.[195,196] Controlled studies with and without antifibrinolytics have failed to show any clearcut differences in CPB hemorrhage.[124,130,171,197,198] Gomes and McGoon[178] and Tsuji[173] have shown a definite increase in post-CPB hemorrhage with the empirical use of antifibrinolytics. In fact, the need to use EACA to control CPB hemorrhage is extremely rare;[104,105,109,121] this agent should be used only with clear laboratory evidence of primary fibrinolysis in the severely hemorrhaging CPB patient who has failed to respond to adequate platelet transfusions.

Several investigators finding primary fibrinolysis during CPB have considered it to be inconsequential as a cause of postperfusion hemorrhage,[128,130] whereas others have thought that the syndrome is triggered only by specific events, such as pyrogenicity of equipment, use of rheomacrodex, or induction of anesthesia.[132,199,200] Because primary fibrinolysis occurs in most patients subjected to CPB, activation of the fibrinolytic system in the oxygenation mechanisms seems more likely; alternatively, pump-induced accelerated flow rates may activate the plasminogen-plasmin system or alter endothelial plasminogen activator (or inhibitor) activity. Marked activation of factor XII in patients undergoing CPB surgery, with about 70% of factor XII converted to factor XIIa,[201] is another potential activation pathway for the initiation of a primary fibrinolytic syndrome. However, the pathogenesis of fibrinolytic activation during CPB is unclear. Although many investigators have noted enhanced fibrinolysis during CPB, a few studies have found only elevated fibrinolytic activator activity, with no systemically circulating plasmin.[127,171,175] Moreover, a few studies have failed to find any evidence of primary fibrinolysis in association with CPB.[130,131,175,197]

Other Defects in Cardiac Surgery

Heparin rebound has received significant attention as a potential cause of CPB hemorrhage,[200,202,205] particularly in earlier studies. With currently accepted doses of both heparin and protamine, heparin rebound and inadequate heparinization are rare.[104,109,121,134,140,143,145] Neither heparin rebound nor inadequate heparin neutralization has ever been documented as the actual cause of CPB hemorrhage.[104,105,121,134,135] Similarly, protamine excess has occasionally been incriminated as a cause; however, several studies have failed to note this phenomenon in a single patient undergoing CPB.[109,126,139-141,203,206] In addition, although protamine sulfate is a well-known in-vitro anticoagulant, it is an unlikely cause of clinical hemorrhage.[207]

Several authors have reported that both coagulation defects and significant CPB hemorrhage may be associated with hypothermic perfusion;[130,132,197,200] our experience in comparing normothermic with hypothermic perfusions has led to the same conclusion.[187] Gomes and McGoon[178] and Porter and Silver[129] have found no increased incidence of CPB hemorrhage after hypothermic perfusion. Many patients undergoing CABG for coronary occlusive disease have been on warfarin-type drugs. Verska and associates noted that although the PT returns to normal before CPB, patients previously receiving warfarin therapy hemorrhage more than those not previously on such agents.[197] This observation applies to general surgery patients as well. One study[119] noted that increased hemorrhage was associated with a repeat bypass procedure; others, however, have noted no increased hemorrhage in association with a second procedure.[136,178] In addition, patients undergoing CPB for correction of cyanotic heart disease appear to have more severe derangements in hemostasis during perfusion and a greater propensity to hemorrhage than those operated for noncyanotic heart disease.[128,178] Increased hemorrhagic risk during and after CPB is associated with (1) the prior use of warfarin drugs, (2) hypothermic perfusion, (3) surgery for correction of cyanotic heart disease, (4) repeat bypass procedure, (5) long perfusion times, and (6) preoperative ingestion of drugs interfering with platelet function.[104,105,120,121] Advancing age does not appear to be associated with increased risk.[208,209]

SUMMARY OF HEMOSTATIC PATHOPHYSIOLOGY DURING CARDIOPULMONARY BYPASS

Many conclusions regarding altered hemostasis and resultant hemorrhage during CPB surgery are of questionable significance; for example, overheparinization, heparin rebound, inadequate protamine neutralization, and protamine excess, although receiving at least theoretical attention as potential sources, have not been documented as causes of bleeding associated with bypass surgery. Similarly, thrombocytopenia, almost surely a potential source of hemorrhage, is an inconsistent finding during CPB surgery. The finding of isolated coagulation defects has added little, except confusion, to the understanding of altered hemostasis during CPB; these findings probably represent isolated measurements of the results of fibrinolysis and systemically circulating plasmin.

Most carefully performed studies have not documented DIC during CPB. The significant doses of heparin used during CPB, the absence of consistent thrombocytopenia, and the general correction of hypofibrinogenemia, hypoplasminogenemia, and elevated FDPs after heparin neutralization suggest that the presence of DIC during cardiac surgery is a rare event. DIC may be associated with cardiac surgery in the presence of another triggering event, such as sepsis, shock, massive transfusions, or a frank hemolytic transfusion reaction.

Predisposing factors associated with enhanced cardiac surgery hemorrhage are (1) long perfusion times, (2) prior ingestion of warfarin-type drugs, (3) cyanotic heart disease, (4) hypothermic perfusions, (5) preoperative ingestion of drugs known to interfere with platelet function, and (6) repeat bypass procedure (Table 7). Prevailing evidence suggests that most patients undergoing CPB surgery develop a primary fibrinolytic syndrome; although the exact triggering mechanisms are unclear, activation of factor XII may be implicated. However, the resultant secondary derangements in hemostasis certainly create a potential for CPB hemorrhage. In addition, most patients undergoing CPB develop severe platelet dysfunction. It is unclear if this defect results from coating of platelet surfaces by FDP, membrane damage from the oxygenation mechanism, platelet damage from fast flow rates, or other unrecognized mechanisms. Whatever the triggering mechanism(s), the most significant alterations in hemostasis associated with CPB are defective platelet function and primary fibrinolysis. These two defects alone or in combination certainly account for most nonsurgical and nontechnical hemorrhage in patients undergoing CPB; platelet function defects account for far more hemorrhagic episodes than primary fibrinolysis.

DIAGNOSIS OF BYPASS HEMORRHAGE

When bleeding occurs during or after bypass, it is obviously extremely important to define the defect as quickly as possible; only then can specific and effective therapy be delivered.[105,109,121,126,210] As mentioned earlier, many instances of CPB hemorrhage clearly result from inadequate surgical technique, but alterations of hemostasis may also be responsible. This discussion is limited to nontechnical causes of CPB hemorrhage. The types of hemorrhage that occur during CPB are depicted in Table 8 in descending order of probability.

TABLE 7. Factors Predisposing to Hemorrhage During Cardiopulmonary Bypass

Long perfusion times	Hypothermic perfusion
Prior use of warfarins	Preoperative ingestion of antiplatelet drugs
Cyanotic heart disease	Repeat bypass procedure

TABLE 8. Hemorrhagic Syndromes Seen with Cardiopulmonary Bypass Surgery (Descending Order of Probability)

Severe platelet dysfunction	Thrombocytopenia
Cardiopulmonary bypass-induced	Hyperheparinemia or rebound??
Drug-induced	Disseminated intravascular coagulation
Primary fibrinolytic syndrome	(exceedingly rare)

The primary distinction to be made is between strictly surgical bleeding and defects in hemostasis—or a combination of the two. This distinction becomes more difficult and more important after the patient has left the operating room; a decision must be made regarding reexploration and the adequacy of hemostasis for reexploration. In distinguishing between surgical and nonsurgical bleeding, many physical findings are helpful; for example, is the bleeding localized or systemic? If the patient is already in the recovery room, hematuria in association with petechiae and purpura, oozing from intravenous sites in conjunction with increased chest-tube blood loss, and oozing from surgical sites, including the sternotomy wound and saphenous vein harvest site, means a defect in hemostasis. But increased chest-tube blood loss alone often signifies a technical bleeding problem. When the patient is in the operating room, these same findings hold true; the surgeon usually notes bleeding or oozing throughout the surgical field in nontechnical bleeding. Communication between the surgeon and the hematologist or internist is therefore important. Clinical suggestions of a systemic rather than local cause of CPB hemorrhage are depicted in Table 9.

When CPB hemorrhage is seen or suspected, the following laboratory tests are ordered: PT, APPT, complete blood and platelet counts, examination of a peripheral smear, levels of FDP and D-dimer, heparin assay by synthetic substrate, thrombin or reptilase time, and levels of plasminogen/plasmin by synthetic substrate methods.[106,120,121,126] Evaluation of the heparin level provides rapid information about the status of heparin and its potential effects on other tests of hemostasis. The resultant clot from the thrombin or reptilase time, always observed for 5 minutes for evidence of lysis, supplies rapid additional information about the presence or absence of a clinically significant primary fibrino(geno)lytic syndrome. More evidence for or against primary lysis is obtained by noting the FDP and D-dimer level.[180,211-213] A peripheral blood smear and platelet count are invaluable to evaluate rapidly the potential for thrombocytopenic bleeding. Assessment of plasminogen and plasmin levels by synthetic substrate technique is not time-consuming, and although not useful for immediate diagnosis, it is invaluable in making later decisions about

TABLE 9. Clinical Evaluation of Hemorrhage in the Patient Undergoing Cardiopulmonary Bypass

Chest-tube blood loss only?	
Or associated with:	
Petechiae, purpura, or ecchymoses	Oozing from sternotomy wound
Hematuria	Oozing from saphenous vein graft
Oozing from Intraarterial sites	Other systemic bleeding sites
Oozing from intravenous sites	Clots forming in chest tube
Oozing from venipunctures	

antifibrinolytic therapy.[106,120,121,126] If significant primary fibrinolysis is present, FDPs are significantly elevated, the D-dimer level is normal or near-normal, and both hypoplasminogenemia and circulating plasmin are detected. Fibrinopeptide A levels are not elevated, but B-beta 15-42–related peptides are elevated. Excess heparin as a potential problem is noted by the heparin assay and marked prolongation of the thrombin time. If no significant clot lysis is observed, if the clot forms during measurement of the thrombin time, and if FDP elevation is not significant, primary fibrinolysis should not be a concern.

All patients undergoing CPB have a platelet function defect; when bleeding occurs, this author assumes that the defect is always present; although it may not be the primary reason for hemorrhage, platelet dysfunction can be assumed to be additive to any other defect, whether related to surgery or to altered hemostasis. No tests of platelet function are routinely performed, but platelet tests are immediately ordered for any patient who demonstrates intra- or postbypass hemorrhage.[104,105,121] The time period when hemorrhage occurs— that is, intraoperatively, after heparin neutralization, or in the recovery room— appears to bear little relationship to the etiology of the primary hemostatic defect responsible for hemorrhage. Exceptions are thrombocytopenic bleeding, which usually occurs after the patient is in the recovery room, and a significant drug-induced defect in platelet function, which is usually manifest as significant oozing immediately after the operative procedure is started. Tests ordered for the differential diagnosis of the etiology of hemorrhage during CPB surgery are listed in Table 10.

MANAGEMENT OF BYPASS HEMORRHAGE

When first encountering a patient with CPB hemorrhage, whether intraoperative or postoperative, it is of prime importance (1) to note the type of bleeding (systemic vs. local), (2) to order an immediate (stat) laboratory screen as outlined above, and (3) to administer 6-8 units of platelet concentrates as quickly as possible. Although the use of platelet concentrates is somewhat empirical at this point, it is based on two sound reasons: (1) all patients have a significant platelet function defect, which may be the primary reason for hemorrhage and usually is if the bleeding is nontechnical; and (2) this defect is likely to accentuate bleeding from other causes, whether it be a surgical defect or defective hemostasis. The quick administration of platelet concentrates while awaiting the results of laboratory evaluation often stops or significantly reduces most instances of nontechnical CPB hemorrhage.[104,105,121] Recently, a fibrin glue in paste or spray form has been applied, with reasonable success,

TABLE 10. Laboratory Evaluation of Bypass Hemorrhage (Ordered STAT)

Platelet count and complete blood count	D-dimer assay
Peripheral blood smear evaluation	Heparin assay*
Prothrombin time	Thrombin time†
Partial thromboplastin time	Plasminogen assay*
Fibrinogen degradation product titer	Plasmin assay*

* Synthetic substrate assay.
† Observe for clot lysis × 5 min.
STAT = immediate.

to bleeding sites in patients experiencing CPB hemorrhage; the source of this fibrin glue may be autologous or allogeneic.[214-217]

When bleeding begins immediately upon initiation of surgery, a platelet function defect, usually drug-induced, can be assumed to be present until further laboratory investigation can be completed. In this instance, the patient should be given 6-8 units of platelet concentrates as quickly as possible, and the surgical wound should be closed, if feasible. If a platelet function defect is responsible for the hemorrhage (no laboratory evidence of significant fibrinolysis or hyperheparinemia), 6-8 units of platelet concentrates should be repeated the evening after surgery and for 2 postoperative mornings. Thrombocytopenic CPB hemorrhage should be controlled in the same manner, although greater numbers of platelet concentrates may be needed, as dictated by the initial platelet count, the site and severity of hemorrhage, and the response to platelet transfusions. Hyperheparinemia and heparin rebound, if thought to be a real clinical problem as documented by synthetic substrate assays, are managed by delivering 25% of the original calculated dose of protamine sulfate; this dose is repeated every 30-60 minutes until bleeding stops. Hyperheparinemia and heparin rebound, however, are unlikely to be responsible for bleeding and should not be of concern unless concrete laboratory proof of hyperheparinemia is present and evidence of primary fibrinolysis is clearly absent. This author has seen many instances of excessive heparinization resulting from mistakes in calculations and preparation of the solution; none of these instances was associated with significant cardiac surgical hemorrhage. Similarly, protamine excess is rarely, if ever, a clinical problem. This situation never calls for therapy and should not be dwelled upon at the risk of ignoring other potential defects in hemostasis.

Primary fibrinolysis is commonly present and may or may not be responsible for hemorrhage. This syndrome should not be treated empirically; antifibrinolytic therapy should be considered if the patient has failed to respond to platelet concentrates and if there is documented laboratory evidence for this syndrome, such as the presence of hypoplasminogenemia, circulating plasmin, and elevated FDPs. In addition, for those having appropriate testing systems available, the absence of elevated fibrinopeptide A, the absence of elevated D-dimer, and the presence of elevated B-beta 15-42-related peptides offer further evidence for primary lysis. Primary fibrino(geno)lytic bleeding is generally treated with epsilon aminocaproic acid given as an initial dose of 5-10 grams slow intravenous push followed by 1-2 g/hr until bleeding stops or slows to a non-life-threatening level. Because EACA may be associated with ventricular arrhythmias (tachycardia or fibrillation), hypotension, hypokalemia, localized or diffuse thrombosis, and frank DIC, it should be injected slowly, and patients should be monitored carefully for cardiac status, renal output, blood pressure, and electrolytes. A newer and more potent antifibrinolytic agent now available is tranexamic acid, which is usually delivered intravenously at a dose of about 3-6 g/24 hr.[218]

HEMOSTASIS AND PROSTHETIC HEART VALVES

The use of prosthetic heart valves has become common and has greatly reduced morbidity and mortality in patients with valvular heart disease.

However, complications of these devices, which include thromboembolism, infection, hemolysis, and detachment, may also significantly alter morbidity and mortality.[219] Of these complications, thromboembolism is the most common and often the most serious; the likeliest sites of embolism are the central nervous system, coronary arteries, retinal vessels, and extremities.[220] Early in the history of cardiac valve placement, it was found that warfarin could decrease but not eliminate the thromboembolic events occurring with mitral and aortic valves.[221] Thromboembolism is more common with mitral valves than aortic valves, especially if atrial fibrillation or left atrial enlargement is present.[219,221-223] Early valves with metal exposed to blood were associated with a 50% chance of thromboembolism, which could be reduced to 13% with the use of warfarin.[224] Original aortic valves were associated with a 35% chance of thromboembolism, which was reduced to 8% with the use of warfarin.[225] Valvular thromboemboli arise from platelets; after valve replacement, platelets adhere to the foreign surface by adhesion and aggregation.[105,120,121,219,226-228] Another impetus for platelet aggregation may come from ADP, liberated during red cell hemolysis.[226] Because of platelet consumption on valvular surfaces, many patients with prosthetic valves demonstrate decreased platelet survival and increased platelet turnover; the decreased survival appears to correlate well with the incidence of thromboemboli.[229-231] However, patients with rheumatic valve disease without prosthetic valves also show decreased platelet survival, increased platelet consumption, and an increased chance of thromboembolism.[232] Valvular platelet consumption has decreased progressively with new valve design but still has not been totally eliminated. Platelet deposits and thromboemboli were most pronounced with the early metal valves and decreased in incidence with second-generation cloth-bound valves that induced neoendothelialization of the valve surface and a hopefully inert valve. New xenograft (porcine) valves are associated with an even greater reduction in thromboembolic complications. Despite this improvement, however, chance of serious thromboembolism in patients with prosthetic aortic or mitral valves is still significant, and most are committed to long-term or life-long anticoagulation of some type.

Both dipyridamole and sulfinpyrazone normalize decreased platelet survival in patients with prosthetic valves, but aspirin alone does not demonstrate this effect.[229,233] However, aspirin potentiates the effect of dipyridamole in normalizing platelet survival.[229] The mechanisms are unclear, as the doses of dipyridamole and sulfinpyrazone that normalize platelet survival are lower than doses needed to alter platelet aggregation in vitro. In addition, sulfinpyrazone normalizes decreased platelet survival in patients with rheumatic mitral valvular disease who do not have prosthetic valves.[232] These observations led to interest in antiplatelet drugs for the control of thromboembolism associated with prosthetic heart valves, and many clinical trials have proved the efficacy of several agents, including aspirin and dipyridamole.[234-238] One early trial showed a reduction in incidence of thromboemboli from 14 to 1.3% with the addition of dipyridamole to a warfarin regimen.[234] Another early trial showed that the addition of aspirin to the warfarin regimen decreased the chance of thromboembolism by 80%.[235] The efficacy of antiplatelet agents alone is unclear; one trial has found aspirin plus dipyridamole alone (no warfarin) to be effective,[239] but another trial found the same regimen to be ineffective.[240]

Although the role of antiplatelet agents alone is unclear, an antiplatelet agent should be used with warfarin in patients with prosthetic valves. At the present time, there is no uniformity in anticoagulant regimens for patients with prosthetic cardiac valves. One theory suggests that the chance of thromboembolism decreases with time; thus, after a given period, an anticoagulant is no longer needed in selected patients.[156,241,242] Another recommendation is to use adequate doses of warfarin (2.5 times control time) plus aspirin or dipyridamole.[228] Yet another regimen uses warfarin in patients with mitral or double valve replacement but antiplatelet agents alone in patients with aortic valves.[223] Another author suggests only a combination of antiplatelet agents in prosthetic valve patients, with thrice daily doses of both aspirin (330 mg) and dipyridamole (75 mg).[230] Probably the safest recommendation is that of Frankl: patients with aortic valves should receive adequate doses of aspirin and dipyridamole, whereas patients with mitral valve replacement or double valve replacement should be treated with aspirin, dipyridamole, and warfarin.[219]

Recently specific anticoagulant regimens for patients with mechanical or bioprosthetic heart valves have been recommended by a national panel conference of the National Heart, Lung, and Blood Institute and the American College of Chest Physicians.[243] The following recommendations apply to mechanical prosthetic heart valves: (1) all patients should be anticoagulated with long-term warfarin at a dose appropriate to prolong the PT from 1.5 to 2.0 times control (using rabbit brain thromboplastin), with the addition of dipyridamole an acceptable option; (2) if the patient suffers systemic embolization, then dipyridamole, at a dose of 400 mg/day, should be added to the aforementioned warfarin dose; (3) antiplatelet agents alone are not considered adequate protection; and (4) when a major bleeding episode occurs in a patient treated with long-term warfarin, doses of warfarin should be lowered to give a PT ratio of 1.2-1.5 times control. The following recommendations apply to bioprosthetic heart valves: (1) all patients with bioprosthetic heart valves in the mitral position should be treated for the first 3 months with appropriate warfarin to render a PT ratio of 1.3-1.5 times control; similarly, if patients have been implanted with bioprosthetic valves in the aortic position and remain in normal sinus rhythm, warfarin therapy may be considered optional; (2) patients who have a history of systemic embolization, who demonstrate a left atrial thrombus at surgery, or who have atrial fibrillation should be treated with long-term warfarin therapy, although ideal doses are unclear; and (3) patients in regular sinus rhythm may be treated with long-term aspirin at 500 mg/day.

CONCLUSION

This chapter provides a review of altered hemostasis associated with CPB surgery. The key to prevention of CPB hemorrhage is an adequate preoperative work-up. Of extreme importance is an adequate history for bleeding and thrombotic tendencies in both patient and family; of equal importance is a careful history of use of drugs affecting hemostasis, especially those known to interfere with platelet function. A careful physical examination, searching for clues of a real or potential bleeding diathesis, may also prevent catastrophic cases of hemorrhage. An adequate presurgical screen must be performed in

CPB candidates. In addition to the usual PT, PTT, and platelet count, a standardized template bleeding time and thrombin time should be assessed. The use of these simple testing modalities guards against significant defects in vascular and platelet function. Most instances of nontechnical cardiovascular surgical hemorrhage are due to several well-defined defects in hemostasis, which should be easily controlled if approached in a logical manner and as a team effort among cardiac surgeons, pathologists, and hematologists.

REFERENCES

1. Bick RL: Physiology of hemostasis. In Disorders of Thrombosis and Hemostasis: Clinical and Laboratory Practice. Chicago, ASCP Press, 1992, p 1.
2. Bick RL: Basic physiology of hemostasis and thrombosis. In Disorders of Hemostasis and Thrombosis: Principles of Clinical Practice. New York, Thieme, Inc., 1985, p 1.
3. Crawford T: Blood and lymphatic vessels. In Anderson WAD, Kissane JM (eds): Pathology. St. Louis, C.V. Mosby, 1977, p 879.
4. Harker LA, Ross R: Pathogenesis of arterial vascular disease. Semin Thromb Hemost 5:274, 1979.
5. Lie JT, Brown AL: Normal structure of the vascular system and general reactive changes of the arteries. In Fairbairn JF, Ivergens JL, Spittel JA (eds): Peripheral Vascular Diseases. Philadelphia, W.B. Saunders, 1972, p 45.
6. O'Brian JR: The adhesiveness of native platelets and its prevention. J Clin Pathol 14:140, 1961.
7. Sheppard B, French JE: Platelet adhesion in the rabbit abdominal aorta following the removal of endothelium: A scanning and transmission electron microscopic study. Proc R Soc Lond 176:427, 1971.
8. McCoy L: Vascular function in hemostasis. In Murano G, Bick RL (eds): Basic Concepts of Hemostasis and Thrombosis. Boca Raton, FL, CRC Press, 1980, p 5.
9. Harlan JM: Consequences of leukocyte-vessel wall interactions in inflammatory and immune reactions. Semin Thromb Hemost 13:434, 1987.
10. Bevilacqua MP, Gimbrone MA: Inducible endothelial functions in inflammation and coagulation. Semin Thromb Hemost 13:425, 1987.
11. Nawroth PP, Stern DM: Endothelial cell procoagulant properties and the host response. Semin Thromb Hemost 13:391, 1987.
12. Henry RL: Platelet function. Semin Thromb Hemost 4:93, 1977.
13. Droller MJ: Ultrastructure of the platelet release reaction in response to various aggregating agents and their inhibitors. Lab Invest 29:595, 1973.
14. Stuart MJ: Inherited defects of platelet function. Semin Hematol 12:233, 1975.
15. White JG: Identification of platelet secretion in the electron microscope. Ser Haematol 6:429, 1973.
16. White JG: Interaction of membrane systems in blood platelets. Am J Pathol 66:295, 1972.
17. Born GVR, Cross MJ: The aggregation of blood platelets. J Physiol 168:178, 1963.
18. Bull BS, Zucker MB: Changes in platelet volume produced by temperature, metabolic inhibitors, and aggregating agents. Proc Soc Exp Biol Med 120:296, 1965.
19. McLean JR, Veloso N: Changes of shape without aggregation caused by ADP in rabbit platelets at low pH. Life Sci 6:1983, 1967.
20. Zucker MB, Peterson J: Serotonin, platelet factor 3 activity and platelet aggregating agent released by adenosine diphosphate. Blood 30:556, 1967.
21. Davis RB, Mecker WR, Bailey WL: Serotonin release after injection of *E. coli* endotoxin in the rabbit. Fed Proc 20:261, 1961.
22. Des Prez RM, Horowitz HI, Hook EW: Effects of bacterial endotoxin on rabbit platelets. I. Platelet aggregation and release of platelet factors in vitro. J Exp Med 114:857, 1961.
23. Mueller-Eckhardt C, Luscher EF: Immune reactions of human blood platelets. I. A comparative study on the effects on platelets of heterologous antiplatelet antiserum, antigen-antibody complexes, aggregation gamma-globulin, and thrombin. Thromb Diath Haemorrh 20:155, 1968.
24. Pfueller SL, Luscher EF: The effects of immune complexes on blood and their relationship to complement activation. Immunochemistry 9:1151, 1972.

25. Gerrard JM, White JG: Prostaglandins and thromboxanes: "Middlemen" modulating platelet function in hemostasis and thrombosis. Prog Hemost Thromb 4:87, 1978.
26. Hinman JW: Prostaglandins. Annu Rev Biochem 41:161, 1972.
27. Nalbandian RM, Henry RL: Platelet-endothelial cell interactions: Metabolic maps of structure and actions of prostaglandins, prostacycline, thromboxane, and cyclic AMP. Semin Thromb Hemost 5:87, 1979.
28. Day CE: On the newly discovered role of prostaglandins in arteries and its implications for the control of atherosclerosis, platelets, and thrombosis. Artery 2:480, 1976.
29. Gryglewski RJ, Bunting S, Moncada S, et al: Arterial walls are protected against deposition of platelet thrombi by a substance (prostaglandin X) which they make from prostaglandin endoperoxides. Prostaglandins 12:685, 1976.
30. Moncada R, Gryglewski R, Bunting S, Vane JR: A lipid peroxide inhibits the enzyme in blood vessel microsomes that generate from prostaglandin endoperoxides the substance (prostaglandin x) which prevents platelet aggregation. Prostaglandins 12:715, 1976.
31. Gryglewski RJ, Szczklik A, Nizankowski R: Antiplatelet action of intravenous infusion of prostacyclin in man. Thromb Rcs 13:153, 1978.
32. Hensby CN, Lewis PJ, Hilgard P, et al: Prostacyclin deficiency in thrombotic thrombocytopenic purpura. Lancet 2:748, 1979.
33. Turpie AGG: Antiplatelet therapy. In Prentice CRM (ed): Thrombosis. Clin Haematol 10:497, 1981.
34. Berndt MC, Caen JP: Platelet glycoproteins. Prog Hemost Thromb 7:111, 1984.
35. Bick RL, Baker WF: Disseminated intravascular coagulation syndromes. Hematol Pathol 6:1–24, 1992.
36. Coleman RW, Bagdasarian A, Talmo RC, et al: Williams trait: Human kininogen deficiency with diminished levels of plasminogen proactivator and prekallikrein associated with abnormalities of the Hageman factor dependent pathway. J Clin Invest 56:1650, 19xx.
37. Habel FM, Movat HZ: Kininogens of human plasma. Semin Thromb Hemost 3:27, 1976.
38. Murano G: The "Hageman connection" interrelationships of blood coagulation, fibrino(geno)lysis, kinin generation, and complement activation. Am J Hematol 4:303, 1978.
39. McKusick VA: Mendelian Inheritance in Man: Catalogs of Autosomal Dominant, Autosomal Recessive and X-linked Phenotypes, 9th ed. Baltimore, Johns Hopkins University Press, 1990.
40. Schriver CR, Beaudet AL, Sly WS: Blood and blood forming tissue (part 14). In Stanbury JB (ed): The Metabolic Basis of Inherited Disease. New York, McGraw-Hill, 1989, p 2107.
41. Kaplan AJ, Meier HL, Mandle R: The Hageman factor dependent pathways of coagulation, fibrinolysis, and kinin-generation. Semin Thromb Hemost 3:1, 1976.
42. Kaplan AP: Initiation of the intrinsic coagulation and fibrinolytic pathways of man: The role of surfaces, Hagemen factor, prekallikrein, high molecular weight kininogen, and factor XI. Prog Hemost Thromb 4:127, 1978.
43. Meyer KL, Pierce JV, Coleman RW, Kaplan AV: Activation and function of human Hageman factor. J Clin Invest 60:18, 1977.
44. Ratnoff OD, Saito H: Coagulation factors and the role of surfaces in their activation. Ann NY Acad Sci 283:88, 1977.
45. Griffin JH, Cochrane CG: Recent advances in the understanding of contact activation reactions. Semin Thromb Hemost 5:254, 1979.
46. Wiggins RC, Bouma BN, Cochrane CG, Griffin JH: Role of high-molecular-weight kininogen in surface-binding and activation of coagulation Factor XI and prekallikrein. Proc Natl Acad Sci (USA) 74:4636, 1977.
47. Seegers WH: Enzymes in blood clotting. J Med Enzymol (Japan) 2:68, 1977.
48. Irwin JF, Seegers WH, Andary TJ, et al: Blood coagulation as a cybernetic system: Control of autoprothrombin C (Xa) formation. Thromb Res 6:431, 1975.
49. Seegers WH, Murano G: Blood coagulation: A cybernetic system. Pol Arch Med Wewn 55:1, 1976.
50. Seegers WH, Hassouna HI, Hewett-Emmett D, Andary TJ: Prothrombin and thrombin: Selected aspects of thrombin formation, properties, inhibition, and immunology. Semin Thromb Hemost 1:211, 1975.
51. Seegers WH, Sakuragawa N, McCoy LE, et al: Prothrombin activation: ac-globulin, lipid, platelet membrane, and autoprothrombin c (Xa) requirements. Thromb Res 1:293, 1972.
52. Denson KWE: The levels of Factor II, VII, IX, and X by antibody neutralization techniques in the plasma of patients receiving phenindione therapy. Br J Haematol 20:643, 1971.
53. Pereira M, Couri D: Studies on the site of action of dicoumarol on prothrombin synthesis. Biochem Biophys Acta 237:348, 1971.

54. Stenflo T: Vitamin K, prothrombin, and gamma-carboxy-glutamic acid. N Engl J Med 296:624, 1977.
55. Mackie MJ, Douglas AS: Drug-induced disorders of coagulation. In Ratnoff OD, Forbes CD (eds): Disorders of Hemostasis. Philadelphia, W.B. Saunders, 1991, p 493.
56. Huseby RM: Conformational structure of the fibrinopeptides related during fibrinogen to fibrin conversion. Physiol Chem Phys 5:1, 1973.
57. Walz DA, Seegers WH, Reuterby J, McCoy LE: Proteolytic specificity of thrombin. Thromb Res 4:713, 1974.
58. Alami SY, Hampton JW, Race GH, Speer RH: Fibrin stabilizing factor (Factor XIII). Am J Med 44:1, 1968.
59. Ratnoff OD: The molecular basis of hereditary clotting disorders. Prog Hemost Thromb 1:39, 1972.
60. Winman B, Hamsten A: The fibrinolytic enzyme system and its role in the etiology of thromboembolic disease. Semin Thromb Hemost 16:207, 1990.
61. Aoki N, Harpel PC: Inhibitors of the fibrinolytic enzyme system. Semin Thromb Hemost 10:24, 1984.
62. Bick RL: The clinical significance of fibrinogen degradation products. Semin Thromb Hemost 8:302, 1982.
63. Castellino FJ: Biochemistry of human plasminogen. Semin Thromb Hemost 10:18, 1984.
64. Bang NU: Physiology and biochemistry of the fibrinolytic system. In Bang NU, Beller KF, Deutch E, Mammen EF (eds): Thrombosis and Bleeding Disorders. New York, Academic Press, 1971, p 292.
65. Bick RL, Kunkel L: Disseminated intravascular coagulation syndromes. Int J Haematol 55:1-26, 1992.
66. Bick RL, Scates S: Disseminated intravascular coagulation syndromes. Lab Med 23:161-165, 1992.
67. Ratnoff OD, Naff GB: The conversion of C'1s to C'1 esterase by plasmin and trypsin. J Exp Med 125:337, 1967.
68. Robbins KM: Present status of the fibrinolytic system. In Fareed J, Messmore HL, Fenton J, Brinkhous KM (eds): Perspectives in Hemostasis. New York, Pergamon Press, 1980, p 53.
69. Bachmann F, Kruithof KO: Tissue plasminogen activator: Chemical and physiological aspects. Semin Thromb Hemost 10:6, 1984.
70. Kaplan AP, Austin F: The fibrinolytic pathway of human plasma. Isolation and characterization of the plasminogen proactivator. J Exp Med 135:1378, 1972.
71. Robbins KC, Barlow GH, Hguyen G: Comparison of plasminogen activators. Semin Thromb Hemost 13:131, 1987.
72. Bick RL: Thrombolytic therapy. In Disorders of Thrombosis and Hemostasis: Clinical and Laboratory Practice. Chicago, ASCP Press, 1992, p 313.
73. Schreiber AD: Plasma inhibitors of the Hageman factor dependent pathways. Semin Thromb Hemost 3:43, 1976.
74. Loskutoff DJ, Sawdey M, Mimuro J: Type 1 plasminogen activator inhibitor. Prog Hemost Thromb 9:87, 1989.
75. Astedt B, Lecander I, Ny T: The placental type plasminogen activator inhibitor: PAI-2. Fibrinolysis 1:203, 1987.
76. Sprengers ED, Verheijen JH, van Hinsbergh VMW, et al: Evidence for the presence of two different fibrinolytic inhibitors in human endothelial cells culture medium. Biochem Biophys Acta 801:163, 1984.
77. Sprengers ED, Princen HMG, Kooistra T, et al: Inhibition of plasminogen activators by conditioned medium of human hepatocytes and hepatoma cell line. J Lab Clin Med 105:751, 1985.
78. Booth NA, Anderson JA, Bennett B: Platelet release protein which inhibits plasminogen activators. J Clin Pathol 38:825, 1985.
79. Laug EW: Vascular smooth muscle cells inhibit the plasminogen activators secreted by endothelial cells. Thromb Res 53:165, 1985.
80. Philips M, Juul AG, Thorsen S, et al: Purification and characterization of reactive and nonreactive plasminogen activator inhibitor-1 from human placenta. Thromb Haemost 58:2, 1987.
81. Kopitar M, Rozman B, Babnik J, et al: Human leukocyte urokinase inhibitor—purification, characterization and comparative studies against different plasminogen activators. Thromb Haemost 54:750, 1985.
82. Vasalli JD, Dayer JM, Wohlwend A, et al: Concomitant secretion of prourokinase and of plasminogen activator-specific inhibitor by cultured human monocytes-macrophages. J Exp Med 159:1653, 1984.

83. Rosse WF: Complement. In Williams WJ, Beutler E, Erslev AJ, Rundles RW (eds): Hematology. New York, McGraw-Hill, 1977, p 87.
84. Ruddy S, Gigli I, Austen KF: The complement system in man. I. Activation, control, and products of the reaction sequences. N Engl J Med 278:489, 1972.
85. Mayer MM: The component system. Sci Am 229:54, 1973.
86. Muller-Eberhard HJ: Complement. Annu Rev Biochem 44:667, 1975.
87. Muller-Berghaus G: Pathophysiologic and biochemical events in disseminated intravascular coagulation: Dysregulation of procoagulant and anticoagulant pathways. Semin Thromb Hemost 15:58, 1989.
88. Bennett B, Ogston D: Role of complement, coagulation, fibrinolysis, and kinins in normal haemostasis and disease. In Bloom AL, Thomas DP (eds): Haemostasis and Thrombosis. London, Churchill-Livingston, 1981, p 236.
89. Ryan JW, Ryan US: Biochemical and morphological aspects of the actions and metabolism of kinins. In Pisano JJ, Austen KF (eds): Chemistry and Biology of the Kallikrein-Kinin System in Health and Disease. DHEW Publ No. 76-791, Bethesda, MD, U.S. Department of Health, Education, and Welfare, 1974, p 315.
90. Van Arman CG, Bohidar HR: Role of the kallikrein-kinin system in inflammation. In Pisano JJ, Austin KF (eds): Chemistry and Biology of the Kallikrein-Kinin System in Health and Disease. DHEW Publ No. 76-791. Bethesda, MD, U.S. Department of Health, Education and Welfarre, 1974, p 471.
91. Comp PC: Hereditary disorders predisposing to thrombosis. Prog Hemost Thromb 8:71, 1986.
92. Joist JH: Hypercoagulability: Introduction and perspective. Semin Thromb Hemost 16:151, 1990.
93. Esmon CT: Protein-C: Biochemistry, physiology, and clinical implications. Blood 62:1155, 1983.
94. Seegers WH: Protein C and autoprothrombin II-A. Semin Thromb Hemost 7:257, 1981.
95. Scully MF, Ellis V, Kakkar VV: Studies of anti-Xa activity. Thromb Res 29:387, 1983.
96. Bick RL: Clinical relevance of antithrombin III. Semin Thromb Hemost 8:276, 1982.
97. Rosenberg RD: The effect of heparin on Factor XIa and plasmin. Thromb Diath Haemorrh 33:51, 1975.
98. Rosenberg RD, Damus P: The purification and mechanism of action of human antithrombin-heparin cofactor. J Biol Chem 248:6490, 1973.
99. Jaques LB, McDuffie NM: The chemical and anticoagulant nature of heparin. Semin Thromb Hemost 4:277, 1978.
100. Rosenberg RD: Biologic actions of heparin. Semin Hematol 14:427, 1977.
101. Seegers WH: Antithrombin-III theory and clinical applications. Am J Clin Pathol 69:367, 1978.
102. Bick RL: Assessment of patients with hemorrhage. In Disorders of Thrombosis and Hemostasis: Clinical and Laboratory Practice, Chicago, ASCP Press, 1992, p 27.
103. Bick RL, Tse N: Hemostasis abnormalities associated with prosthetic devices and organ transplantation. Lab Med 3:462–486, 1992.
104. Bick RL: Hemostasis defects with cardiac surgery, general surgery, and prosthetic devices. In Disorders of Thrombosis and Hemostasis: Clinical and Laboratory Practice. Chicago, ASCP Press, 1992, p 195.
105. Bick RL: Hemostasis defects in general surgery, cardiac surgery, transplantation, and the use of prosthetic devices. In Disorders of Hemostasis and Thrombosis: Principles of Clinical Practice. New York, Thieme, Inc., 1985, p 223.
106. Mielke CH, Kaneshiro MM, Maher LA, et al: The standardized normal Ivy bleeding time and is prolongation by aspirin. Blood 34:204, 1969.
107. Bick RL: Platelet defects. In Disorders of Hemostasis and Thrombosis: Principles of Clinical Practice. New York, Thieme, Inc., 1985, p 65.
108. Bick RL, Murano G: Primary hyperfibrino(geno)lytic syndromes. In Murano G, Bick RL (eds): Basic Concepts of Hemostasis and Thrombosis. Boca Raton, FL, CRC Press, 1980, p 181.
109. Bick RL: Syndromes associated with hyperfibrino(geno)lysis. In Disseminated Intravascular Coagulation. Boca Raton, FL, CRC Press, 1983, p 105.
110. Shahian DM, Wallach SR, Bern MM: Open heart surgery in patients with cold-reactive proteins. Surg Clin North Am 65:315, 1985.
111. Landymore R, Isom W, Barlam B: Management of patients with cold agglutinins who require open-heart surgery. Can J Surg 26:79, 1983.

112. Guena L, Kwabena KA, Addei A: Intraoperative hypothermia in a patient with cold agglutinin disease. JAMA 74:691, 1982.
113. Klein HG, Faltz LL, McIntosh CL, et al: Surgical hypothermia in a patient with a cold agglutinin. Transfusion 20:354, 1980.
114. Leach AB, Van Hasselt GL, Edwards JC: Cold agglutinins and deep hypothermia. Anaesthesia 38:140, 1983.
115. Moore RA, Geller EA, Mathews ES, et al: The effect of hypothermic cardiopulmonary bypass on patients with low-titer, non-specific cold agglutinins. Ann Thorac Surg 37:233, 1984.
116. Brecker G, Cronkite EP: Morphology and enumeration of human blood platelets. J Appl Physiol 3:365, 1950.
117. Hougie C: Fundamentals of Blood Coagulation in Clinical Medicine. New York, McGraw-Hill, 1963, p 241.
118. Proctor RR, Rapaport SI: The partial thromboplastin time with kaolin. A simple screening test for first stage plasma clotting factor deficiencies. Am J Clin Pathol 36:212, 1961.
119. Quick AJ, Stanley-Brown M, Bancroft FW: A study of the coagulation defect in hemophilia and in jaundice. Am J Med Sci 190:501, 1935.
120. Bick RL: Alterations of hemostasis associated with surgery, cardiopulmonary bypass surgery, prosthetic devices and transplantation. In Ratnoff OD, Frobes CD (eds): Disorders of Hemostasis, 2nd ed. Philadelphia, W.B. Saunders, 1991, p 382.
121. Bick RL: Hemostasis defects associated with cardiac surgery, prosthetic devices, and other extracorporeal circuits. Semin Thromb Hemost 11:249, 1985.
122. Beall C, Yow EM, Blodwell RD, et al: Open heart surgery without blood transfusion. Arch Surg 94:567, 1967.
123. Cordell AR: Hematological complications of extracorporeal circulation. In Cordell AR, Ellison RG (eds): Complications of Intrathoracic Surgery. Boston, Little, Brown, 1979, p 27.
124. Mammen EF: Natural proteinase inhibitors in extracorporeal circulation. Ann NY Acad Sci 146:754, 1968.
125. Koets MH, Washington BC, Wolk LW, et al: Hemostasis changes during cardiovascular bypass surgery. Semin Thromb Hemost 11:281, 1985.
126. Bick RL: Pathophysiology of hemostasis and thrombosis. In Sodeman T: Sodeman's Pathologic Physiology, Mechanisms of Disease, 7th ed. Philadelphia, W.B. Saunders, 1985, p 705.
127. Kevy SV, Glickman RM, Bernhard WF, et al: The pathogenesis and control of the hemorrhagic defect in open-heart surgery. Surg Gynecol Obstet 123:313, 1966.
128. Signori EE, Penner JA, Kahn DR: Coagulation defects and bleeding in open heart surgery. Ann Thorac Surg 8:521, 1969.
129. Porter JM, Silver D: Alterations in fibrinolysis and coagulation associated with cardiopulmonary bypass. J Thorac Cardiovasc Surg 56:869, 1968.
130. Tice DA, Worth MH: Recognition and treatment of postoperative bleeding associated with open heart surgery. Ann NY Acad Sci 146:745, 1968.
131. Wright TA, Darte J, Mustard WT: Postoperative bleeding after extracorporeal circulation. Can J Surg 2:142, 1959.
132. von Kaulla KN, Swan H: Clotting deviations in man during cardiac bypass: Fibrinolysis and circulating anticoagulants. J Thorac Surg 36:519, 1958.
133. Blomback M, Noren I, Senning A: Coagulation disturbances during extracorporeal circulation and the postoperative period. Acta Chir Scand 127:433, 1964.
134. Deiter RA, Neville WE, Pifarre R, Jasuja M: Preoperative coagulation profiles and posthemodilution cardiopulmonary bypass hemorrhage. Am J Surg 121:689, 1971.
135. Penick GD, Averette HE, Peters RM, Brinkhous KM: The hemorrhagic syndrome complicating extracorporeal shunting of blood: An experimental study of its pathogenesis. Thromb Diath Haemorrh 2:218, 1958.
136. Trimble AS, Herst R, Grady M, Crookston J: Blood loss in open heart surgery. Arch Surg 93:323, 1966.
137. Bick RL, Arbegast NR, Holtermann N, et al: Platelet function abnormalities in cardiopulmonary bypass. Circulation 50(Suppl):301, 1974.
138. Bick RL, Schmalhorst WR, Crawford L, et al: The hemorrhagic diathesis created by cardiopulmonary bypass. Am J Clin Pathol 63:588, 1975.
139. Bick RL, Arbegast NR, Crawford L, et al: Hemostatic defects induced by cardiopulmonary bypass. Vasc Surg 9:228, 1975.
140. Bick RL, Schmalhorst WR, Arbegast NR: Alterations of hemostasis associated with cardiopulmonary bypass. Am J Clin Pathol 63:588, 1975.

141. Castenada AR: Must heparin be neutralized following open heart operations? J Thorac Cardiovasc Surg 52:716, 1966.
142. deVries SI, von Creveld S, Green P, et al: Studies on the coagulation of the blood in patients treated with extracorporeal circulation. Thromb Diath Haemorrh 5:426, 1961.
143. Muller N, Popov-Cenic S, Buttner W, et al: Studies of fibrinolytic and coagulation factors during open-heart surgery. II. Postoperative bleeding tendencies and changes in the coagulation system. Thromb Res 7:589, 1975.
144. Bick RL: Alterations of hemostasis during cardiopulmonary bypass: A comparison between membrane and bubble oxygenators. Am J Clin Pathol 73:300, 1980.
145. Bick RL, Schmalhorst SW, Arbegast NR: Alterations of hemostasis associated with cardiopulmonary bypass. Thromb Res 8:285, 1976.
146. Holswade GR, Nachman RL, Killip T: Thrombocytopathies in patients with open-heart surgery. Preoperative treatment with corticosteroids. Arch Surg 94:365, 1967.
147. Salzman WE: Blood platelets and extracorporeal circulation. Transfusion 3:274, 1963.
148. Bick RL, Adams T, Schmalhorst WR: Bleeding times, platelet adhesion, and aspirin. Am J Clin Pathol 65:69, 1976.
149. Bowie EJW, Owen CA, Thompson JH: Platelet adhesiveness in von Willebrand's disease. Am J Clin Pathol 52:69, 1969.
150. Bowie EJW, Owen CA: The value of measuring platelet adhesiveness in the diagnosis of bleeding diseases. Am J Clin Pathol 60:302, 1973.
151. Hirsh J: Laboratory diagnosis of thrombosis. In Coleman RW, Hirsh J, Marder VJ, Salzman EW (eds): Basic Principles and Clinical Practice. Philadelphia, J.B. Lippincott, 1982, p 789.
152. Zimmerman TS, Meyer D: Factor VIII-von Willebrand factor and the molecular basis of von Willebrand's disease. In Coleman RW, Hirsh J, Marder VJ, Salzman EW (eds): Hemostasis and Thrombosis: Basic Principles and Clinical Practice. Philadelphia, J.B. Lippincott, 1982, p 54.
153. Adams T, Schutz L, Goldberg L: Platelet function abnormalities in the myeloproliferative disorders. Scand J Haematol 13:215, 1975.
154. Mustard JF, Packham MA: Factors influencing platelet function: Adhesion, release, and aggregation. Pharmacol Rev 23:97, 1970.
155. Bick RL: The clinical significance of fibrinogen degradation products. Semin Thromb Hemost 8:302, 1982.
156. Sarin CL, Yalav E, Clement AJ, Braimbridge MV: Thromboembolism after Starr valve replacement. Br Heart J 33:111, 1971.
157. Hellem AJ: The advances of human blood platelets in vitro. Scand J Clin Lab Invest 51(Suppl):1, 1960.
158. Bick RL, Fekete LF: Cardiopulmonary bypass hemorrhage: Aggravation by pre-op ingestion of antiplatelet agents. Vasc Surg 13:277, 1979.
159. Kowalski E, Kopec M, Wegrzynowicz Z: Influence of fibrinogen degradation products (FDP) on platelet aggregation, adhesiveness, and viscous metamorphosis. Thromb Diath Haemorrh 10:406, 1963.
160. Kowalski E: Fibrinogen derivatives and their biologic activities. Semin Hematol 5:455, 1968.
161. Harker LA, Malpass TW, Branson HE, et al: Mechanisms of abnormal bleeding in patients undergoing cardiopulmonary bypass: Acquired transient platelet dysfunction associated with selective alpha-granule release. Blood 56:824, 1980.
162. Stass S, Bishop C, Fosberg R, et al: Platelets as affected by cardiopulmonary byapss. Trans Am Soc Clin Pathol, 1976, p 35 [abstract].
163. Saunders CR, Carlisle L, Bick RL: Hydroxyethyl starch versus albumin in cardiopulmonary bypass prime solutions. Ann Thorac Surg 36:53282.
164. Salzman EW, Weinstein MJ, Weintraub RM, et al: Treatment with desmopressin acetate to reduce blood loss after cardiac surgery. N Engl J Med 314:1402, 1986.
165. Weinstein M, Ware JA, Troll J, Salzman EW: Changes in von Willebrand Factor during cardiac surgery: Effect of desmopressin acetate. Blood 71:1648, 1988.
166. Rocha E, Llorens R, Paramo JA, et al: Does desmopressin acetate reduce blood loss after surgery in patients on cardiopulmonary bypass? Circulation 77:1319, 1988.
167. Mannucci PM: Desmopressin (DDAVP) for treatment of disorders of hemostasis. Prog Hemost Thromb 8:19, 1986.
168. Warrier I, Lusher JM: DDAVP: A useful alternative to blood components in moderate hemophilia A and von Willebrand's disease. J Pediatr 102:228, 1983.
169. Mariani G, Ciavarella N, Mazzuconni MG: Evaluation of the effectiveness of DDAVP in surgery and in bleeding episodes in hemophilia and von Willebrand's disease: A study of 43 patients. Clin Lab Haematol 6:229, 1984.

170. De La Fuente B, Kasper CK, Rickles FR: Response of patients with mild hemophilia A and von Willebrand's disease to treatment with desmopressin. Ann Intern Med 103:6, 1985.
171. Derman UM, Rand PW, Barker N: Fibrinolysis after cardiopulmonary bypass and its relationship to fibrinogen. J Thorac Cardiovasc Surg 51:223, 1966.
172. Bachmann F, McKenna R, Cole ER, Maiafi HJ: The hemostatic mechanisms after open-heart surgery. I. Studies on plasma coagulation factors and fibrinolysis in 512 patients after extracorporeal circulation. J Thorac Cardiovasc Surg 70:76, 1975.
173. Tsuji HK, Redington JV, Kay JH, Goesswald RK: The study of fibrinolytic and coagulation factors during open heart surgery. Ann NY Acad Sci 146:763, 1968.
174. Woods JE, Kirklin JW, Owen CA, et al: The effect of bypass surgery on coagulation sensitive clotting factors. Mayo Clin Proc 42:724, 1967.
175. Gans H, Subramanian V, John S, et al: Theoretical and practical (clinical) considerations concerning proteolytic enzymes and their inhibitors with particular reference to changes in the plasminogen-plasmin system during assisted circulation in man. Ann NY Acad Sci 146:721, 1968.
176. Palester-Chlebowzyk M, Strzyzewska E, Sitowski W, Olender K: Detection of the intravascular coagulation of blood clotting. II. Results of the paracoagulation test in patients undergoing o pen-heart surgery, with extracorporeal circulation. Pol Med J 11:59, 1972.
177. Kladetsky RG, Popov-Cenic S, Buttner W, et al: Studies of fibrinolytic and coagulation factors during open-heart surgery with ECC. Thromb Res 7:579, 1975.
178. Gomes MM, McGoon D: Bleeding patterns after open heart surgery. J Thorac Cardiovasc Surg 60:87, 1970.
179. Bick RL: Disseminated intravascular coagulation. In Disorders of Thrombosis and Hemostasis: Clinical and Laboratory Practice. Chicago, ASCP Press, 1992, p 137.
180. Bick RL: Disseminated intravascular coagulation and related syndromes: A clinical review. Semin Thromb Hemost 14:299, 1988.
181. Bick RL: Clinical hemostasis practice: The major impact of laboratory automation. Semin Thromb Hemost 9:139, 1983.
182. Bick RL, Kovacs I, Fekete LF: A new two stage functional assay for antithrombin III (heparin cofactor): Clinical and laboratory evaluation. Thromb Res 8:745, 1976.
183. Lackner H, Javid JP: The clinical significance of the plasminogen level. Am J Clin Pathol 60:175, 1973.
184. Tsitouris G, Bellet S, Eilberg R, et al: Effects of major surgery on plasmin-plasminogen systems. Arch Intern Med 108:98, 1961.
185. Wuelfing D, Brandau KP: Fibrinolytic activity after surgery. Minn Med 51:1503, 1968.
186. Ygge J: Changes in blood coagulation and fibrinolysis during the postoperative period. Am J Surg 119:225, 1970.
187. Bick RL, Bishop RC, Warren M, Stemmer E: Changes in fibrinolysis and fibrinolytic enzymes during extracorporeal circulation. Trans Am Soc Hematol 109, 1971.
188. Graeff H, Beller FK: Fibrinolytic activity in whole blood, dilute blood, and euglobulin lysis time tests. In Bang N, Beller FK, Deutsch E (eds): Thrombosis and Bleeding Disorders, Theory and Methods. New York, Academic Press, 1970, p 328.
189. Menon IS: A study of the possible correlation of euglobulin lysis time and dilute blood clot lysis in the determination of fibrinolytic activity. Lab Pract 17:334, 1968.
190. Bick RL, Bishop RC, Shanbrom ES: Fibrinolytic activity in acute myocardial infarction. Am J Clin Pathol 57:359, 1972.
191. Bishop RC, Ekert H, Gilchrist G, et al: The preparation and evaluation of a standardized fibrin plate for the assessment of fibrinolytic activity. Thromb Diath Haemorrh 23:202, 1970.
192. Fareed J: New methods in hemostatic testing. In Fareed J, Messmore H, Fenton J (eds): Perspectives in Hemostasis. New York, Pergamon Press, 1981, p 310.
193. Fareed J, Messmore HL, Bermes EW: New perspectives in coagulation testing. Clin Chem 26:1380, 1980.
194. Huseby RM, Smith RE: Synthetic oligopeptide substrates: Their diagnostic application in blood coagulation, fibrinolysis, and other pathologic states. Semin Thromb Hemost 6:173, 1980.
195. Naeye RL: Thrombotic state after a hemorrhagic diathesis: A possible complication of therapy with epsilon aminocaproic acid. Blood 19:694, 1962.
196. Ratnoff OD: Epsilon aminocaproic acid: A dangerous weapon. N Engl J Med 280:1124, 1969.
197. Verska JJ, Lonser ER, Brewer LA: Predisposing factors and management of hemorrhage following open-heart surgery. J Cardiovasc Surg (Torino) 13:361, 1972.
198. Verska J: Letter to the editor. Ann Thorac Surg 13:87, 1972.

199. Brooks DH, Bahnson HT: An outbreak of hemorrhage following cardiopulmonary bypass. J Thorac Cardiovasc Surg 63:449, 1972.
200. O'Neill JA, Ende N, Collins IS, Collins HA: A quantitative determination of perfusion fibrinolysis. Surgery 60:809, 1966.
201. Bick RL, Frazier BL, Saunders CL, Arbegast NR: Alterations of hemostasis during cardiopulmonary bypass: The potential role of Factor XII activation in inducing primary fibrino(geno)lysis. Blood 64:926, 1984.
202. Akkerman JW, Runne WC, Sixma JJ, Zimmerman AE: Improved survival rates in dogs after extracorporeal circulation by improved control of heparin levels. J Thorac Cardiovasc Surg 68:59, 1974.
203. Ellison N, Betty CP, Blake DR, et al: Heparin rebound: Studies in patients and volunteers. J Thorac Cardiovasc Surg 67:723, 1974.
204. Gollub S: Heparin rebound in open-heart surgery. Surg Gynecol Obstet 124:337, 1967.
205. Jaberi M, Bell WR, Benson DW: Control of heparin therapy in open-heart surgery. J Thorac Cardiovasc Surg 67:133, 1974.
206. Ellison N, Ominsky AJ, Wollman H: Is protamine a clinically important anticoagulant? A negative answer. Anesthesiology 35:621, 1971.
207. Ollendorff P: The nature of the anticoagulant effect of heparin, protamine, Polybrene, and toluidine blue. Scand J Clin Lab Invest 14:267, 1962.
208. Tsai TP, Matloff JM, Gray RJ, et al: Cardiac surgery in the octagenarian. J Thorac Surg 91:924, 1986.
209. Horneffer PJ, Gardner TJ, Manolio TA, et al: The effects of age on outcome after coronary bypass surgery. Circulation 76:5-6, 1987.
210. Soloway HB, Cornett BM, Donahoo JV, Cox SP: Differentiation of bleeding diathesis which occurs following protamine correction of heparin anticoagulation. Am J Clin Pathol 60:188, 1973.
211. Lewis JH, Wilson HJ, Brandon JM: Counterelectrophoresis test for molecules immunologically similar to fibrinogen. Am J Clin Pathol 58:400, 1972.
212. Salzman EW: The events that lead to thrombosis. Bull NY Acad Med 48:225, 1972.
213. Bick RL, Baker WF: Diagnostic efficacy of the D-Dimer assay in DIC and related disorders. Blood 68:329, 1986.
214. Rousou JA, Engelman RM, Breyer RH: Fibrin glue: An effective hemostatic agent for nonsuturable intraoperative bleeding. Ann Thorac Surg 38:409, 1984.
215. Rousou J: Randomized clinical trial of fibrin glue sealant in patients undergoing resternotomy or reoperation after cardiac operations: A multicenter study. J Thorac Surg 97:194, 1989.
216. Garcia-Rinaldi R, Simmons P, Salcedo V, Howland C: A technique for spot application of fibrin glue during open heart operations. Ann Thorac Surg 47:59, 1989.
217. Dresdale A, Bowman FO, Malm JR, et al: Hemostatic effectiveness of fibrin glue derived from single-donor fresh frozen plasma. Ann Thorac Surg 40:385, 1985.
218. Verstraete M: Clinical application of inhibitors of fibrinolysis. Drugs 29:236, 1985.
219. Frankl WS: Indications for anticoagulants in cardiovascular disease. In Jepson JH, Frankl WS (eds): Hematological Complications in Cardiac Practice. Philadelphia, W.B. Saunders, 1975, p 182.
220. Kaltman AJ: Late complications of heart valve replacement. Annu Rev Med 2:343, 1971.
221. Fraser RS, Waddell J: Systemic embolization after aortic valve replacement. J Thorac Cardiovasc Surg 54:81, 1967.
222. Effler DB, Favaloro R, Groves LK: Heart valve replacement: Clinical experience. Ann Thorac Surg 1:4, 1965.
223. Mason RG, Chuang HYK, Mohammad SF, Saba HI: Thrombosis and artificial surfaces. In van de Loo J, Prentice CRM, Beller FK (eds): The Thromboembolic Disorders. Stuttgart, Schattauer Verlag, 1983, p 533.
224. Akbarian M, Austen WG, Yurchak PM, Scannel JG: Thromboembolic complications of prosthetic cardiac valves. Circulation 37:826, 1968.
225. Duvoisin GE, Brandenburg RO, McGoon DC: Factors affecting thromboembolism associated with prosthetic heart valves. Circulation 35:70, 1967.
226. Forbes CD: Thrombosis and artificial surfaces. In Prentice CRM (ed): Thrombosis. Clin Haematol 10:653, 1981.
227. Berger S, Salzman EW: Thromboembolic complications of prosthetic devices. Prog Hemost Thromb 2:273, 1974.
228. Weiss HJ: Antiplatelet drugs in clinical medicine. In Platelets: Pathophysiology and Antiplatelet Drug Therapy. New York, Alan R. Liss, Inc., 1982, p 75.

229. Harker LA, Slichter SJ: Studies of platelet and fibrinogen kinetics in patients with prosthetic heart valves. N Engl J Med 282:1302, 1970.
230. Harker LA, Hirsh J, Gent M, Genton E: Critical evaluation of platelet-inhibiting drugs in thrombotic disease. Prog Hematol 9:229, 1975.
231. Weily HS, Steele PP, Davies H, et al: Platelet survival in patients with substitute heart valves. N Engl J Med 290:534, 1974.
232. Steele PP, Weily HS, Davies H, Genton E: Platelet survival in patients with rheumatic heart disease. N Engl J Med 290:537, 1974.
233. Weily HW, Genton E: Altered platelet function in patients with prosthetic mitral valves. Effects of sulfinpyrazone therapy. Circulation 42:967, 1970.
234. Sullivan JM, Harken DE, Gorlin R: Pharmacologic control of thromboembolic complications of cardiac-valve replacement. N Engl J Med 284:1391, 1971.
235. Dale J, Myhre E, Storstein A, et al: Prevention of arterial thromboembolism with acetylsalicylic acid. Am Heart J 94:101, 1977.
236. Dale J, Myhre E, Lowe D: Bleeding during acetylsalicylic acid and anticoagulant therapy in patients with reduced platelet reactivity after aortic valve replacement. Am Heart J 99:746, 1980.
237. Altman R, Boullon F, Rouvier J, et al: Aspirin and prophylaxis of thromboembolic complications in patients with substitute heart valves. J Thorac Cardiovasc Surg 72:127, 1976.
238. Arrants JE, Hairston E: Use of persantine in preventing thromboembolism following valve replacement. Ann Surg 38:432, 1972.
239. Taguchi K, Matsumura H, Washizu T, et al: Effect of athrombogenic therapy, especially high dose therapy of dipyridamole, after prosthetic valve replacement. J Cardiovasc Surg 16:8, 1975.
240. Bjork VO, Henz A: Management of thrombo-embolism after aortic valve replacement with the Bjork-Shiley tilting disc valve. Scand J Thorac Cardiovasc Surg 9:183, 1975.
241. Gadboys HL, Litwak RS, Niemetz J, Wisch N: Role of anticoagulants in preventing embolization from prosthetic heart valves. JAMA 202:282, 1967.
242. Friedli B, Aerichide N, Grondin P, Campeau L: Thromboembolic complications of heart valve prostheses. Am Heart J 81:702, 1971.
243. Dalen JE, Hirsh J: American College of Chest Physician and the National Heart, Lung, and Blood Institute National Conference on Antithrombotic Therapy. Chest 95:107, 1989.

Chapter 3

Protocol for Anticoagulation During Cardiopulmonary Bypass

Roque Pifarré, M.D., Maher Istanbouli, C.C.P., and Jamal Sinno, C.C.P.

The first repair of an atrial septal defect was performed by Gibbons[12] in 1953 under direct vision using cardiopulmonary bypass (CPB). Many technical and mechanical advances made possible that milestone in cardiac surgery; however, CPB was possible only with anticoagulation with heparin. Systemic anticoagulation is required to prevent coagulation of the blood when it comes in contact with the foreign surfaces of the heart-lung machine. Heparin is used for this purpose because it inhibits thrombin, thus preventing the creation of fibrin. McLean[19] discovered heparin fortuitously in 1916 while trying to isolate the procoagulant thromboplastin in Howell's laboratory. Howell reported his preliminary communication on heparin as an anticoagulant in 1922.[17] The discovery of the anticoagulant effect of heparin and the subsequent finding that protamine reverses this effect made possible the routine use of CPB in cardiac surgery.

The complexity of hemostatic control during CPB needs to be emphasized. The cardiovascular surgeon must have a good understanding of the variables associated with the therapeutic use of heparin, its neutralization with protamine, and the individual nature of these responses. The protocol for anticoagulation during CPB has varied greatly from institution to institution. Lately, with the use of the activated clotting time (ACT) (Hemochron mode 400, International Technidyne, Edison, NJ) and the heparin analyzer (Hepcon HMS, Medtronic Hemotec, Inc.), the control of anticoagulation has become more uniform and the neutralization of heparin with protamine more accurate.

The importance of ascertaining the proper dose of heparin during CPB cannot be overemphasized. The amount of heparin given must be carefully calculated. Too high a dose can lead to bleeding, whereas too low a dose can lead to clotting.

HEPARIN

Heparin, a polysaccharide sulfuric acid ester found in the liver, lung, and other tissues, prolongs the clotting time of blood by preventing the formation of fibrin. Heparin exerts its anticoagulant action via a plasmaprotein called antithrombin III (AT-III). By binding to AT-III, heparin effects an accelerated reaction with thrombin and leads to the formation of an inactive complex of the two proteins.

Heparin is the anticoagulant of choice during CPB surgery, because of its immediate anticoagulant action, ease of administration, and rapid reversal with protamine. However, the changes in coagulation parameters that take place during CPB vary significantly among individuals as well as with time. The high concentration of heparin required during CPB precludes the use of most standard monitoring techniques, because of the length of time required to perform such tests and the difficulty in determining the endpoint of the clotting assays.[3] At the present time, the ACT and the Hepcon are used to monitor the level of anticoagulation during bypass. The Hepcon is used to calculate the amount of protamine needed to neutralize the heparin at the end of bypass.

Complications of heparin include allergic reactions, thrombocytopenia, thrombosis, bleeding, and disseminated intravascular coagulation (DIC).

Heparin Administration Protocol

In order to have a baseline value, the ACT is calculated with Hemochron model 400 at 200 U/kg of body weight (Table 1). The heparin is administered directly into the right atrium of the heart by the surgeon before cannulation of the aorta and right atrium for CPB. This method of administration accomplishes two objectives: (1) it ensures that the heparin has entered the central circulation, and (2) it ensures that the full dose of heparin has been administered. Heparin administered in a peripheral line may not reach the central circulation; the result could be catastrophic. During CPB the ACT is maintained above 400 seconds. Several doses of 2000-3000 units of heparin are added to the oxygenator, if needed, to maintain the ACT above the level of 400 seconds.

Other teams use an initial dose of 300-400 U/kg of body weight. During bypass, heparin is added at a rate of 50-100 U/kg/hour. Monitoring anticoagulation with the ACT and the heparin analyzer (Hepcon) has convinced us that the lower dosage is safe and the higher unnecessary. Our findings[2,24] agree with those of Metz and Keats.[20]

Once CPB is discontinued, the dose of protamine for heparin reversal is calculated with use of the Hepcon HMS heparin analyzer system (Fig. 1). The procedure is as follows: A 3-ml blood sample from an unheparinized line is withdrawn from the patient. Then blood is injected automatically into each of the 6 chambers of the Heparin Assay cartridge, which determines quantitatively

TABLE 1. Loyola University Medical Center Anticoagulation Protocol

Heparin total dose: 2 mg (200U) × kg
Add: 2000-3000U as required to maintain ACT at 400 sec.

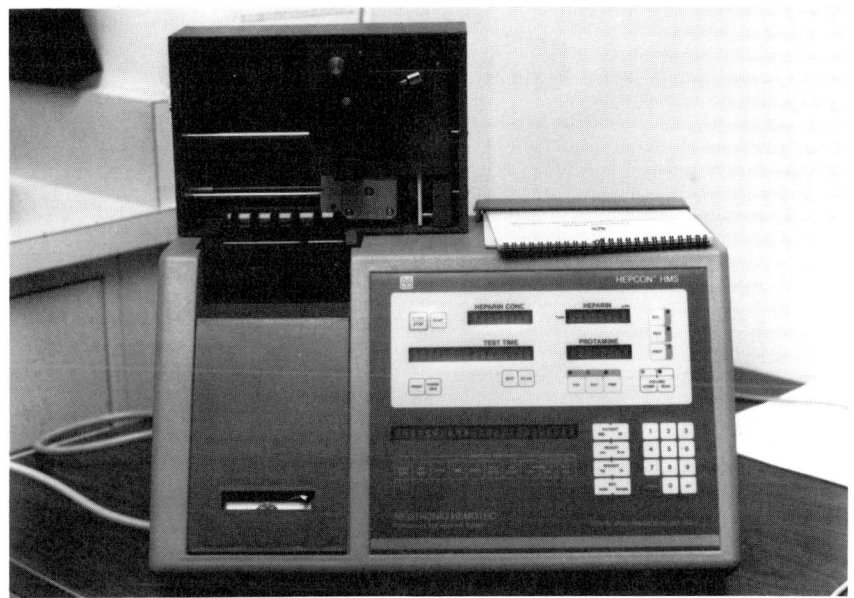

FIGURE 1. The Hepcon HMS Heparin Analyzer.

the amount of United States Pharmacopeia (USP) anticoagulant heparin in a blood sample by protamine titration (heparin/protamine titration or HPT). The method involves addition of known quantities of protamine to an unknown heparinized sample and measuring the clotting time. The quantity of protamine that neutralizes the heparin has the shortest clotting time. The concentration of heparin can be calculated on the basis of the known protamine. Dilute thromboplastin is added to HMS Heparin Assay cartridges to hasten reaction time.

The HPT is performed in a 4- or 6-channel cartridge. Each channel contains a different level of protamine sulfate and an equal amount of dilute thromboplastin. A heparin assay consists of injecting 0.2 ml of fresh whole blood into each channel of the assay cartridge. At the initiation of the test, the reagents are mixed with the blood sample, activating blood coagulation. The protamine in each channel neutralizes a specific amount of heparin. In the HMS Heparin Assay cartridges, both excess heparin and excess protamine act as anticoagulants when fresh whole blood is assayed. The first channel to clot is the channel in which the amount of protamine most closely neutralizes all of the heparin in the blood without an excess of either agent.

The endpoint of the test is the detection of clot formation. The Hepcon HMS coagulation instrument detects clot formation by measuring the rate of fall of the plunger mechanism contained in each cartridge channel. The plunger assembly falls rapidly through an unclotted sample, but the fibrin web formed during clotting impedes the rate of descent. The rate of fall is detected by a photooptical system located in the actuator assembly of the instrument.

HMS Heparin Assay cartridges are formulated from USP protamine sulfate with a 1:1 ratio of protamine to heparin (mg). The activator is thromboplastin diluted with a buffered solution. At the termination of the test the protamine sulfate required to neutralize the heparin concentration is calculated.

The total amount of protamine to be given is divided into two doses: (1) 75% of the dose is given to the patient by intravenous drip, and (2) the other 25% is given once the blood from the oxygenator and the cell saver has been reinfused into the patient. The blood from the oxygenator is centrifuged with the cell saver. In spite of this procedure, some heparin remains and has to be neutralized. For that reason 25% of the dose is given when the retrieved blood has been reinfused. Fifteen minutes after the entire amount of protamine is administered, a second sample of blood is withdrawn and analyzed with the Hepcon to determine if additional protamine is needed.

Heparin Rebound

After CPB, satisfactory hemostasis is not accomplished if the reversal of heparin is only temporary. The rate at which heparin is metabolized, the amount of protamine necessary for its reversal, and the patient's response to heparin are subject to wide variations. The reappearance of hypocoagulability after adequate neutralization of heparin has been called heparin rebound. After investigating this phenomenon, Gollub[13] concluded that the hypocoagulability was due to reappearance of heparin in the circulating blood.

The incidence of heparin rebound varies significantly in the literature. In a study of 50 patients, prior to the present neutralization protocol, we found that 26 (52%) required an additional dose of protamine 1 hour postoperatively, after adequate intraoperative heparin neutralization.[25] An average of 70 mg of additional protamine (range: 5-180 mg) was required to reverse rebounded circulating heparin. After adoption of the present neutralization protocol (Table 2), the incidence of heparin rebound has been reduced significantly.

The etiology of heparin rebound has not been clarified satisfactorily. It is likely that heparin is deposited in extravascular tissues and reappears intravascularly after the neutralizing heparin has disappeared. However, many other etiologies have been suggested (Table 3).

Regardless of the exact pathophysiology, heparin rebound seems to be due to the heparin effect that reappears after heparin neutralization with protamine. It has been suggested that enough protamine should be given to prevent heparin rebound and to ensure adequate neutralization.[8] We, like others,[1] believe that it is not necessary to give a high dose of protamine. The dose of protamine can be calculated with the Hepcon and administered in the usual two doses. Heparin rebound may happen up to 6 hours later, according to our experience;[24] however, it most commonly takes place within the first 1-3 hours after administration of protamine. We recommend, therefore, that the Hepcon

TABLE 2. Heparin Neutralization

Protamine dose calculated with the Hepcon
Give: 75% of the dose after cardiopulmonary bypass is discontinued. 25% once all the cell saver blood has been reinfused.
Usual dose: 1 to 1 or less. Repeat Hepcon once all the protamine is in. Repeat in 1 hour to rule out heparin rebound.

TABLE 3. Etiology of Heparin Rebound

1957	Heparin may be released by breakdown of red blood cells.[11]
1958	Heparin may escape from the circulation into the extravascular space and return via the lymphatics and thoracic duct to the circulation many hours later, after protamine has been administered and cleared.[12]
1959	Heparin may be injected into tissues instead of intravenously, forming a depot source for prolonged absorption.[13]
1961	A part of the heparin level may be temporarily neutralized by an endogenous antagonist, not otherwise specified. When this antagonist is cleared from the blood, heparin activity is then demonstrated.[14]
1962	Protamine may be metabolized or combined with other plasma proteins before heparin is removed.[15]
1966	Protamine chloride does not produce heparin rebound, although protamine sulfate does. This may be due in part to the more rapid metabolism of protamine sulfate.[16]
1970	Heparin rebound is seen more commonly with hypothermia.[17] It has previously been shown that heparin levels do not decay as rapidly during hypothermic perfusions.[18]
1974	For a given heparin level, low levels of platelets result in a more pronounced effect of that heparin level on the coagulation mechanism.[19]
1981	Monitoring postcardiopulmonary bypass with an automated protamine titration will detect heparin rebound more frequently.[4]

Adapted from Ellison N, Beatty CP, Blake DR, et al: Heparin rebound: Studies in patients and volunteers. J Thorac Cardiovasc Surg 67:723–729, 1974.

be repeated several times during that period, especially if the patient shows signs of oozing after a period of dryness in the operative field.

Heparin Resistance

Heparin resistance is decreased sensitivity to heparin. Excessive doses of heparin must be administered to a patient to prolong ACT to a therapeutic level. Profound cases of heparin resistance are rare. The mechanisms for heparin resistance are not well understood; it may be due to decreased levels of AT-III or increased levels of platelet factor 4.[9] Patients on preoperative heparin therapy are at increased risk of inadequate anticoagulation during CPB. In these cases, the importance of prebypass ACT and proper adjustment of the heparin dose needs to be emphasized. Other causes of heparin resistance are listed in Table 4.

Anticoagulation during CPB has to be adequate to prevent excessive consumption of clotting factors, yet it has to be reversible with protamine at the completion of bypass. The consequences of inadequate anticoagulation during CPB is a low-level activation of the hemostatic system, leading to platelet and coagulation factor consumption.[25] This consumption can manifest as bleeding in the postoperative period. To avoid these potential complications, it is important to be aware of conditions associated with heparin resistance and to ensure adequate anticoagulation before initiating cardiopulmonary bypass.

TABLE 4. Causes of Heparin Resistance

Antithrombin III deficiency	Presence of thrombois
Prolonged preoperative heparin therapy	Disseminated intravascular coagulation
Heparin-induced thrombocytopenia	Oral contraceptive therapy

According to Soloway and Christiansen,[28] fresh frozen plasma was used successfully to reverse heparin resistance in a patient with AT-III deficiency. Although its mechanism of action is not clear, fresh frozen plasma appears to neutralize heparin resistance.

PROTAMINE

Protamine is obtained from salmon milt, which is the secretion-laden gonads of the male salmon fish. In 1936 Hagedorn[14] used protamine to delay absorption of insulin by combining the two and creating protamine-zinc insulin. In 1937 Chargoff and Olson[5] discovered that protamine neutralized heparin, and it became the routinely used antidote.

Protamine has a significant amount of positively charged arginine. Apparently an ionic attraction binds protamine to heparin. Administered intravenously, it distributes primarily in extracellular fluid. Protamine forms large complexes with heparin that are digested by cells of the reticuloendothelial system. Macrophages in the lung perform this function when protamine is given intravenously. This fact may explain some of the recognized side effects of protamine administration.

The appropriate dose of protamine for heparin neutralization has varied widely and has involved great controversy. Castaneda advocated that heparin neutralization with protamine was not necessary.[4] Most cardiovascular surgeons use a dose of 1-1.5 mg/100 U of heparin. In our institution we calculate the dose of protamine to be given with the Hepcon. The calculated dose is given as a split dose (Table 2), with which we have been able both to reduce the total amount of protamine given and to prevent heparin rebound.

Adverse Responses to Protamine

At the present time, protamine is the only agent to neutralize heparin. This neutralization takes place in thousands of cases without difficulty. However, once in a while an adverse response to protamine occurs that may be life threatening. Cardiovascular surgeons and anesthesiologists should be familiar with these adverse reactions in order to make prompt and adequate response.

There are three major types of adverse response to protamine. Type I, the most common, is a hypotensive reaction that results from administering the protamine too rapidly. Apparently related to the release of histamine,[10] it is characterized by hypotension, a decrease in systemic vascular resistance, and an increase in cardiac output.[22] In most cases these hemodynamic alterations are well tolerated and require no further action. If an adverse reaction is recognized, the protamine drip should be stopped and restarted slowly. Antihistaminic medication may be indicated.

Type II adverse reaction is a true anaphylactic response mediated by immunoglobins. It occurs more frequently among patients with a history of fin-fish allergy. Release of histamine and leukotrienes results in systemic and pulmonary capillary leak. If the adverse reaction is allowed to continue, systemic hypotension, angioedema, anasarca, and noncardiac pulmonary edema will appear.[16] Type II reaction requires vigorous treatment. Oxygen and fluids should be administered, and peak end-expiratory pressure (PEEP) should be instituted. Antihistaminics and steroids are the drugs of choice.

Type III reactions are related to heparin-protamine complexes.[15] Pulmonary macrophages activate complement and leukocyte aggregation, resulting in release of free radicals and activation of the arachidonic acid pathway, which lead to the formation of thromboxane. The release of thromboxane into the pulmonary circulation causes intense vasoconstriction, which results in pulmonary hypertension and low left atrial pressure. The end result is right-heart dilatation and right-heart failure. Fortunately, this type of reaction is rare. When it occurs, the administration of protamine should be stopped and a drip of isoproterenol initiated. Epinephrine may be necessary; calcium may be useful. The administration of pulmonary vasodilators (prostacyclin) via the central venous line has also been recommended.

To prevent these reactions, protamine should be given slowly. The dose, which should be the minimum required, is best calculated with the Hepcon. Heparin rebound should always be considered. Monitoring the ACT and the Hepcon at regular intervals results in the diagnosis of unusual responses to heparin or to its neutralization with protamine.

CONCLUSIONS

1. The use of heparin as an anticoagulant and its neutralization with protamine have made possible CPB for open-heart surgery.

2. Enough heparin is administered to maintain the ACT above 400 seconds.

3. Protamine is administered in a split dose: 75% at the end of the bypass and the other 25% when all the blood from the oxygenator and the cell saver has been reinfused.

4. Heparin rebound is prevented with the split dose.

5. Adverse reactions to protamine may be prevented by (1) slow administration of protamine, (2) use of minimal dose required, and (3) attention to heparin rebound.

REFERENCES

1. Aren C, Feddersen K, Radegran K: Comparison of two protocols for heparin neutralization by protamine after cardiopulmonary bypass. J Thorac Cardiovasc Surg 94:539-541, 1987.
2. Babka R, Colby C, El-Etr A, Pifarre R: Monitoring of intraoperative heparinization and blood loss following cardiopulmonary bypass surgery. J Thorac Cardiovasc Surg 73:780-782, 1977.
3. Bull BS, Huse WM, Brauer FS, Korpman RA: Heparin therapy during extracorporeal circulation. II. The use of a dose-response curve to individualize heparin and protamine dosage. J Thorac Cardiovasc Surg 69:685-689, 1975.
4. Castaneda AR: Must heparin be neutralized following open heart operation? J Thorac Cardiovasc Surg 52:716-719, 1966.
5. Chargaff E, Olson KB: Studies on the chemistry of blood coagulation, part VI. J Biol Chem 122:153-167, 1937.
6. Conley CL, Hartman RC, Lalley JJ: The relationship between heparin activity and platelet concentration. Proc Soc Exp Biol Med 69:284-290, 1948.
7. Dodrill FD, Marshall N, Nybour J, et al: The use of the heart-lung apparatus in human cardiac surgery. J Thorac Surg 33:60-67, 1957.
8. Ellison N, Beatty CP, Blake DR, et al: Heparin rebound. Studies in patients and volunteers. J Thorac Cardiovasc Surg 67:723-729, 1974.

9. Esposito RA, Culliford HT, Colvin SB, et al: Heparin resistance during cardiopulmonary bypass: The role of heparin pretreatment. J Thorac Cardiovasc Surg 85:346-353, 1983.
10. Frater RWM, Oka Y, Hong Y, et al: Protamine induced ciculatory changes. J Thorac Cardiovasc Surg 97:687-692, 1984.
11. Frick DG, Brogh H: The mechanism of heparin rebound after extracorporeal circulation for open cardiac surgery. Surgery 59:721-726, 1966.
12. Gibbon JH Jr: Application of a mechanical heart and lung apparatus to cardiac surgery. Minn Med 37:171-178, 1954.
13. Gollub S: Heparin rebound in open heart surgery. Surg Gynecol Obstet 124:337-346, 1967 [abstract].
14. Hagedorn HC, Jensen BN, Karup NB, et al: Protamine insulate. JAMA 106:177-180, 1936.
15. Horrow JC: Heparin reversal of protamine toxicity: Have we come full circle? J Cardiothorac Vasc Anesth 4:539-542, 1990.
16. Horrow JC: Protamine allergy. J Cardiothorac Anesth 2:225-242, 1988.
17. Howell WH: Heparin: An anticoagulant. Preliminary communication. Am J Physiol 63:434-435, 1922.
18. Hyun BH, Pence RE, Davila JC, et al: Heparin rebound phenomenon in extracorporeal circulation. Surg Gynecol Obstet 115:191, 1971.
19. McLean J: The discovery of heparin. Circulation 19:75-78, 1959.
20. Metz S, Keats AS: Low activated coagulation time during cardiopulmonary bypass does not increase postoperative bleeding. Ann Thorac Surg 49:440-444, 1990.
21. Pardamani DS, Roy G, Semr PK: Heparin rebound. J Postgrad Med 16:26, 1970.
22. Perkins HA, Acra DJ, Rolfs MR: Estimation of heparin levels in stored and traumatized blood. Blood 18:807, 1961.
23. Perkins HS, Osborn JJ, Gerbode F: The management of abnormal breathing following extracorporeal circulation. Ann Intern Med 5:650, 1959.
24. Pifarre R, Babka R, Sullivan HJ, et al: Management of postoperative heparin rebound following cardiopulmonary bypass. J Thorac Cardiovasc Surg 81:378-381, 1981.
25. Pifarre R, Sullivan HJ, Montoya A, et al: Management of blood loss and heparin rebound following cardiopulmonary bypass. Semin Thromb Hemost 15:173-177, 1989.
26. Schreiner R: Discussion of Nakamoto S and Holmes JH: Our experience in regional heparinization. ASAIO Trans 4:63, 1958.
27. Shapiro N, Schaff HV, Piehler JM, et al: Cardiovascular effects of protamine sulfate in man. J Thorac Cardiovasc Surg 84:505-514, 1982.
28. Soloway H, Christiansen TW: Heparin anticoagulation during cardiopulmonary bypass in an antithrombin III deficiency patient. Am J Clin Pathol 73:723, 1980.
29. Wright JS, Osborne JJ, Perkins HA, et al: Heparin level during and after hypothermic perfusion. J Cardiovasc Surg 5:244, 1964.

Chapter 4

Monitoring Systemic Anticoagulation in Cardiovascular Surgery

*Clara I. Traverso, M.D., Ph.D., and
Joseph A. Caprini, M.D., FACS*

Cardiopulmonary bypass (CPB) is a surgical procedure associated with thrombogenic changes that simulate a whole-body inflammatory reaction. This reaction results from the contact of blood with nonbiologic oxygenators, mechanical trauma from the pump and tubing, gases and fluids, alterations in temperature, infusion of whole-blood and plasma products, and administration of drugs.[11,95] Knowledge of the body's response to this blood-perfused artificial organ has notably improved in recent years, and the effector systems of the inflammatory reaction are well-identified.[20,98] Within these effector systems, the coagulation and fibrinolytic systems are humoral and the platelets are cellular.[98] Activation of the hemostatic system is one of the consequences of CPB.

Since CPB was introduced more than 30 years ago, outstanding improvements have taken place, and its use has increased in recent years. However, several unsolved issues remain and are still under investigation,[71] including oxygenators that mimic the surface of biological membranes to avoid an adverse body response.[14,45,97] Other topics for discussion include major changes in the hemostatic system associated with CPB; various anticoagulant and drug reversal protocols in common use; and monitoring of drugs as well as overall level of anticoagulation.

As a result of an unbalanced coagulation-anticoagulation equilibrium, clotting or bleeding complications may ensue.[4,48,65,73,90] In fact, postoperative hemorrhage remains a serious cause of morbidity after CPB in spite of technical advances and improved surgical procedures.[47,57] In addition, the anticoagulant drug must induce an adequate level of anticoagulation to prevent clotting without increasing blood loss.[2,13,67] Therefore, assessing the coagulation-anticoagulation level during and following CPB is crucial. However, in spite of the immense literature regarding CPB monitoring, there is no agreement on which hemostatic test should be selected.

This chapter attempts to establish a guideline for monitoring systemic anticoagulation during and after CPB by addressing and integrating different proposed approaches. Unfortunately, study of this complex issue still has significant room for improvement, and several considerations will remain unanswered until further studies are carried out.

HEMOSTATIC CHANGES, ANTICOAGULATION, AND BLOOD LOSS

Anticoagulation is required to prevent clot formation due to the thrombogenic nature of CPB. To date, heparin is the anticoagulant drug of choice. Nevertheless, routine systemic heparinization has been reported to be ineffective in totally suppressing the ongoing activation process,[35,87] which may lead to clotting; at the same time, heparin is known to increase the risk of hemorrhage from 1 to 35%.[57] Thus suitable monitoring of the coagulation-anticoagulation balance during and after CPB is crucial. Unfortunately, these facts are not as simple as they appear to be. In addition to the dosages of heparin administered, blood loss is influenced by other circumstances,[47] mainly mechanical causes attributable to the surgical procedure[82] and duration of intervention.[25] Protocols for heparin administration and neutralization are not conclusive[37]; heparin response varies widely not only among patients,[15] but also within each patient,[40] and heparin- as well as protamine-related complications are well-documented.[54,56,59] Accordingly, monitoring of the hemostatic changes induced by CPB, heparin, and protamine, as well as heparin and protamine protocols, is a complex issue that needs to be settled. In addition, investigation of alternative anticoagulant drugs, especially in recent years, raises the question of whether the same tests used for monitoring heparin therapy will be effective for alternative drugs.

Several changes in the hemostatic system associated with CPB have been considered to have pathophysiologic implications in terms of postoperative blood loss. A better understanding of these changes is important not only for preventing bleeding complications, but also for developing improved methods for monitoring CPB. About 3% of patients undergoing open-heart surgery require reexploration of the chest because of excessive postoperative blood loss[4]; this figure, which seems quite high in itself, becomes more important in view of the recently increased concern about the risk of transfusion-transmitted diseases.[24]

The changes in the coagulation and fibrinolytic systems most frequently identified include thrombocytopenia and platelet dysfunction, decreased clotting factor activity, increased fibrinolysis, and disseminated intravascular coagulation.[9,48,65,73] In addition, excessive doses of heparin and protamine, as well as unneutralizated heparin, have been reported to provoke hemorrhagic complications.[9,90] However, the exact mechanisms of some of these alterations remain either unclear or incompletely recognized; this fact is responsible, at least in part, for the lack of a suitable CPB monitor.

Ten to thirty percent of patients exposed to heparin develop an immediate, transient, and moderate decrease in platelet count (PLT) that has no clinical consequences and is not considered to be an immune-mediated effect of heparin.[60] This syndrome, which is dose-dependent, has been more frequently reported with the use of bovine lung heparin.[7] In addition to this syndrome, heparin-induced thrombocytopenia, which has an immune basis, is associated with high morbidity and mortality.[56,96] Thrombocytopenia has been reported as a protamine-related effect as well.[59] Platelet dysfunction has also been associated with administration of heparin and with duration of the surgical procedure, although its mechanism remains unclear.[25,51] Another important reported disadvantage of heparin is poor response. This resistance, although unpredictable within each patient, is influenced by preoperative administration of heparin.[21,35] In addition, some hemodynamically adverse effects, previously attributed to administration of protamine, have been recognized as a result of the protamine-heparin interaction.[39,86] These problems have created continuous interest in developing alternative drugs to heparin for anticoagulation in CPB.

Adequate reversal of the anticoagulant effect of heparin after CPB is of equal importance to suitable monitoring in reducing bleeding complications. Since 1939, protamine has been the reversal drug of choice because of its proven effectiveness in neutralizing the effect of heparin anticoagulation.[53] Although in clinical practice 1–1.3 mg of protamine is used to neutralize 100 IU of heparin, the protocol is not definitely established, and administration in divided doses, instead of a single bolus, has been proposed to achieve complete heparin neutralization.[2] In addition, a faster rhythm of bolus infusion than that classically used has been suggested.[83] Furthermore, as with heparin, individual response to protamine is variable, and previous exposure to the drug influences the adverse effects.[39,54] Protamine itself may also cause dosage-independent complications, such as hemodynamic effects, which are not preventable by preinjection of calcium chloride.[83] Anaphylactoid reactions have also been reported, and a need either for an alternative drug to protamine or for adjustment of dosage has been suggested.[42,54,103] Finally, data regarding protamine's activation of the classical complement pathway are contradictory.[59,100]

Especially in the last decade, alternative means of anticoagulation during CPB in heparin-sensitive (documentation or suspicion of heparin-induced thrombocytopenia) or heparin-resistant patients have been studied. The new approaches involve either alternative drug implementation or two other methods that have been analyzed in experimental models with promising results: omission of heparin and reduction of dosage by modifying the extracorporeal circuits.[33,68,99] A low-molecular-weight heparinoid (Org 10172) has proved to be effective in dogs,[49] and one investigation verified its efficacy in humans.[80] Ancrod has also been proposed as an alternative to heparin in humans.[108] The association of aprotinin with diminished heparin dosages has been suggested as effective,[31] although a clotting trend has been stressed.[47,64] Experimental studies with hirudin in dogs have also provided favorable results.[101] To date, however, the experience is limited, and further studies are necessary to reach any conclusion. Accordingly, this analysis of the laboratory role in monitoring CPB focuses on anticoagulation with heparin and reversal with protamine.

ROLE OF LABORATORY TESTING IN HEPARIN MONITORING

Preliminary Considerations

As documented, assessment of the coagulation-anticoagulation level during and after CPB is mandatory. In fact, there is a consensus on the need for laboratory monitoring in open-heart surgery, which differs from other surgical procedures in that routine testing results may not modify the surgeon's opinion or perioperative care.[69,70] Unfortunately, a suitable monitor has not been clearly established.

Certain considerations should be reviewed before analyzing the different tests proposed and the reasons for their advocacy. First, regardless of the test selected, the optimal protocol is established by assuming that the risk of both clotting and bleeding complications is low if the test values are maintained within a determined range. For this reason, each laboratory has to establish a reference range, and each surgical team should adjust the heparin monitoring to the laboratory's experience.[81] Second, a trend that should be avoided is overuse of laboratory testing because of the availability of rapid screening.[70] On the contrary, the first question in selecting a test should be what kind of information one is looking for; i.e., what do the test results mean in relation to the complications that one hopes to avoid? Third, it is important to select the proper intervals for repeating the test during and after the surgical procedure.

In addition to these general considerations, the test employed for heparin monitoring should reflect abnormalities in the entire hemostatic system rather than in a selected portion.[84] In fact, the most informative tests appear to be those that are performed on whole blood, that record all phases of the coagulation-fibrinolytic system, and that, at the same time, evaluate the different components involved in clot formation.[10,63] Finally, a combination of information from two tests is expected to be more complete and more useful in obtaining the optimal doses of heparin.

Integrated Experience with the Available Tests

A balanced coagulation-anticoagulation level that avoids underheparinization without causing bleeding complications requires a suitable monitor, which does not seem to be established. To date, there is no consensus on which hemostatic test is the best for monitoring CPB. Lack of an exact monitor and significantly increased use of CPB make laboratory testing a cardinal issue.

The activated clotting time (ACT) is the generally accepted test for monitoring CPB.[6,15,37,77] The ACT measures the time required for fibrin to form; because it is easy to perform and rapid, it can be employed inside the operating room.[85] However, the use of the ACT in open-heart surgery has well-defined, yet limited indications; thus ACT should not be recommended as the proper monitor for the entire surgical procedure, i.e., before and during CPB, as well as after administration of protamine.

The role of ACT is certainly defined for monitoring dosages of heparin during CPB.[6,13,22,37,44] The test must be generated before the surgical procedure, and the endpoint has to be exactly defined by each laboratory before performance.[22] Apart from this indication, no evidence suggests that ACT is an appropriate monitor before CPB[21] or that the test provides useful information on protamine adjustment and blood losses.[2,13,38]

In addition, a very important issue still remains unsolved: the minimal ACT value for adequate anticoagulation during CPB.[67] Young et al.,[106] after studying 5 patients, stated that 400 seconds is the optimal minimal value; their conclusion has been widely accepted, but it has never been validated. ACT values between 350 and 500 seconds seem an appropriate range[44]; it has also been suggested that this range reduces the degree of platelet dysfunction.[35] In any case, values have to be <500 seconds for ACT to be reliable.[22]

As mentioned above, ACT is considered useless for the adjustment of protamine after CPB, because the test is highly influenced by technique[12,34] and is not heparin-specific.[74] Because the ACT has failed to predict excessive bleeding after CPB,[37,85,102] some authors have seen no advantage to adjusting heparin dosage to ACT values during CPB.[27,32,67] The failure of ACT to diagnose and manage bleeding problems during CPB has also been reported.[93] Finally, a reduction in PLT from 20 to 30% seems to be needed before ACT reflects thrombocytopenia.[51]

Studies evaluating the other generally accepted test, the heparin concentration ([H]) in plasma or blood, have provided contradictory results. Some authors have reported a strong correlation between increased [H] and excessive postoperative blood loss,[43] whereas others have found the test of little use in identifying either bleeding complications or clotting.[67] Likewise, whereas some authors have found this test heparin-specific, and thus effective in determining both the level of circulating heparin and the dosages of protamine required for neutralizing the heparin effect,[74] others maintain that it does not reflect the degree of anticoagulation.[81] No report suggests that these assays have a role in predicting the anticoagulant effect of heparin.[38] In addition, the test requires an experienced technologist and is more expensive than ACT. It may have some role, but only when combined with ACT.[81]

Use of the activated partial thromboplastin time (APTT) in CPB has been recommended by some authors.[13,25] However, this test is considered inappropriate because it is time-consuming and usually performed outside the operating room.[92] In addition, APTT assesses only a selected portion of the hemostatic system and therefore does not reflect the coagulation changes that occur in CPB.[66,107] APTT's inability to predict potential hemostatic changes has also been reported.[58] A main disadvantage of the test is the fact that it is significantly influenced by technique[12,41] and remains far from standardization.[28] For all these reasons, routine use of APTT in open cardiac surgery seems inadvisable.

In regard to bleeding time (BT), a recent review[79] concluded that no evidence supports its use for prognosis or for monitoring heparin. Moreover, results are significantly influenced by both technique and numerous drugs. Finally, although BT is prolonged in a very high number of patients undergoing CPB, bleeding complications associated with abnormal values are recorded infrequently.[4]

Introduced by Hartert in 1948[46] and extensively used in Europe since then, thromboelastography (TEG) has recently gained advocates in the U.S. In fact, it is becoming a widely selected test because of studies that have provided more than promising results in evaluating several aspects of CPB. TEG is a test for a global study of coagulation that displays information on extrinsic and intrinsic pathways, the common pathway, and fibrinolysis. TEG measures the time needed for clot generation, as the other hemostatic tests do, by using the reaction time (R) and the clot formation time (K). R measures from the beginning of coagulation to the formation of the first fibrin strands; i.e., it corresponds to the invisible phase of coagulation and is influenced by all factors that belong to the intrinsic pathway. It is often employed for monitoring intravenous administration of heparin.[62] K is related to the speed of the clot formation; it corresponds to the beginning of the visible phase of coagulation and is influenced by factor II, thrombin formation, fibrin precipitation, fibrinogen concentration, and hematocrit.[16,52] In addition, TEG provides information on the strength of the clot,[3,75] a characteristic that is not recorded by other hemostatic tests; this, in fact, is considered to be the major advantage of TEG. This valuable information on the dynamics of coagulation is provided by the maximal amplitude (Ma), which reflects the overall competence of the clot and is influenced by PLT and platelet function, fibrinogen and thrombin concentrations, fibrin, factor XIII, and hematocrit.[16,17,29,50,52] Because of the kind of information it provides, Ma is considered the most important thromboelastographic parameter. Over the years, several parameters have been proposed as additions to those introduced by Hartert.[46] In analyzing native whole blood, however, the evaluation and interpretation of the thromboelastogram is still based essentially on the original constants, R, K, and Ma.

Native whole blood is used in performing TEG for monitoring of heparinized patients as well as for cardiac surgery. The TEG information resembles that which occurs in the patient's blood,[26,63,75,76,85] because it reflects the interaction of all the components of the clotting process.[55,62,107] The experience related to monitoring of intravenous heparin therapy is excellent.[3,18,62,75,76] Because the response of each patient to heparin is depicted by TEG, the individualization of heparin administration, which is especially important in heparin-resistant patients, is possible.[63,88] As mentioned above, TEG is becoming an optimal monitor in CPB. In cardiac surgical procedures, the maximal amplitude calculated at a predetermined time after Ma—usually 30, 60, and 120 minutes, is another parameter (Ma + x) frequently employed[72]; it, too, has been shown to be useful.[75] Finally, the alpha angle (α) measures the rate of fibrin polymerization, thus indicating the relation between the strength of the clot and the speed at which it is formed; it is also often used.

All of these measurable parameters are obtained from an uninterrupted tracing that is recorded as the thromboelastogram. TEG information is thus objective and permanent, providing information on the coagulation-fibrinolytic process during the surgical procedure and allowing review of results. These data are not provided by the other tests.[8,30,76] The TEG is also rapid; the tracing can be obtained in about 15–20 minutes[50,55,78,92] or less. Our modified technique using celite (diatomacious earth) reduces the recording time with native whole blood[17] and enables TEG to detect a contaminated blood specimen that may commonly occur during venipuncture or in manipulating the collection apparatus, tubes, and reagents. Some authors have communicated good results with this modified technique.[23,91] In addition, a first look at the graphic during the surgical procedure provides a global appraisal of the coagulation-anticoagulation state, which is of enormous concern in cardiac surgery, because exact and uninterrupted monitoring is required in the operating room. The duration of the recording should be adjusted to the information required and the patient's condition.

These and other advantages—such as the analysis of the fibrinolytic system,[52,104] the detection of variations in clot formation that are unrecognized by other coagulation tests,[30,107] and ease and low cost of performance in standard laboratories—have made TEG an especially interesting tool to be tested in various surgical procedures that demand exact and uninterrupted monitoring, including cardiac procedures. TEG analyses in cardiovascular surgery have focused on the study of the coagulation state, anticoagulant drugs and response to reversal drugs, as well as postoperative blood losses and their causes.[42,66,93,94] TEG has also been used for testing hemocompatible biomaterials for application in CPB.[1,19,45] The role of TEG in open heart surgery is singularly valuable in terms of information about the anticoagulation state induced by anticoagulant drugs, the effect of protamine, platelet dysfunction, and blood losses.[42,85,93]

Thromboelastography has been reported as a satisfactory test for facilitating the identification of alterations in coagulation caused by different factors involved in cardiac surgery.[5,85] In contrast, neither ACT nor heparin assays can fully evaluate the complex interactions of the hemostatic system.[94] In fact, because TEG is able to measure variables generated after onset of clotting, the endpoint of many standard hematologic tests, it gives more clinically useful information about coagulation than other hemostatic tests.[85,107] Furthermore, TEG not only evaluates conventional heparin, but also provides good results for monitoring low-molecular-weight heparinoids[36]; this aspect would be valuable if heparinoids become alternatives to unfractionated heparin because neither ACT nor APTT reflects the level of anticoagulation they induce.[80] Consequently, in comparison with other tests, TEG seems superior for monitoring before and during cardiac surgery. Nevertheless, a lack of correlation between TEG and blood loss during surgery has been reported,[85] and our results in experimental models confirm this fact; however, an adequate relation to clotting was found, whereas ACT failed in this regard.[89] TEG appears to be a suitable test for assessing the different treatments proposed for management of patients undergoing CPB,[13,42,92,103,105] which is probably its best role during the surgical procedure.

After CPB, a relationship between TEG results and postoperative bleeding complications has been documented,[85] although Wang et al.[102] have recently reported a laboratory failure, in which both TEG and ACT were included. Other authors have also seen ACT failures when using the test for this purpose.[13,37,85] Gillies and Spiess[42] have found TEG able to distinguish surgical bleeding from bleeding due to other reasons; as a result, the use of TEG may be followed by a decreased number of reoperations. After experimental analyses in dogs, we concluded that TEG is well correlated with postoperative bleeding.[89]

One of the most interesting pieces of information provided by the maximal amplitude (Ma) concerns platelet function.[29] In fact, TEG has been reported to depict not only platelet number,[66] but also platelet function, and it has been found to be significantly correlated with platelet aggregometry.[91] In contrast, ACT seems to require a significant reduction in platelet number to reflect a decrease, and it provides no information on platelet function.[51] These findings are valuable because in CPB both heparin and protamine may generate platelet alterations and a decreased PLT; these alterations make a large contribution to bleeding after surgery. Finally, promising results have been recently reported in the use of TEG for adjustment of the protamine dosage,[42] which has also been noted experimentally.[89] No role for ACT in this regard has been reported.

Final Considerations and Proposed Guidelines for Laboratory Monitoring

Proper blood sample collections are an important part of laboratory testing. A two-syringe technique is best and perhaps the only method to ensure reliable test results. As mentioned above, the combined analysis of native whole blood and celite-activated TEGs displays a contaminated blood specimen, which can avoid not only altered TEG results, but also altered ACT values if both tests are used together. The optimal timing of blood collections has not been established, although it has been suggested after sternotomy.[105] In any case, the fact that a trend to hypercoagulability usually occurs after opening of the thorax must be considered in analyzing the results. After the surgical procedure, intervals for sample collection are not specifically defined; they should be adjusted to every patient. However, in the absence of complications, a minimum of once every 30 minutes seems reasonable.

After combining the experience reported in regard to cardiovascular surgery monitoring, our opening statement is confirmed; i.e., this complex issue still has significant room for improvement, and more studies are needed to establish a conclusive guideline. Nevertheless, two tests seem to be the most useful: the activated clotting time and thromboelastography.

TEG seems to be a better monitor than ACT before and after CPB, and ACT seems to be a better monitor than TEG during the surgical procedure. Spiess et al.[85] advocated the combined use of both tests. In our opinion, TEG could be complementary to ACT during surgery, and ACT could be complementary to TEG afterward. Therefore, until other studies are carried out, the use of both tests before (because baseline values are always needed), during, and after open cardiac surgery is recommended. Heparin assays add no further information. We do not recommend any test that does not provide useful information; we advocate selection of tests on the basis of laboratory experience.

We believe that monitoring by TEG requires more experienced personnel who know well both the technique and the meaning of the results and who are able to adjust heparin and protamine dosages to the TEG tracings. Monitoring by ACT seems less flexible, and its protocol is easier to set; therefore, it can be conducted by a technician without hematologic experience. Accordingly, we recommend TEG at those institutions at which the interpretation of the results is well-known. In any case, the experience of each surgical team should be the guide for selecting a monitor. If we assume the combined use of both tests, ACT values <500 seconds seem to be appropriate. After CPB, protamine should be adjusted on the basis of TEG results to obtain a rapid yet progressive return to baseline values.

REFERENCES

1. Affeld K, Berger J, Muller R, Bucherl ES: A new method for an in vitro test of blood-contact materials. Proc Eur Soc Artif Organs 1:26-29, 1974.
2. Aren C, Fedderson K, Radegran K: Comparison of two protocols for heparin neutralization by protamine after cardiopulmonary bypass. J Thorac Cardiovasc Surg 94:539-541, 1987.
3. Audier M, Serradimigni A: Savoir interpreter un thrombo-elastogramme ou l'exploration precise de la coagulation sanguine. Paris, Maloine, 1962.
4. Bachmann F, McKenna R, Cole ER, Najafi H: The hemostatic mechanism after open heart surgery. I. Studies on plasma coagulation factors and fibrinolysis in 512 patients after extracorporeal circulation. J Thorac Cardiovasc Surg 70:76-85, 1975.
5. Baeuerle JJ, Mongan PD, Hosking MP: An assessment of the duration of Cephapirin-induced coagulation abnormalities as measured by the thromboelastograph. Anesthesiology 75:A70, 1991.

6. Baugh RF, Deemar KA, Zimmermann JJ: Heparinase in the activated clotting time assay: Monitoring heparin-independent alterations in coagulation functions. Anesth Analg 74:201-205, 1992.
7. Bell W, Royal R: Heparin associated thrombocytopenia: A comparison of three heparin preparations. N Engl J Med 303:902-907, 1980.
8. Bernard J, Levy J, Varet B: Hemostase, coagulation et fibrynolise: Physiologie et exploration. In Bernard J (ed): Hematologie. Paris, Masson, 1981, pp 291-306.
9. Bick RL: Hemostasis defects associated with cardiac surgery, prosthetic devices, and other extracorporeal circuits. Sem Thromb Hemost 11:249-280, 1985.
10. Bird R, Hall B, Hobbs KEF, Chapman D: New haemocompatible polymers assessed by thromboelastography. J Biomed Eng 11:231-234, 1989.
11. Blackstone EH, Kirklin JW, Steward RW, Chenoweth DE: Damaging effects of cardiopulmonary bypass. In Wu KK, Rossi EC (eds): Prostaglandins in Clinical Medicine: Cardiovascular and Thrombotic Disorders. Chicago, Year Book, 1982, pp 355-369.
12. Bode AP, Castellain WJ, Hodges ED, Yelverton S: The effect of lysed platelets on neutralization of heparin in vitro with protamine as measured by the Activated Clotting Time. Thromb Hemost 66:213-217, 1991.
13. Boldt J, Zickmann B, Herold CH, et al: Heparin management during cardiac surgery with respect to various blood-conservation techniques. Surgery 111:260-265, 1992.
14. Boonstra PW, Vermeulen FEE, Leusink JA, et al: Hematological advantage of a membrane oxygenator over a bubble oxygenator in long perfusions. Ann Thorac Surg 41:297-300, 1986.
15. Bull HS, Huse WN, Brauer FS, Korpman RA: Heparin therapy during extracorporeal circulation. The use of a dose-response curve to individualize heparin and protamine dosage. J Thorac Cardiovasc Surg 69:685-689, 1975.
16. Butler MJ: Thromboelastography during and after elective abdominal surgery. Thromb Hemost 39:488-495, 1978.
17. Caprini JA, Eckenhoff JB, Ramstack JM, et al: Contact activation of heparinized plasma. Thromb Res 5:379-400, 1974.
18. Caprini JA, Vagher JP, Rabidi SJ, Mitchell JE: Laboratory monitoring of continuous intravenous heparin therapy. Thromb Res 29:91-94, 1983.
19. Carr SH, Zuckerman L, Caprini JA, Vagher JP: In vitro testing of surface thrombogenicity using the thromboelastograph. Res Comm Chem Path Pharm 13:507-519, 1976.
20. Chenoweth DE, Cooper W, Hugli TE, et al: Complement activation during cardiopulmonary bypass. Evidence for generation of C3a and C5a anaphylatoxins. N Engl J Med 304:497-503, 1981.
21. Cloyd GM, D'Ambra MN, Akins CW: Diminished anticoagulant response to heparin in patients undergoing coronary artery bypass grafting. J Thorac Cardiovasc Surg 94:535-538, 1987.
22. Cohen JA: Activated coagulation time method for control of heparin is reliable during cardiopulmonary bypass. Anesthesiology 60:121-124, 1984.
23. Confino E, El-Roeiy A, Friberg J, Gleicher N: The thromboelastogram and circulating lupus anticoagulant. J Reprod Med 4:289-291, 1989.
24. Consensus Conference: Perioperative red blood cell transfusion. JAMA 260:2700-2703, 1988.
25. Copeland JG, Harker LA, Joist JH, De Vries WC: Circulatory support 1988 Bleeding and anticoagulation. Ann Thorac Surg 47:87-95, 1989.
26. Coppola L, Giunta R, Spiezia R, et al: Accentuata ed irregolare deflessione postmassimale nei tracciati tromboelastografici: Incidenza in varie patologie. Boll Soc It Biol Sper 61:263-270, 1985.
27. Culliford AT, Gitel SN, Starr N: Lack of correlation between activated clotting time and plasma heparin during cardiopulmonary bypass. Ann Surg 193:105-111, 1981.
28. D'Angelo A, Seveso MP, Vigano S, et al: Effect of clot-detection methods and reagents on activated partial thromboplastin time (APTT). Am J Clin Pathol 94:297-306, 1990.
29. De Gaetano G, Vermylen J: Effect of aspirin on the thromboelastogram of human blood. Thromb Diath Haemorrh 30:494-498, 1973.
30. De Nicola P: Thromboelastography. Springfield, IL, Charles C Thomas, 1957.
31. De Smet AAEA, et al: Increased anticoagulation during cardiopulmonary bypass by aprotinin. J Thorac Cardiovasc Surg 100:520-527, 1990.
32. Dauchot PJ, Berzina L, Rabinovitch A, Ankeney JL: Activated coagulation and activated partial thromboplastin times in assessment and reversal of heparin-induced anticoagulation for cardiopulmonary bypass. Anesth Analg 62:710-719, 1983.
33. DelRossi AJ, et al: Heparinless extracorporeal bypass for treatment of hypothermia. The Journal of Trauma 30:79-82, 1990.

34. Dhir AK: Heparin dose-response: In vitro versus in vivo technique. Anaesthesia 46:232-233, 1991 [letter].
35. Dietrich W, Spannagl M, Schramm W, et al: The influence of preoperative anticoagulation on heparin response during CPB. J Thorac Cardiovasc Surg 102:505-514, 1991.
36. Edwards CM, Peacock B, Donnelly PK: Differential effects of unfractionated versus low molecular weight heparin in post-operative anticoagulant prophylaxis. Br J Hematol 80(Suppl 1):21, 1992 [abstract].
37. Esposito RA, et al: The role of the activated clotting time in heparin administration and neutralization for cardiopulmonary bypass. J Thorac Cardiovasc Surg 85:174-185, 1983.
38. Esposito RA, Culliford AT, Colvin SB, et al: Heparin resistance during cardiopulmonary bypass. The role of heparin pretreatment. J Thorac Cardiovasc Surg 85:346-353, 1983.
39. Fiser WP, Fewell JE, Hill DE, et al: Cardiovascular effects of protamine sulfate are dependent on the presence and type of circulating heparin. J Thorac Cardiovasc Surg 89:63-70, 1985.
40. Friesen RH, Clement AJ: Individual responses to heparinization for extracorporeal circulation. J Thorac Cardiovasc Surg 72:875-879, 1976.
41. Gawoski JM, Arkin ChF, Bovill T, et al: The effects of heparin on the activated partial thromboplastin time of the College of American Pathologists survey specimens. Arch Pathol Lab Med 111:785-790, 1987.
42. Gillies BSA, Spiess BD: Cardiopulmonary bypass coagulation management, education, and transfusion practice at the University of Washington. Am Soc Anesthesiol October, 1991 [abstract].
43. Gravlee GP, et al: Predicting the pharmacodynamics of heparin: A clinical evaluation of the Hepcon System 4. J Cardiothorac Anesth 5:379-387, 1987.
44. Gravlee GP, et al: Heparin dosing and monitoring for cardiopulmonary bypass. A comparison of techniques with measurement of subclinical plasma coagulation. J Thorac Cardiovasc Surg 99:518-527, 1990.
45. Hall B, Bird RR, Kojima M, Chapman D: Biomembranes as models for polymer surfaces. V. Thrombelastographic studies of polymeric lipids and polyesters. Biomaterials 10:219-224, 1989.
46. Hartert H: Blutgerinnungsstudien mit der Thrombelastographie einem neuen Untersuchingsverfahren. Klin Wochenschir 26:577-583, 1948.
47. Havel M, et al: Effect of intraoperative aprotinin administration on postoperative bleeding in patients undergoing cardiopulmonary bypass operation. J Thorac Cardiovasc Surg 101:968-972, 1991.
48. Hennesy VL, et al: Function of human platelets during extracorporeal circulation. Am J Physiol 232:626-628, 1977.
49. Henny CP, et al: A randomized blind study comparing standard heparin and a new low molecular weight heparinoid in cardiopulmonary bypass surgery in dogs. J Lab Clin Med 106:187-196, 1985.
50. Howland WS, et al: Hypercoagulability, thrombelastographic monitoring during extensive hepatic surgery. Arch Surg 108:605-608, 1974.
51. Inada E: Blood coagulation and autologous blood transfusion in cardiac surgery. J Clin Anesth 2:393-406, 1990.
52. Jaulmes A, Querangal D, Delga J: Hematologia. In Practica de laboratorio. Bacelona, Toray-Masson, 1972, pp 591-721.
53. Jorpes E, Edman P, Thaning T: Neutralisation of activation of heparin by protamine. Lancet 2:975, 1939.
54. Just-Viera JO, Fischer CR, Gago O, Morris JD: Acute reaction to protamine. Its importance to surgeons. Am Surg 50:52-60, 1984.
55. Kang Y, Borland LM, Picone J, Martin LK: Intraoperative coagulation changes in children undergoing liver transplantation. Anesthesiology 71:44-47, 1989.
56. Kappa JR, Horn MDK, Fisher CA, et al: Efficacy of iloprost (36374) versus aspirin in preventing heparin induced platelet activation during cardiac operations. J Thorac Cardiovasc Surg 94:405-413, 1987.
57. Kelton JG, Hirsh J: Bleeding associated with antithrombotic therapy. Semin Haematol 17:259-291, 1980.
58. Kitchens CS: Prolonged activated partial thromboplastin time of unknown etiology: A prospective study of 100 consecutive cases referred for consultation. Am J Haematol 27:38-45, 1988.
59. Kirklin JK, et al: Effects of protamine administration after cardiopulmonary bypass on complement, blood elements, and the hemodynamic state.. Ann Thorac Surg 41:193-199, 1986.

60. Laster J, et al: The heparin induced thrombocytopenic syndrome: An update. Surgery 102:763-770, 1987.
61. Lee BY, Thoden WR, Del Guercio LRM, et al: Monitoring coagulation dynamics with thrombelastography. Contemp Surg 24:19-24, 1984.
62. Lee BY, Thoden WR, McCann WJ, et al: Intraoperative anticoagulation during arterial reconstructive procedures. Surg Gynecol Obstet 155:809-812, 1982.
63. Lee BY, Trainor FS, Kavner D, McCann WJ: Monitoring of heparin therapy with thromboelastography. Surg Gynecol Obstet 149:843-846, 1979.
64. Levy JH, Salmenpera MT: Increased anticoagulation during cardiopulmonary bypass by aprotinin. J Thorac Cardiovasc Surg 102:802, 1991 [letter].
65. Mammen EF, et al: Hemostasis changes during cardiopulmonary bypass surgery. Semin Thromb Hemost 11:281-292, 1985.
66. Martin P, Horkay F, Rajah SM, Walker DR: Monitoring of coagulation status using thrombelastography during paediatric open heart surgery. J Clin Monitor 6:183-187, 1991.
67. Metz S, Keats AS: Low activated coagulation time during cardiopulmonary bypass does not increase postoperative bleeding. Ann Thorac Surg 49:440-444, 1990.
68. Mottaghy K, Oedekoven B, Schaich-Lester D, et al: Application of surfaces with end point attached heparin to extracorporeal circulation with membrane lungs. ASAIO Trans 35:146-152, 1989.
69. Mozes B, Lubin D, Modan B, et al: Evaluation of an intervention aimed at reducing inappropriate use of preoperative blood coagulation tests. Arch Intern Med 149:1836-1838, 1989.
70. Narr BJ, Hansen TR, Warner MA: Preoperative laboratory screening in healthy Mayo patients: Cost-effective elimination of tests and unchanged outcomes. Mayo Clin Proc 66:155-159, 1991.
71. Nose Y: The need for a second-generation pump oxygenator. Artif Organs 13:89-90, 1989.
72. Owen CA, et al: Hemostatic evaluation of patients undergoing liver transplantation. Mayo Clin Proc 62:761-772, 1987.
73. Páramo JA, Rifón J, Llorens R, et al: Intra- and postoperative fibrinolysis in patients undergoing cardiopulmonary bypass surgery. Haemostasis 21:58-64, 1991.
74. Pifarre R, et al: Management of blood loss and heparin rebound following cardiopulmonary bypass. Semin Thromb Hemost 15:173-177, 1989.
75. Raby C: Exploración del tiempo trombodinámico. In Hemorragias y trombosis. Barcelona, Toray-Masson, 1968, pp 190-211.
76. Raby C: Coagulaciones intravasculares diseminadas y localizadas. Barcelona, Toray-Masson, 1976.
77. Reich DL, Zahl K, Perucho MH, Thys DM: An evaluation of two activated clotting time monitors during cardiac surgery. J Clin Monit 8:33-36, 1992.
78. Rettke SR, et al: Hemodynamic and metabolic changes in hepatic transplantation. Mayo Clin Proc 64:232-240, 1989.
79. Rodgers RPCH, Levin J: A critical reappraisal of the bleeding time. Semin Thromb Haemostas 16:1-20, 1990.
80. Rowlings PA, et al: The use of a low molecular weight heparinoid for extracorporeal procedures in patients with heparin dependent thrombocytopenia and thrombosis. Aust NZ J Med 21:52-54, 1991.
81. Saleem A, Shenaq SS, Yawn DH, et al: Heparin monitoring during cardiopulmonary bypass. Ann Clin Lab Sci 14:474-479, 1984.
82. Schwartz S, Silver D: What routine preoperative tests for bleeding tendencies? JAMA 236:2547, 1976.
83. Shapira N, Schaff HV, Piehler JM, et al: Cardiovascular effects of protamine sulfate in man. J Thorac Cardiovasc Surg 84:505-514, 1982.
84. Soloway HB, Cox SP: In vitro comparison of the thrombin time and activated partial thromboplastin time in the laboratory control of heparin therapy. Am J Clin Pathol 60:648-650, 1973.
85. Spiess BD, Tuman KJ, McCarthy RJ, et al: Thromboelastography as an indicator of postcardiopulmonary bypass coagulopathies. J Clin Monit 3:25-30, 1987.
86. Stefaniszyn HJ, Novick RJ, Salerno TA: Toward a better understanding of the hemodynamic effects of protamine and heparin interactions. J Thorac Cardiovasc Surg 87:678-686, 1984.
87. Tanaka K, et al: The role of the protein C-thrombomodulin system in physiologic anticoagulation during CPB. ASAIO Trans 35:373-375, 1989.

88. Traverso CI: Valoración del test de tolerancia a la heparina intravenosa realizado con tromboelastografía en la predicción de la enfermedad tromboembólica venosa tras cirugía general electiva. Granada, Spain, Granada University School of Medicine, doctoral thesis, 1989.
89. Traverso CI, et al: Role of thromboelastography when compared to other hemostatic tests for monitoring heparin and new synthetic peptide (DUP-714) protocols used as anticoagulants in cardiopulmonary bypass. Experimental study in dogs (in press).
90. Trimble AS, Herst R, Grady M, Crookston H: Blood loss in open heart surgery. Correlation with laboratory tests of hemostatic function. Arch Surg 93:323-326, 1966.
91. Tuman KJ, McCarthy RJ, Patel RV, et al: Comparison of thromboelastography and platelet aggregometry. Anesthesiology 75:A433, 1991.
92. Tuman KJ, Spiess BD, Schoen RE, Ivankovich AD: Use of thrombelastography in the management of von Willebrand's disease during cardiopulmonary bypass. J Cardiothorac Anesth 1:321-324, 1987.
93. Tuman KJ, Spiess BD, McCarthy RJ, Ivankovich AD: Effects of progressive blood loss on coagulation as measured by thrombelastography. Anesth Analg 66:856-863, 1987.
94. Tuman KJ, Spiess BD, McCarthy RT, Ivankovich AD: Comparison of viscoelastic measures of coagulation after cardiopulmonary bypass. Anesth Analg 69:69-74, 1989.
95. Utley JR: Early development of cardiopulmonary bypass. Perfusion 1:14, 1986.
96. Van-Damme H, Damas P, David JH, Limet R: Heparin-induced thrombocytopenia: A case report. Angiology 41:1075-1081, 1990.
97. Videm V, Fosse E, Mollnes TE, Garred P, Svennevig JL: Complement activation with bubble and membrane oxygenators in aortocoronary bypass grafting. Ann Thorac Surg 50:387-391, 1990.
98. Volanakis JE: Invited letter concerning complement activation caused by different oxygenators. J Thorac Cardiovasc Surg 98:292-295, 1989.
99. Von Segesser LK, Turina M: Cardiopulmonary bypass over 24 hours without systemic anticoagulation: New horizons? Helv Chir Acta 57:389-393, 1990.
100. Wakefield TW, Kirsh MM, Till GO, et al: Absence of complement-mediated events after protamine reversal of heparin. J Surg Res 51:72-76, 1991.
101. Walenga JM, Bakhos M, Messmore HL, et al: Potential use of recombinant hirudin as an anticoagulant in a cardiopulmonary bypass model. Ann Thorac Surg 51:271-277, 1991.
102. Wang JS, et al: Thromboelastogram fails to predict postoperative hemorrhage in cardiac patients. Ann Thorac Surg 53:435-439, 1992.
103. Weiss ME, Adkinson NF Jr: Allergy to protamine. Clin Rev Allergy 9:339-355, 1991.
104. Whitten CW, et al: Thromboelastographic fibrinolysis does not correlate with levels of D-Dimers after cardiopulmonary bypass. Anesthesiology 75:A432, 1991.
105. Wong CA, Jones JH, Wade L: Comparison of ACT and TEG in patients receiving autologous platelet-rich-plasma during cardiac surgery. Anesthesiology 75:A434, 1991.
106. Young JA, Kisker CT, Doty CB: Adequate anticoagulation during cardiopulmonary bypass determined by activated clotting time and the appearance of fibrin monomer. Ann Thorac Surg 26:231-240, 1978.
107. Zuckerman L, Cohen E, Vagher JP, et al: Comparison of thrombelastography with common coagulation tests. Thromb Haemost 46:752-756, 1981.
108. Zulys VJ, et al: Ancrod (Arvin) as an alternative to heparin anticoagulation for cardiopulmonary bypass. Anesthesiology 71:870-877, 1989.

Chapter 5

Blood Preservation in Cardiac Surgery at Loyola University Medical Center

Jeanine M. Walenga, Ph.D., and Roque Pifarré, M.D.

Surgical procedures for cardiac disorders have become routine and are practiced around the world with increasing frequency. Although optimal surgical technique can minimize or prevent any significant postoperative bleeding, certain patients and pathologies do not always allow for low postoperative bleeding. Moreover, the patient is often older, with a previous history of surgery and more severe disease that requires more complex surgeries with a higher incidence of postoperative bleeding. Thus the more routine cases are becoming less and less frequent.

Because blood bank resources have been strained and are currently under additional stress due to the AIDS epidemic, measures need to be taken to reduce the requirements of blood bank products. In addition, in view of the general rising cost of health care and the high cost of blood bank product processing (e.g., $100 for 1 unit of whole blood; $525 for 10 units of platelets)[6] attempts should be made to reduce expenses.

Many factors affect the degree of postoperative blood loss, including extracorporeal bypass pump time, experience of the surgical team, use of heparin/protamine sulfate, presurgical coagulation status of the patient, prior injection of anticoagulant (Coumadin, heparin) or antiplatelet (aspirin) drugs, and prior treatment with thrombolytic agents. This chapter describes the procedure used at the Loyola University Medical Center in the cardiovascular surgery service to help reduce postoperative bleeding. This protocol takes into account the preoperative status and intraoperative techniques as well as drug dosing and administration regimens.

BLOOD PRESERVATION PROTOCOL

The protocol followed in our cardiopulmonary bypass surgical patients has evolved over several years, beginning with our experiences in 1981, and incorporates our own ideas as well as other new techniques as they are

TABLE 1. Blood Preservation Protocol at Loyola Medical Center

Preoperative evaluation to identify bleeding disorders and current drug use.
Preoperative donation by patient of own blood, whenever possible.
Autologous transfusion during operation.
Use of cell saver intraoperatively.
Use of the ACT (400-450 seconds) to adjust proper heparin level intraoperatively.
Use of the Hepcon to titrate exact dose of protamine sulfate required.
Split injections of protamine sulfate.

developed (Table 1). According to data reported in 1981, our average postoperative blood loss was 450 cc/24 hr.[16] Today the average is 350 cc/24 hr, primarily because of the cell saver device and split injection of the dose of protamine sulfate. Compared with published reports of postoperative blood loss from numerous other groups, our rate is typically lower—even lower than the best-case scenario, in which specific drug treatments (e.g., aprotinin) were used.[2,10,12]

Preoperative Evaluation

A careful history is taken preoperatively to identify the recent use of any antiplatelet or anticoagulant medication or the tendency to bleed. For the 7-10 preoperative days, patients are requested not to ingest antiplatelet drugs (aspirin) and to take nonaspirin compounds such as Tylenol for pain. The use of heparin, while not restricted if medically indicated, is carefully monitored preoperatively. Patients on Coumadin are weaned from their medication and placed on heparin during the 5-7 preoperative days. All patients undergo preoperative coagulation testing, including prothrombin time (PT), activated partial thromboplastin time (APTT), bleeding time test, and platelet count.

Preoperative Blood Preservation

Whenever possible patients are asked to donate blood for their own use during surgery. This practice is associated with a decreased likelihood of viral transmission, transfusion reactions, and postoperative infections as well as a shorter hospital stay,[17] whereas homologous transfusions are immunosuppressive.[14] However, because many patients require emergency surgery or are too ill to donate blood, presurgical donations cannot always be planned.

Autologous Transfusion

Unless contraindicated, we routinely preserve 300-700 cc of heparinized whole blood from the patient at the start of surgery before going on pump. Because this blood does not go through the rigors of the cardiopulmonary bypass (CPB) pump, the clotting mechanism is preserved. Immediately after coming off pump, this blood is transfused back into the patient, who thus should normalize more rapidly to preoperative status. Our group reported that this technique requires a greater amount of heparin to reach the same level of activated clotting time (ACT) than in patients from whom blood has not been removed.[13] Therefore, more frequent determination of ACT levels was recommended to prevent underheparinization in patients receiving autotransfused blood.

Cell Saver

In all patients, the cell saver device (Haemonetics; American Bentley, Irvine, CA) is used to salvage intraoperatively lost blood that can be aspirated from the chest cavity. This practice has been important in the reduction of transfusion needs.

Because of concern that different collection techniques may result in leukocyte and platelet activation with subsequent thrombotic complications of pulmonary damage,[5] we conducted a study to determine whether the material was in fact thrombogenic and which factors may contribute to the amount of material deposited on the surface of the cell saver bowl.[4] In 63 cases the various amounts of material deposited in the bowls appeared to be correlated with the collection of all fluid (watery material) rather than only high hematocrit fluid (bloody material). However, the quantity of deposit suggested no correlation with any of the following clinical variables: patient's presurgical hematocrit, platelet count, PT, APTT, or bleeding time. It also showed no correlation with estimated intrasurgical blood loss, hematocrit of bloody fluid collected, extracorporeal bypass (pump) time, pump suction, waste volume, amount of heparin administered during the procedure, or volume of concentrated red blood cells returned to the patient.

The deposit collected from the cell saver bowl did not reveal any procoagulant activity when tested by routine clotting assays such as the PT and APTT. However, these test systems are relatively insensitive and indicate only major abnormalities. In the F1.2 prothrombin fragment and the chromogenic assays for measuring thrombin generation, which were chosen for the sensitivity and specificity of the assay endpoints, the deposit had a weak but nonsignificant thromboplastic effect (Fig. 1). Thrombin was generated from plasma by the deposit in a manner and with an efficacy suggestive of a dilute standard rabbit-brain thromboplastin similar to the reagent used in the PT assay. The clinical relevance of this activity could not be proved; nevertheless, returning this deposit could be potentially harmful in a patient predisposed to thrombosis.

The anticoagulation during cardiovascular procedures may be an important factor in reducing the amount of these deposits and/or their potential thromboplastinlike activity. Earlier reports were from general surgery or procedures other than those of cardiovascular surgery, in which patients are highly heparinized.[5] For example, repair of aortic aneurysm typically involves total administration of approximately 5000 U heparin which represents 0.5 mg/kg vs. 2-4 mg/kg in the cardiovascular cases studied here. Heparin inhibits not only coagulation but also platelet function. This may have accounted for the low amount and the low thromboplastinlike activity of the deposit obtained from the surgical cases evaluated in this study.

Thus, in cardiovascular surgery with high-dose heparin, there appears to be no clear advantage to restricting blood salvage to only fluids with a high hematocrit. However, because high-dose heparin may be the protective mechanism in this setting, one should not assume a general absence of risk with the use of the cell saver. The thromboplastic activity of the deposit should be further studied for its clinical relevance.

EFFECT OF CELL SAVER DEPOSIT ON THROMBIN GENERATION

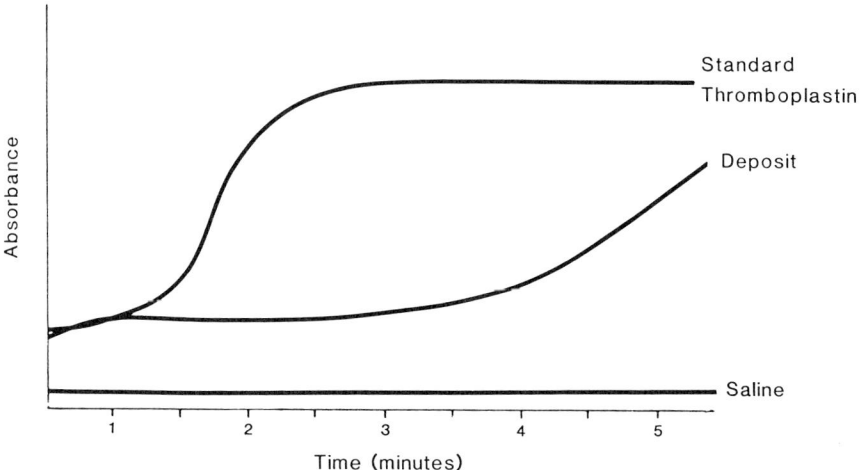

FIGURE 1. Results of thrombogenic activity using a representative specimen of deposit from the cell saver bowl. The three curves reflect the saline control, undiluted standard thromboplastin, and the weak thromboplastin effect of the cell saver bowl deposit material, roughly equivalent to a 1:128 dilution of standard thromboplastin. The tracing illustrates increasing absorbance (y-axis) over a period of 5 minutes (x-axis) as the generated thrombin caused by the action of the bowl deposit on human plasma cleaves the chromogenic substrate specific for thrombin.

Heparin Titration with the ACT

In our experience, the heparin dose that provides adequate anticoagulation is approximately 2.0-2.5 mg/kg (200-250 U/kg), which corresponds to an activated clotting time (ACT; International Technidyne, Edison, NJ) of 400-450 seconds. Higher dosages provide no further benefit, yet additional protamine sulfate, which can produce severe side effects (including hypotension and shock), is required to neutralize the excess heparin.[1] During the course of the surgery the initial heparin bolus is naturally metabolized, as demonstrated by decreasing ACT values. Periodic injections of approximately 0.2-0.4 mg/kg heparin are given to maintain the ACT at a 400-450 second level.

We have previously reported that incorporation of the ACT into the heparin dosing regimen rather than empirical administration of heparin by the standard protocol (i.e., 3.0 mg/kg to all patients) with periodic supplements of 0.3 mg/kg and no monitoring of the heparin blood level can reduce postoperative blood loss because heparin is not overdosed[16] (Fig. 2). On the other hand, over the years it has become obvious that patients have distinctly individual responses to heparinization. Thus a titration method, such as the one described above, provides a more meaningful approach to avoid both over- and underheparinization.

Protamine Sulfate Titration with the Hepcon

Because intravenously administered heparin is rather rapidly metabolized and because several injections are given throughout the course of surgery, it is

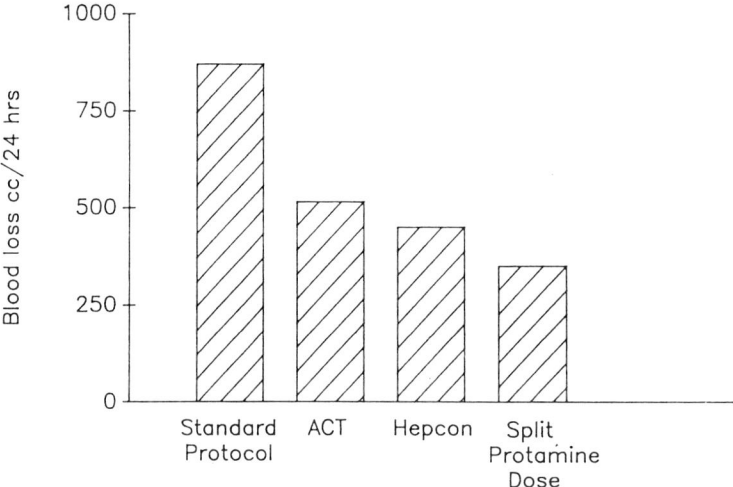

FIGURE 2. The average 24-hour postoperative blood loss in cardiac surgery patients at Loyola University Medical Center using the standard protocol (equivalent heparin dosing to all patients without monitoring); monitoring heparin blood levels with the ACT to maintain consistent heparinization; use of the ACT combined with determining an exact protamine sulfate dose based on the heparin blood level with the Hepcon; use of the ACT and the Hepcon, combined with splitting the administration of the protamine dose.

unclear exactly how much heparin is on board at the time of administering protamine sulfate. We have, therefore, incorporated the use of the Hepcon (HemoTec, Englewood, CO) to titrate the dose of protamine sulfate to exactly what is needed for the patient, thus avoiding overdose (Fig. 2). Reduced dosages of protamine sulfate decrease the possibility of side effects. In addition, protamine sulfate is itself an anticoagulant at high dosages. We have used the Hepcon system for effective reduction of postoperative blood loss.

Split Injections of Protamine Sulfate

Probably the most important part of our protocol for blood preservation in the cardiac surgery patient is the two-injection administration of protamine sulfate. After the appropriate dose of protamine is determined with the Hepcon system, the patient is given 75% of the dose. After all the pump blood and the autotransfused blood has been returned to the patient, the remaining 25% is administered, and the blood level of heparin is checked again with the Hepcon. Additional protamine is administered, if needed. This technique avoids the phenomenon of heparin rebound, which we used to observe in our patients and which often contributed to significant postoperative bleeding (Fig. 2).

In a study conducted at Loyola in 1991, we evaluated the occurrence of heparin rebound in our cardiac surgery patients as a ten-year follow-up to our 1981 study.[16] With the development of our blood preservation protocol to its current format, we were unable to detect any heparin rebound in 60 patients, whereas two cases of heparin rebound occurred in patients of two other surgeons who did not follow the same blood preservation protocol.[7] In general, we have rarely observed heparin rebound since institution of the blood preservation protocol.

SUMMARY

The concept of blood conservation in cardiac surgery is not new and has gone through many developments and modifications over the past years. New devices specifically designed for blood preservation, such as the cell saver devices, have also become available. However, the basic aspects of cardiac surgery that employ the extracorporeal circuit of the heart-lung machine have remained relatively constant. Our focus in developing a blood preservation protocol was to take into account the presurgical state of the patient, the techniques used in surgery, and the new blood conservation devices. This approach provides an integrated, comprehensive method of reducing postoperative blood loss.

The Loyola protocol for blood preservation in cardiac surgery incorporates the following elements: careful presurgical screening of the patient for coagulation abnormalities; reducing the presurgical use of aspirin; autologous blood transfusions (pre- and intraoperative); use of a cell saver device; titration of both heparin and protamine sulfate by laboratory assays; minimizing the total heparin dose so as not to exceed the needed level; and split administration of protamine sulfate to avoid heparin rebound. In all patients an 8.0 gm/dl hemoglobin is used to define the limit of when to transfuse. This protocol has proved to be cost-effective. The additional expenses incurred by the use of the cell saver, the ACT and the Hepcon are far outweighed by the possible expenses that a bleeding patient can incur through blood bank charges and longer hospital stays.

A review of other blood conservation programs in the literature included many of the above techniques in various forms and to various degrees.[3,8,9,11,15,18] We have not included in our protocol the technique of reinfusing into the patient the postoperative blood drainage. Several institutions use this procedure, which in some centers covers the entire 18-hour postoperative period.[15] Although this procedure was demonstrated to be safe in one study,[11] we have chosen to avoid it because of the possibility of thromboplastic (blood clotting) or fibrinolytic (bleeding) substances that may contaminate the blood. We do, however, reinfuse the blood into patients who severely bleed during the first 2 or 3 postoperative hours.

The future will bring further changes in methods to reduce blood loss after cardiac surgery. In development are drugs such as aprotinin, tranexamic acid, and recombinant plasminogen activator inhibitor-1 (r-PAI-1), which are designed specifically to reduce fibrinolytic activation, to protect platelets from damage, and to reverse thrombolytic therapy. Anticoagulant alternatives to heparin, which act through different physiologic mechanisms (such as r-hirudin and peptides), which may have reduced platelet interactions and which may not require neutralization with protamine sulfate are also in development. Finally, computer models may play a role in predicting the patient who is at risk of bleeding.

REFERENCES

1. Babka R, Colby C, El Etr A, Pifarre R: Monitoring of intraoperative heparinization and blood loss following cardiopulmonary bypass surgery. J Thorac Cardiovasc Surg 73:780–782, 1977.
2. Bidstrup BP, Royston D, Sapsford RN, et al: Reduction in blood loss and blood use after cardiopulmonary bypass with high dose aprotinin (Trasylol). J Thorac Cardiovasc Surg 97:364–372, 1989.

3. Boldt T, Zickmann B, Herold C, et al: Heparin management during cardiac surgery with respect to various blood-conservation techniques. Surgery 111:260-265, 1992.
4. Birdsong BA: Personal communication, 1991.
5. Bull MH, Bull BS, VanArsdell GS, Smith LL: Clinical implications of procoagulant and leukoattractant formation during intraoperative blood salvage. Arch Surg 123:1073-1078, 1988.
6. Chavez AM, Cosgrove DM III: Blood conservation. Semin Thorac Cardiovasc Surg 2:358-363, 1990.
7. Chettur V: Personal communication, 1991.
8. Cosgrove DM: Evaluation of perioperative risk factors. J Cardiovasc Surg 5(Suppl 3):227-230, 1990.
9. Dietrich W, Barankay A, Dilthey G, et al: Reduction of blood utilization during myocardial revascularization. J Thorac Cardiovasc Surg 97:213-219, 1989.
10. Dietrich W, Spannagl M, Jochum M, et al: Influence of high-dose aprotinin treatment on blood loss and coagulation patterns in patients undergoing myocardial revascularization. Anesthesiology 73:1119-1126, 1990.
11. Fuller JA, Buxton BF, Picken J, et al: Haematological effects of reinfused mediastinal blood after cardiac surgery. Med J Aust 154:737-740, 1991.
12. Havel T, Teufelsbauer H, Knöbl P, et al: Effect of intraoperative aprotinin administration on postoperative bleeding in patients undergoing cardiopulmonary bypass operation. J Thorac Cardiovasc Surg 101:968-972, 1991.
13. Mummaneni N, Istanbouli M, Pifarre R, El-Etr AA: Increased heparin requirements with autotransfusion. J Thorac Cardiovasc Surg 86:446-447, 1983.
14. Murphy P, Heal JM, Blumberg N: Infection or suspected infection after hip replacement surgery with autologous or homologous blood transfusions. Transfusion 31:212-217, 1991.
15. Ovrum E, Holen EA, Abdelnoor M, Oystese R: Conventional blood conservation techniques in 500 consecutive coronary artery bypass operations. Ann Thorac Surg 52:500-505, 1991.
16. Pifarre R, Babka R, Sullivan HJ, et al: Management of postoperative heparin rebound following cardiopulmonary bypass. J Thorac Cardiovasc Surg 81:378-381, 1981.
17. Pineo GF, Raskob GE, Hull RD, et al: Autologous blood transfusion: What are the advantages? International Society of Hematology 24th Congress, London. Blackwell, 1992, Abstract 756, p 197.
18. Scott WJ, Rode R, Castlemain B, et al: Efficacy, complications, and cost of a comprehensive blood conservation program for cardiac operations. J Thorac Cardiovasc Surg 103:1001-1006, 1992.

Chapter 6

Cardiopulmonary Bypass and the Salvaged Blood Syndrome

Brian S. Bull, M.D., and Maureen H. Bull, M.D.

Intraoperative salvage of red cells during cardiopulmonary surgery is commonplace. Blood shed into the thoracic cavity is aspirated and diluted with physiologic saline containing heparin. The red cells are then:

1. batch-concentrated in a continuous-flow, disposable centrifuge bowl;
2. washed with 4–6 volumes of physiologic saline;
3. resuspended in saline at a hematocrit of 0.50–0.65; and
4. reinfused.

The oxygen-carrying power of the aspirated blood is preserved, but all plasma proteins, including coagulation factors, are lost. The majority of the white cells and platelets are also lost.

Often, at the conclusion of bypass, additional red cells are salvaged from the diluted blood remaining in the bypass circuit. This decreases the need for autologous blood transfusions.

SALVAGED BLOOD SYNDROME

The reinfusion of the salvaged red-cell preparation may, on rare occasions, be associated with a marked worsening of the patient's condition. The close, temporal association of this syndrome with the reinfusion of salvaged red cells has led to the descriptive term **salvaged blood syndrome** (SBS).[1]

Patients with SBS may show any or all of the following:

1. decreased pulmonary compliance;
2. decreasing PaO_2 on 100% oxygen;
3. pulmonary infiltrates on x-ray consistent with adult respiratory distress syndrome (ARDS);
4. widespread bleeding with laboratory findings suggestive of disseminated intravascular coagulopathy (DIC);
5. marked left shift in circulating neutrophils without other evidence of sepsis; and
6. whole body edema (anasarca).

The incidence of SBS is difficult to estimate because only the most severe cases are commonly recognized. Fortunately, the syndrome is encountered only rarely after cardiopulmonary bypass. The circumstances that exist during a normal bypass procedure often deactivate the elements that can produce SBS. However, the reasons for this happy coincidence are well worth delineating so that cardiothoracic surgeons may keep them in mind when exploring new frontiers where circumstances differ from those that, at present, confer relative immunity to SBS.

CELL SALVAGE PROCESS

Centrifuge Bowl

All cases of SBS investigated by the authors have been associated with salvage devices that use a rapidly spinning plastic bowl to separate the cellular blood elements and the suspending plasma/diluent. A truncated cone-shaped bowl (sometimes referred to as a Latham bowl, after the design engineer, Jack Latham) is most common. Other bowl shapes (e.g., squat cylindrical or pear-shaped bowls) are also used. The upper end of the Latham bowl is usually equipped with a rotating seal traversed by an exit port and an entrance port. The entrance port funnels incoming blood down the center of the spinning bowl to the base. At the base the blood encounters a spinning disk-shaped chamber occupying the space between the outside bottom of the centrifuge bowl and the bottom of the inside chamber (Fig. 1a).

The Process of Blood Separation

The cell separation device functions like a typical centrifuge in that it uses an increased gravity (g) field to separate more dense, suspended particulate matter from the less dense suspending medium. The denser elements are held by centrifugal force against the outer bowl wall, whereas the less dense medium floats inward toward the core of the spinning bowl. On reaching the core, the less dense medium rises as more fluid is pumped into the bowl. Eventually it encounters the centrally located exit port, traverses the rotating seal once more, and is discarded.

The cells of blood are considerably more dense than the suspending plasma:[5]

Saline	~1.006
Plasma	~1.026
Platelets	~1.065
White cells	~1.075
Red cells	~1.094

Thus the red cells, white cells, and platelets are held against the outer bowl wall. The less dense plasma or saline diluent moves upward and eventually exits the bowl.

Fill Cycle

Salvaged blood mixed with other fluids recovered from the operative field or from the bypass circuit is pumped through the rotating seal and down the

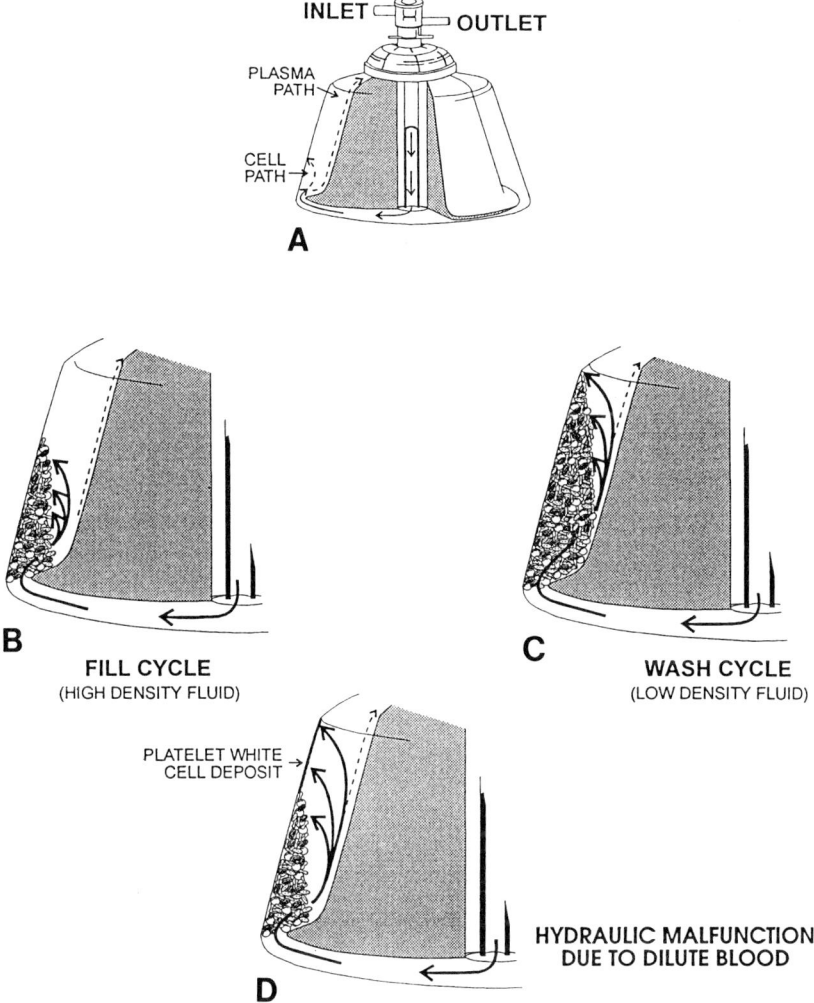

FIGURE 1. A, A cutaway view of the centrifuge bowl with the path taken by the incoming salvaged blood and the outgoing plasma stream; B, a normal fill cycle; C, a normal wash cycle; D, a malfunction due to excessively dilute salvaged blood. The hydraulic malfunction depicted in D combines the cell plume of the wash cycle with the exposed bowl wall of the fill cycle.

center of the spinning bowl. As it enters the disk-shaped, false-bottom chamber at the lower end of the inlet port, it is spun outward, accelerating rapidly as it reaches the entrance ports situated around the lower outer edge of the bowl. The centrifugal force experienced by the blood rises from zero as it leaves the lower end of the entrance tube to ~1,650 g as it is forced through the entrance ports into the lower outer edge of the centrifuge chamber proper.

The incoming blood is considerably more dense than the plasma/diluent occupying the center of the rotating bowl. Under these circumstances the dense, incoming blood is detained in the parts of the bowl most distant from the axis of rotation—where the g force is highest. The cellular burden is left behind as the plasma separates and moves inward and upward to the exit port (Fig. 1b).

Eventually the retained cells completely fill the outer portions of the rotating bowl. The addition of more cells to the lower portion of the cell deposit merely pushes the other cells inward and upward toward the exit port. Because platelets and white cells are less dense than red cells, they are typically the first elements to spill over and be discarded. But if the salvage process is not stopped at this point, red cells will be lost as well.

Wash Cycle

Once the bowl is full of red cells, the fill cycle ends and the wash cycle begins. The inlet port is now switched so that large volumes of physiologic saline are introduced. This saline follows the same path previously taken by the salvaged blood. The saline enters the bowl proper at the lower outer corner, as did the blood. Saline, however, is of no greater density than the fluid occupying the center of the bowl. Indeed, it may be less dense if undiluted plasma was the suspending medium for the red cells.

When no difference in density exists between the fluid entering the bowl and the fluid filling the bowl's core, the incoming fluid is unaffected by the g field. Although it enters the bowl at the outer edge, it rapidly traverses the dense cellular accumulations filling the outer part of the bowl on its way to the centrally located discard port. In so doing it stirs up the cells, producing turbid currents in the cell deposit and a cell plume that erupts from the surface of the accumulated red cells. The cells in this plume travel upward toward the exit port for a short distance before they are moved outward again by the g field and rain down on the surface of the cell accumulation. This process contributes further to the effectiveness of the wash cycle (Fig. 1c).

Virtually all of the anticoagulant in the originally salvaged blood is removed by the washing process. Any hemoglobin from lysed cells is also diluted and removed. The process is not as efficient in removing the less dense cellular elements, such as white cells and platelets. However, 30–60% of these cells are also washed out because of their decreased density relative to the underlying red-cell layer.

At the conclusion of the wash cycle the bowl rotation is stopped. The contents of the bowl are then pumped into a flexible plastic container for immediate or delayed reinfusion.

Hydraulic Malfunction, the Origin of Salvaged Blood Syndrome

The function of the blood salvage device is determined by the density of the material pumped into the centrifuge bowl. If the incoming fluid is sufficiently dense compared with the fluid already occupying the inner part of the chamber, a normal fill cycle ensues. This is the case whenever whole blood is salvaged; centrifugal force holds the relatively dense whole blood against the outer wall of the chamber until the plasma separates from the cells and moves inward.

If there is little difference in density between the incoming fluid and the fluid in the inner portion of the centrifuge chamber, the hydraulic flow pattern approximates a wash cycle. The incoming fluid merely traverses the bowl, diluting and thus washing out any dissolved substances. Because the incoming fluid is no heavier than the fluid already in the bowl, centrifugal force does not detain it in the outer portion of the bowl.

The stage is set for SBS whenever the density difference between the salvaged blood and the fluid in the spinning bowl drops below a certain critical difference. This condition exists whenever whole blood has been excessively diluted. Under such circumstances the fill cycle no longer functions properly. The incoming fluid is no longer detained by the g field in the outer portions of the centrifuge bowl until it has separated into cells and plasma.

The incoming fluid pushes rapidly inward through the accumulated red cells and raises a cell plume. The cells carried in this plume move upward and slowly outward. When they eventually reach the outside of the bowl wall, they are higher than the cushioning layer of accumulated red cells. Thus they encounter an unyielding polycarbonate surface. The cells strike the angled surface and roll downward until they join the red cell layer.

During this journey the cells are exposed to unphysiologically high shear forces. Red cells are deformable enough to escape serious harm. Platelets are activated by the process and adhere. White cells are unable to adhere to a bare plastic surface when also subjected to a downward vector from centrifugal force; however, they are able to stick to an adherent platelet layer. Thus, as the platelet layer deepens, it attracts white cells. These two cell types then interact with each other. This interaction is capable of generating substances that, when reinfused into the patient along with the red cells, cause the salvaged blood syndrome.

PLATELET AND WHITE CELL PATHOPHYSIOLOGY DURING SALVAGED BLOOD SYNDROME

Platelet/White Cell Interactions

It is surprising that so simple a matter as the salvaging of excessively dilute blood can set in motion a series of events that may prove fatal to a patient. That so simple a cause can have such profoundly damaging results is due to the complexities of platelet physiology, white cell physiology, and the unique response that each cell type manifests when, after activation, it is exposed to the other.

The salvage of dilute blood raises a cell plume, which may deposit platelets on the upper reaches of the bowl wall that are not yet covered by the rising red-cell layer. These platelet deposits are of little significance if they merely stick to the bowl wall and do not become fully activated and thus attractive to white cells.

The SBS process begins when adherent platelets attract white cells. This attraction occurs when, during platelet activation, a basic protein contained in the platelet alpha granule, GMP-140, is transported to the platelet surface. GMP-140 functions as an integrin, a white-cell adhesion molecule. In a region of inflammation it appears on the surface of nearby endothelial cells and causes white cells to marginate, traverse the endothelium, and enter the inflamed area. When GMP-140 is exposed on the surface of the layer of activated platelets lining the centrifuge bowl, it induces a similar response in the nearby white

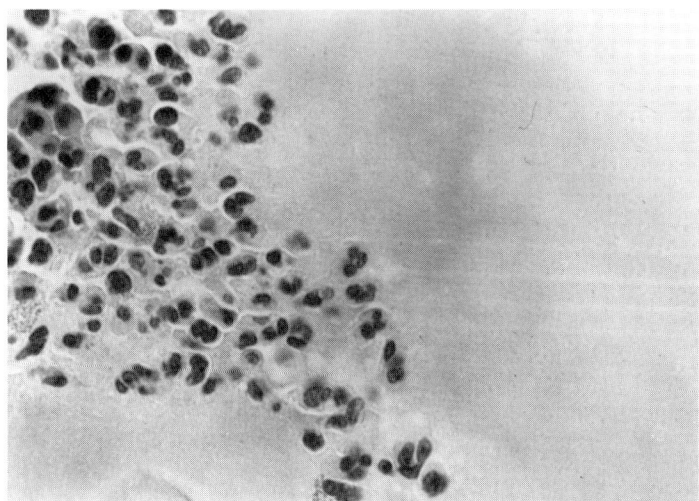

FIGURE 2. Accumulation of white cells in the platelet layer. The majority of these cells are of a single type—neutrophils.

cells. Aided by centrifugal force, they marginate on the surface of the deposit and attempt to burrow into the platelet layer in order to reach the presumed region of inflammation beneath. The process results in accumulations of unusually well-segregated white cells. Some consist entirely of neutrophils (Fig. 2), whereas others consist largely of monocytoid cells (Fig. 3). The evidence suggests that the exposed adhesion molecules are specific for type of white cell and can distinguish between monocytoid cells and neutrophils.

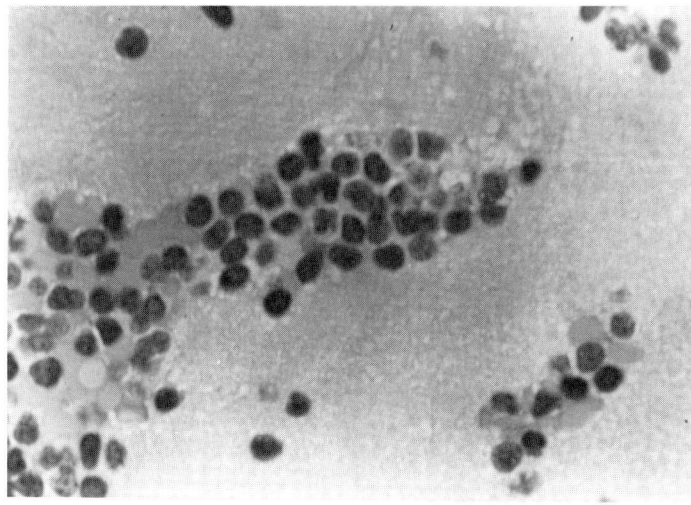

FIGURE 3. White-cell accumulation in a different region of the platelet layer. These are all mononuclear cells with very few trapped red cells; no neutrophils are present.

Activated platelets are capable of other actions in addition to the simple expression of adhesion molecules for neutrophils and monocytes. Platelets also contain a specific neutrophil-activating peptide (NAP-2)[2] capable of stimulating the respiratory burst enzymes of phagocytes as they roll downward over the platelet mat. Arachidonic acid and the high-energy metabolites adenosine triphosphate (ATP), adenosine diphosphate (ADP), and adenosine monophosphate (AMP), also present in abundance, are capable of neutrophil activation and stimulation of respiratory burst enzymes.[4,6,8]

The materials known to be released by this activated platelet/granulocyte combination include a variety of leukotrienes capable of impairing vascular integrity[3] as well as substances capable of potentiating the damage produced by activated monocytes and neutrophils.[7] Furthermore, because the deposit contains white cells, it is rich in proteolytic enzymes and undergoes partial autodigestion with dissolution within 60–100 minutes if simply incubated in vitro. Thus further use of the same bowl for processing subsequent units of salvaged red cells potentially exposes those units to large numbers of activated white cells and considerable platelet/white cell debris.

Cellular Pathophysiology Leading to Salvaged Blood Syndrome

Whenever dilute blood is salvaged, the above chain of events may be set in motion, resulting in the reinfusion of activated white cells and thromboplastic platelet debris along with salvaged red cells. The first and usually the most obvious result of such a reinfusion is damage to the lungs because the pulmonary microvasculature is the first capillary bed encountered by the white cells in the infusate.

Although the aspiration of dilute blood is a necessary cause of SBS, it is not in itself a sufficient cause. Aspiration of dilute blood merely ensures that platelets and white cells are exposed to high wall shear forces as they strike the bowl wall well above the cushioning red-cell layer. The cellular deposit can become harmful only when platelets are fully capable of

1. adhesion;
2. layer formation;
3. the release of ADP, arachidonic acid, NAP-2, and other elements; and
4. the transport of GMP-140 from internal stores to the surface of the platelet layer.

Refractory Platelets After Bypass: A Happy Coincidence

Most platelets are refractory in the later stages of cardiopulmonary bypass. Although a remnant of normal function remains (the bleeding time is long but fortunately not infinite), the platelet alpha granules and storage pools are depleted as a result of exposure to the multiple artifical surfaces of the bypass equipment. Thus, despite the routine salvage of highly dilute blood at the close of bypass, fully developed SBS is rarely seen.

However, very short pump runs, hyperactive platelets, and reactive thrombocytosis still place some patients at risk. Likewise, cardiovascular operations that do not require bypass leave the platelets fully functional and increase the risk that the patient may suffer from SBS. These possibilities should be kept in mind when cardiothoracic surgeons use cell salvage in circumstances other than after bypass.

SUMMARY

During cardiopulmonary bypass the salvage and processing of blood with a hematocrit value ≤0.20 should be avoided. Blood low in hematocrit presents such a minimal increase in density over the plasma/saline already occupying the center of the centrifuge bowl that it exceeds the design limits of the centrifuge and leads to hydraulic malfunction during the fill cycle (Fig. 4). This malfunction is likely to deposit a layer of platelets over much of the inner surface of the centrifuge bowl. If these platelets are physiologically intact, they can activate the respiratory burst enzymes of neutrophils and monocytes. When these activated neutrophils and monocytes are reinfused, they may produce ARDS. The accompanying platelet/white cell debris may initiate DIC, and leukotrienes produced by the activated white cells may result in anasarca.

Some protection agains SBS is afforded by the refractory state of most platelets after cardiopulmonary bypass. Other steps can and should be taken to decrease the risk of SBS, including the following:

1. The use of two suckers in the operative field whenever blood salvage is underway. One sucker should be used to discard irrigation fluids, cell debris, and any other particulate matter as well as to maintain a clear operating field. A second sucker should always be used for blood salvage. Blood salvage should be undertaken only with the constant awareness that the salvaged blood should be of as high a density (hematocrit) as possible.

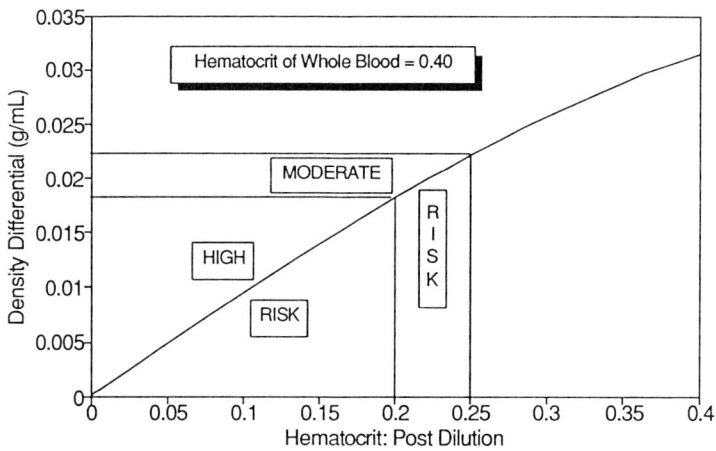

FIGURE 4. Density difference between the incoming salvaged blood and the plasma occupying the central portion of the centrifuge bowl. This difference is due to the red-cell content of the salvaged material. Below a hematocrit of approximately 20% the incoming material is of too low a density to allow the centrifuge to function properly.

2. Particular care should be exercised when the pump run has been unusually short, when platelet transfusions have been administered during surgery, or when the patient has an unusually high platelet count.

Finally, a deposit on the bowl wall may not be harmful; the platelets must attract and activate white cells before SBS will ensue. However, bowls that are completely deposit-free will not produce SBS. Deposit-free bowls can be achieved routinely if the centrifugal salvage devices are operated within design limits. This is an achievable goal and should be pursued by all who undertake the process of red-cell salvage.

REFERENCES

1. Bull BS, Bull MH: The salvaged blood syndrome: A sequel to mechanochemical activation of platelets and leukocytes? Blood Cells 16:5-23, 1990.
2. Detmers PA, Powell DE, Walz A, et al: Differential effects of neutrophil-activating peptide 1/IL-8 and its homologues on leukocyte adhesion and phagocytosis. J Immunol 147:4211-4217, 1991.
3. Ford-Hutchinson AW, Bray MA, Doig MV, et al: Leukotriene B, a potent chemokinetic and aggregating substance released from polymorphonuclear leukocytes. Nature 286:264-265, 1980.
4. Freyer DR, Boxer LA, Axtell RA, Todd RF III: Stimulation of human neutrophil adhesive properties by adenine nucleotides. J Immunol 141:580-586, 1988.
5. Geigy Scientific Tables, vol. 3. Basle, Ciba Geigy Ltd., 1984, p 67.
6. Kuhns DB, Wright DG, Nath J, et al: ATP induces transient elevations of $[Ca2+]_i$ in human neutrophils and primes these cells for enhanced O_2-generation. Lab Invest 58:448-453, 1988.
7. McCulloch KK, Powell J, Johnson KJ, Ward PA: Enhancement by platelets of oxygen radical mediated damage. Fed Proc 45:380A, 1986.
8. McPhail LC, Shirley PS, Clayton CC, Snyderman R: Activation of the respiratory burst enzyme from human neutrophils in a cell-free system. J Clin Invest 75:1735-1739, 1985.

Chapter 7

Antithrombotic Therapy in Cardiology and Cardiovascular Surgery

Ik-Kyung Jang, M.D., Ph.D., and Valentin Fuster, M.D., Ph.D.

Vascular injury is divided into three types (Fig. 1), depending upon the severity of the damage[1]: type I represents functional alterations without obvious morphologic changes; type II consists of superficial endothelial denudation and intimal injury without penetration into internal elastic lamina; and type III is a deeper injury involving both intima and media.

Intimal injury of varying degrees (type I) as a result of turbulent blood flow and motion and contraction of the artery is the initiating event in atherogenesis.[2,3] The damaged areas are covered with platelets and fibrin mural thrombus (type II). Platelets and thrombin in the thrombus stimulate not only formation of macrophages and foam cells but also proliferation and migration of smooth muscle cells, thereby accelerating the progression of atherosclerotic plaques.[4-6] Smooth muscle cells and fibroblasts also synthesize connective tissue and incorporate lipid into the cells. These processes lead to the formation of a fibromuscular lesion or fibrous capsule of lipid-rich plaque; rupture leads to type III injury with thrombus formation (Fig. 2). Once a plaque reaches a certain size, coronary flow may be compromised, as in stable angina. In contrast, plaque disruption with associated thrombosis may cause an abrupt reduction in coronary perfusion, leading to unstable angina, myocardial infarction, or ischemic sudden death.

Macrophages (originated from circulating monocytes), lipid-laden smooth muscle cells, and extracellular lipid contribute to atherogenesis by enhancing transport and oxidation of low-density lipoprotein, secreting mitogenic factors, and generating toxic products, such as free radicals.[7-10] Macrophages also release proteases, such as elastase and collagenase, which may lead to the formation of abscesses that make the plaque prone to rupture.[11]

The progression of venous coronary bypass graft disease can be divided into three phases[12]: (1) acute thrombotic phase, (2) intimal hyperplasia, and (3) atherosclerosis (Fig. 3). Acute thrombotic process occurs within the first month after surgery and is mainly mediated by platelets. Between 1-12 months, smooth muscle cells begin to proliferate, and synthesis of connective tissue

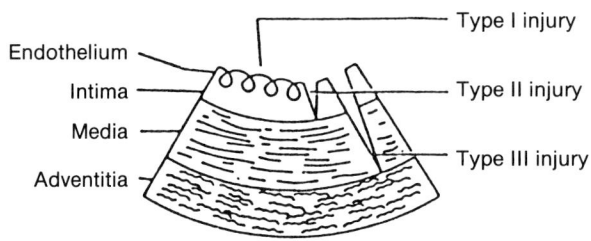

	Lipid Accumulation and Monocyte Adhesion	Platelet Deposition and Thrombosis	Proliferation of Smooth-Muscle Cells
Type 1	Moderate	No	Mild
Type 2	?	Minor	Moderate: capsule surrounding atheroma
Type 3	?	Moderate	Extensive, with organization of thrombus

FIGURE 1. Three types of vascular injury and response. (From Ip H et al: J Am Coll Cardiol 15:1667–1687, 1990, with permission).

increases. After 3 years, atherosclerotic lesions progress further, and the natural history of venous bypass grafts resembles that of native coronary arteries with advanced atherosclerosis.

Endothelial injury (type II) is induced by multiple factors, such as handling of the vein during harvest, ischemia due to disruption of vasa vasorum and delay before anastomosis, the type of preservation solution used during the procedure, and rheologic factors after restoration of blood flow. The injury leads to the exposure of collagen in the subendothelium, which, in combination with thrombin generated by the extrinsic and intrinsic coagulation pathways and adenosine diphosphate (ADP) from red blood cells, activates platelets.[13,14]

MECHANISM OF THROMBOSIS

Platelet Adhesion

When superficial endothelial cell injury occurs, platelets adhere to the subendothelium. This process depends on the interaction among platelet membrane receptors, adhesive glycoproteins, and the substrate formed by collagen, subendothelial microfibrils, and other proteins. One of the platelet membrane receptors, the glycoprotein (GP) Ib, serves as the binding site for von Willebrand's factor (vWF), particularly at high shear rates, and is necessary for the initial contact of platelets with the subendothelial surface. Another platelet membrane receptor, the GP IIb/IIIa, not only binds fibrin during platelet aggregation but also serves as an additional binding site for vWF in the process of adhesion (Fig. 3).[15]

Once platelets adhere to the subendothelium, they spread over the surface. Under appropriate conditions, such as high shear rates or turbulent blood flow, additional platelets reach the area of injury, become activated, and form

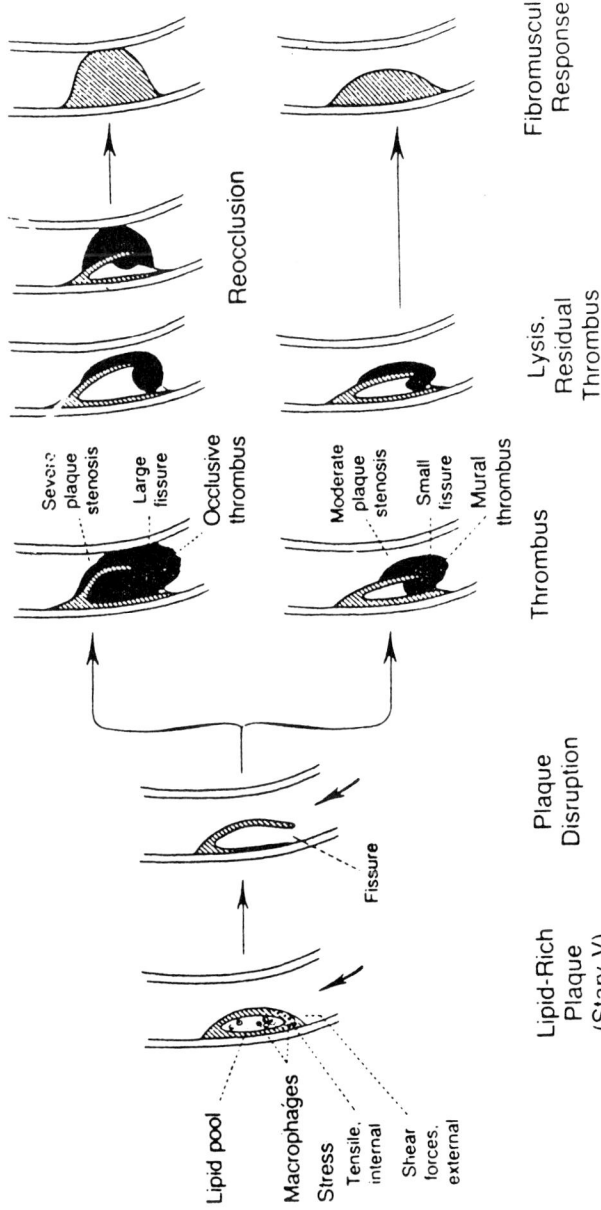

FIGURE 2. Rapid evolution of the atherosclerotic plaque. (From Fuster V et al: N Engl J Med 326:242–250, 1992, with permission).

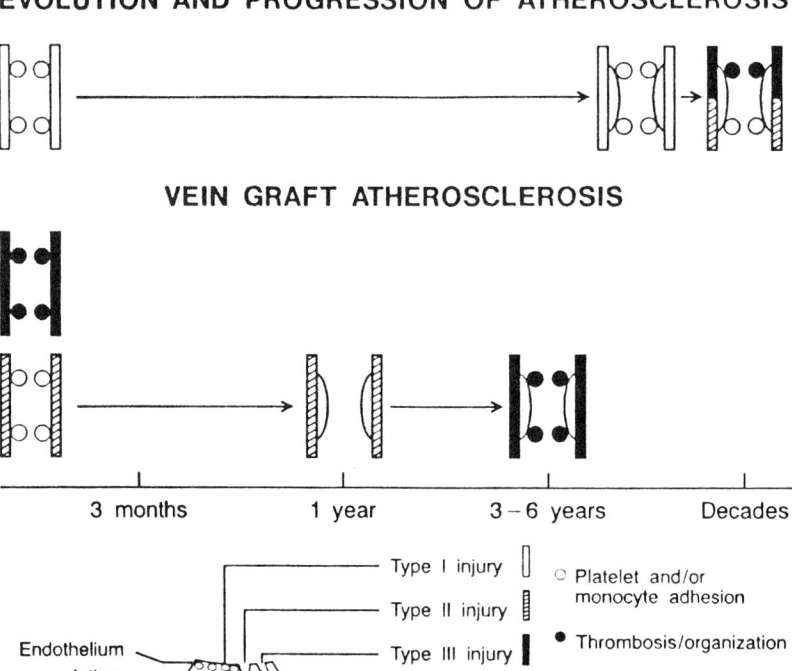

FIGURE 3. Pathogenesis of plaque formation and occlusion of venous bypass graft as compared with that of native vessel.

aggregates. Adherent platelets may contribute to atherosclerosis by the release of three mitogens: platelet-derived growth factor (PDGF), epidermal growth factor, and transforming growth factor-beta.[16] Of these, PDGF appears to be the most important. Under the influence of this polypeptide, smooth muscle cells migrate from the media into the intima and proliferate.

Platelet Aggregation

Deep injury to the vessel wall, such as occurs after rupture of an atherosclerotic plaque, leads to the exposure of fibrillar collagen (type I), which is more abundant in the deeper layers of the vessel wall.[17] This results in activation of platelets, which leads to the exposure of surface receptor GP IIb/IIIa and subsequent binding of fibrinogen, vWF, and fibronectin. These adhesive macromolecules, which form links between platelets, are essential to the process of aggregation (Fig. 4).

Platelets are activated via three different metabolic pathways (Fig. 5).[18] The first pathway depends on ADP and serotinin, which are released from the platelet dense granules. In addition, ADP is released from erythrocytes during lysis in conditions of high turbulent flow. These compounds act as potent

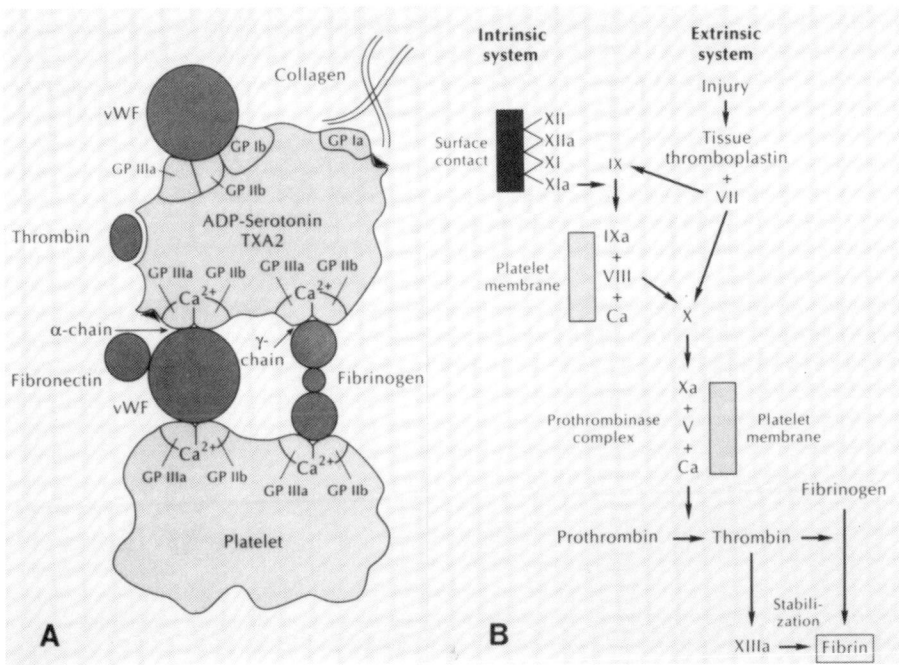

FIGURE 4. A, Platelet membrane receptors and their interaction with adhesive macromolecules. B, The intrinsic and extrinsic coagulation pathways. (From Fuster V et al: Circulation 82(Suppl II):II-47–II-59, 1990, with permission.)

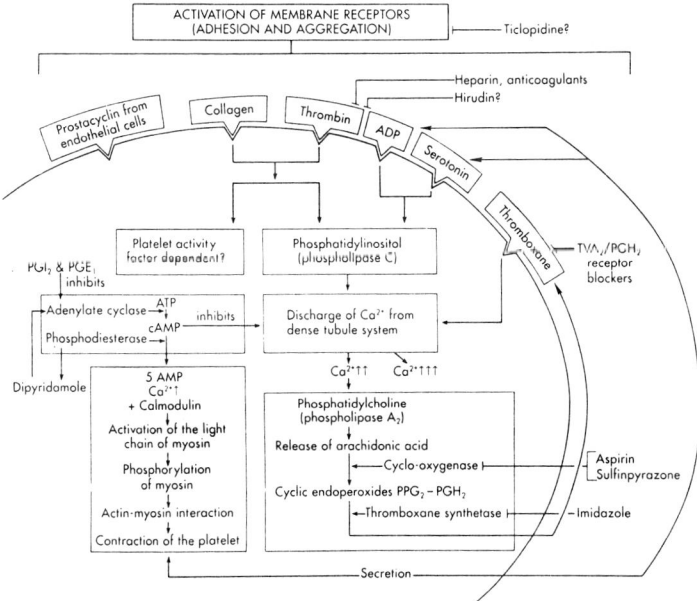

FIGURE 5. Three different pathways of platelet activation. ADP-adenosine diphosphate, ATP-adenosine triphosphate. PG-prostaglandin. (From Stein B et al: J Am Coll Cardiol 14:813–836, 1989, with permission.)

inducers of platelet aggregation by promoting the exposure of the platelet-binding site (GP IIb/IIIa) for fibrin and vWF, which is an essential step in the process of aggregation.[19] The second pathway depends on the release of thromboxane A_2 (TXA_2) through the action of cyclooxygenase and thromboxane synthase on arachidonic acid and prostaglandin endoperoxide intermediates (PGH_2 and PGG_2), respectively. TXA_2 promotes the mobilization of intracellular calcium and leads to a conformational change in the GP IIb/IIIa receptor, which results in the exposure of previously occult fibrin-binding sites.[20] TXA_2 is not only a potent platelet agonist but also induces vasoconstriction. In addition, cyclooxygenase leads to the generation of prostaglandin I_2 (PGI_2) by acting on vessel wall arachidonic acid and on platelet-derived PGG_2. PGI_2 powerfully inhibits platelet aggregation by increasing platelet cyclic adenosine monophosphate (cAMP) and reducing the mobilization of calcium.[21] The third pathway of platelet activation is mediated by collagen and thrombin, which may directly stimulate the release of a platelet-activating factor and favors the interaction of fibrin and vWF with the receptor GP IIb/IIIa. During rupture of atherosclerotic plaque, thrombin and exposed collagen may be more important in promoting platelet aggregation than the physiologically low concentrations of ADP and TXA_2. This may partially explain why thrombosis still occurs even when patients are treated with platelet-inhibitor drugs.

Activation of Coagulation System and Thrombus Formation

Deep injury to the vessel wall, which occurs during disruption of an atherosclerotic plaque, results not only in platelet adhesion to the exposed surface and subsequent aggregation but also in marked activation of the coagulation system via the intrinsic (surface-activated) and extrinsic (tissue factor-dependent) pathways (Fig. 4). This leads to the generation of thrombin, which, in addition to being a powerful platelet activator, catalyzes the conversion of fibrinogen to fibrin and promotes its polymerization. Consequently, the growing thrombotic mass composed of platelets, fibrin, and erythrocytes is able to withstand the force of blood flow.[22]

ANTITHROMBOTIC THERAPY IN CARDIAC AND CARDIOVASCULAR DISEASE

Acute Coronary Syndromes

Acute ischemic coronary syndromes (unstable angina pectoris, acute myocardial infarction [AMI], and sudden ischemic death) have, as their common underlying pathology, rupture of atherosclerotic plaque with intraluminal thrombus formation.[1,23-27] This thrombus may embolize and cause sudden ischemic death[28-31] or progressively encroach the coronary arterial lumen to cause unstable angina pectoris[25,31,32] or AMI (Fig. 2).[33-35] The rupture is caused by a tear of the thin fibrous cap separating the fatty material of a soft atheromatous plaque or abscess from the arterial lumen. The exact mechanism of plaque rupture is unknown; it may include ulceration by shear forces engendered by hypertension, changes in coronary tone or turbulent flow at the stenosis, or disruption of ingrown vasa vasorum, which causes intraplaque hemorrhage and plaque expansion.[27] It may also be simply an incidental event in the evolution and growth of the atherosclerotic plaque, which occurs when the cap has become thinned to the extent that normal hemodynamic stresses result in fragmentation.[25] It has also been suggested that macrophages release enzymes that digest collagen and elastin and thereby weaken the cap.

Several events may then occur: (1) the contents of the atheromatous abscess may discharge into the lumen and embolize distally; (2) blood from the lumen may enter into the plaque and cause intraplaque hemorrhage; (3) platelet aggregation may occur at the site of the rupture, leading to peripheral embolization of platelet clumps or progression toward luminal occlusion; and (4) the occlusive thrombus may propagate both proximally and distally.[25,27,34] The composition of the intraluminal thrombus formed in association with plaque rupture depends to a significant degree on whether blood leaks into the abscess cavity or whether plaque material extends into the lumen.[34] In the first case, the thrombi usually appear to be homogeneous in structure and consist of red cells with a few atheromatous elements, platelets, and fibrin strands. In the second case the thrombus usually consists of distinct zones, a head and body and frequently also a tail. The body, which is contiguous to the area of plaque rupture, consists predominantly of aggregated platelets with scattered red cells, components derived from the atheroma, and strands of fibrin. The head, which occupies the lumen proximally to the area of wall fracture, and the distally extending tail are composed almost entirely of red cells and fibrin.

Unstable Angina Pectoris

The initial pathogenetic mechanism of unstable angina is a plaque rupture that leads to an acute change in plaque configuration, with superimposed thrombosis that results in a reduction in coronary blood flow. The role of platelets and fibrin is suggested by the multiple platelet emboli to the distal vessels,[31] angiographic findings,[36] and a recent angioscopic study.[37] In addition, Fitzgerald et al. reported increased levels of thromboxane and prostacyclin metabolites in patients with unstable angina, indicating activation of platelets in this syndrome.[38]

The effect of aspirin and heparin on unstable angina pectoris has been tested in four large, randomized, placebo-controlled, double-blind studies. In the Veterans Administration Cooperative Study[39] 1266 men with unstable angina were randomized to either buffered aspirin (324 mg/day) or placebo. During a 12-week period the incidence of AMI and death was reduced from 10.1% to 5% in the aspirin-treated group with a risk reduction of 51%. The overall benefits of aspirin were maintained during the 1-year follow-up period. In the Canadian Multicenter Trial[40] 555 patients (73% men) with unstable angina were randomized to aspirin (1300 mg/day), sulfinpyrazone (800 mg/day), the combination of both, or placebo. After 18 months the incidence of AMI and death was reduced from 17% to 8.6% in the aspirin group with a risk reduction of 51%; sulfinpyrazone conferred no benefit. In the Montreal Heart Institute Study[41] 479 patients (71% men) were randomized to aspirin (325 mg twice daily), intravenous heparin, the combination of both, or placebo. Over a period of 6 days aspirin significantly reduced the rate of AMI by 72% from 11.9% to 3.3%, and heparin reduced the rate by 93% from 11.9% to 0.8%. However, the difference among patients treated with aspirin, heparin, or the combination of both was not statistically significant. The European RISC Study Group[42] randomized 794 men with unstable angina or non-Q wave infarction to aspirin (75 mg/day) for 3 months, intravenous heparin for 5 days, both, or neither. In 3 months the risk of AMI or death was significantly reduced by aspirin and to an even greater degree by the combination of aspirin and heparin.

In summary, convincing data support the role of aspirin and heparin in the reduction of AMI or death in patients with unstable angina. Available data suggest that combination therapy is probably more beneficial than either agent alone in patients with unstable angina.

Acute Myocardial Infarction

In more than 85% of patients, AMI is caused by intracoronary thrombosis.[43] Thrombus formation is initiated by the activation of platelets at the site of plaque rupture.[34] In these patients, spontaneous reperfusion occurs in more than 50%,[44,45] followed by reocclusion in about 5-15%.[46] Patients treated with thrombolytic therapy also have a high incidence of reocclusion. The reocclusion is also mainly mediated by platelets. In regard to the role of platelets in the progression of coronary atherosclerosis, preliminary evidence[47] suggests that aspirin (975 mg/kg) plus dipyridamole (225 mg/day) reduces the incidence of AMI from 12% to 4% (67% reduction) in patients with stable angina during a 5-year follow-up period. In a study of 333 men with stable angina, aspirin alone (325 mg every other day) reduced the incidence of AMI by 87%.[48] Therefore, aspirin may be helpful for the inhibition of thrombus growth in AMI and for the prevention of early reinfarction.

The possible benefit of aspirin in **primary prevention of myocardial infarction** was tested in two large randomized studies: the British Physicians' Primary Prevention Studies[49] and the United States Physicians' Health Study.[50,51] In the British study two-thirds of more than 5000 male physicians, aged 50-78 years, were randomly assigned to aspirin (500 mg/day) and one-third to no aspirin (no placebo used). No significant difference in the incidence of AMI or cardiovascular death was observed between the groups. Aspirin led to an overall 33% reduction in nonfatal AMI, but at the price of increased risk of stroke (0.35%/year vs. 0.20%/year). The American study recruited more than 22,000 male physicians, aged 40-84. Aspirin reduced the incidence of AMI from 0.4% to 0.2% during the 5-year period, a 44% reduction. No difference in cardiovascular death was found between the groups. Again, aspirin was associated with an increase in hemorrhagic stroke (0.2% vs. 0.1% in the placebo group).

For the **treatment of acute myocardial infarction** with or without thrombolytic therapy, both aspirin and heparin are prerequisite. The most convincing evidence for the efficacy of aspirin alone in AMI came from a single large trial, ISIS-2.[52] More than 17,000 patients with suspected AMI within 24 hours were randomized to intravenous streptokinase, oral aspirin, both, or neither. Aspirin alone reduced mortality by 23%, nonfatal AMI by 49%, and nonfatal stroke by 46%—levels that are comparable to those achieved by intravenous streptokinase. The combination of streptokinase and aspirin further reduced mortality by 42% compared with a control group. An even more striking 53% reduction in mortality occurred when combination therapy was initiated within 6 hours of the onset of symptoms; it was also associated with a significantly lower reinfarction rate (1.8% vs. 3.8% in the streptokinase group). The role of anticoagulant therapy in patients with AMI has not been settled. However, retrospective meta-analysis of 6 randomized trials clearly shows a significant 21% reduction in mortality in treated patients.[53]

Reinfarction is one of the important factors for cardiac morbidity and mortality following infarction, together with left ventricular dysfunction and ventricular arrhythmia. Aspirin has been widely tested for the **secondary prevention of myocardial infarction** in patients surviving AMI. Six randomized, placebo-controlled, double-blind trials[54-59] have been conducted with different doses of aspirin (from 300–1500 mg/day). The entry window varied from days to 60 months after infarction and the mean follow-up from 12–41 months. Although none of the results reached a statistical significance, aspirin showed a tendency to benefit survivors of AMI. The reduction of cardiac mortality was between 5% and 42%; nonfatal infarction was reduced between 12% and 57%. Meta-analysis of these studies is not possible because of various study designs. Despite the absence of difference in coronary morbidity and mortality between aspirin plus dipyridamole and aspirin alone in PARIS I,[59] the combination of aspirin and dipyridamole was compared with placebo in PARIS II.[60] The rate of coronary events was significantly lower in the combination group than the placebo group (30% reduction at 1 year and 24% reduction at the end of the study). Although multiple studies[61-63] suggested a beneficial effect of anticoagulation on the secondary prevention of AMI, only 1 study reached statistical significance.[63] A pooled analysis of 9 trials[64] showed that anticoagulation in postinfarction patients decreased mortality by 20%.

The effect of dipyridamole on secondary prevention after AMI was studied in 120 patients within 2 weeks after infarction.[65] In this placebo-controlled, randomized study, dipyridamole (400 mg) was given daily for 4 weeks. Mortality was 15.7% in the dipyridamole group and 5.8% in the placebo group.

In summary, current data suggest that aspirin is not recommended for the primary prevention of AMI. Based on risk/benefit analysis, use of prophylactic aspirin seems prudent in patients over 50 years of age with clear cardiac risk factors or with evidence of cerebrovascular or peripheral vascular disease. However, aspirin in combination with heparin should be part of the standard therapy for AMI, especially in patients with a contraindication for thrombolytic therapy who may or may not undergo coronary angioplasty. Aspirin, rather than anticoagulation, is recommended in survivors of infarction for secondary prevention.

Percutaneous Transluminal Coronary Angioplasty

Atheromatous plaque, when torn by an angioplasty balloon, exposes its contents as well as subendothelial tissues that are rich in tissue factor and collagen. This leads to platelet adhesion and aggregation, which subsequently stimulates migration and proliferation of smooth muscle cells. Not until 1987 was there a uniform antiplatelet therapy for percutaneous transluminal coronary angioplasty (PTCA). In 1987 a retrospective study[66] showed a significant effect of antiplatelet therapy before PTCA on the intracoronary thrombus. Comparing the groups with and without antiplatelet therapy after PTCA, the rates of intracoronary thrombus were 12% and 22%, respectively; the group pretreated with aspirin and dipyridamole showed no thrombus. Accordingly, 376 patients were randomized either to aspirin plus dipyridamole or placebo in a prospective study.[67] The treated group showed a significant reduction in periprocedural Q-wave myocardial infarction (1.6%) compared with the placebo group (6.9%). No difference, however, was seen in restenosis rate after 6 months between the two groups. In a separate study,[68] dipyridamole conferred no additional benefit.

The role of heparin alone in prevention of acute thrombotic occlusion during PTCA has not been properly tested, but an inverse relationship between the dose of heparin and platelet deposition was shown in a pig carotid angioplasty preparation. In addition, in a small number of patients with unstable angina, heparin treatment several days before PTCA reduced the incidence of thrombotic occlusion.[69]

Current practice is to give a high-dose bolus of intravenous heparin (10,000 or 15,000 IU) in the beginning of the procedure, followed by a continuous infusion throughout the procedure (1000 IU/hr). Aspirin should be given to all patients except those with an allergy or intolerance, in whom ticlopidine can be used as an alternative.

Coronary Artery Bypass Graft Surgery

The occlusion rate of saphenous venous graft after surgery is 5–15% per distal anastomosis at 1 month, 15–25% at 12 months, 2–4% annually for the next few years, and up to 50% at the end of 10 years.[70,71] Platelets seem to play an important role in venous graft occlusion during the first postoperative year, either by acute thrombus formation or by stimulating intimal hyperplasia.[72]

Aspirin at a wide range of doses (100–1300 mg/day), either alone or in combination with dipyridamole, has been tested in multiple studies.[73-84] The mean follow-up period was from 8 days to 21.5 months. The benefits of aspirin with or without dipyridamole were observed only when the therapy was started within 24 hours postoperatively.

Chesebro et al.[76] studied the effect of the combination of dipyridamole (beginning 2 days preoperatively) and aspirin (975 mg daily beginning 7 hours postoperatively) on saphenous vein graft patency in 407 patients. Within 6 months of the operation, distal anastomosis occlusion was decreased from 15% in the placebo group to 4% in the treated group. The proportion of patients with one or more occluded distal anastomoses decreased from 30% in the placebo group to 10% in the treated group. No significant difference in bleeding was observed between the groups. This benefit of combined aspirin and dipyridamole therapy was maintained up to 12 months after surgery.[77] Distal anastomosis was occluded in 11% of the treated group and 25% of the placebo group after 12 months. The proportion of patients with occlusion of distal anastomosis decreased from 47% in the placebo group to 22% in the treated group.

In the Veterans Administration Cooperative Study[81] 5 groups were compared: (1) aspirin (325 mg daily), (2) aspirin (975 mg daily), (3) aspirin (975 mg daily) plus dipyridamole (225 mg daily), (4) sulfinpyrazone (801 mg daily), and (5) placebo. Aspirin was started 12 hours preoperatively and other therapies 24 hours preoperatively. After 9 days the aspirin groups (with and without dipyridamole) had a significantly higher patency rate than the placebo group (90% vs. 85%). This benefit was maintained up to 1 year (graft patency rate of 84% in the aspirin groups vs. 77% in the placebo group). No difference was found between the high- and low-dose aspirin groups, and dipyridamole offered no additional benefit. However, the aspirin groups had significantly higher bleeding rates, which were probably related to the earlier administration of the drug.

In summary, antiplatelet therapy with aspirin and dipyridamole appears effective for the prevention of saphenous vein graft occlusion. Dipyridamole should be started 2 days before surgery and aspirin within 12 hours after surgery. This combination therapy should be continued at least 1 year and probably indefinitely. Finally, low-dose aspirin (100 mg/day) may be as effective as high-dose for the prevention of vein graft occlusion.

Prosthetic Heart Valve

Morbidity and mortality after prosthetic heart valve surgery are usually related to thromboembolism. The incidence is influenced by the type of valve implanted, heart rhythm (atrial fibrillation or sinus rhythm), size of left atrium, presence of thrombus at the time of surgery, history of previous embolism, and tightness of anticoagulation control.

Changes in rheology and prosthetic valve material as a foreign body probably contribute to the thromboembolic complications. In addition, several studies showed that platelet survival time was shortened in patients with a mechanical valve[85-87]; a relationship between platelet survival time and incidence of thromboembolic events was reported by Harker et al.[88]

On the basis of the above findings, anticoagulation is clearly prerequisite. Aspirin with or without dipyridamole has been tested in 5 studies.[89,93] In all 5 aspirin without anticoagulation significantly increased the thromboembolic complications, and one study[89] was prematurely terminated because of the unacceptably high incidence of thromboembolism. In the direct comparison anticoagulation was significantly better than either aspirin or dipyridamole alone.[92] The role of aspirin as an adjunctive agent to anticoagulation was tested in 5 studies.[89,94-97] Although initial results showed conflicting results, a recent study showed a definitive beneficial effect of the combination of anticoagulation and aspirin without increased risk for bleeding.

In summary, antiplatelet therapy alone without anticoagulation is not sufficient for the prevention of thromboembolic complications in patients with a mechanical prosthetic heart valve. As adjunctive therapy to anticoagulation, aspirin is recommended over dipyridamole. For those patients at high risk for bleeding, dipyridamole may be substituted for aspirin.

NEW SELECTIVE THROMBIN INHIBITORS

Recently it was shown that thrombin plays a key role in platelet-mediated arterial thrombosis.[98] Because thrombin formation is a final common pathway in the coagulation system and fibrinolysis is a phenomenon of continuous clot lysis and new clot formation, mainly by platelets, blocking thrombin may conceivably enhance fibrinolysis and prevent reocclusion. Hirudin has been shown to be effective in both enhancement of thrombolysis and prevention of reocclusion.[99,100] Another synthetic selective thrombin inhibitor, Argatroban— (2R,4R)-4-methyl-1-[N^2-(3-methyl-1,2,3,4-tetrahydro-8-quinolinesulfonyl)-1-arginyl]-2-piperidinecarboxylic acid monohydrate—is also effective in accelerating thrombolysis and preventing reocclusion.[101,102] Recombinant tick anticoagulant peptide (r-TAP), a selective inhibitor of factor Xa, was comparable to hirudin in terms of reperfusion rate and time in a canine model of coronary artery thrombosis.[103]

For the primary prevention of platelet-mediated arterial thrombosis, not followed by fibrinolysis, several selective thrombin inhibitors have been tested. The synthetic irreversible thrombin inhibitor, D-phenylalanyl-L-prolyl-L-arginyl chloromethyl ketone (FPRCH$_2$Cl), was shown to be effective for the prevention of platelet-rich thrombosis in the nonhuman primate with vascular graft[98] and endovascular stent.[104] Recombinant hirudin almost abolished platelet deposition in the pig carotid angioplasty model, in which heparin was much less effective.[100] Argatroban also maintained patency free from occlusive platelet-rich thrombosis in the rabbit model of femoral artery eversion graft, especially when administered intraarterially.[102] In this study high local intraarterial concentration of the thrombin inhibitor was much more potent than intravenous delivery. Moreover, vessel patency was maintained even when the effect of Argatroban disappeared from the circulation, which suggests that the thrombogenecity of the surface may have been altered after a 1-hour infusion of the thrombin inhibitor. This finding was subsequently confirmed in a 24-hour experiment with the same animal model.[105] A 60-aminoacid polypeptide that selectively inhibits factor Xa, r-TAP, compared with heparin, significantly reduced platelet and fibrin deposition on the Dacron graft in the baboon.[104] A peptide containing a boronic acid derivative of arginine, DuP 714 (Ac-[D]-Phe-Pro-boroArginine), was also shown to be highly effective for the prevention of both venous and arterial thrombosis in the rabbit.[106]

REFERENCES

1. Fuster V, Badimon L, Badimon JJ, Chesebro J: The pathogenesis of coronary artery disease and the acute coronary syndrome. N Engl J Med 326:242–250, 1992.
2. Davies MJ, Woolf N, Rowles PM, Pepper J: Morphology of the endothelium over atherosclerotic plaques in human coronary arteries. Br Heart J 60:459–464, 1988.
3. Davies MJ, Bland MJ, Hartgartner WR, et al: Factors influencing the presence or absence of acute coronary thrombi in sudden ischemic death. Eur Heart J 10:203–208, 1989.
4. Schwartz CJ, Valente AJ, Kelly JL, et al: Thrombosis and the development of atherosclerosis: Rokitansky revisited. Semin Thromb Hemost 14:189–195, 1988.
5. Cunningham DD, Farrell DH: Thrombin interaction with cultured fibroblasts: Relationship to mitogenic stimulation. Ann NY Acad Sci 485:240–244, 1986.
6. Shuman MA: Thrombin-cellular interactions. Ann NY Acad Sci 485:228–239, 1986.
7. Steinberg D, Parthasarathy S, Carew TE, et al: Beyond cholesterol: Modifications of low-density lipoprotein that increase its atherogenicity. N Engl J Med 320:915–924, 1989.
8. Schwartz CJ, Valente AJ, Sprague EA, et al: The pathogenesis of atherosclerosis. Clin Cardiol 14(Suppl I):I-1–I-16, 1991.
9. Mitchinson MJ, Ball RY: Macrophages and atherogenesis. Lancet 2:146–148, 1987.
10. Gown AM, Tsukada T, Ross R: Human atherogenesis. II. Immunocytochemical analysis of the cellular composition of human atherosclerotic lesions. Am J Pathol 125:191–207, 1986.
11. Richardson PD, Davies MJ, Born GVR: Influence of plaque configuration and stress distribution on fissuring of coronary artery atherosclerotic plaques. Lancet 2:941–944, 1989.
12. Chesebro JH, Goldman S: Coronary artery bypass surgery: Antithrombotic therapy. In Fuster V, Verstraete M (eds): Thrombosis in Cardiovascular Disorders. Philadelphia, W.B. Saunders, 1992, pp 375–388.
13. Fuster V, Chesebro JH: Role of platelets and platelet inhibitors in aortocoronary artery-vein graft disease. Circulation 73:227–232, 1986.

14. Josa M, Lie JT, Bianco RL, Kaye MP: Reduction of thrombosis in canine coronary bypass vein grafts with dipyridamole and aspirin. Am J Cardiol 47:1248-1254, 1981.
15. Hawiger J: Formation and regulation of platelet and fibrin hemostatic plug. Hum Pathol 18:111-122, 1987.
16. Ross R: The pathogenesis of atherosclerosis—An update. N Engl J Med 314:488-500, 1986.
17. Mayne R: Collagenous proteins of blood vessels. Arteriosclerosis 6:585-593, 1986.
18. Vermylen J, Verstraete M, Fuster V: Role of platelet activation and fibrin formation in thrombogenesis. J Am Coll Cardiol 8(Suppl B):2B-9B, 1986.
19. Peerschke EIB: The platelet fibrinogen receptor. Semin Hematol 22:241-259, 1985.
20. Coller BS: Activation affects access to the platelet receptor for adhesive glycoproteins. J Cell Biol 103:451-456, 1986.
21. Moncada S, Vane JR: Arachidonic acid metabolites and the interactions between platelets and blood-vessel walls. N Engl J Med 300:1142-1147, 1979.
22. Fuster V, Badimon L, Cohen M, et al: Insight into the pathogenesis of acute ischemic syndromes. Circulation 77:1213-1220, 1988.
23. Friedman M: The coronary thrombus: Its origin and fate. Hum Pathol 2:81-128, 1971.
24. Ridolfi RL, Hutcins GM: The relationship between coronary artery lesions and myocardial infarct: Ulceration of atherosclerotic plaques precipitating coronary thrombosis. Am Heart J 93:468-486, 1977.
25. Falk E: Plaque rupture with severe pre-existing stenosis precipitating coronary thrombosis: Characteristics of coronary atherosclerotic plaques underlying fatal occlusive thrombi. Br Heart J 50:127-134, 1983.
26. Falk E: Unstable angina with fatal outcome: Dynamic coronary thrombosis leading to infarction and/or sudden death. Autopsy evidence of recurrent mural thrombosis with peripheral embolization culminating in total vascular occlusion. Circulation 71:699-708, 1985.
27. Davies MJ, Thomas AC: Plaque fissuring: The cause of acute myocardial infarction, sudden ischemic death, and crescendo angina. Br Heart J 53:363-373, 1985.
28. Haerem JW: Platelet aggregates in intramyocardial vessels of patients dying suddenly and unexpectedly of coronary artery disease. Atherosclerosis 5:199-213, 1972.
29. El-Maraghi N, Genton E: The relevance of platelet and fibrin thromboembolism of the coronary microcirculation with special reference to sudden cardiac death. Circulation 62:936-944, 1980.
30. Davies MJ, Thomas A: Thrombosis and acute coronary artery lesions in sudden cardiac ischemic death. N Engl J Med 310:1137-1140, 1984.
31. Davies MJ, Thomas AC, Knapman PA, Hangartner JR: Intramyocardial platelet aggregation in patients with unstable angina suffering sudden ischemic cardiac death. Circulation 73:418-427, 1986.
32. Levin DC, Fallon JT: Significance of the angiographic morphology of localized coronary stenoses: Histopathologic correlations. Circulation 66:316-320, 1982.
33. Davies MJ, Woolf N, Robertson WB: Pathology of acute myocardial infarction with particular reference to occlusive coronary thrombi. Br Heart J 38:659-664, 1976.
34. Friedman M, Van den Bovenkamp GJ: The pathogenesis of a coronary thrombus. Am J Pathol 48.19-44, 1966.
35. Erhardt LR, Lundman T, Mellstedt H: Incorporation of ^{125}I-labelled fibrinogen into coronary arterial thrombi in acute myocardial infarction in man. Lancet 1:387-390, 1973.
36. Ambrose JA, Israel DH: Angiography in unstable angina. Am J Cardiol 68:78B-84B, 1991.
37. Mizuno K, Satomura K, Miyamoto A, et al: Angioscopic evaluation of coronary-artery thrombi in acute coronary syndrome. N Engl J Med 326:287-291, 1992.
38. Fitzgerald DJ, Roy L, Catella F, FitzGerald GA: Platelet activation in unstable angina. N Engl J Med 315:983-989, 1986.
39. Lewis HD, Davis JW, Archibald DG, et al: Protective effects of aspirin against acute myocardial infarction and death in men with unstable angina. Results of a Veterans Administration Cooperative Study. N Engl J Med 309:396-403, 1983.
40. Cairns JA, Gent M, Singer J, et al: Aspirin, sulfinpyrazone, or both in unstable angina. N Engl J Med 313:1369-1375, 1985.
41. Theroux P, Ouimet H, McCans J, et al: Aspirin, heparin, or both to treat acute unstable angina. N Engl J Med 319:1105-1111, 1988.
42. The RISC Group: Risk of myocardial infarction and death during treatment with low dose aspirin and intravenous heparin in men with unstable coronary artery disease. Lancet 1:827-830, 1990.

43. DeWood MA, Spores J, Notske R, et al: Prevalence of total coronary occlusion during the early hours of transmural myocardial infarction. N Engl J Med 303:897–902, 1980.
44. Jang IK, Vanhaecke J, De Geest H, et al: Coronary thrombolysis with recombinant tissue-type plasminogen activator: Patency rate and regional wall motion after 3 months. J Am Coll Cardiol 8:1455–1460, 1986.
45. Raynaud PL, Desveaux B: Reocclusion après traitment par L'Actilyse. Arch Mal Coeur 81(Suppl 1):25–32, 1988.
46. Fuster V, Badimon L, Badimon JJ, Chesebro JH: Mechanism of disease: The pathogenesis of coronary artery disease and the acute coronary syndromes (Part II). N Engl J Med 326:310–318, 1992.
47. Chesebro JH, Webster MWI, Smith HC, et al: Antiplatelet therapy in coronary disease progression: Reduced infarction and new lesion formation. Circulation 80:II-266, 1989 [abstract].
48. Ridker PM, Manson JE, Gaziano M, et al: Low-dose aspirin therapy for chronic stable angina: A randomized placebo-controlled clinical trial. Ann Intern Med 114:835–839, 1991.
49. Peto R, Gray R, Collins R, et al: Randomized trial of prophylactic daily aspirin in British male doctors. Br Med J 296:313–316, 1988.
50. The Steering Committee of the Physicians' Health Study Research Group: Preliminary report: Findings from the aspirin component of the ongoing Physicians' Health Study. N Engl J Med 318:262–264, 1988.
51. American Steering Committee of the Physicans' Health Study Research Group: Final report on the aspirin component of the ongoing Physicians' Health Study. N Engl J Med 321:129–135, 1989.
52. ISIS-2 (Second International Study of Infarct Survival) Collaborative Group: Randomised trial of intravenous streptokinase, oral aspirin, both, or neither among 17187 cases of suspected acute myocardial infarction: ISIS-2. Lancet 2:3491–1360, 1988.
53. Chalmers TC, Matta RJ, Smith H, Kunzler AM: Evidence favoring the use of anticoagulation in the hospital phase of acute myocardial infarction. N Engl J Med 297:1091–1096, 1977.
54. Elwood PC, Cochrane ASL, Burr ML, et al: A randomized controlled trial of acetyl salicylic acid in the secondary prevention of mortality from myocardial infarction BMJ 1:436–440, 1974.
55. Coronary Drug Project Group: Aspirin in coronary heart disease. J Chronic Dis 29:625–642, 1976.
56. Breddin K, Loew D, Lechner K, et al: Secondary prevention of myocardial infarction: Comparison of acetylsalicylic acid, phenoprocoumon and placebo: A multicenter two-year prospective study. Throm Haemost 40:225–236, 1979..
57. Elwood PC, Sweetnam PM: Aspirin and secondary mortality after myocardial infarction. Lancet 2:1213–1315, 1979.
58. Aspirin Myocardial Infarction Study Research Group: A randomized controlled trial of aspirin in persons recovered from myocardial infarction. JAMA 243:661–669, 1980.
59. Persantine-Aspirin Reinfarction Study Research Group: persantine and aspirin in coronary heart disease. Circulation 62:449–461, 1980.
60. Klimt CR, Knatterud GL, Stamler J, Meier P: Persantine-aspirin reinfarction study. Part II. Secondary coronary prevention with Persantine and aspirin. J Am Coll Cardiol 7:251–269, 1986.
61. Kannel WB, Wolf PA, Garrison RJ: Survival following initial cardiovascular events: Framingham study: Section 35, Publ. No. PB 88-204049. U.S. Department of Health and Human Services, National Institute of Health, U.S. Department of Commerce. Washington, DC, U.S. Government Printing Office, 1988.
62. Ebert RV, Borden CW, Hipp HR, et al: Long-term anticoagulant therapy after myocardial infarction: Final report of the Veterans Administration Cooperative Study. JAMA 207:2263–2267, 1969.
63. Breddin K, Loew D, Lechner K, et al: The German-Austrian Aspirin trial: A comparison of acetylsalicylic acid, placebo and phenprocoumon in secondary prevention of myocardial infarction. Circulation 62(Suppl 62):V63–V72, 1980.
64. International Anticoagulation Review Group: Collaborative analysis of long-term anticoagulation administration after acute myocardial infarction. Lancet 1:203–209, 1970.
65. Gent AE, Brook GD, Foley TH, et al: Dipyridamole: A controlled trial of its effect in acute myocardial infarction. BMJ 4:366–368, 1968.
66. Barnathan ES, Schwartz JS, Taylor L, et al: Aspirin and dipyridamole in the prevention of acute coronary thrombosis complicating coronary angioplasty. Circulation 76:125–134, 1987.

67. Schwartz L, Bourassa MG, Lesperance J, et al: Aspirin and dipyridamole in the prevention of restenosis after percutaneous transluminal coronary angioplasty. N Engl J Med 318:1714-1719, 1988.
68. Lembo NJ, Black AJR, Roubin GS, et al: Effect of pretreatment with aspirin versus aspirin plus dipyridamole on frequency and type of acute complications of percutaneous transluminal coronary angioplasty. Am J Cardiol 65:422-426, 1990.
69. Laskey MAL, Deutsch E, Barnathan E, Laskey WK: Influence of heparin therapy on percutaneous transluminal coronary angioplasty outcome in unstable angina pectoris. Am J Cardiol 65:1425-1429, 1990.
70. Stein PD, Kantrowitz A: Antithrombotic therapy in mechanical and bilogical prosthetic heart valves and saphenous vein bypass graft. Chest 95(Suppl):107S-117S, 1989.
71. Henderson W, Goldman S, Copeland J, et al: Antiplatelet or anticoagulant therapy after coronary artery bypass surgery: A meta-analysis of clinical trials. Ann Intern Med III:743-750, 1989.
72. Fuster V, Chesebro JH: Role of platelets and platelet inhibitors in aortocoronary artery vein-graft disease. Circulation 73:227-232, 1986.
73. Pantely GS, Goodnight SH, Rahimtoola SH, et al: Failure of antiplatelet and anticoagulant therapy to improve patency of grafts after coronary artery bypass. A controlled, randomized study. N Engl J Med 301:962-966, 1979.
74. Mayer JE, Lindsay WG, Castaneda W, et al: Influence of aspirin and dipyridamole on patency of coronary artery bypass grafts. Ann Thorac Surg 31:204-210, 1981.
75. McEnany MI, Salzman EW, Mundth ED, et al: The effect of antithrombotic therapy on patency rates of saphenous vein coronary artery bypass grafts. J Thorac Cardiovasc Surg 83:81-89, 1982.
76. Chesebro JH, Clements IP, Fuster V, et al: A platelet-inhibitor drug trial in coronary artery bypass operations. Benefit of perioperative dipyridamole and aspirin therapy on early postoperative vein graft patency. N Engl J Med 307:73-78, 1982.
77. Chesebro JH, Fuster V, Elveback LR, et al: Effect of dipyridamole and aspirin on late vein graft patency after coronary bypass operation. N Engl J Med 310:209-214, 1984.
78. Lorenz RL, Weber M, Kotzur J, et al: Improved aortocoronary bypass patency by low-dose aspirin (100 mg daily). Lancet 1:1261-1264, 1984.
79. Brown B, Cukingnan RA, DeRouen T, et al: Improved graft patency in patients treated with platelet-inhibiting therapy after coronary bypass surgery. Circulation 72:138-146, 1985.
80. Rajah SM, Slater MCP, Donaldson DR, et al: Acetylsalicylic acid and sipyridamole improve the early patency of aortocoronary bypass grafts. J Thorac Cardiovasc Surg 90:373-377, 1985.
81. Goldman S, Copeland J, Moritz T, et al: Improvement in early saphenous vein graft patency after coronary artery bypass surgery with antiplatelet therapy: Results of a Veterans Administration Cooperative Study. Circulation 77:1324-1332, 1988.
82. Goldman S, Copeland J, Moritz T, et al: Saphenous vein graft patency 1 year after coronary artery bypass surgery and effects of antiplatelet therapy. Circulation 80:1190-1197, 1989.
83. Pfisterer M, Burkart F, Jockers G, et al: Trial of low-dose aspirin plus anticoagulants for prevention of aortocoronary vein graft occlusion. Lancet 2:1-7, 1989.
84. Goldman S, Copeland J, Moritz T, et al: Starting aspirin therapy after operation. Effects on early graft patency. Circulation 84:520-526, 1991.
85. Dale J. Prevention of arterial thromboembolism with acetylsalicylic acid in patients with prosthetic heart valves. Thromb Haemost 38:66, 1975 [abstract].
86. Weily HS, Steele PP, Davies H, et al: Platelet survival in patients with substitute heart valves. N Engl J Med 290:534-537, 1974.
86. Steele PP, Weily H, Davies H, et al: Platelet survival time following aortic valve replacement. Circulation 51:358-362, 1975.
88. Harker LA, Slichter SJ: Studies of platelet and fibrinogen kinetics in patients with prosthetic heart valves. N Engl J Med 283:1302-1305, 1970.
89. Dale J, Myhre E, Rootwelt K: Effects of dipyridamole and acetylsalicylic acid on platelet function in patients with aortic ball-valve prosthesis. Am Heart J 89:613-618, 1975.
90. Moggio RA, Hammond CL, Stansel HC, et al: Incidence of emboli with cloth-covered Starr-Edwards valves without anticoagulation and with varying forms of anticoagulation. J Thorac Cardiovasc Surg 75:296-299, 1978.
91. Brott WH, Zaytchuk R, Bowen TE, et al: Dipyridamole-aspirin as thromboembolic prophylaxis in patients with aortic valve prosthesis. J Thorac Cardiovasc Surg 81:632-635, 1981.

92. Mok CK, Boey J, Wang R, et al: Warfarin versus dipyridamole-aspirin and pentoxifylline-aspirin for the prevention of prosthetic heart valve thromboembolism: A prospective randomized clinical trial. Circulation 72:1059-1063, 1985.
93. Ribeiro PA, Zaibag M, Idis M, et al: Antiplatelet drugs and the incidence of thromboembolic complications of the St. Jude Medical aortic prosthesis in patients with rheumatic heart disease. J Thorac Cardiovasc Surg 91:92-98, 1986.
94. Altman R, Boullon F, Rouvier J, et al: Aspirin and prophylaxis of thromboembolic complications in patients with substitute heart valves. J Thorac Cardiovasc Surg 72:127-129, 1976.
95. Chesebro JH, Fuster V, Elveback LR, et al: Trial of combined warfarin plus dipyridamole or aspirin therapy in prosthetic heart valve replacement: Danger of aspirin compared with dipyridamole. Am J Cardiol 51:1537-1541, 1983.
96. Sullinvan JM, Harken DE, Grolin R: Pharmacologic control of thromboembolic complications of cardiac-valve replacement. N Engl J Med 284:1391-1394, 1971.
97. Turpie AGG, Gent M, Laupacis A, et al: Reduction in mortality by adding aspirin (100 mg) to oral anticoagulants in patients with heart valve replacement. J Am Coll Cardiol 19(Suppl A):103A, 1992 [abstract].
98. Hanson SR, Harker LA: Interruption of acute platelet-dependent thrombosis by the synthetic antithrombin D-phenylalanyl-L-prolyl-L-arginyl chloromethyl ketone. Proc Natl Acad Sci USA 85:3184-3188, 1988.
99. Haskel EJ, Prager NA, Sobel BE, Abendschein DR: Relative efficacy of antithrombin compared with antiplatelet agents in accelerating coronary thrombolysis and prevention of reocclusion. Circulation 83:1048-1056, 1991.
100. Heras M, Chesebro JH, Penny WJ, et al: Effects of thrombin inhibition on the development of acute platelet-thrombus deposit or during angioplasty in pigs. Heparin vs. hirudin, as specific thrombin inhibitor. Circulation 79:657-665, 1989.
101. Jang IK, Gold HK, Leinbach RC, et al: In vivo thrombin inhibition enhances and sustains arterial recanalization with recombinant tissue-type plasminogen activator. Cir Res 67:1552-1561, 1990.
102. Jang IK, Gold HK, Ziskind AA, et al: Prevention of platelet-rich arterial thrombosis by selective thrombin inhibition. Circulation 81:219-225, 1990.
103. Schaffer LW, Davidson JT, Vlasuk GP, Siegel PKS: Antithrombotic efficacy of recombinant tick anticoagulant peptide: A potent inhibitor of coagulation factor Xa in a primate model of arterial thrombosis. Circulation 84:1741-1748, 1991.
104. Krupski WC, Bass A, Kelly AB, et al: Heparin-resistant thrombus formation by endovascular stents in baboons. Interruption by a synthetic antithrombin. Circulation 81:570-577, 1990.
105. Jang IK, Gold HK, Leinbach RC, et al: Persistent inhibition of arterial thrombosis by a 1-hour intravenous infusion of argatroban, a selective thrombin inhibitor. Coronary artery disease 3:407-414, 1992.
106. Knabb RM, Kettner CA, Timmermans PBMEM, Reilly TM: In vivo characterization of a new synthetic thrombin inhibitor. Thromb Haemost 67:56-59, 1992.

Chapter 8

An Overview of Current Anticoagulant and Antithrombotic Drugs

Jawed Fareed, Ph.D., Debra Hoppensteadt, M.S., MT(ASCP), Jeanine M. Walenga, Ph.D., and Roque Pifarré, M.D.

Many significant developments in the understanding of the hemostatic process have occurred recently, including the role of plasmatic components, platelets, white cells, endothelial cells, and cytokines.[16,21] The blood coagulation system is thus no longer perceived to be the sole mechanism of the clotting process. Although thrombin, which is one of the main targets of the new anticoagulant and antithrombotic drugs, plays an important role in the regulation of clotting, other processes involving cells and nonthrombin proteases are also considered important contributing factors.[21] Thus, the development of new anticoagulants now focuses on multiple targeting of the hemostatic system.[22] Although heparin remains the major anticoagulant and antithrombotic agent for treatment of the thrombotic process, its efficacy as a surgical anticoagulant is being questioned for various reasons related to both safety and efficacy. Many newer drugs currently under development are being compared with heparin in the surgical setting. Furthermore, postsurgical prophylaxis of deep venous thrombosis and related disorders is now considered an essential element in the management of patients. Several new drugs are also currently under development for this purpose.

ANTICOAGULANT VS. ANTITHROMBOTIC DRUGS

Because many drugs produce an antithrombotic effect without producing an anticoagulant effect, it is important to differentiate between these two processes. The commonly used anticoagulant agents, such as heparin, exhibit both anticoagulant and antithrombotic actions (Table 1). The anticoagulant actions of heparin can be assessed in vitro. Blood drawn from patients given heparin exhibits an anticoagulant action. In contrast, aspirinized blood does not exhibit an anticoagulant action; however, patients treated with aspirin do not have arterial thrombosis. The anticoagulant effects of a drug are mainly

TABLE 1. Anticoagulant vs. Antithrombotic Actions of Drugs

Anticoagulant	Antithrombotic
In vitro phenomenon	In vivo phenomenon
Blood does not clot	Blood may or may not clot
Primarily a plasmatic process	Plasmatic and cellular components involved
Direct effect on thrombin	Both direct and indirect effects on thrombin
Heparin, hirudin, and anticoagulant peptides	Aspirin, dextrans, and prostaglandin derivatives
Whole blood clotting time prolonged	No effect on clotting assays

due to its plasmatic effect. On the other hand, antithrombotic actions may be due to effects on the plasmatic and/or cellular elements. Anticoagulants such as heparin and hirudin directly inhibit the action of thrombin, whereas antithrombotic drugs inhibit the generation of thrombin.[19] Aspirin, dextrans, and many eicosanoids produce antithrombotic action without producing any anticoagulant action.

The whole-blood assays, such as the activated clotting time (ACT), are significantly prolonged in patients who are given heparin. However, patients administered low-molecular-weight heparins do not exhibit a marked prolongation of the clot-based assays. Heparin is a polycomponent drug. Some of its components exhibit both anticoagulant and antithrombotic actions, whereas many of the components exhibit only antithrombotic actions. Single-component drugs such as hirudin exhibit only an anticoagulant action and as antithrombotic agents are not as effective as low-molecular-weight heparins and related drugs that inhibit thrombin generation.

Most surgical anticoagulants exhibit a stronger anticoagulant component and may not have a comparable antithrombotic action. During a surgical procedure, an effective drug should have a balance of antithrombotic and anticoagulant components. This is particularly important if the surgical procedure results in the activation of the clotting process.

Heparin, which has remained the anticoagulant of choice for over three decades, is a naturally derived, polycomponent sulfated mucopolysaccharide that is usually obtained from mammalian tissues such as the lung or mucosa. Figure 1 depicts the molecular heterogeneity of heparin, which consists of various chains of sulfated mucopolysaccharides with molecular weights ranging from 2–50 kd. Besides producing anticoagulant effects, heparin can also inhibit proliferation of smooth muscle cells, enhance fibrinolysis, and modulate lipoprotein lipase.[17-19] Heparin also releases several endogenous factors, such as the tissue factor pathway inhibitor (TFPI), which facilitates the anticoagulant and antithrombotic actions.

Heparin can be fractionated into high- and low-molecular-weight fractions. Low-molecular-weight heparins (LMWHs), which represent depolymerized heparins, are usually obtained by chemical or enzymatic digestion of heparin (Fig. 2). Usually the resulting product is significantly lower in mean molecular weight and exerts different pharmacologic actions. These agents have been successfully used in the prophylaxis of deep venous thrombosis and offer several advantages over heparin, including (1) better bioavailability, (2) lower risk of bleeding and osteoporosis, and (3) requirement of only one injection per day for prophylactic actions.

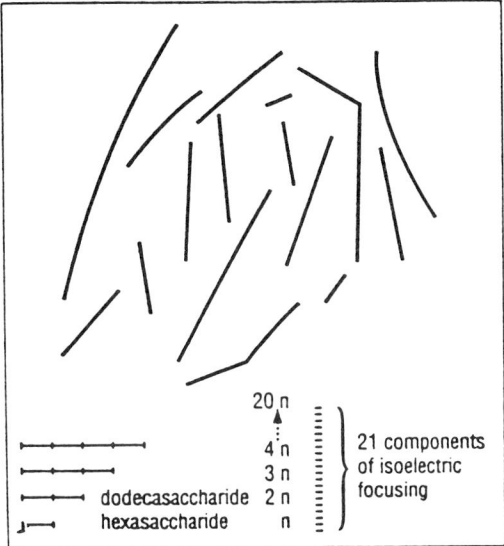

FIGURE 1. The polycomponent nature of unfractionated heparin. Note the differences in the molecular range of various components. Heparin is composed of low-, medium-, and high-molecular-weight components. The mean molecular weight of this polycomponent drug is 15,000 daltons.

Heparin produces its anticoagulant actions mainly by inhibiting both thrombin and factor Xa, whereas the LMWHs inhibit factor Xa and the generation of thrombin. Both are capable of prolonging the ACT, activated partial thromboplastin time (APTT), and thrombin time (albeit at different dosages). Table 2 shows the circulating levels of heparin required for various surgical procedures. For the common procedures, a circulating level of 0.5-1.0 U/ml is adequate; however, a surgeon uses his or her judgment to determine the exact level of anticoagulation needed. High thrombotic risk as well as cardiac catheterization and other interventions require 1.5-2.5 U/ml of heparin. Open-heart surgery, cardiac transplantation, and other major procedures require 3.0-5.0 U/ml. Common APTT methods are not useful in the management of anticoagulation at such high levels of heparinization, but the ACT assay can be adequate. Several other assays based on protamine titration and other measures can also be used to monitor levels of heparin.

The same degree of anticoagulation is achievable with LMWHs, although much higher dosages are needed. At the present time only limited data are available on the feasibility of LMWHs for surgical purposes, including isolated reports of differing conclusions on their use as a surgical anticoagulant during extracorporeal circulation.

The introduction of newer heparins has added another dimension to the medical and surgical management of thrombotic disorders. Although many of these agents have been primarily developed and used in Europe, more recently other continents, including North America, have started to evaluate their usefulness. Among the newer heparins the LMWHs have been widely accepted for various clinical indications. Well-designed clinical trials have been carried out for different indications with several of these agents. In comparison with other anticoagulant drugs, such as aspirin and the oral anticoagulants, the LMWHs appear to exhibit an improved safety/efficacy profile for postsurgical prophylaxis of thrombosis.

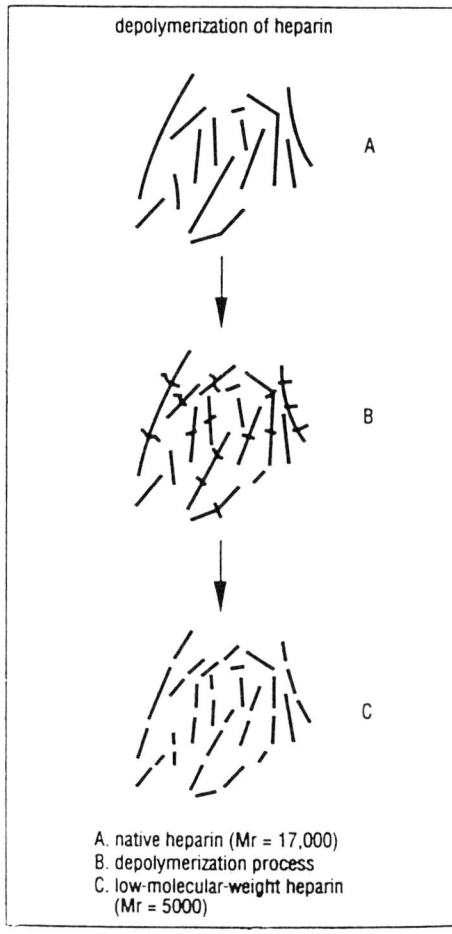

FIGURE 2. Chemical or enzymatic depolymerization of heparin into low-molecular-weight heparins (LMWHs). Porcine/beef mucosal heparin is subjected to a depolymerization process. This results in the formation of LMWHs, which exhibit different biochemical or pharmacologic properties.

A. native heparin (Mr = 17,000)
B. depolymerization process
C. low-molecular-weight heparin (Mr = 5000)

Besides the currently available LMWH preparations, some 14 other agents are under development.[19] Although both the original and newer products have similar basic characteristics, differences in the physicochemical properties and pharmacologic actions have been reported. However, only results from valid clinical trials will show if the individual agents are, in fact, similar or different for a given indication. Many significant developments of LMWHs will take place in the coming years. In addition to their use for the prophylaxis of venous thrombosis, LMWHs are currently under development as therapy for established thromboembolic conditions. Furthermore, they may also be

TABLE 2. Circulating Heparin Levels During Surgical Anticoagulation

Surgical Procedures	Heparin U/ml
Common surgical procedures	0.5–1.0
Cardiac catheterization angioplasty	1.5–2.5
Open-heart surgery, cardiac transplantation	3.0–5.0

developed as presurgical anticoagulants for prophylaxis against postsurgical thrombosis and for treatment of established thromboembolic conditions.

Heparin has been widely used for surgical anticoagulation and for the prevention of postoperative thromboembolism. However, its undesirable side effects include bleeding, heparin-induced thrombocytopenia, and heparin-induced thrombosis. In addition, prolonged administration of heparin has been shown to induce osteoporosis.

Heparin is usually obtained from either porcine or beef mucosa or from beef lung preparations. Usually these products are standardized by the United States Pharmacopoeia (USP) method; however, significant compositional difference have been noted in products obtained from various species. If heparin is used at a circulating level of <0.5 U/ml for various indications, very few, if any, differences are noted. However, at levels of >1.0 U/ml, anticoagulant responses may vary with different heparins because of their molecular composition. Heparin from beef lung is usually richer in high-molecular-weight fractions, whereas the porcine mucosal heparin has a lower-molecular-weight profile. Differences in the anticoagulant responses are obvious in the ACT test. Thus, it is important to have a consistent product for a given procedure. It may be necessary to adjust the dosage if a different product is substituted.

During the 1970s several investigators studied the structure of heparin to identify its active component(s). This work, coupled with recognition of the clinical problems with heparin, resulted in the development of LMWHs and other derivatives. Experimental studies revealed that the major difference is the bioavailability by the subcutaneous route of about 100% for LMWHs compared with 15–25% for heparin.

Advantages of LMWHs as surgical anticoagulants are listed in Table 3. All of the LMWHs produce a strong antithrombotic action at a lower anticoagulant level than heparin. Thus, the activation process during surgical procedures can be controlled without major compromise of the hemostatic system. Despite the higher safety index due to lesser anticoagulant action, LMWHs have not yet been evaluated as a substitute anticoagulant in all surgical considerations. Because they exhibit less anticoagulant action than heparin, it is likely that a very high dose of LMWHs is needed for achieving comparable anticoagulant levels; however, because of their higher bioavailability, delivery will be easier to control; combined approaches, therefore, may be developed.

Patients who are deficient in antithrombin III (AT III) are poor responders to heparin. However, because LMWHs produce their actions via some of the non-AT III pathways, they are more useful in the management of heparin-resistant patients. LMWHs also produce sustained anticoagulant and antithrombotic actions. Thus, reheparinization may not be necessary with use of

TABLE 3. Advantages of Low-molecular-weight Heparins as Surgical Anticoagulants

High antithrombotic–low anticoagulant index
Nonantithrombin III-mediated anticoagulant and antithrombotic actions
Sustained antithrombotic actions
Can be administered via subcutaneous route
Lesser platelet interaction than heparin
Lesser neutralization by endogenous antiheparin agents
Monitoring may not be necessary in prophylaxis

LMWHs. Because of higher bioavailability, they can be administered via the subcutaneous route, thus adding a new approach to surgical anticoagulation. In addition, LMWHs produce less thrombocytopenia and platelet activation than heparin. Endogenous heparin-neutralizing agents, such as platelet factor 4 and histidine-rich glycoproteins, do not neutralize the actions of LMWHs. Thus they may be of special benefit in patients with compromised platelet function.

NEWER ANTICOAGULANTS FOR SURGICAL INDICATIONS: FUTURE CONSIDERATIONS

In the past, attempts to replace heparin with other anticoagulants have not been successful. However, with the development of many newer agents, it is now possible to use alternate approaches[22,44] (Table 4).

Synthetic antithrombin peptides with potent anticoagulant actions have been developed. On a gravimetric basis, these agents are 3–5 times more potent than heparin. They require no endogenous cofactors for mediation of their anticoagulant actions, nor are they neutralized by endogenous antiplatelet agents such as platelet factor 4 and histidine-rich glycoproteins. The synthetic peptide, D-Me-Phe-Pro-Arginal, is currently under development as an anticoagulant by the Eli Lilly Pharmaceutical Company (Indianapolis, MN). Such peptides produce minor effects on platelet activation and inhibit platelet release. The inhibitory effects of peptides vary in their action and have been only partially explored. At the present time, only phase I human studies of D-Me-Phe-Pro-Arginal have been completed. Several other pharmaceutical companies, such as Dupont-Merck Pharmaceuticals (Wilmington, DE) and Sandoz Pharmaceuticals (Basel, Switzerland), are actively developing newer peptide anticoagulant agents.

Synthetic analogs of heparin, which act by indirect mechanism, are also being developed as anticoagulant drugs. Aprosulate, a sulfated derivative of lactobionic acid developed by Luitpold Pharma (Munich, Germany), is currently in phase II trials.[36] Several other synthetic agents are under development by numerous U.S. pharmaceutical companies, including Genelabs (Redwood City, CA) and Glycomed (San Francisco, CA).

Peptide conjugates represent antithrombin peptides coupled to other peptide moieties. In comparison with pure antithrombin peptides, their anticoagulant actions are weaker. One such agent, currently under development by Biogen Laboratories (Cambridge, MA), is Hirulog, a derivative of antithrombin peptide that is coupled with other amino acids joined by a linker group. The developers claim that it has a novel mechanism of anticoagulant action, but it is capable of producing only a direct antithrombin action and is devoid of many of the other actions produced by heparin. The primary target

TABLE 4. Alternative Surgical Anticoagulants

Synthetic antithrombin peptides	Venoms
Synthetic antithrombin nonpeptide agents	Enzymes
Peptide conjugates	Recombinant antithrombin agents
Glycosaminoglycan-derived drugs	

for Hirulog is currently in cardiovascular areas such as percutaneous transluminal coronary angioplasty (PTCA) and treatment of angina. Because of its anticoagulant actions, however, it can be used as a surgical anticoagulant. The short half-life of Hirulog requires adjustment of dosing by controlled delivery systems, but no endogenous modulators (e.g., AT III) are needed to produce its anticoagulant action. Currently several clinical trials to test the anticoagulant efficacy of Hirulog are underway.

The glycosaminoglycan-derived agents, such as heparan, dermatan, and chondroitin sulfates, are relatively weaker anticoagulants than heparin.[53,54] Although these agents may not produce stronger anticoagulant actions than heparin, they are often devoid of antiplatelet actions.[29] Thus some have been experimentally used as anticoagulants at very high doses, and some have been used in conjunction with heparin and other agents. Because of these limitations, nonheparin glycosaminoglycans may be of limited value as anticoagulants in surgical indications.

Many of the naturally derived agents, such as defibrinating venoms, specific enzymes, and recombinant antithrombin drugs (e.g., hirudin and antistatin), have been developed as surgical anticoagulants for various indications. Of these, hirudin is now under development by several pharmaceutical companies as an anticoagulant for surgical indications. The original form was extracted from medicinal leeches, but several variants are currently produced by recombinant technology at Ciba Geigy (Basel, Switzerland), Hoechst (Frankfurt, Germany), Mitsui Company (Minoh, Japan), and Transgene (Strasbourg, France). At many other companies, hirudin is in the preclinical developmental stages.

Recombinant hirudin is 3–5 times more potent than heparin in its anticoagulant actions. For acute anticoagulation, it has several advantages over heparin: (1) it does not produce side effects such as heparin-induced thrombocytopenia and heparin-induced thrombosis[44,45]; (2) it does not require protamine for neutralization; and (3) because the anticoagulant actions last for a short period, it can be given by controlled delivery systems. Although some concern over the generation of antihirudin antibodies has been raised, for short-term use (as in cardiac surgery) this agent can be given without problems. Several clinical trials are currently in progress to evaluate recombinant hirudin as a surgical anticoagulant.

Table 5 compares recombinant hirudin and synthetic peptides as anticoagulants for surgical indications. Although both groups are strong anticoagulants and exhibit certain similarities, the differences in biochemical and pharmacologic systems are significant. Recombinant hirudin is a specific anticoagulant agent that targets thrombin.[44] The synthetic antithrombin agents

TABLE 5. Recombinant Hirudins vs. Synthetic Peptides as Surgical Anticoagulants

Recombinant Hirudins	Synthetic Peptides
Specific antithrombin agents	Antithrombin peptides with multiple inhibitory actions; also inhibit nonthrombin proteases
Short half-life	Ultrashort half-life
Minimal effect on platelets	Significant inhibitory effect on platelets
No modulation of fibrinolysis	Inhibition of fibrinolysis
Minor antigenic effect	No significant antigenic effect

exhibit a broad-spectrum antiprotease action; in addition to thrombin, they can also inhibit many other proteases. Although hirudins have a short half-life, the half-life of peptides is much shorter. Because both groups of drugs can be given by controlled delivery systems, their actions can be readily controlled.

One of the major side effects of heparin during surgical procedures is bleeding due to the activation of fibrinolysis. Recombinant hirudin is not known to induce fibrinolytic activation during surgery. However, because recombinant hirudin is a potent inhibitor of thrombin, it may also inhibit the activation of protein C by thrombin. Endogenous activation of fibrinolysis by this pathway may be inhibited in the presence of recombinant hirudin. The exact implications of this process are not known at this time. The antithrombin peptides are potent inhibitors not only of thrombin, but also of other serine protease enzymes, including plasmin. Therefore, whereas the activation of fibrinolysis by heparin may lead to facilitation of bleeding, similar complications may not result from the use of peptides and hirudin. To what extent endogenous activation of fibrinolysis contributes to the safety and efficacy of heparin and other anticoagulants is not known at this time. The effect on final clinical outcome of the inhibition of the fibrinolytic process by antithrombotic agents is also unclear.

Both the peptides and hirudins are expected to be used as surgical anticoagulants at concentrations ranging from 10-50 µg/ml for periods of up to 3-5 hours. During this period it is unlikely that they will produce any generation of antibodies. The peptides are small in size and readily cleared through the renal system. Hirudin, however, may bind to endogenous sites and thus cause antibody formation, although this is yet to be proved.

Drug interaction plays a key role in the mediation of the overall anticoagulant actions of various agents.[14] Table 6 lists some of the drug interactions that may result in a modulation of responses. The potentiation of the anticoagulant actions can be observed in patients taking other anticoagulant agents or nonsteroidal antiinflammatory drugs. Many patients undergoing surgical procedures have been treated previously with aspirin and oral anticoagulants. Heparinization may result in a synergism of the anticoagulant responses in these patients. When the newer antithrombin-type anticoagulants are introduced for clinical use, a similar outcome may be observed. Thus, a careful review of the anticoagulant medications given to a patient before beginning treatment may be helpful in optimizing the responses.

Fibrinolytic action during surgical procedures facilitates the anticoagulant response. Because activation of fibrinolysis is often observed in patients undergoing cardiovascular bypass (CPB) surgery, antifibrinolytic agents have been used to counteract the undesirable effects of heparin. More recently, aprotinin has been used with success in the management of surgical bleeding complications associated with CPB surgery.

TABLE 6. Drug Interactions Resulting in the Alteration of the Hemostatic System During Surgical Procedures

Potentiation of the anticoagulant actions of heparin	Modulation of endothelial function
Activation of the fibrinolytic system	Reduction of blood viscosity
Inhibition of platelet function	Volume expansion

Many drugs used during surgical procedures are also capable of impairing platelet function, including dextran sulfate, calcium channel blockers, anesthetics, and plasma expanders. Furthermore, additives and crystalloids in solution contribute to the overall anticoagulant and antiplatelet responses. Thus, such agents should be used with caution during surgical procedures. To what extent these interactions will come into play with the new antithrombotic agents is not clear at this time.

Many of the newer anticoagulants exert specific actions on endothelial functions, which play a pivotal role in the mediation of the antithrombotic and anticoagulant responses. Thus, the plasmatic responses for the anticoagulant actions are often augmented by endothelial effects, which are not easily neutralized by the conventional means and last for a longer period of time than the plasma effects.

Volume expansion and reduction in viscosity also play a role in the anticoagulant response during surgery. Many of these effects are not monitorable by conventional laboratory methods. Thus, new methods must be developed for proper assessment of global anticoagulant effects of these newer drugs.

The activation of fibrinolysis and the inhibition of platelet function facilitate the hemorrhagic response during CPB surgery. Other factors, such as vascular dysfunction, also contribute to the syndrome. Protease inhibitors such as aprotinin have been used to control bleeding during CPB surgery. Table 7 lists various mechanisms by which aprotinin restores hemostatic function. This agent inhibits certain fibrinolytic enzymes, such as plasmin/plasminogen activators. Aprotinin also maintains platelet function by both direct and indirect processes. Because plasmin can impair platelet function, its inhibition may result in improved platelet function; moreover, aprotinin restores platelet function by membrane stabilization. Aprotinin also inhibits some of the nonthrombin proteases and may have a modulatory effect on the leukocytes. Thus, the mechanisms by which aprotinin restores hemostasis may be multicomponent.

Aprotinin produces an independent anticoagulant effect at high dosages and has been shown to interact with heparin. Thus, routinely used methods for monitoring the anticoagulant effects of heparin during CPB surgery may result in false elevation of the degree of anticoagulation. For patients administered aprotinin, a different calibration curve is needed to adjust the effects of heparin and thus to optimize the anticoagulant action of combined heparin and aprotinin treatment. A definite synergistic interaction is obtained in both clinical and experimental trials. The newer anticoagulants, such as hirudin, antithrombin peptides, and related agents, do not activate fibrinolysis and therefore may not require administration of aprotinin.

Hypothermia, which is commonly used during CPB surgery, should also be considered an important factor contributing to the anticoagulant action of newer drugs. Hypothermia prolongs the half-life of heparin and other drugs used during surgical procedures. The physiologic effects of hypothermia are rather complex; the known effects are listed in Table 8. Hypothermia may

TABLE 7. Hemostatic Restoration by Aprotinin in Cardiovascular Surgery

Inhibition of fibrinolysis	Inhibition of nonthrombin serine proteases
Maintenance of platelet function	Interaction with leukocytes

TABLE 8. Hypothermia and Anticoagulation

Effect of hypothermia on the clotting process	Effect of hypothermia on the fibrinolytic process
Heparin-AT III interactions in hypothermic conditions	Anticoagulant dosing in hypothermia

inhibit or augment the components of the hemostatic system. Predisposing factors such as infection, hemodynamic compromise, and disseminated intravascular coagulation (DIC) also play an important role.

Hemodilution during surgical procedures is routinely accomplished by administering physiologic solutions. Although these solutions replace the electrolytes and other nutrients, they usually result in the dilution of plasma proteins, with a decrease in coagulation factors, activators, inhibitors, and albumin/globulin. This decrease is particularly important with the use of heparin, which requires several endogenous cofactors for its anticoagulant action, such as AT III, heparin cofactor II, and TFPI. At the same time, heparin-neutralizing proteins, including factor VIII and platelet factor 4 as well as others, are also released. Although the outcome of the anticoagulant effects is patient-dependent, hemodilution results in a significantly altered environment that in turn alters the expected anticoagulant response. This may not be the case with the newly developed synthetic and recombinant agents, because their anticoagulant actions are not modulated by plasmatic and cellular factors.

PROPHYLAXIS OF POSTSURGICAL THROMBOEMBOLISM

Surgeons and physicians worldwide witness a large number of cases of venous thromboembolism, particularly after surgery. With the availability of several newer drugs, these incidents can be avoided by correct prophylaxis. With more education, better understanding of risk factors, and the introduction of newer and more efficacious agents, a prophylactic approach is likely to become routine for all patients undergoing surgery.[27,31,33,50,59]

Of the many prophylactic agents, heparin has a long history of use in both deep vein thrombosis (DVT) and pulmonary embolism (PE).[2,5,32,33] Many studies have shown that in moderate- and high-risk patients, heparin can prevent postoperative DVT and PE.[10,31,32,50] Now, with the introduction of LMWH, these benefits are accompanied by easier dosing and potentially less risk of bleeding complications.

However, certain objective considerations remain in regard to the use of new antithrombotic agents for thromboprophylaxis.[11,27] One of the most common fears is bleeding. Major issues requiring clarification include litigation if the outcome of surgery is not considered to be satisfactory; concern about the cost of protection; and the real benefits of prophylaxis.

If heparin is not used in correct doses, there may indeed be a risk of bleeding. Adjusted-dose heparin thus has clear advantages over fixed-dose heparin.[39] An ideal approach for pharmacologic prophylaxis is to produce an antithrombotic effect without marked anticoagulant effects. This ideal is achievable with the use of LMWH and related agents.[27] Definition of crucial terms is worth repeating: an anticoagulant prevents in vivo thrombosis and can be monitored by prolongation of a clotting assay, whereas an antithrombotic prevents in vivo thrombosis but may not be able to be monitored by known assays.

Bleeding is a complex problem that involves several processes, including the patient's predisposing factors, type and extent of surgery, and postsurgical complications. No single definition of bleeding applies in all cases; what some surgeons regard as minor, others may view more seriously. The LMWHs have less of an anticoagulant effect than heparin but retain antithrombotic potential; thus the risks of bleeding are lower when LMWHs are properly used.[28,47,56,60,63]

The awareness of venous thrombosis and its prevention is likely to increase. Nowadays patients take an active interest in the prevention of heart disease and arterial thrombosis; they understand the significance of cholesterol and prophylactic aspirin. Although the problem of DVT and PE is likely to remain an individual rather than a public concern, particular patient groups probably will become more knowledgeable and vociferous in the 1990s. Already in some European countries, acceptance of pharmacologic prophylaxis is so high that regimens for patients who have just undergone surgery are continued for longer periods, extending into the time when the patient has returned home.[37] With the arrival of LMWHs the knowledge at both the medical and public levels has greatly increased.

Postsurgical and medical thromboembolic disorders that require hospitalization affect nearly one million Americans. Approximately 10% of these patients develop serious PE. Recognizing this major public health problem, the National Institutes of Health called a consensus meeting in March 1986 to discuss the magnitude of thromboembolic disorders and the need for prophylactic therapy.[11] The following key questions were raised before a panel of U.S. and international physicians, surgeons, and public representatives:

1. What is the level of risk of DVT and embolism in various patient groups?
2. What are the efficacy and safety of various forms of prophylaxis in these groups?
3. What are the recommended forms of prophylaxis in these groups?
4. What questions remain to be answered about prophylaxis of various thromboembolic conditions?

After discussion, the panel reached the following conclusions:

1. DVT and PE constitute major health hazards in the United States.
2. Patients can be grouped according to risk.
3. High-risk groups can be identified.
4. Prophylaxis can reduce DVT and PE in high-risk patients.
5. Low-dose heparin, dextran, warfarin, and compression devices can be used for prophylaxis. Aspirin should not be used.
6. Optimization of prophylaxis is desirable.
7. Elective prophylactic regimens differ; the patient's status and degree of risk should be considered.
8. More than one effective prophylactic regimen may be required for some patients.

The consensus conference was effective in identifying the magnitude of medical and postsurgical thromboembolic disorders and made a strong recommendation in favor of prophylactic measures. Although various pharmacologic and physical methods for the prophylaxis of thromboembolic disease

were reviewed, low-dose heparin therapy received specific attention. The following recommendations were made:
1. Low-dose heparin can be used for the prophylaxis of DVT in general surgical patients (patients with medium risk).
2. Individualized dosages of low-dose heparin should be given to high-risk patients (trauma and orthopedic surgery).
3. None of the available (as of 1986) prophylactic regimens was considered optimal.

At the time these recommendations were made, only one LMWH was commercially available in France, and limited information was available in the U.S. on these drugs. Today the LMWHs are commonly used in many European countries for the prophylaxis of thromboembolic disorders in both surgical and medical patients. Several LMWHs are currently under evaluation in phase II and III trials in the U.S.; a LMWH preparation is expected to be available commercially in the early part of 1993.

Available clinical data indicate that LMWHs can be substituted for low-dose heparin. Several comparative trials of low-dose heparin and LMWHs are now in progress throughout the world. In several European clinical trials, the efficacy of the LMWHs in the prevention of postsurgical DVT has now been proved; they are considered to be the drugs of choice.[3,13,27,34,59] Because of patient compliance and outpatient usage, they are comparable to other outpatient parenteral drugs. When used for prophylactic treatment (subcutaneous), the different LMWHs mediate their actions in a similar manner; however, their safety/efficacy profiles differ markedly, as do the recommended dosages for different products.[15,24]

Despite significant clinical developments for LMWHs, their mechanisms of action, pharmacologic behavior, endogenous interaction, and dosimetry remain questionable issues that require clarification. Each product exhibits a certain degree of individuality in biochemical and pharmacologic tests.[17,18,23,24] Although their molecular weight is generally lower than that of heparin, marked differences in patterns of molecular component distribution are evident.[23,24] Variations in the end groups and internal structures have also been found.[23,24] In biochemical assays, affinities for AT III and heparin cofactor II (HC II), neutralization profiles of platelet factor 4 and protamine, cellular interactions, inhibition of protease generation, and susceptibility to various enzymes have varied from product to product.[12,14,16,20,21,24,30,38,40-49,53,54,57]

LMWHs may eventually replace unfractionated heparin for prophylaxis of thromboembolic disorders in both surgical and medical patients, attaining the status of drug of choice. Several commercial products, currently under development, will be available in the near future; however, they should be considered as different drugs, and their clinical performance should be determined by data obtained in independent clinical trials for a given indication. The recognition of the individuality of each of the LMWHs is extremely important and will have a major impact on their prophylactic and therapeutic use. The claimed improvements in efficacy and safety indices are valid only when dosage studies and basic pharmacologic data are considered.

For the prophylaxis of medical and surgical thromboembolic disorders, several pharmacologic and physical methods have been used in addition to heparin and LMWH.[48,52,55,58] Table 9 compares the various drugs/devices in current use for the prophylaxis of postsurgical thrombosis.

TABLE 9. Comparison of Various Methods for Prophylaxis of Postsurgical and Medical Thromboembolism

Method	Advantage	Disadvantage
Heparin	Subcutaneous administration (2–3 dosages)	Dosage adjustment, bleeding, inefficient
Low-molecular-weight heparin	Single, subcutaneous administration, sustained actions, outpatient usage	Dosage adjustment in high-risk patients, bleeding, products not readily interchangeable
Warfarin	Oral administration	Bleeding, delayed action, need for laboratory monitoring
Dextran	High efficacy	Hypervolemia, bleeding, cost, intravenous administration
Aspirin	Low cost, ease of administration	Questionable efficacy, bleeding
Compression devices	Few complications/side effects	Low compliance, rehabilitation, ineffective in high-risk patients

Heparin is generally administered 2–3 times a day. Although subcutaneous administration has a definite advantage in safety over intravenous administration, a bleeding risk still exists and dose adjustment may be necessary.[7,15,49] The LMWHs have proved to be more beneficial than heparin. LMWHs can be administered as a single daily dose via the subcutaneous route, even on an outpatient basis. However, dosage adjustment in high-risk patients may be desirable. The bleeding risk appears to be less with LMWHs than with heparin.[7,15] One drawback of LMWHs is the differences among products, which preclude direct interchange during treatment.[7,19,22,23]

Oral anticoagulants, which are often used for the prophylaxis of thrombosis, demonstrate good patient compliance, because one oral dose is sufficient for the daily prophylaxis of thrombotic complications. Drawbacks to this mode of therapy include bleeding, necrosis, delayed action, and the needs for laboratory monitoring and dosage adjustment.[1,8,26,51] Dextrans are generally administered via the intravenous route. Prolonged use of dextrans often results in hypervolemia, bleeding, and defects in platelet function.[4,35] Although aspirin is useful for prophylaxis of arterial thrombosis, it has questionable value for the prophylaxis of venous thrombosis. Furthermore, its use may result in bleeding or gastric ulcers.[1,9]

More recently, sequential compression devices have been used for the prophylaxis of postsurgical thrombosis.[52,55] Advantages include minor or no side effects, no pharmacologic manipulation, and activation of the patient's own physiologic systems. However, the devices are bulky, patient compliance is not as high as desired, and efficacy in high-risk patients is questionable.

Beside the above approaches, several newer drugs to prevent thromboembolic disorders have been developed (Table 10). Because most of these drugs are in the early phase of development, it will take some time before clinical efficacy is proved.

It is now known that ultra-LMWH fractions can also produce antithrombotic actions. An example is CY 222, which has been developed for clinical trials. This agent, which acts through multiple mechanisms, produces no bleeding and no anticoagulant activity but exhibits high bioavailability.

One of the major breakthroughs in the development of antithrombotic agents is the identification of AT-III binding sites of heparin. A pentasaccharide

TABLE 10. Comparison of Various Newer Methods for the Prophylaxis of Postsurgical and Medical Thromboembolism

Drug	Advantage	Disadvantage
Ultra-low-molecular-weight heparins	Better bioavailability, promote endogenous fibrinolysis	Polycomponent GAGs, mechanism of action is unknown
Pentasaccharide	Synthetic well-defined antithrombotic agent	Cost, mechanism of action is unknown, efficacy is not yet proved
Dermatan sulfate and derivatives	No effect on platelets, do not require AT III	Polycomponent GAGs with poor bioavailability; mechanism of action is unknown
Heparan sulfate and derivatives	Modulate endogenous cellular and plasmatic functions, independent of HC II and AT III	Poorly defined agents whose mechanism of action is unknown, poor bioavailability
Synthetic lactobionic acid derivatives	Synthetic, homogeneous antithrombotic agents	Hypersulfated agents may bind to endogenous sites
Depolymerized heparinoids	Contain mixtures of GAGs with multiple sites of action	Polycomponent drugs with several activities
Polydeoxyribonucleotide derivatives	DNA-derived agents with endogenous modulatory actions on blood/vascular cells	Mechanism of action is unknown, poor bioavailability via SC route
Synthetic peptides and related drugs	Specific inhibitors of thrombin and other proteases, good bioavailability characteristics	Short-half life, pharmacologic antagonist is unknown
Recombinant hirudin and related anticoagulants	Specific antithrombotic agents, extremely potent inhibitors	Highly specific inhibitors of thrombin, limited bioavailability

GAG = glycosaminoglycan.

with a high affinity for AT III has recently been synthesized. This well-defined antithrombotic agent, which specially inhibits factor Xa (not thrombin), may prove to be very useful.[60,63]

Recently several dermatan sulfates have been developed for the prophylaxis of venous thromboembolism. Although similar in structure to heparin, these agents produce no effect on platelets.[29] Furthermore, they are poorly absorbed via the subcutaneous route. More recently low-molecular-weight dermatans have been developed. Regardless of their state of development, the currently available dermatan sulfate preparations should not be considered as optimal agents for prophylaxis of thrombosis.

Heparan sulfates have also been developed as prophylactic antithrombotic agents. Although they are not homogeneous and contain other chondroitin sulfates, they produce their antithrombotic action without major interaction with AT III or HC II.[6,25] Some of the heparin-derived drugs (e.g., ORG 10172) have been used for the prophylaxis of postsurgical thromboembolism.[4,26] However, large dosages are needed for effective treatment.

A totally synthetic hypersulfated lactobionic acid amide (Aprosulate) has also been developed for thrombotic prophylaxis. This agent produces it action by interacting with HC II and by inhibiting protease generation.[36] Its bioavailability is better than that of the dermatan and heparan sulfates.

Many other glycosaminoglycans have also been developed for the prophylaxis of thromboembolism. Some represent mixtures of glycosaminoglycans with varying molecular weight profiles. Noteworthy are Lomoparan (Organon) and Suleparoide (Syntex), which are depolymerized heparan preparations that exert antithrombotic actions by unknown mechanisms; however, they are clinically effective drugs. Other agents such as Hemoclar (Bene) and Arteparon (Luitpold-Werk) are sulfated polymers of natural origins with antithrombotic activities. Although these agents have been in existence for some time, data about their prophylactic actions is unavailable at this time.

Defibrotide (Crinos) is a derivative of polydeoxyribonucleotide that has been used for the prophylaxis of both venous and arterial thrombosis.[58] This agent acts primarily by modulating endothelial/cellular function, but much more work is needed to understand the exact mechanism.

One of the major breakthroughs in the development of antithrombotic drugs is application of the techniques of molecular biology to develop naturally occurring anticoagulants. One of these is recombinant hirudin, which is three times as potent as heparin for producing anticoagulant activity.[33,43,45] Although this agent may be useful as an anticoagulant, its limited bioavailability and extreme specificity suggest that it may not be an effective prophylaxis of thromboembolism.[43-45] Additional studies are needed to modify its structure and to obtain desirable biologic behavior.

CONCLUSION

In view of the novel mechanisms of action of recently developed anticoagulant and antithrombotic drugs, newer methods to evaluate their effect in surgical and therapeutic indications is needed. A multiparametric laboratory profile of individual drugs will be developed for each individual agent.[61,52] Applicable methods can then be chosen for each form of therapy.

The recent developments in prophylactic antithrombotic therapy have warranted a revision of educational and training programs, at the level of both physician and allied health personnel. Education and training will play a major role in the development and use of newer anticoagulant and antithrombotic drugs. It is projected that current approaches for the management of thrombotic and atherosclerotic disorders will undergo major transitions in the near future.

REFERENCES

1. Andersen P, Smith P, Ourebo J: Prevention of thrombosis with warfarin or acetylsalicylic acid related to the risk of hemorrhage. Tidsskr Nor Laegeforen 112:1222-1223, 1992.
2. Becher D: Venous thromboembolism: Epidemiology, diagnosis, prevention. J Gen Intern Med 1:401-411, 1986.
3. Bergqvist D, Matzsch T, Burmark US, et al: Low molecular weight heparin given the evening before surgery compared with conventional low-dose heparin in prevention of thrombosis. Br J Surg 74:888-891, 1988.
4. Bergqvist D, Kettunen K, Fredin H, et al: Thromboprophylaxis in patients with hip fractures: A prospective randomized, comparative study between Org 10172 and dextran 70. Surgery 109:617-622, 1991.
5. Bergqvist D: Frequency of thromboembolic complications. In Postoperative Thromboembolism: Frequency, Etiology and Prophylaxis. Berlin, Springer Verlag, 1982, pp 8-32.
6. Bianchini P, Osima B, Parma B, et al: Lack of correlation between "in vitro" and "in vivo" antithrombotic activity of heparin function and related compounds. Heparan sulfate as an antithrombotic agent "in vivo." Thromb Res 40:597-607, 1985.

7. Breddin HF: Low molecular weight heparins and bleeding. Semin Thromb Hemost 15:401-404, 1989.
8. Brooks LW Jr, Blais FX: Coumadin-induced skin necrosis. J Am Osteopath Assoc 91:601-605, 1991.
9. Buring JC, Hennekens CH: Overt gastrointestinal bleeding in the course of chronic low-dose aspirin administration for secondary prevention of arterial occlusive disease. Am J Gastroenterol 86:1279-1280, 1991.
10. Collins R, Scrimgcour A, Yusuf S, et al: Reduction in fatal pulmonary embolism and venous thrombosis by perioperative administration of subcutaneous heparin. N Engl J Med 318:1162-1173, 1988.
11. Consensus Conference NIH: Prevention of venous thrombosis and pulmonary embolism. JAMA 256:744-749, 1986.
12. Doutremepuich C, Bonini F, Masse A, et al: Protamine neutralization of a very low molecular weight heparin fragment CY 222 in vitro and in vivo study. Thromb Res Suppl VI:88, 1986 [abstract].
13. European Fraxiparin Study Group: Comparison of low molecular weight heparin and unfractionated heparin for the prevention of deep vein thrombosis in patients undergoing abdominal surgery. Br J Surg 75:1058-1063, 1988.
14. Fareed J, Hoppensteadt DA, Bick RL, Bacher P: Drug-induced alterations of hemostasis and fibrinolysis. Hematol Oncol Clin North Am 6:1229-1245, 1992.
15. Fareed J, Bick RL, Squillaci G, et al: Implications in the diagnosis and therapeutic management of thrombotic and bleeding disorders. Clin Chem 29:1641-1658, 1983.
16. Fareed J: New methods in hemostatic testing. In Fareed J (ed); Perspectives in Hemostasis. New York, Pergamon Press, 1981, pp 310-348.
17. Fareed J: Development of heparin fractions: Some overlooked considerations. Semin Thromb Hemost 11:227-236, 1985.
18. Fareed J, Kumar A, Walenga JM, et al: Antithrombotic actions and pharmacokinetics of heparin fragments. Nouv Rev Fr Hematol 26:267-275, 1984.
19. Fareed J, Walenga JM, Racanelli A, et al: Validity of the newly established low molecular weight heparin standard in cross-referencing low molecular weight heparins. Haemostasis 18:33-47, 1988.
20. Fareed J: Heparin, its fractions, fragments and derivatives. Semin Thromb Hemost 11:1-9, 1985.
21. Fareed J, Baker WH, Walenga JM, et al: Molecular markers of pathophysiological activation of hemostasis: Current perspectives and future trends. In Ulutin ON, Vinazzer H (eds): Thrombosis and Hemorrhagic Diseases. Istanbul, Gozlem Matbaachk Koll. Sto., 1986, pp 83-88.
22. Fareed J, Walenga JM, Breddin K, et al: Newer avenues in antithrombotic therapy. Semin Thromb Hemost 15(1 & 2), 1989.
23. Fareed J, Walenga JM: Biochemical and pharmacological considerations in the development of heparin and its depolymerized derivatives. Med J Aust 144:21-30, 1986.
24. Fareed J, Walenga JM, Hoppensteadt DA, et al: Chemical and biologic heterogeneity in low molecular weight heparins: Implications in clinical use and standardization. Semin Thromb Hemost 15:440-463, 1989.
25. Gallagher J, Lyon M, Stewart W: Structure and function of heparan sulfate proteoglycans. Biochem J 236:313-325, 1986.
26. Gerhart TN, Yeh HS, Robertson LK, et al: Low-molecular-weight heparinoid compared with warfarin for prophylaxis of DVT in patients who are operated on for fractures of the hip: A prospective, randomized trial. J Bone Joint Surg 73:494-502, 1991.
27. Hirsh J, Levine M: The development of low molecular weight heparins for clinical use. In Verstraete M et al (eds): Thrombosis and Haemostasis. Leuven, Leuven University Press, 1987, pp 425-448.
28. Holmer E, Mattson C, Nilsson S: Anticoagulant and antithrombotic effects of heparin and low molecular weight heparin fragments in rabbits. Thromb Res 25:475-485, 1982.
29. Hoppensteadt D, Walenga JM, Fareed J: Effect of dermatan sulfate and heparan sulfate on platelet activity compared to heparin. Semin Thromb Hemost 17:60-64, 1991.
30. Jaques LB, Kavanaugh LW: Protamine neutralization factors for heparin. Can J Pharmacol Sci 12:44-47, 1977.
31. Kakkar VV, Corrigan TP, Fossard DP: Prevention of fatal post-operative pulmonary embolism by low doses of heparin: An international multicentre trial. Lancet 2:45-51, 1975.
32. Kakkar VV, Fok PJ, Murray WJG, et al: Heparin and dihydroergotamine prophylaxis against thromboembolism after hip arthroplasty. J Bone Joint Surg 67B:539-542, 1985

33. Kakkar VV, Howe C, Flane C, et al: Natural history of post-operative deep vein thrombosis. Lancet 2:230-232, 1969.
34. Kakkar VV, Murray WJG: Efficacy and safety of low molecular weight heparin (CY 216) in preventing postoperative venous thromboembolism: A cooperative study. Br J Surg 72:786-791, 1985.
35. Kitzigeri KJ, Sanders WE, Andrews CP: Acute pulmonary edema associated with the use of low molecular weight dextran for the prevention of microvascular thrombosis. J Hand Surg 15:902-905, 1990.
36. Klauser RJ: Interaction of the sulfated lactobionic acid amide LW 10082 with thrombin and its endogenous inhibitors. Thromb Res 62:557-565, 1991.
37. Laerstedt CI, Fagher B, Olsson C, Oqvist BW: Need for long-term anticoagulant treatment in symptomatic calf vein thrombosis. Lancet 2:515-518, 1985.
38. Lane DA, Denton J, Flynn AM, et al: Anticoagulant activities of heparin oligosaccharides and their neutralization by platelet factor 4. Biochem J 218:725-732, 1984.
39. Leyvarz PF, Richard J, Bachmann F, et al: Adjusted versus fixed subcutaneous heparin in the prevention of deep vein thrombosis after total hip replacement. N Engl J Med 309:954-958, 1983.
40. Lindahl U, Hook M: Glycosaminoglycans and their binding to biological macromolecules. Annu Rev Biochem 47:385-417, 1978.
41. Lindahl U, Backstrom G, Hook M, et al: Structure of the antithrombin-binding sites in heparin. Proc Natl Acad Sci USA 76:3198-3302, 1979.
42. Lindahl U, Backstrom G, Thunberg L, et al: Evidence for a 3-0 sulfated D-glucosamine residue in the antithrombin-binding sequence of heparin. Proc Natl Acad Sci USA 77:6551, 1980.
43. Markwardt F: Pharmacology of hirudin: One hundred years after the first report of the anticoagulant agent. Biomed Biochim Acta 44:1007-1013, 1985.
44. Markwardt F: Pharmacological approaches to thrombin regulation. Ann NY Acad Sci 485:204,214, 1986.
45. Markwardt F, Fink E, Kaiser B, et al: Pharmacological survey of recombinant hirudin. Pharmazie 43:202-207, 1988.
46. Messmore HL, Walenga JM, Fareed J: Molecular markers of platelet activation. Semin Thromb Hemost 10:264-269, 1984.
47. Ockelford PA, Carter CJ, Mitchell L, et al: Discordance between the anti-Xa activity and antithrombotic activities of an ultra-low molecular weight heparin fraction. Thromb Res 28:401-409, 1982.
48. Petitti DB, Strom B, Melmon K: Duration of warfarin anticoagulant therapy and the probabilities of recurrent thromboembolism and hemorrhage. Am J Med 81:255-259, 1986.
49. Racanelli A, Fareed J, Walenga JM, et al: Biochemical and pharmacologic studies on the protamine interactions with heparin, its fractions and fragments. Semin Thromb Hemost 11:176-189, 1985.
50. Reilly DT: Prophylactic methods against thromboembolism. Acta Chir Scand Suppl 550:115-118, 1988.
51. Ritchie AJ, Hart NB: Massive tissue necrosis can be induced by heparin or warfarin. Ulster Med J 60:248-250, 1991.
52. Scurr JH, Coleridge-Smith PD, Hasty JH: Regimen for improved effectiveness of intermittent pneumatic compression in deep venous thrombosis prophylaxis. Surgery 103:816-820, 1987.
53. Sie P, Ofosu F, Fernandez F, et al: Respective role of antithrombin III and heparin cofactor II in the in vitro anticoagulant effect of heparin and various sulphated polysaccharides. Br J Haematol 64:707-714, 1986.
54. Sie P, Ailluap MF, deProst D: Measurement of low molecular weight heparin ex vivo activities in clinical laboratories using various anti-Xa assays: Interlaboratory variability and requirements for an agreed upon low molecular weight heparin standard. Thromb Haemost 56:879-883, 1987.
55. Summaria L, Caprini JA, McMillan R, et al: Relationship between postsurgical fibrinolytic parameters and deep vein thrombosis in surgical patients treated with compression devices. Am Surg 54:156-160, 1988.
56. Thomas DP, Barrowcliffe TW, Merton RE, et al: In vivo release of anti-Xa clotting activity by heparin analogue. Thromb Res 17:831-840, 1980.
57. Tollefsen DM, Majerus DW, Blank MK: Heparin cofactor II: Purification and properties of a heparin-dependent inhibitor of thrombin in human plasma. J Biol Chem 257:2167-2169, 1982.

58. Ulutin ON, Fareed J, Kumar A, et al: Pharmacologic profiling of the action of defibrotide in animal models of hemostatic and thrombotic disorders. In Ulutin ON, Vinazzer H (eds): Thrombosis and Hemorrhagic Diseases. Istanbul, Gozlem Matbaachk Kol. Sto., 1986, pp 101-110.
59. Verstraete M: Pharmacotherapeutic aspects of unfractionated and low molecular weight heparins. Drugs 40:498-530, 1990.
60. Walenga JM, Petitou M, Lormeau JC, et al: Antithrombotic activity of a synthetic heparin pentasaccharide in a rabbit stasis thrombosis model using different thrombogenic challenges. Thromb Res 46:187-198, 1987.
61. Walenga JM, Fareed J, Messmore HL: Newer avenues in the monitoring of antithrombotic therapy: The role of automation. Semin Thromb Hemost 9:346-354, 1983.
62. Walenga JM, Fareed J, Hoppensteadt D, et al: Laboratory monitoring of heparin: Old vs. new methods. CRC Crit Rev Lab Sci 22:361-389, 1986.
63. Walenga JM, Bara L, Petitou M, et al: The inhibition of the generation of thrombin and the antithrombotic effect of a pentasaccharide with sole-factor Xa activity. Thromb Res 51:23-33, 1988.

Chapter 9

Effect of Aprotinin on Blood Loss and Blood Use after Cardiopulmonary Bypass

Kenneth M. Taylor, M.D., FRCS (Eng), FRCS (Glasg), FSA

Aprotinin is a low-molecular-weight protease inhibitor that has been used for many years in a number of inflammatory conditions (notably acute pancreatitis) with variable effect. Recently it was discovered that high-dose aprotinin had a dramatic effect in reducing bleeding in patients undergoing open-heart surgery. The effect was particularly striking in patients at high risk of bleeding (e.g., reoperative and septic patients, patients treated with aspirin and/or streptokinase). This chapter reviews the background to the discovery of aprotinin as a blood-conserving therapy and considers the data related to efficacy and safety that have accumulated after extensive clinical experience in the United Kingdom and Europe.

CARDIAC SURGERY AND HEMOSTASIS

From the earliest days of cardiac surgery excessive bleeding has been recognized as a major complication. The risk of excessive bleeding is known to be greater in certain categories of patients such as those undergoing reoperation after previous cardiac surgery, acutely septic patients with uncontrolled infective endocarditis, and patients maintained on drugs that interfere with the hemostatic process (e.g., aspirin, thrombolytic agents). In such high-risk categories, excessive bleeding may at worst lead to operative death or at least influence postoperative morbidity.

Even in routine primary cardiac operations, the requirement for transfusion of blood and blood products is not inconsiderable. In a recent review of experience in a large cardiac surgical unit, Murphy et al.[1] reported the use of 3-5 units (U) of blood per patient, according to the nature of the procedure. In addition, the use of blood products (platelets, cryoprecipitate, and fresh frozen plasma) raised total transfusion requirements to 13.5 units in valve rereplacement surgery (Table 1).

In addition to the need to conserve blood as a potentially scarce resource, the recent increased emphasis on blood conservation in all areas of medicine

TABLE 1. Blood Transfusion in Cardiac Surgery

Primary CABS	3 units/case
Re-op CABS	4 units/case
Primary valve	4 units/case
Re-op valve	5 units/case

Data derived from Murphy et al.[1]

and surgery relates to awareness of the risks of transfusion (Table 2). In particular, the unacceptably high risk of transmission of infective agents (hepatitis and human immunodeficiency virus) have made blood conservation a priority in cardiac surgery.[2]

Effects of Cardiopulmonary Bypass on the Hemostatic System

The feature that distinguishes cardiac surgery from other types of major surgery is the inevitable use of cardiopulmonary bypass (CPB). The pathophysiology of CPB is a complex subject. CPB requires the use of systemic anticoagulation with heparin, but also modifies hemostasis by inducing major changes in blood cells and their activity levels (Fig. 1). Contact activation of factor XII occurs when the patient's blood contacts the artificial materials of the extracorporeal circuit at the onset of CPB. Activated factor XII stimulates a number of important cascade mechanisms, including coagulation, fibrinolysis, release of kallikrein, and complement activation.[3,4] The final result of contact activation is thought to be the production of a systemic inflammatory response, which may be detected in many internal organs but is particularly well visualized in the lung.[5-7]

Platelet dysfunction is also known to occur during CPB, including change in shape of circulating platelets, release of activation factors,[8-10] and reduction in glycoprotein surface receptor populations, such as the GpIb and GpIIb/IIIa complexes.[11,12]

In summary, the complex effects of CPB on hemostatic function during cardiac surgery include (1) heparin anticoagulation and protamine reversal, (2) fibrinolysis, and activation of kallikrein and complement (via activated factor XII, and (3) platelet dysfunction. In view of this complexity, therapy designed to prevent or at least attenuate the hemostatic disorder in cardiac patients has previously been varied (according to target mechanism) and only of limited efficacy.

TABLE 2. Blood and Blood Product Transfusions: Incidence of Adverse Reactions per Unit Transfusion

Hazard		Incidence per Unit Transfusion
Transmission of infective agent	hepatitis	1:100
	HIV	1:40,000 –10^6
	CMV	–
	HTLV I/II	–
Immunologic reactions	fever, urticaria	1:100
	hemolysis	1:6,000
	fatal hemolysis	1:100,000

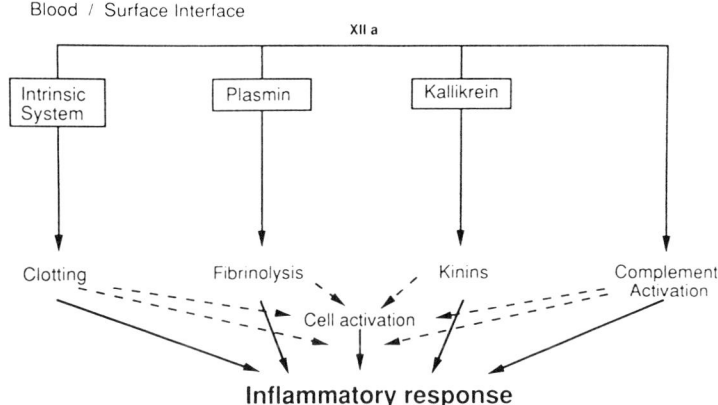

FIGURE 1. Contact activation pathways, including stimulation of coagulation, fibrinolysis, and complement activation, leading to a systemic inflammatory response.

PHARMACOLOGIC AGENTS TO REDUCE BLOOD LOSS IN CARDIAC SURGERY

Epsilon-amino-caproic Acid. Epsilon-amino-caproic acid (EACA) is a lysine analogue that exerts an antifibrinolytic effect by blocking the lysine binding sites at which plasminogen and plasmin bind to fibrin.[13] EACA has been used successfully to reduce blood loss in several clinical situations (for example, transurethral prostatectomy,[14] but its efficacy in cardiac surgery is controversial.[15,16] Thrombotic complications have been reported,[17,18] and, despite 25 years of availability, its value in cardiac surgical practice remains dubious.

Tranexamic Acid. Tranexamic acid is also a lysine analogue with a reported increase in plasminogen binding 6 times that of EACA. Despite the anticipated increase in efficacy, studies have shown little increase in clinical benefit.[19]

Desmopressin Acetate (DDAVP). Desmopressin is a synthetic vasopressin analogue with reduced vasoconstrictor effects. Its mode of action in hemostasis is thought to be related to improved platelet adhesion, mediated through release of von Willebrand's factor (vWF) from endothelial cells.[20,21] DDAVP is particularly effective in reducing bleeding times in patients with von Willebrand's disease and in hemophiliacs. In recent studies using DDAVP therapy (0.3 μg/kg) in cardiac surgery, some authors reported significant reductions in blood loss, whereas others failed to demonstrate any real effect on bleeding.[22,23] In a randomized, double-blind trial of patients undergoing heart valve surgery with or without coronary grafting, Salzman and associates showed a reduction in blood loss of almost 1 L over 24 hours in the treated group.[24] Transfusion requirements in the first 24 hours were not, however, significantly different for treated and control groups.

Prostacyclin and Other Prostaglandin Derivatives. Prostacyclin (PGI2) is a naturally occurring prostaglandin that inhibits platelet activation by increasing the levels of platelet cyclic adenosine monophosphate (AMP); this effect is mediated by stimulation of adenyl cyclase.[25] Although PGI2 has a short duration of action, it is a relatively potent vasodilator. Resultant arterial hypotension, which has been a feature in several reported studies, limits delivery of the drug and compromises its usefulness.[26,27] The potential role for prostacyclin in cardiac surgery—to preserve platelet numbers and function without impairing the coagulation process—led to its use in several clinical studies. Although several authors reported the expected effect of platelet preservation, evidence of reduced bleeding was neither consistent nor convincing. Interpretation of the studies was complicated by great variability in dosage, which ranged from 10-100 mg/kg/min. The variability in dosage may reflect the problem of excessive vasodilation and consequent hypotension at higher dose levels.[26-30] More recently, carbacyclin and oxycyclin derivatives of prostacyclin have been developed in an attempt to reduce the hypotensive side effects of the parent compound.[31] Reported experience with these analogues has, however, been disappointing.[32]

Aprotinin and Serine Protease Inhibition. Aprotinin, a serine protease inhibitor (molecular weight = 6512) isolated from bovine lung, is a nonspecific inhibitor of several proteinases, including trypsin, plasmin, and kallikrein. The drug must be given by intravenous injection; its half-life is around 2 hours. In the past, aprotinin has been used in acute pancreatitis, septic and hemorrhagic shock, and adult respiratory distress syndrome (ARDS). In view of its antiplasmin effect, it has also been used as an antifibrinolytic agent. Indeed, as long ago as 1964, Tice and coworkers used low dose aprotinin in cardiac surgical patients to reduce excessive bleeding.[33] Other reports followed,[34,35] but equivocal efficacy led to failure to recognize the drug's potential role.

Interest in the use of aprotinin in cardiac surgery revived after the serendipitous discovery by the Hammersmith group that high-dose aprotinin showed remarkable efficacy in reducing bleeding in cardiac surgical patients. The discovery was truly by chance; the drug was in fact used to reduce the kallikrein-induced lung inflammation that occurs during CPB. The potential effects of aprotinin on the contact activation process are shown in Figure 2. In addition to its inhibition of kallikrein, aprotinin also inhibits the fibrinolytic pathway and complement activation.

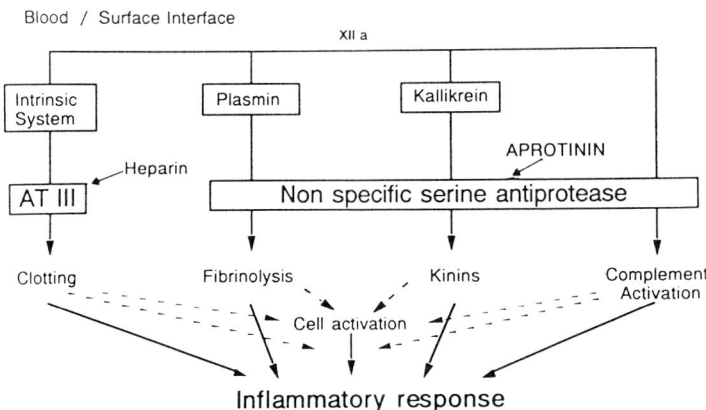

FIGURE 2. Effects of nonspecific protease inhibition (such as aprotinin therapy) on contact activation pathways.

INITIAL CLINICAL STUDIES AND DOSAGE REGIMEN FOR APROTININ THERAPY

For the initial Hammersmith studies, an empirical dosage regimen was calculated on the basis of a 4-μM plasma concentration of aprotinin, which effectively blocks kallikrein. Aprotinin dosage is expressed in kallikrein-inhibitory units (KIU); 100,000 KIU is equivalent to 14 mg of protein. The actual dosage regimen for aprotinin (Trasylol-Bayer AG) in the initial studies was as follows: (1) loading dose of 2×10^6 KIU (280 mg); (2) CPB pump prime dose of 2×10^6 KIU (280 mg); and (3) maintenance infusion of 0.5×10^6 KIU/hr until the end of the operation (70 mg/hr).

When the blood-conserving effect of aprotinin was recognized, a series of 3 initial clinical studies was undertaken by the Hammersmith group: study 1 focused on primary coronary artery surgery; study 2 on reoperative cardiac surgery; and study 3 on acute infective endocarditis surgery.

After these initial clinical studies, confirmatory multicenter studies were carried out, and extended clinical use of aprotinin was investigated in patients taking aspirin and in patients treated acutely with thrombolytic therapy.

Initial Study 1: Primary Coronary Artery Surgery[36]

Study 1, which was placebo-controlled, randomized, and double-blinded, involved 80 patients undergoing primary coronary artery surgery. Standard protocols for anesthesia, CPB, and perioperative transfusion of blood and blood products were observed. The results are summarized in Table 3. Total blood loss was reduced from around 600 ml/patient in the placebo group to around 300 ml/patient in the aprotinin group. Measurement of hemoglobin loss (a better way to assess actual blood loss than overall loss of tissue fluid) was reduced from 37 gm in controls to 12 gm in the aprotinin group. Seventy-five units of blood were transfused in controls, compared with 13 units in treated patients. This reduction in blood transfusion was not achieved at the expense of creating normovolemic hemodilution in the aprotinin patients, whose hemoglobin levels on the seventh postoperative day were identical to control values.

Initial Study 2: Reoperative Cardiac Surgery[37]

Study 2, which was prospective and randomized, included 22 patients undergoing reoperative cardiac surgery after at least 1 previous open-heart procedure through a median sternotomy. The anesthetic, CPB, and transfusion

TABLE 3. Aprotinin Study 1 Results: Primary Coronary Surgery

	Aprotinin (n = 40)	Control (n = 40)
Post-op blood loss (ml)	309 ± 133	573 ± 166 (p <0.01)
Post-op hemoglobin loss (gm)	12 ± 12.6	37.1 ± 18.3
Total no. of blood units transfused	13	75
% of patients transfused	20%	95%
Average no. of grafts	3.88 ± 0.5	3.86 ± 0.8

(Results expressed as mean ± S.D.)

TABLE 4. Aprotinin Study 2 Results: Re-do Cardiac Surgery

	Aprotinin (n = 11)	Control (n = 11)
Post-op blood loss (ml)	286 ± 48	1509 ± 388 (p <0.001)
Post-op hemoglobin loss (gm)	8.3 ± 2.4	78 ± 23 (p <0.001)
Total no. of blood units transfused	5	41
% of patients transfused	36%	100%

(Results expressed as mean ± S.D.)

protocols were standardized, as in Study 1. The results in patients known to be at greater risk of excessive bleeding were particularly striking (Table 4). Total blood loss was reduced from around 1,500 ml in the control group to less than 300 ml in the aprotinin group. Hemoglobin loss was reduced almost 10-fold. These differences were highly significant statistically. Blood transfusion requirements were reduced from 41 units in the control group (around 4 U/patient) to 5 units in the aprotinin group (<0.5 U/patient). Seven of the 11 treated reoperative patients required no intra- or postoperative blood or transfusion of blood products. As in Study 1, hemoglobin levels on discharge were the same for both groups. Another interesting statistic is that chest closure times were halved in the aprotinin group (from 60 min in controls to 30 min), reflecting the dryness of the operating field at the end of CPB.

Initial Study 3: Acute Infective Endocarditis Surgery[38]

Study 3, which was open and uncontrolled, involved a group of patients who were actively septic with acute infective endocarditis, uncontrolled at the time of emergency surgery. Such patients present an exceptionally high risk of torrential post-CBP bleeding, because many of them have severe hemostatic disorders as a result of acute sepsis. Aprotinin therapy was administered to 15 such patients, the vast majority of whom were undergoing reoperation because the infection had settled on a previously implanted valve or valves. In this particularly high-risk group, total blood loss was 388 ml/patient, and blood transfusion requirements were <1 U/patient.

The results of the three initial studies indicated that high-dose aprotinin had remarkable efficacy in reducing blood loss and blood transfusion requirements in cardiac surgical patients. The effect was particularly impressive in patients considered to be at high risk of excessive bleeding. Although safety was not a priority in the initial studies, aprotinin therapy appeared to be very safe, with no adverse reactions reported. The presentation and publication of these data prompted further studies, including a large number of multicenter studies as well as studies of extended use.

EXPERIENCE IN MULTICENTER STUDIES OF APROTININ THERAPY

Experience with aprotinin therapy in cardiac surgical patients is now considerable in many European countries, where the drug was available or where authorities permitted compassionate use before full licensing of the drug

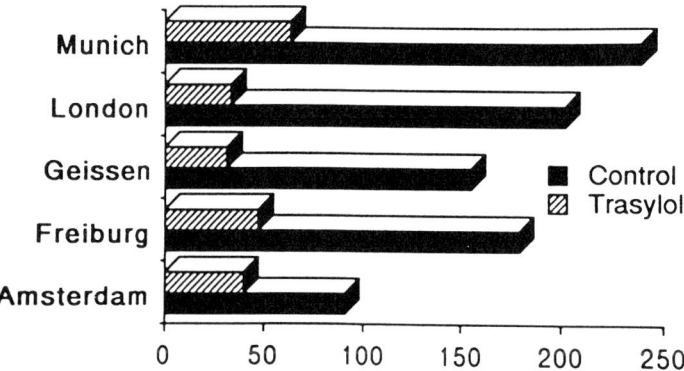

FIGURE 3. Effect of high-dose aprotinin therapy on blood transfusion requirements (calculated per 100 cases in 5 European cardiac surgical centers in primary coronary surgery operations). (From Royston D: Aprotinin in open-heart surgery. Perfusion 5(Suppl):63–72, 1990, with permission.)

in high-dose formulation. In Germany, in particular, aprotinin has been used extensively. In addition to the earlier studies of Fraedrich et al.[39] and Deitrich et al.[40] in both primary surgery and reoperations, it is estimated that the majority of all cardiac surgical cases in Germany are performed with the use of aprotinin.

A large five-center study of aprotinin in primary coronary surgery patients was reported by Royston.[41] The results are summarized in Figure 3. This prospective, randomized, double-blind study involved 350 patients. The 174 patients who received aprotinin (using the dosage regimen of the initial Hammersmith studies) had a highly significant reduction in postoperative blood loss and in blood transfusion requirements. Data were also collected on the occurrence of adverse events: 61 events were reported in the control group and 52 in the aprotinin group. The incidence of cardiovascular adverse events (perioperative myocardial infarction or neurologic deficit) showed no significant differences between the groups.

More recently, the author and colleagues[42] reported the results of an open study of 671 patients who received aprotinin therapy in 40 United Kingdom cardiac surgical centers. This study was limited to high-risk patients, defined as those undergoing reoperation, acute septic cases, and patients with preexisting coagulopathy or known tendency toward excessive bleeding. Of the 671 patients, over 450 underwent reoperation, and an additional 79 patients had acute septic endocarditis at the time of surgery. Data related to postoperative blood loss are shown in Figure 4; data related to perioperative blood transfusion in Figure 5. Despite a small number of patients in whom blood loss and transfusion requirements were enormous (up to 7,585 ml and 65 units, respectively), the median blood loss for this high-risk population was around 400 ml (250–690 interquartile range) and the median blood transfusion requirement was around 2 units (1–4 interquartile range). The reporting of any adverse event was mandatory in the open study protocol. The incidence of reported adverse events was remarkably low (Table 5).

Confirmatory data on the efficacy of aprotinin has recently been reported from the Cleveland Clinic by Cosgrove and colleagues.[43] They carried out a prospective, randomized, double-blind, placebo-controlled trial of 169 patients

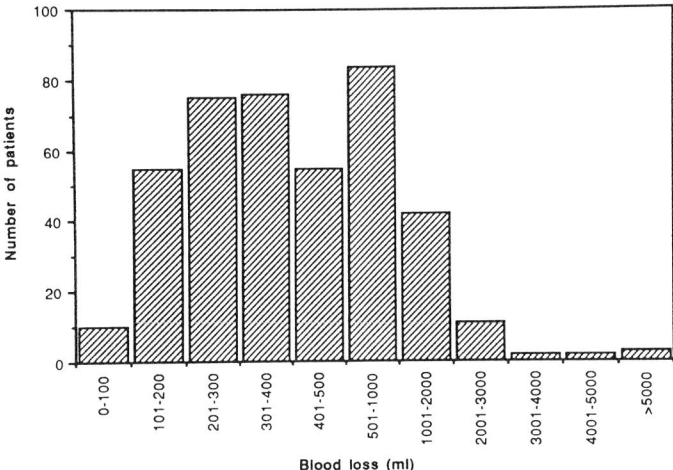

FIGURE 4. Chest-tube drainage volumes (blood loss in ml) in United Kingdom open study of 671 patients receiving high-dose aprotinin therapy during cardiac surgery.

undergoing reoperative coronary surgery. Treated patients received either high-dose (the original Hammersmith dosage) or low-dose aprotinin (50% of the original Hammersmith dosage). Both high- and low-dose groups had significant reductions in postoperative blood loss (720 ml and 866 ml compared with 1,121 ml in the control group); significant reduction in transfusion requirements, however, were seen only in the high-dose group (2.1 units compared with 4.8 units and 4.1 units for the low-dose and control groups, respectively). The Cleveland data are summarized in Table 6.

Although the Cleveland study raises safety issues, which are considered later in this chapter, the data provide interesting confirmatory evidence for the

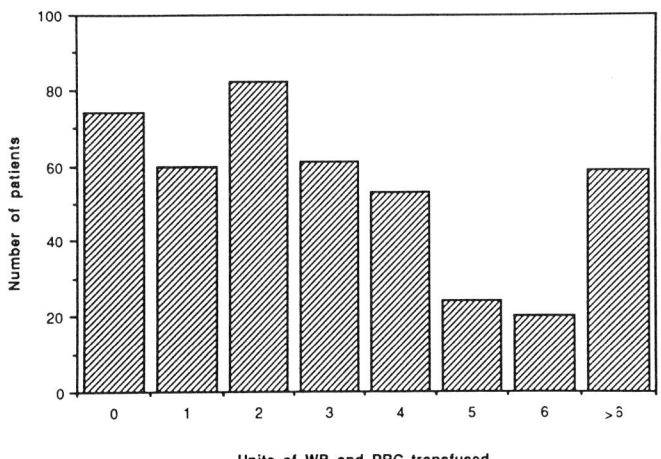

FIGURE 5. Blood transfusion requirements (volumes of whole blood and packed red cells) in United Kingdom open study of 671 patients receiving high-dose aprotinin therapy during cardiac surgery.

TABLE 5. Aprotinin—United Kingdom Multicenter Data

Number of patients	671	
Reported adverse events	20	(3.0%)
Allergic reactions	4	(0.6%)
Renal failure	3	(0.4%)
Graft thrombosis	1	(0.1%)

efficacy of aprotinin in reoperative cases, particularly in the high-dose group. Cosgrove also comments that patients receiving aprotinin had lower requirements for additional hemostatic agents such as EACA and platelet transfusions.

EXTENDED USE IN CARDIAC SURGERY OF APROTININ THERAPY

Aspirin-treated Patients

Soon after completion of the initial studies, Bidstrup et al. carried out a prospective study of aprotinin in patients maintained on aspirin therapy to the time of cardiac surgery. Such patients are known to bleed excessively, an effect thought to be related to the effect of aspirin in blocking platelet cyclooxygenase and in partially inhibiting platelet aggregatory function. Previous studies have reported increased blood loss in aspirin-treated patients and have recommended discontinuance of aspirin theapy 7–10 days before cardiac surgery.[44-46]

In Bidstrup's study,[47] 44 patients who had taken aspirin therapy for over 2 weeks before surgery were randomly allocated to the aprotinin (at the initial study dosage) or the control group. Mean preoperative bleeding time was 9.6 minutes in the aprotinin group and 7.4 minutes in controls. The blood loss data are summarized in Figure 6. Total chest drainage was 352 ml in the aprotinin group, compared with 1393 ml in controls. Transfusion requirements were reduced from 2.7 units/patient for controls to 0.8 units/patient in the treated group. These results are of considerable clinical significance because

TABLE 6. Transfusion Requirements for Re-do CABS—Cleveland Clinic Study

	High Dose	Low Dose	Placebo	p value
Entire group (n = 169)				
No. of patients	57	56	56	NS
Red cells (units)	2.1 ± 4.2	4.8 ± 11.8	4.1 ± 6.2	0.001
Platelets (units)	1.6 ± 6.3	3.3 ± 15.4	5.4 ± 14.6	0.006
Patients transfused	26	29	44	0.001
Aspirin pre-treated group (n = 36)				
No. of patients	17	7	12	NS
Red cells (units)	1.9 ± 3.3	3.7 ± 2.9	3.8 ± 2.6	0.03
Patients transfused	8	5	12	0.006

Tests of statistical significance, aspirin verses placebo. NS = Not significant. Randomized to high-dose and low-dose aprotinin therapy and placebo. Data from Cosgrove.[43]

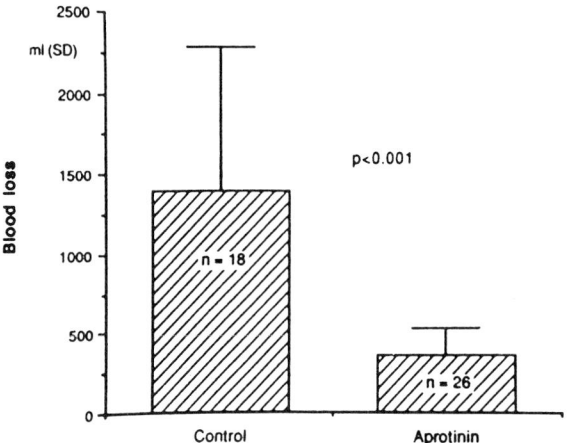

FIGURE 6. Chest-tube drainage volumes in aspirin pretreated patients (control and aprotinin groups). (From Bidstrup BP, Royston D, McGuiness C, Sapsford RN: Aprotinin in aspirin pre-treated patients. Perfusion 5(Suppl):77–81, 1990, with permission.)

continuation of preoperative aspirin therapy is now feasible, without discontinuance 7–10 days before surgery.

Although Bidstrup's study used the high-dose regimen, the present author, on a purely empirical basis, has used a low-dose regimen in aspirin-treated patients without obvious loss of efficacy. This dosage (only in primary cases) includes a loading dose of 1×10^6 KIU (140 mg) and a pump prime dose of 1×10^6 KIU (140 mg). No maintenance infusion is given during the operation.

Patients Given Thrombolytic Therapy

The increasing application of thrombolytic therapy (e.g., streptokinase tissue-type plasminogen activator) in coronary patients led the author and colleagues at Hammersmith to use aprotinin therapy in patients transferred for emergency surgery soon after receiving systemic or intracoronary thrombolytic agents. Our first experience was with a patient referred for emergency coronary surgery less than 60 minutes after receiving thrombolytic therapy. Aprotinin therapy was completely effective in restoring satisfactory hemostasis. The patient underwent multiple bypass grafts (left internal mammary artery plus vein grafts) with low postoperative loss of blood and minimal blood transfusion. Since that initial published report,[48] we have continued to use aprotinin in such cases, as have others, with similar success.[49]

SAFETY ISSUES IN APROTININ THERAPY

Thus far, this chapter has focused on the efficacy of aprotinin; both the level and the consistency of its efficacy are quite remarkable. Without doubt, high-dose aprotinin reduces blood loss and transfusion requirements during cardiac surgery. It is important, however, to assess the safety data of this new therapy, particularly when the drug is clearly exerting a powerful biologic effect. Three safety issues are discussed: (1) allergic reactions; (2) renal function effects; and (3) prothrombolic effects.

Allergic Reactions to Aprotinin Therapy

Because aprotinin is derived from bovine lung, a significant incidence of allergic reactions may be expected. In addition, the question of previous exposure to the drug and the production of a hypersensitivity reaction on subsequent exposures should be considered.

The reported incidence of primary allergic reactions to high-dose aprotinin has been surprisingly low. In the United Kingdom open study, allergic reactions were reported in 4 cases (0.6%); only 1 (0.1%) involved a significant early reaction requiring cessation of the infusion. Other workers have also reported a low incidence of allergic reactions. No mention of allergic reactions was made in the discussion of morbidity in the Cleveland Clinic study.[43]

The question of second or subsequent exposure has not been formally studied. However the clinical experience of the author and of colleagues who have had several years' experience with aprotinin confirms that patients receiving the drug on a second or subsequent occasion show no increased incidence of hypersensitivity or other allergic reactions. *A test dose, however, is recommended before giving the entire loading dose in all patients.*

Although allergic reactions do not appear to be a significant safety issue, the development of genetically-engineered protease inhibitor compounds may remove all concerns about the allergic potential of the current animal-based product.

Renal Function Effects of Aprotinin Therapy

Some concerns have been expressed about a potential nephrotoxic effect of high-dose aprotinin. Previous noncardiac studies of the pharmacology of aprotinin suggested a possible renal effect, although the relevance of species and dose in these experimental studies is difficult to assess.[50,51] The more recent and more relevant clinical study of Blauhut et al.[52] failed to demonstrate any nephrotoxic effect in cardiac surgery patients. The larger European studies have reported no significant increase in perioperative renal dysfunction. In the United Kingdom open study, pre- and postoperative levels of blood urea and creatinine showed only the small rise anticipated in cardiac surgery patients. The Cleveland study[43] reported no significant differences in the rise in serum creatinine or the creatinine clearance levels between the aprotinin and control groups.

Prothrombotic State and Aprotinin Therapy

The fear that aprotinin therapy, so obviously effective in stopping bleeding, might be prothrombotic seems almost inevitable. The author has lectured on the subject of aprotinin therapy since its discovery at Hammersmith around 7 years ago, and from the outset, this has been the ubiquitous question. If aprotinin stops bleeding, does it clot bypass grafts? Although my colleague, Dr. David Royston, deals with this topic from another perspective in the succeeding chapter, a brief review of the studies reporting on this issue, is beneficial.

The large United Kingdom and European studies have reported no increase in incidence of premature coronary graft occlusion, myocardial infarction, or pulmonary thromboembolism. In the United Kingdom open study,[42] only 1 case of coronary vein graft occlusion was reported among 671 patients, and that case was attributed by the surgical team to technical factors. A large European series involving over 2,000 cases recently reported no increased incidence of premature graft closure. More specifically, a recent study focused on postoperative graft patency in coronary surgery patients randomized to aprotinin or control groups found no significant difference in graft patency[53] (Table 7). These data appear to provide consistent reassurance that thrombosis is not associated with aprotinin therapy.

However, within the Cleveland Clinic study, despite the clear demonstration of efficacy, the data raised concern in the minds of the investigators. Although the overall mortality was not different between aprotinin and control groups, the incidence of perioperative myocardial infarction was 15.8% in the high-dose aprotinin group, 8.9% in the low-dose aprotinin group, and 7.1% in the control group. The differences did not reach statistical significance, but the authors conclude that "these complications bear further investigation."[43] Cosgrove and colleagues are quite correct in their concerns and in their call for further investigations. Because cardiac surgeons will always have a low threshold of concern over graft patency, the clear disparity between the Cleveland Clinic data and the United Kingdom and European data in regard to this safety issue demands further elucidation.

This, in the present author's opinion, is the one safety issue related to aprotinin therapy that has to be resolved. The therapy is highly effective, transforms high-risk reoperations, and dramatically reduces transfusion requirements; it is poised to extend throughout cardiovascular surgery, transplant procedures, major hepatic surgery, and beyond. The only cloud on the horizon is the prothrombotic concern. If it were to be resolved, the discovery of aprotinin therapy might well be regarded as the most important breakthrough in major surgery for many years. The closing section of this chapter indicates ways in which this issue may be better understood and perhaps ultimately resolved.

RISK/BENEFIT CONSIDERATIONS IN APROTININ THERAPY

Hematologic Effects of Aprotinin

Although the precise mechanism(s) of action of aprotinin in reducing excessive bleeding is not fully understood, the potential for a direct prothrombotic effect seems, on the basis of available evidence, unlikely.

TABLE 7. Coronary Artery Bypass Graft Patency with Aprotinin and Placebo

	Aprotinin	Placebo
No. of grafts patent	126 (96.2%)	134 (97.1%)
No. of grafts occluded	5 (3.8%)	4 (2.9%)
No. of patients with all grafts patent	38 (88.4%)	43 (91.5%)
No. of patients with one or more grafts occluded	5 (11.6%)	4 (8.5%)

From Bidstrup et al.[53]

Prentice has described aprotinin as an agent with mild anticoagulant rather than prothrombotic effects.[54] Certainly, aprotinin therapy reduces both thrombin-antithrombin III complexes and the release of fibrinopeptide A from fibrinogen.[55] With regard to platelet function, although studies have shown a preservation of platelet glycoprotein surface receptors,[56] aprotinin therapy induces an inhibition of platelet aggregation similar to the effect of aspirin. Rather more evidence exists for the antifibrinolytic effects of aprotinin,[48,57] which have been recognized for many years. Although this subject is complex, at present no evidence suggests that aprotinin has an intrinsic, direct prothrombotic effect.

Heparin Dosage and Activated Clotting Time with Aprotinin Therapy

The initial Hammersmith studies provided interesting data in relation to ACT in patients who were given high-dose aprotinin. ACT was substantially increased compared with controls, despite use of a standard heparin dose (3 mg/kg) in all patients. This finding was also reported in early European studies[58,59] (Fig. 7). The increase in ACT was dose-related but was corrected to preheparin levels by the standard reversal dosage of protamine. This finding may have been misinterpreted by some workers as indicating that aprotinin therapy was heparin-sparing and that lower-dose systemic heparin might be safe.

The author cannot overemphasize that in the context of high-dose aprotinin therapy, full systemic heparinization must be maintained and that an ACT >700-800 seconds should be expected during CPB. An ACT of 400-500 seconds in patients receiving high-dose aprotinin should be considered evidence of inadequate heparinization and should be treated in the same way as when an ACT <400 seconds is encountered in patients on CPB without aprotinin. Cosgrove et al.[43] rightly raise the possibility of inadequate anticoagulation as

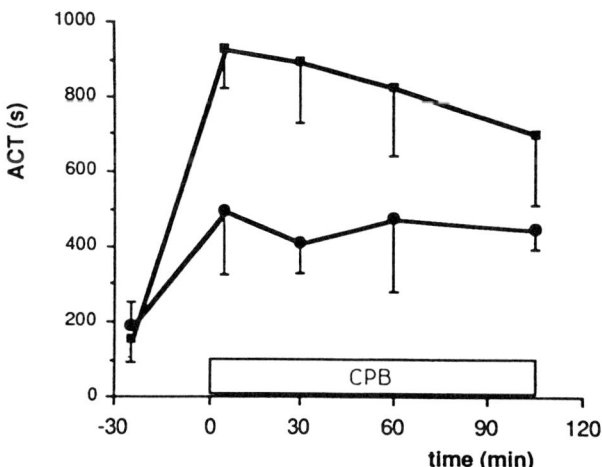

FIGURE 7. Activated clotting times (ACT) in patients treated with aprotinin (squares) and controls (circles) during cardiopulmonary bypass. Standard heparinization regimen was used in all patients. (From Harder et al: Ann Thorac Surg 51:936-941, 1991, with permission.)

an explanation for the trend toward an increased rate of infarct. The more recent data presented by Mills et al.[60] in aortic surgery patients managed by deep hypothermic circulatory arrest also hint at the possibility of lower heparin dosage and suboptimal ACT in patients receiving aprotinin. These data emphasize the needs to maintain full systemic heparin anticoagulation in patients receiving aprotinin and to achieve and maintain increased ACT (>700–800 sec) throughout the period of CPB.

Patient Variability and the Thrombotic/Hemorrhagic Spectrum

Our attitude toward anticoagulation and hemostatic responses is altogether too simplistic. We take virtually no account of variability from the norm in individual patients. If we consider the issue of postimplant anticoagulation for patients with a prosthetic heart valve, we currently medicate all patients to an accepted level of anticoagulant control. We know, however, that some patients have thrombosis or embolic complications, whereas others have hemorrhagic complications, despite apparently good anticoagulant control. We also know of patients who have stopped anticoagulant therapy without complications, even over several years.

These differences clearly reflect the variability of individual patients in regard to hemostasis. We have to assume that a spectrum exists, with patients positioned from the prothrombotic to the prohemorrhagic ends, perhaps in a normal distribution curve. Currently, we have no simple and reliable way to identify the intrinsic prothrombotic or prohemorrhagic status of individual patients. Such information would obviously be helpful in postoperative anticoagulation for heart-valve patients, but it would be of even wider benefit in assessing all patients before cardiac surgery.

Some workers have suggested that elevated levels of factor VII may be a marker of hypercoagulability.[61] The potential exists, therefore, for preoperative identification of patients who may be inherently prothrombotic. Better protocols should be designed for the management of anticoagulation and aprotinin or other hemostatic therapies in such patients.

The Risk/Benefit Equation of Aprotinin Therapy

Clinicians make risk/benefit assessments whenever they make clinical decisions. No therapy is completely free from risk. The availability of aprotinin presents cardiothoracic surgeons with precisely such an equation (Fig. 8). The therapy is highly effective in preventing excessive bleeding and the need for high-volume transfusions of blood and blood products. Such a powerful therapy may seem likely to have a negative side, with the risk of prothrombotic trends at the forefront of the coronary surgeon's mind. The decisions to use or not to use—and in which patients, at what dosage, and at what time—must ultimately be made by the individual clinician.

The author has had the benefit of experience with aprotinin since its discovery. We began using the drug routinely, according to the indications that eventually became the licensed indications for use in the United Kingdom: (1) reoperation, (2) acute septic cases, (3) patients expected to bleed excessively because of intrinsic coagulopathy or drug therapy, and (4) patients in

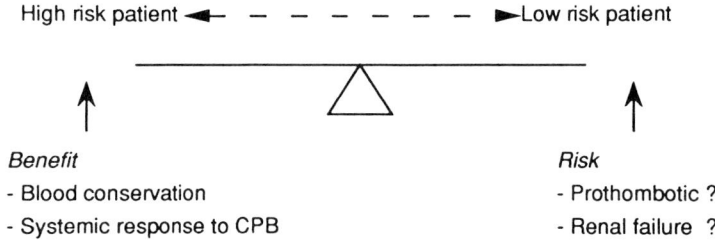

FIGURE 8. Risk/benefit analysis applied to clinical use of aprotinin therapy.

whom blood transfusion(s) is contraindicated (e.g., severe mismatch, Jehovah's Witnesses).

The author and his colleagues have continued to use aprotinin therapy in all such patients for over 6 years. We have been careful to maintain adequate anticoagulation with high ACTs during CPB. We are fully satisfied that the therapy is both highly effective and acceptably safe. We believe that aprotinin therapy has revolutionized blood conservation, particularly in patients at high risk of excessive bleeding. We also believe that aprotinin therapy will be extended into other forms of major surgery and that, in addition to obvious hemostatic effects, protease inhibition may well provide additional benefits in cardiac patients by modification of the systemic inflammatory response during CPB.

REFERENCES

1. Murphy JA, Smith H, Walker ID, et al: Blood transfusion in cardiac surgery. Perfusion 5(Suppl):1-7, 1990.
2. Bove JR: Transfusion-associated hepatitis and AIDS—what is the risk? N Engl J Med 317:242-245, 1987.
3. Kluft C, Dooijewaard G, Emeis JJ: Role of the contact system in fibrinolysis. Semin Thromb Hemost 13:50-68, 1987.
4. Kirklin JK, Westaby S, Blackstone EH, et al: Complement and the damaging effects of cardiac surgery. J Thorac Cardiovasc Surg 86:845-852, 1983.
5. Ratliff NB, Young WG, Hacket DB, et al: Pulmonary injury secondary to extracorporeal circulation. J Thorac Cardiovasc Surg 65:425-431, 1973.
6. Royston D, Fleming JS, Desai JB, Taylor KM: Increased peroxide product generation associated with open heart surgery: Evidence for free radical generation. J Thorac Cardiovasc Surg 91:759-766, 1986.
7. Braude S, Nolop KB, Fleming JS, Taylor KM: Increased pulmonary transvascular protein flux after canine cardiopulmonary bypass: Association with lung neutrophil sequestration and tissue peroxidation. Am Res Respir Dis 134:867-872, 1986.
8. Harker L, Malpass TW, Branson HE, et al: Mechanism of abnormal bleeding in patients undergoing cardiopulmonary bypass: Acquired transient platelet dysfunction associated with selective granule release. Blood 56:824-834, 1980.
9. Zilla P, Fasol R, Groscurth P, et al: Blood platelets in cardiopulmonary bypass operations. Recovery occurs after initial stimulation, rather than continual activation. J Thorac Cardiovasc Surg 97:379-383, 1989.
10. Addonizio VP Jr, Strauss JF III, Colman RW, Edmunds LH Jr: Effects of prostaglandin E1 on platelet loss during in vivo and in vitro extracorporeal circulation with a bubble oxygenator. J Thorac Cardiovasc Surg 77:119-123, 1979.

11. George JN, Pickett EB, Saucerman S, et al: Platelet surface glycoproteins: Studies on resting and activated platelets and platelet membrane microparticles in normal subjects, and observations in patients during adult respiratory distress syndrome and cardiac surgery. J Clin Invest 78:340-348, 1986.
12. Dechavanne M, French M, Pages J, et al: Significant reduction in the binding of a monoclonal antibody (LYP 18) directed against the IIb/IIIa glycoprotein complex to platelets of patients having undergone extracorporeal circulation. Thromb Haemost 57:106-109, 1987.
13. Verstraete M: Clinical application of inhibitors of fibrinolysis. Drugs 29:236-242, 1985.
14. Madsen P, Stanch A: The effect of aminocaproic acid on bleeding following transurethral prostatectomy. J Urol 96:255-256, 1974.
15. Del Rossi AJ, Cernaianu AC, Botros S, et al: Prophylactic treatment of postperfusion bleeding using EACA. Chest 96:27-32, 1989.
16. Van Der Salm TJ, Ansell JE, Okike ON, et al: The role of epsilon-aminocaproic acid in reducing bleeding after cardiac operation: A double-blind randomized study. J Thorac Cardiovasc Surg 95:538-540, 1988.
17. Hoffman EP, Koo AH: Cerebral thrombosis associated with amicar therapy. Radiology 131:667-672, 1979.
18. Naeye RL: Thrombotic state after a hemorrhagic diathesis: A possible complication of therapy with epsilon-aminocaproic acid. Blood 19:694-698, 1962.
19. Horrow JC, Hlavacek J, Strong MD, et al: Prophylactic tranexamic acid decreases bleeding after cardiac operations. J Thorac Cardiovasc Surg 99:70-75, 1990.
20. Manucci PM, Canciani MT, Rota L, Donovan BS: Response of factor VIII. von Willebrand factor to DDAVP in healthy subjects and patients with haemophilia A and von Willebrand's disease. Br J Haematol 47:283-293, 1981.
21. Takeuchi M, Nagura H, Kaneda T: DDAVP and epinephrine induced changes in the localization of von Willebrand factor antigen in endothelial cells of human oral mucosa. Blood 72:850-854, 1988.
22. Hackmann T, Gascoyne RD, Naiman SC, et al: A trial of desmopressin (1-desamino-8-d-argine vasopressin) to reduce blood loss in uncomplicated cardiac surgery. N Engl J Med 321:1437-1439, 1989.
23. Rocha E, Llorens R, Paramo JA, et al: Does desmopressin acetate reduce blood loss after surgery in patients on cardiopulmonary bypass? Circulation 77:1319, 1988.
24. Salzman EW, Weinstein MJ, Weintraub RM, et al: Treatment with desmopressin acetate to reduce blood loss after cardiac surgery. N Engl J Med 314:1402-1406, 1986.
25. Weskler BB: Platelet interactions with the blood vessel wall. In Coleman RW, Hirsh J, Marder VJ, Salzman EW (eds): Hemostasis and Thrombosis, 2nd ed. Philadelphia, J.B. Lippincott, 1987, pp 793-812.
26. Walker ID, Davidson JF, Faichney A, et al: A double blind study of prostacyclin in cardiopulmonary bypass surgery. Br J Hematol 49:415-419, 1981.
27. Aren C, Feddersen K, Radegran K: Effects of prostacyclin infusion on platelet activation and postoperative blood loss in coronary bypass. Ann Thorac Surg 36:49-53, 1983.
28. Longmore DB, Guerrara D, Bennett G, et al: Prostacyclin: A solution to some problems of extracorporeal circulation: Experiments in greyhounds. Lancet 1:1002-1004, 1979.
29. Disesa VJ, Huval W, Lelcuk S, et al: Disadvantages of prostacyclin infusion during cardiopulmonary bypass: A double-blind study of 50 patients having coronary revascularization. Ann Thorac Surg 38:514-520, 1984.
30. Fish KJ, Sarnquist FH, van Steennis C, et al: A prospective, randomized study of the effects of prostacyclin on platelets and blood loss during coronary bypass operations. J Thorac Cardiovasc Surg 91:436-441, 1986.
31. Addonizio VP Jr, Fisher CA, Jenkin BK, et al: Iloprost (ZK36374), a stable analogue of prostacyclin, preserves platelets during stimulated extracorporeal circulation. J Thorac Cardiovasc Surg 89:926-930, 1985.
32. Blauth C, Brady A, Arnold J, Brannan JJ, Taylor KM: A double blind trial of Iloprost during cardiopulmonary bypass. Perfusion 2:271-276, 1987.
33. Tice DA, Reed GE, Clauss RH, Worth MH: Hemorrhage due to fibrinolysis occurring with open-heart operations. J Thorac Cardiovasc Surg 46:673-676, 1963.
34. Mammen EF: Natural protease inhibitors in extracorporeal circulation. Ann NY Acad Sci 146:754-762, 1968.
35. Ambrus JL, Schimert G, Lajos TZ, et al: Effect of antifibrinolytic agents and estrogens on blood loss and blood coagulation factors during open heart surgery. J Med 2:65-81, 1971.

36. Bidstrup BP, Royston D, Sapsford RN, Taylor KM: Reduction in blood loss and blood use after cardiopulmonary bypass with high dose aprotinin (Trasylol). J Thorac Cardiovasc Surg 97:364-372, 1989.
37. Royston D, Bidstrup BP, Taylor KM, Sapsford RN: Effect of aprotinin on need for blood transfusions after repeat open heart surgery. Lancet ii:1289-1291, 1987.
38. Bidstrup BP, Royston D, Taylor KM, Sapsford RN: Effect of aprotinin on need for blood transfusion in patients with septic endocarditis having open heart surgery. Lancet i:366-367, 1988.
39. Fraedrich G, Weber C, Bernard A, et al: Reduction of blood transfusion requirements in open heart surgery by administration of high dose aprotinin—preliminary results. Thorac Cardiovasc Surg 37:89-91, 1989.
40. Dietrich W, Barankay A, Dilthey G, et al: Reduction in homologous blood requirement in cardiac surgery by intraoperative aprotinin application—clinical experience in 152 cardiac surgical patients. Thorac Cardiovasc Surg 37:92-98, 1989.
41. Royston D: Aprotinin in open heart surgery. Perfusion 5(Suppl):63-72, 1990.
42. Bidstrup B, Harrison J, Royston D, et al: Aprotinin therapy in cardiac surgery. Ann Thorac Surg 1992 (in press).
43. Cosgrove DM: Use of aprotinin in repeat myocardial revascularization: Cleveland Clinic experience. Perfusion 1993 (in press).
44. Goldman S, Copeland J, Moritz T, et al: Improvement in early saphenous vein graft patency after coronary artery bypass surgery with antiplatelet therapy: Results of a Veterans Administration Cooperative Study. Circulation 77:1324-1332, 1988.
45. Michelson E, Morganroth J, Torosian M, MacVaugh H III: Relation of preoperative use of aspirin to increased mediastinal blood loss after coronary artery bypass surgery. J Thorac Cardiovasc Surg 76:694-697, 1978.
46. Ferraris VA, Ferraris SP, Lough FC, Berry WR: Preoperative aspirin ingestion increases operative blood loss after coronary artery bypass grafting. Ann Thorac Surg 45:71-74, 1988.
47. Bidstrup BP, Royston D, McGuinness C, Sapsford RN: Aprotinin in aspirin pretreated patients. Perfusion 5(Suppl):77-81, 1990.
48. Efstratiadis T, Munsch C, Crossman D, Taylor KM: Aprotinin therapy after thrombolytic treatment. Ann Thorac Surg 52:1320-1321, 1991.
49. Flajmo F, Calamai G: High dose aprotinin in emergency coronary artery surgery following thrombolysis. Ann Thorac Surg 1993 (in press).
50. Dudziak R, Kirchhoff PG, Reuter HD, Schumann F: Proteolyse und Proteaseninhibition in der Herz-und Gefässchirurgie. Stuttgart, FK Schattauer, 1985.
51. Verstraete M: Clinical applications of inhibitors of fibrinolysis. Drugs 29:236-261, 1985.
52. Blauhut B, Gross C, Necek S, et al: Effects of high-dose aprotinin on blood loss, platelet function, fibrinolysis, complement, and renal function after cardiopulmonary bypass. J Thorac Cardiovasc Surg 101:958-967, 1991.
53. Bidstrup B: Aorto-coronary bypass graft patency after high-dose aprotinin. J Thorac Cardiovasc Surg 1993 (in press).
54. Prentice CM: Aprotinin: Modes of action. Perfusion 1993 (in press).
55. Dietrich W, Jochum M, Schramm W, et al: Reduction of homologous blood requirement in cardiac surgery using high dose aprotinin. Anesthesiology 71(Suppl):A7, 1989.
56. van Oeveren W, Eijsman L, Roozendaal KJ, Wildevuur Ch RH: Platelet preservation by aprotinin during cardiopulmonary bypass. Lancet i:644, 1988.
57. van Oeveren W, Jansen NJ, Bidstrup BP, et al: Effects of aprotinin on hemostatic mechanisms during cardiopulmonary bypass. Ann Thorac Surg 44:640-645, 1987.
58. deSmet AAEA, Joen MCN, van Oeveren W, et al: Increased anticoagulation during cardiopulmonary bypass by aprotinin. J Thorac Cardiovasc Surg 100:520-527, 1990.
59. von Segesser LK, Weiss BM, Pasic M, et al: Experimental evaluation of heparin-coated cardiopulmonary bypass equipment with low systemic heparinization and high-dose aprotinin. Thorac Cardiovasc Surg 39:251-256, 1991.
60. Sundt TM, Kouchoukos NT, Saffitz JE, et al: Renal dysfunction and intravascular coagulation after use of aprotinin in thoracic aortic operations employing hypothermic cardiopulmonary bypass and circulatory arrest. Ann Thorac Surg 1993 (in press).
61. Miller GJ, Meade TW: Hypercoagulability: In Butchartt E, Bodnar E (eds): Thrombosis, Embolism and Bleeding. London, ICR Publishers, 1992, pp 81-92.

Chapter 10

Controversies in the Practical Use of Aprotinin

David Royston, FFARCS

This chapter discusses recent data related to the use of aprotinin to reduce bleeding associated with cardiac surgery. Although the topic encompasses a number of areas, the particular focus is background to the presently recommended dose regimen, which is based on inhibition of inflammatory cascades associated with contact activation; included are relevant details about the basic chemistry of aprotinin. A second focus is description and discussion of a number of suggestions for possible modifications to this regimen, either by alterations in the dose administered or by timing of administration. Finally, the chapter outlines recent evidence of aprotinin's action to inhibit certain aspects of the coagulation system which have led to problems in controlling anticoagulation during cardiopulmonary bypass (CPB).

It is now well recognized that aprotinin has the effect of reducing bleeding associated with a wide variety of operative procedures. Limitation of discussion to cardiac and vascular surgery alone necessitates the omission of a large quantity of data.

BACKGROUND TO USE OF HIGH-DOSE APROTININ THERAPY IN CARDIAC SURGERY

Serendipity was the basis for the discovery that high-dose aprotinin could dramatically reduce bleeding during cardiac surgery. The drug was being used in studies designed to reduce inflammatory lung injury by inhibiting the contact activation associated with cardiac surgery; the details have been described previously.[43,44]

The contact of blood with the foreign surface of the oxygenator stimulates contact activation systems, which can be thought of as primitive host defense mechanisms, programmed to isolate and, if possible, to destroy a foreign substance or surface which the blood "sees." The contact systems involve a large number of inflammatory cascades that can act through humoral or cellular mechanisms but that are ultimately controlled by amplification cascades of proteolytic enzymes, the vast majority of which are serine proteases. Serine proteases can be thought of as the enzyme controller system found in the plasma and circulation.

The principal event in the activation of these systems is thought to be the activation of factor XII, the so-called Hageman factor, to produce factor XIIa. Factor XIIa, a serine protease, can initiate and amplify a number of other inflammatory systems (Fig. 1).

One of the main mediators produced is kallikrein, which has a number of potential routes for activation of inflammatory cascades. Principally, it is able to act on neutrophil granulocytes to produce other phlogistic agents. Of relevance is its role to initiate the release of proteolytic enzymes, such as elastase and cathepsin. In addition, kallikrein primes polymorphonuclear leucocytes to produce reduced species of oxygen—so-called free radicals—when challenged by a second phlogistic agent.[60]

In addition to the release of factor XIIa, the stimulation at the foreign surface releases factor XIIb, which in turn initiates the stimulation of fibrinolysis by augmenting the conversion of plasminogen to plasmin (a serine protease). Factor XIIb also aids the process of clot formation by stimulating activation of factor V. Kallikrein and bradykinin exert further action on the fibrinolytic system: kallikrein stimulates plasmin production by its action of prourokinase and bradykinin by release of tissue type plasminogen activator (tPA) from the endothelium. The cumulative effects of this initial contact activation and subsequent amplification is to produce a whole-body inflammatory response.

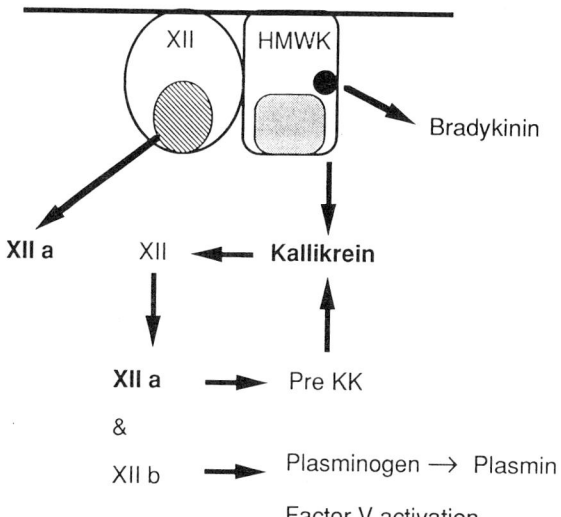

FIGURE 1. Following surface contact, possibly as a result of the recognition of a negatively charged surface, factor XII undergoes a conformational change and becomes attached to high-molecular-weight kininogen (HMWK), which itself has undergone a conformational change. This complex can then bind to the surface. Following limited proteolysis, the HMWK releases kallikrein (a serine protease) and bradykinin. The factor XII portion of the complex can also undergo limited proteolysis to release more factor XIIa. This active proteolytic fragment (again a serine protease) can initiate coagulation through the intrinsic coagulation cascade by direct effects on factor IX, which again binds to the surface. Factor XIIa can also prime factor VII to activate the extrinsic coagulation system. Factor XIIa concentrations are also increased by a feedback system involving kallikrein. Factor XIIa acts on prekallikrein to release kallikrein, which in turn is able to act on factor XII to produce factor XIIa.

This concept was developed by the group working in Birmingham, Alabama, whose focus of attention had been the role of complement activation in this process.[31]

Previously my colleagues and I had studied the lungs and pulmonary circulation as the target organs of this inflammatory process. In humans, it was possible to demonstrate an increase in solute flux into and from the lungs after open-heart surgery.[47,49] In addition, there was evidence of increased oxygen-derived, free-radical activity, probably derived from neutrophils,[48] and of a significant relationship between the degree of free-radical activity produced from the pulmonary circulation and an index of protein leak into the lung.[8] A number of possible therapeutic maneuvers were considered to inhibit or ameliorate this inappropriate stimulation of the inflammatory response. During the period of extracorporeal circulation the only inhibition of these potentially deleterious cascades is the routine administration of heparin to inhibit the intrinsic pathway and to prevent blood clotting. Heparin achieves this effect by activating the naturally occurring serine protease inhibitor, antithrombin III (AT III).

The hypothesis we originally aimed to test was that fibrinolysis, complement, and kallikrein activation could also be inhibited by giving reasonable amounts of an appropriate, additional serine protease inhibitor (serpin), such as aprotinin. From the above discussion of the contact activation system as the initiator of this response, it seemed reasonable to suggest that this cell activation would be reduced or abolished by the use of a serine protease inhibitor that was able to target factor XII and kallikrein activity. The intention of these studies was to show that such therapy would have a significant effect on the indices of cell activation and lung inflammation that we were investigating.

Aprotinin Chemistry

Aprotinin is a basic polypeptide (pKa 10) composed of 58 amino acid residues and has a molecular weight of 6512 Daltons. The amino acid sequence, biochemical structure, and biophysical characteristics have been previously described and categorized.[20] Aprotinin was independently discovered and isolated from bovine lymph nodes in 1930 by Kraut et al.[33] who identified it as a kallikrein inactivator, and in 1936 by Kunitz and Northrop,[34] who defined its ability as a trypsin inhibitor in a preparation obtained from bovine pancreas.

Aprotinin is a member of a family of serpins (*serine protease inhibitors*) which are found in all aspects of nature; as the name implies, they are able to inhibit a range of proteases that have serine residues at their active site. This inhibition is provided by inactivation of the active serine of the protease by the lysine residue at position 15 of the aprotinin molecule.

The activity of aprotinin is expressed in various ways. Historically kallikrein inactivator units (KIU) and trypsin inhibitory units (TIU) are most commonly used. These units rely on measurements of the biologic potency of aprotinin in fixed analytic systems. Over the years the manufacturing and especially the purification processes for this drug have improved, and it is now more usual to discuss the amount of drug in terms of weight (mg) of protein or concentration (micromolar [μM]) of solution. The conversion factors equate 1 mg of protein with 7143 KIU, or 100,000 KIU with 14 mg protein. A 1-μM solution of aprotinin contains 46.5 KIU/ml. Because the majority of efficacy and other data published before 1986 uses the KIU as the unit of measurement, I have maintained this convention throughout most of the current chapter. However, for certain discussions, particularly those of the pharmacologic effects of aprotinin, I have reverted to the use of weight of substance (mg) or strength of solution (μM).

Development of the High-Dose Regimen

Aprotinin was chosen as the serpin for the pilot study aimed at reducing inflammation associated with extracorporeal circulation for two reasons: (1) it was known to have actions to inhibit kallikrein and plasmin at doses that were potentially possible to achieve clinically,[20] and (2) it was the only serine protease inhibitor available at that time in the United Kingdom with sufficiently low toxicity to allow its use in humans at required concentrations.

The concentration of aprotinin thought necessary to block the actions of kallikrein in pure systems and under laboratory conditions is about 4 μM ($\approx$200 KIU/ml of plasma). Inhibition of plasmin is thought to require concentrations of about 1 μM ($\approx$50 KIU/ml) in these same pure chemical systems.

Based on studies of the use of continuous infusions of aprotinin in polytrauma patients,[10] members of the biochemistry department in Munich formulated a dosing schedule aimed at achieving a concentration of 200 KIU/ml throughout the period of extracorporeal circulation during cardiac surgery. The aim was to inhibit the actions of kallikrein and to observe the effects on the inflammatory cascades.

The dose regimen was to give 2×10^6 KIU (280 mg) as a loading dose over a 20-minute period after induction of anesthesia and to follow with a continuous infusion of 500,000 KIU (70 mg) for 1 hour until the patient was returned to the intensive care unit. To overcome the dilution effect of the two liters of crystalloid prime in the oxygenator, a further 1×10^6 KIU (140 mg) was added to the prime volume. The study was designed as a pilot investigation and therefore was neither randomized nor blinded to the observers. All patients had coronary artery bypass grafts performed by one surgeon, with myself as the anesthetist.

At the time of surgery it was obvious that, despite any alterations in biochemical and hematologic variables, the most striking effect of aprotinin therapy was a reduction in the bleeding that had been an accepted consequence of CPB. Published results of this study[55] show a significant reduction in the blood lost into postoperative drains on the day after surgery in patients receiving the trial drug. The reduction was from a mean of 674 ml in the 11 control patients to a mean of 357 ml in the 11 patients treated with aprotinin.

Analysis of plasma samples for concentrations of aprotinin by the group in Munich showed that the target plasma concentration of about 200 KIU/ml was not achieved throughout the time of bypass[44] and that the fall in plasma concentration of aprotinin shortly after the start of the bypass was greater than predicted. To overcome this effect, it was decided to increase the addition to the prime volume by a further 1×10^6 KIU (140 mg) for a total addition of 2×10^6 KIU (280 mg) aprotinin to the oxygenator prime. This is the dose regimen used, and first described, in the studies aimed at investigating aprotinin therapy in reoperative patients.[46]

This regimen, which has been variously described but which I will call the currently recommended dose regimen, has been used in large numbers of patients. In all the studies thus far reported, none has failed to show significant efficacy of the agent in reducing blood loss and the need for donor blood transfusions. These data have been the subject of recent reviews[13,43] and were considered in the preceding chapter.

Two broad issues related to the use of this agent in clinical practice need to be considered: (1) alterations to the currently recommended regimen (a) in the quantity of drug given or (b) in the timing of administration of the drug, and (2) interactions with heparin therapy and the control of anticoagulation during bypass when aprotinin therapy is used.

MODIFICATIONS TO THE DOSE REGIMEN

Alterations in the Amount Given

The currently recommended dose regimen has a number of inconsistencies and problems. The main one is the obvious fact that no account is taken of the size or weight of the patient. The total dose given to a patient over the course of an operation may vary anywhere between 60,000 KIU/kg for a 100-kg patient to 120,000 KIU/kg for a 50-kg patient.

This element has been addressed only with the regimen recommended for use in children. The present suggestion is to give the currently recommended adult dose to children with a body surface area of >1.16 m^2. In children with a smaller surface area, 240 mg/m^2 is given as the loading dose; this amount is also added to the pump prime. The infusion rate is maintained at 56 mg/m^2/hr. This regimen was designed to administer a final total dose of about 75,000 KIU/kg over the time of surgery.[43]

A second problem related to the dose regimen is the kinetics of the drug and the relationship between its action and the plasma level achieved. To rationalize the dose regimen, we would benefit from a knowledge of the drug's mechanism of action. This is a major difficulty because the exact mechanism of action of aprotinin is currently a mystery. Aprotinin has been shown to have biphasic kinetics with an initial elimination half-life of about 45–60 minutes. The secondary phase half-life is about 2 hours. These values have been generated in otherwise normal volunteers.[20]

Our own studies showed that the plasma concentration achieved after the administration of the fixed loading dose was variable and did not depend on the body weight.[43] Similarly, studies from Munich have shown no relationship between the dose administered and the plasma concentration achieved. Of greater importance, the plasma concentrations in both of these studies could not be unequivocally related to any of the measured variables of efficacy.

The kinetics can be altered by a number of interventions commonly associated with open-heart surgery. In particular, aprotinin is highly charged and binds to plastics.[20] The actual amount which is lost to the machine depends on the system used, especially its material of manufacture. This aspect is currently under investigation. Other influences from the mechanics of extracorporeal circulation are use of hemofiltration or cell saving as an adjunct to blood conservation. Aprotinin has a molecular weight of 6512 Daltons and will be freely filtered with all the commercially available systems. The cell saver will wash away the aprotinin from processed shed blood. Aprotinin is removed by renal clearance, and thus the kinetics may be influenced by perioperative urine output, the control of which is highly variable between institutions. Thus far the dose regimen does not take into account losses through any of these mechanisms.

Differences in bypass technology may also explain apparent differences in measured plasma concentrations during the operative period. For example, the plasma concentration of aprotinin fell more quickly in patients studied in Munich[14] compared with patients in London.[43] Both sets of patients underwent myocardial revascularization with the same bubble oxygenator in the bypass equipment. The group in Munich also used a cell saver system, which was not used in London.

An equally obvious problem in trying to define a dose regimen is how the chosen dose, and thus the plasma concentration, can be assessed in terms of efficacy. Studies aimed at defining and optimizing dose administration have thus far concentrated on certain efficacy variables; for example, drain loss and transfusion volumes. However, comparing efficacy from reported studies poses difficulties for two reasons: (1) for a given institute and for a given procedure, the definition of efficacy of aprotinin (or any other) therapy is unlikely to be uniform, and (2) the differences in the definition of an acceptable efficacy may rely almost entirely on the end point(s) chosen and, of greater importance, the values set for those variables. For example, efficacy could be defined as either a reduction in drain loss or a reduction in the need for donor blood.

Drain Loss as Criterion for Efficacy

The choice of drain loss as the criterion of efficacy ignores intraoperative losses, which may be significant. We then have to consider what is normal and what is indeed abnormal. Three factors come easily to mind: (1) The published literature shows that losses vary depending on the type of surgery being performed. It is well recognized that patients with multiple valve replacement are more likely to bleed than those undergoing primary myocardial revascularization. (2) Definition of normal or anticipated drain loss after a standard operation varies among centers. The drain loss in patients allocated to untreated groups in European studies of aprotinin therapy varied threefold from 347 ± 103 ml (mean $\pm$ SD; range = 210-690 ml) in the most successful center to 1185 ± 601 ml (range = 500-3200 ml) in the least successful.[44] Both centers obviously regard their losses as normal for patients undergoing primary coronary artery surgery, despite the threefold difference in magnitude. Similarly, in North America the losses reported by Goodenough et al.[21] in patients undergoing primary surgery ranged from 672 ± 54 ml to 1445 ± 109 ml in the 18 centers with a firm commitment to blood conservation programs. (3) Differences in losses may occur within the same center. As an example, the group in Amsterdam has published a number of papers on the use of aprotinin therapy.[54,59] In one paper they reported postoperative blood losses for untreated (control) patients as 37 ± 12 g of hemoglobin[54] and in the second as 64 ± 6 g.[59] This twofold difference in postoperative blood loss for the same procedure in the same setting presumably reflects alterations in personnel.

With no consensus as to what constitutes the normal loss after routine coronary artery surgery, either between centers or even within a center, the efficacy of any regimen in relation to altered, as opposed to absolute, postoperative losses is difficult to extrapolate to personal practice. These changes and difficulties may also explain the significant differences among studies investigating the use of lower-dose regimens with drain loss as the endpoint.

Nonetheless, most studies have focused on the reduction in drain loss in the postoperative period. Despite these caveats, in all the studies thus far published that use the currently recommended high-dose regimen, the fall in postoperative losses has been significant and biologically relevant. These decreases vary from about 30% to about 50% in primary coronary artery bypass patients.[13,43] The total volume drained after such a procedure would be expected to be about 300–400 ml when aprotinin is used in the currently recommended dose.

It has also been argued that a much smaller total dose is of equal benefit. The rationale is difficult to define from the published literature in humans, but it does follow the adage that a smaller dose for the same efficacy must produce fewer adverse effects. Some literature supports the view that administration of 2×10^6 KIU (280 mg) is as effective as any higher dose in patients undergoing uncomplicated coronary artery surgery. In two studies the lower dose of aprotinin was given into the oxygenator prime as the only therapy.[9,59] Both studies showed the lower-dose regimen to have benefits on postoperative losses equivalent to those obtained with the higher dose. In contrast, other studies show that the lower-dose regimen is not beneficial in patients undergoing primary myocardial revascularization. For example, Vandevelde and colleagues failed to show any effect of 2×10^6 KIU administered to the pump prime on either hemostatic variables or blood loss.[56]

Earlier studies have also reported investigation of the efficacy of aprotinin at a total dose of about 2×10^6 KIU over the period of surgery.[23] In a study by Hannekum and colleagues of patients undergoing primary surgery for valve replacement, the mean postoperative loss into the drains fell from 596 ml in untreated patients to 443 ml with low-dose aprotinin. The difference failed to reach statistical significance.

A continuum of dose response is likely. The shape and upper end of this relationship is unknown. For example, in studies in Tubingen aprotinin was given in doses related to body weight.[27] The doses used (30,000 KIU/kg and 60,000 KIU/kg) correspond to about 1½ times the original higher-dose regimen. The postoperative drain losses are shown in Figure 2. Children also exhibit a complex dose/response relationship. Studies from Munich[40] have used the same doses of 30,000 and 60,000 KIU/kg (Fig. 3).

Use of lower doses of aprotinin in more complex or higher-risk patients has also been reported. In patients receiving aspirin before surgery, aprotinin 2×10^6 KIU (280 mg) was added to the oxygenator as the only therapy. The mean postoperative drain loss fell from 1096 ± 121 ml to 672 ± 65 ml. This reduction to about 60% of the control group loss was statistically significant ($p < 0.05$).[53] These data compare with a 75% reduction in drain loss from 1393 (979) to 352 (138) ml when the high-dose regimen was used.[4]

Similarly, use of half of the presently recommended dose regimen (i.e., a total of 3×10^6 KIU [360 mg]) given over the period of surgery has been reported in patients undergoing repeat open-heart surgery.[50] Statistically significant efficacy was achieved with this lower-dose regimen. The mean postoperative drain loss fell from 1429 ml to 948 ml ($p < 0.05$). This decrease compares with a fall in drain losses from 1509 (388) ml in the control population to 286 (48) ml in patients receiving high-dose aprotinin therapy. Groups who have suggested

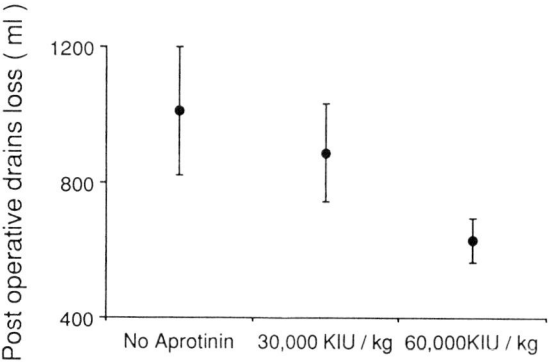

FIGURE 2. Drain loss (mean ± SD) in the first day after myocardial revascularization in adults. Data from Heller et al.[27]

low-dose regimens have not demonstrated efficacy in reoperations but have reported significant efficacy (56% reduction in drain loss) with the high-dose regimen in reoperations.[9]

These reports suggest that lower doses of aprotinin have an effect in reducing drain loss after cardiac surgery; however, the magnitude of effect is far greater when the larger dose is used.

Use of Blood and Blood Products as Criterion of Efficacy

The second criterion for efficacy of the drug is transfusion of blood and blood products. With this criterion of efficacy is the goal to half, quarter, or eliminate transfusion? What are the effects of different dose regimens on use of blood products? This aspect makes the discussion of optimal dose even more complicated because noise in the data will inherently increase due to differences in procedure, patient population, and the institute at which the surgery is performed.

Again, uncomplicated coronary bypass surgery in patients given the high-dose regimen provides a good example. If the percentage of reduction in drain

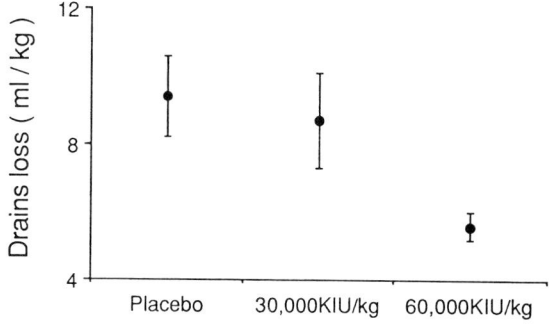

FIGURE 3. Drain loss (ml/kg) in the first 6 hours from infants weighing <10 kg undergoing open-heart surgery. Data from Mössinger et al.[40]

loss is compared with the percentage of reduction in patients requiring donor blood transfusions, the responses among centers varies greatly.[43,44] This difference is difficult to explain. The only simple explanation for this dichotomy is that the amount of hemoglobin in the drains falls by a greater amount than the total drain volume when aprotinin therapy. is used. For example, in the London study of patients undergoing myocardial revascularization, the postoperative drain loss fell by about 50% from 570 to 310 ml. However the hemoglobin loss into the drains was reduced threefold—from 38 to 12 g.[6] These data suggest that aprotinin reduced bleeding, but probably had no effect on the drainage of serosanguinous exudate that occurred in the few hours before the drains were removed. Indeed, the originators of the chest-tube reinfusion technique of blood conservation recognized clearly that the hemoglobin content of the reinfused pericardial drainage fluid is highest in the hours immediately after surgery and becomes progressively less in the later postoperative period.[57]

If we consider the efficacy endpoint for aprotinin therapy as decreased use of blood and blood products or a smaller proportion of patients who require them, then data from the high-dose regimen indicate a reduction in both the number of patients who receive donor blood products and in the total amount of blood products used. For primary myocardial revascularization, blood transfusions are reduced by 40–80%.[13,43] In an uncontrolled study of high-risk patients, such as those with infective endocarditis, about 75% of patients received donor blood products.[3]

For lower-dose regimens, such as the prime only regimen, postoperative transfusions are reduced in comparison with an untreated population. For example, in the reports by van Oeveren and colleagues[54] the total postoperative use of blood products was 60 units (30 units blood, 30 units fresh frozen plasma [FFP]) in the 30 nontreated patients (equivalent to 2 units/patient) and 29 units (9 units blood, 20 units FFP) in the 22 patients allocated to receive aprotinin in the oxygenator alone (1.32 units/patient). Twenty-two units (11 blood, 11 FFP) of blood products were given to the 30 patients receiving aprotinin therapy in the current high-dose regimen (0.73 unit/patient). The proportion of patients who received donor blood postoperatively fell from 68% in the nontreated patients to 38% in patients receiving high-dose aprotinin. Data for the prime-only group are not specifically mentioned.

These data are similar to other reports from the same group for postoperative use of blood and blood products.[24] The difficulties of interpreting the data are highlighted, however, when intraoperative use of blood and blood products is considered. In this center intraoperative use is higher than postoperative use; only 1 in 4 patients did not receive intraoperative transfusions.[24]

In one study using a lower-dose regimen, Hannekum et al.[23] reported a small but statistically significant reduction in use of donor blood. Similarly, Scott and Au[50] reported that all patients receiving half the current high-dose regimen for reoperation required transfusions.

On a number of occasions I have argued that the data published thus far show a continuum of activity of aprotinin therapy: the higher the dose, the greater the effect in a particular circumstance. Undoubtedly, the lower doses have some effect, but it is equally clear that the magnitude of effect is greater with larger doses. Unfortunately, at this time analysis of effect does not include even higher doses than those currently used.

At present no evidence suggests any consistent detrimental effect of the currently recommended regimen; thus the use of a lower-dose regimen seems somewhat illogical. If the lower dose is administered routinely, then a proportion of the patients will bleed sufficiently to require transfusions—at the expense of being challenged by a drug that may have antigenic potential. The end result of this technique of administration may therefore compromise the chance of using aprotinin for a future procedure while failing to prevent the need for transfusion of donor blood or blood products.

Timing of Administration of Aprotinin Therapy

Controversy includes not only the amount of aprotinin but also the timing of administration. Much of this debate has been fueled by the fact that the drug has been actively marketed to cardiac surgeons as having some protective action against the deleterious effects of the contact of blood with the bypass system. This claim is absolutely true, but it does not explain the hemostatic properties of the drug. Aprotinin reduces bleeding in a number of areas in which extracorporeal circulation is never used; for example, during liver transplantation as well as vascular, orthopedic, gynecologic and plastic/cosmetic surgery. To advocate the use of aprotinin to protect the patient from the damaging effects of the inflammatory process associated with the period of bypass seems sensible. This aspect could turn out to be one of the positive indications for use of aprotinin therapy in addition to prevention of bleeding.

Aprotinin, however, improves hemostasis unrelated to the period of extracorporeal support. Our earliest reports on its use commented on the dry operating field achieved prior to administration of heparin.[50] Therefore, in certain cases, such as reoperations or use of both internal thoracic arteries as conduits for myocardial revascularization, administration of the drug during CPB alone fails to take advantage of its ability to produce a dry field during a difficult and possibly prolonged dissection before CPB.

Of greater interest is the postoperative use of aprotinin in patients who bleed excessively. The first studies of administration at the end of CPB used a dose of 10,000 KIU/kg but did not measure aspects of efficacy to reduce bleeding.[32]

Angelini and colleagues reported their anecdotal experiences in patients bleeding excessively after return to the intensive care unit.[33] The authors describe the results of administration of a bolus of 2×10^6 KIU aprotinin, followed by a continuous infusion of 500,000 KIU/hr, in 6 patients who were bleeding in the hours after cardiac surgery. The effects were to produce a fall in the rate of drain loss from a mean of 490 (range: 250-1146)) ml/hr to a mean of 90 (range: 29-193) ml/hr during and up to the 6 hours of therapy.

This report is supported by more recent data from a controlled trial of the same regimen in patients who were bleeding excessively after routine coronary artery bypass surgery.[28] The investigators randomly allocated aprotinin therapy to 60 patients in the intensive care unit who had excessive postoperative bleeding (defined as >400 ml in 3 hours). Results showed a highly significant reduction in drain loss in the next 10 hours from a mean of 1205 to 835 ml. Unfortunately, the administration of aprotinin was delayed until the study criteria of excess bleeding were met. This probably explains the absence of effect on the use of donor blood or blood products. The mean use in patients allocated to aprotinin treatment was 4.3 units compared with 4.4 units in the controls.

Currently no test of preoperative hemostatic function is able to predict which patients will bleed excessively. Some evidence indicates that the thromboelastogram (TEG) may be a sensitive indicator of the likelihood of postoperative bleeding.[52] Perhaps aprotinin therapy could be withheld in certain low-risk circumstances until after the period of extracorporeal circulation. Administration immediately after the TEG has developed (about 20 minutes) rather than three hours later, when bleeding becomes clinically evident and defined as excessive, may benefit the patient by reducing exposure to blood and blood products. It has always been my practice to modify the dose and to continue administration of aprotinin into the postoperative period in patients at particular risk of bleeding, especially those with deranged hemostatic mechanisms due to infection and sepsis at the time of surgery.[5]

CONTROL OF ANTICOAGULATION WHEN APROTININ IS USED

An early observation in patients receiving aprotinin therapy was the effect on the measured activated clotting time (ACT). The Haemochron method of determining ACT is widely used during cardiac surgery.[35] ACT is markedly prolonged in heparinized blood from patients treated with high-dose aprotinin.[12,14,45] Three questions need to be addressed: (1) Why is the ACT prolonged? (2) What might be the effects of reducing the amount of heparin when aprotinin therapy is used? (3) Is it possible to recommend a safe value of ACT?

What Increases the ACT with Aprotinin?

A number of factors are known to be associated with prolonged ACT, particularly hemodilution, hypothermia,[11] and altered platelet number and function.[39] Administration of drugs, such as prostacyclin, that affect platelet function also prolong the ACT.[17]

As a general rule, all of the serine protease inhibitors can inhibit various aspects of platelet function.[36] Aprotinin is no exception, it has been shown to have a large number of direct and indirect actions on platelets. The second phase response of platelet aggregation (associated with the release of thromboxane A_2 and serotonin) after stimulation with adenosine diphosphate (ADP) is effectively inhibited by aprotinin at concentrations of about 100–400 KIU/ml.[2,25] This effect has been used to great advantage in preserving platelets in donor blood. In addition, reports indicate that the use of an intravenous bolus dose of 20,000 KIU/kg prevents platelet aggregation and thereby reduces the incidence of venous thrombosis in major surgery. This dose significantly reduced the platelet adhesion and aggregation associated with hip replacement operations.[29,30]

Evidence also indicates that administration of aprotinin leads to inhibition of the adhesion of platelets to glass beads.[26,29] Other evidence shows that aprotinin acts in the same way as aspirin to inhibit aggregation and the release of thromboxane from platelets. Serpins are able to inhibit phospholipase A_2 and thus the release of lipid mediators, such as platelet activating factor and thromboxane.[19] This mechanism probably accounts for the data in humans that show a reduction in plasma concentrations of thromboxane B_2 during CPB when aprotinin therapy is used.[7]

However, the most likely cause of the effects of aprotinin therapy on the ACT are directly related to its ability to inhibit the serine proteases in the coagulation cascade. Heparin acts by complexing with the naturally occurring serpin AT III. This activated heparin-AT III complex is able to inhibit factors XIIa, XIa, IXa, Xa and IIa and possibly plasmin and kallikrein but not factor VII (Fig. 4).[41] Clinically achieved concentrations of aprotinin inhibit factor XIIa by 50%, factor XIa by 20%, and factor IXa by 80%.[44] Factor VIII was also inhibited but at concentrations unlikely to be found during clinical open-heart surgery. Aprotinin had no inhibitory effects on factors VII, IIa or Xa at concentrations up to 10 times those measured clinically. These data can be explained by the known actions of aprotinin as a serpin, although the major target enzymes for inhibition by aprotinin are trypsin, plasmin, and tissue kallikrein.[20]

The ACT is intended to test the integrity of the intrinsic coagulation system and in a simplistic approach can be thought of as mimicking the process of contact activation at the foreign surface of the oxygenator system. From the known inhibitory actions of aprotinin on platelets and factors in the coagulation cascade, it is easy to understand its effect of increasing the duration of the ACT.

The effects of aprotinin on the ACT are additive to those of heparin. The response of the ACT to the administration of heparin is widely variable;[16] the additional response induced by aprotinin is equally so.

The data in Figure 5a are the mean (± SEM) of ACT times from duplicate measurements of the blood of 11 patients. Three values are indicated: baseline, after the addition of heparin (2 IU/ml), and after the further addition of aprotinin (2 μM [100 KIU/ml]). The response appears additive and linear. However, if the individual data in Figure 5b are examined, it is easy to appreciate the variability of the response. These data show that it will be

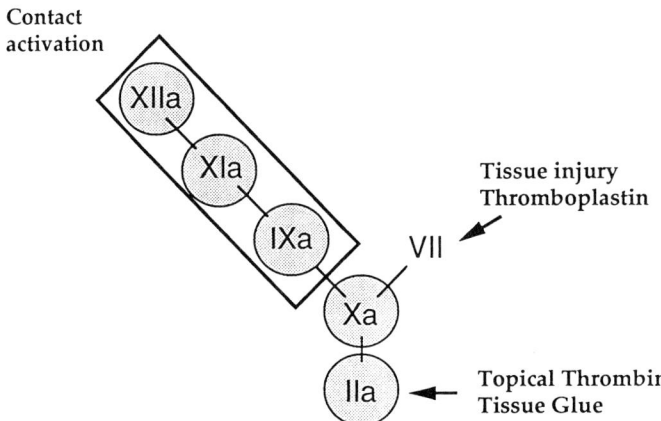

FIGURE 4. Diagrammatic representation of factors in the coagulation cascades (all of which are serine proteases) to show factors inhibited by aprotinin (inside solid box) and heparin-AT III complex (inside shaded circles). Stimuli and points of stimulation for activation of coagulation are also shown.

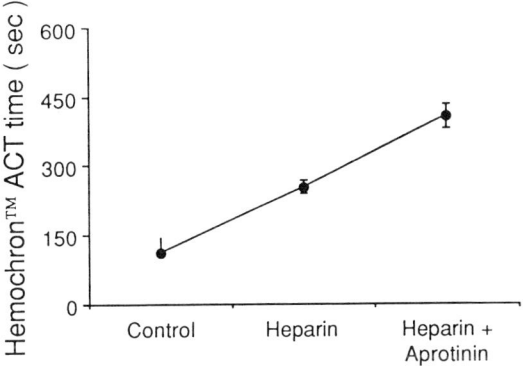

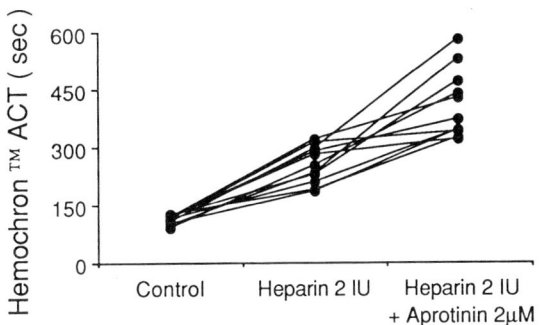

FIGURE 5. Results for the ACT measured with the Hemochron system in blood from 11 patients. Data are mean ± SEM in upper panel; individual data are in lower panel. Measurements were made in blood alone and after the addition of heparin (2 IU/ml final concentration) and heparin and aprotinin (2 IU/ml and 2 μM, respectively). These figures show that although the overall response appears linear, response to heparin and the subsequent addition of aprotinin varies greatly among individuals.

impossible using such current technologies to predict the response of any patient to the administration of heparin and aprotinin in combination.

Possible Effects of Reducing the Amount of Heparin When Aprotinin Is Used

Some investigators suggest that the prolonged ACT represents a heparin-sparing action of aprotinin. More worrying is the fact that a reduction in administration of heparin has been suggested.[12] I cannot stress strongly enough that in my view this approach is extremely dangerous. Certain of the problems associated with heparin, especially reports of abnormal clot formation, result from inappropriate and inadequate dosage.

This stance can be understood most easily when Figures 4 and 5 are considered. As Figure 5 indicates, the ACT can be at 400 seconds despite the fact that the contribution from the heparin-AT III complex is to prolong the ACT to 250 seconds. This is true protection against coagulation initiated by all the mechanisms recognized to occur during open-heart surgery.

In a patient undergoing extracorporeal membrane oxygenation (ECMO), it is common practice to maintain an ACT of about 180-200 seconds. With this value for the ACT the oxygenator system does not develop any significant clot formation over a period of 24-48 hours. However, if the same patient were transferred to the operating theater for an open-heart procedure, then we would anticipate administration of extra heparin to extend the ACT to >400 seconds. We know by experience that clot formation is likely during surgery when the ACT is not above this duration. The reason is likely to be that clot formation is initiated through a factor VII-dependent process, such as tissue trauma and release of thromboplastin. The only inhibition of this process is by heparin-AT III action on factor Xa and thrombin. Maintaining an ACT of 400-500 seconds with aprotinin alone, therefore, must be associated with concentrations of heparin that are inadequate to prevent factor VII-dependent initiation of clot formation. As aprotinin is an antifibrinolytic, in addition to being a mild anticoagulant, then any clot thus formed undergoes lysis more slowly. In such circumstances, persistent microthrombi may be formed in the circulation. These in turn obviously have the potential to affect adversely organ functions. This leads to the last and most difficult issue to address.

The Appropriate Value for the ACT in the Presence of Aprotinin

This question is currently impossible to answer with a definite value based on sound scientific and experimental evidence. The reason is to a certain extent related to what would be regarded as the gold standard for administration of heparin during routine cardiac surgery. The majority of centers that use an automatic system aim to maintain the ACT at 350-500 seconds.[22] This goal is confounded by two factors when aprotinin is used: (1) the effects of aprotinin itself and (2) the effects of the system (and therefore activator) used.

As demonstrated in Figure 4 and outlined in the above discussion, it is possible to have an ACT of 350-500 seconds when aprotinin is given, even though the patient is insufficiently heparinized to prevent coagulation initiated by tissue trauma. If blood is anticoagulated with heparin to produce an ACT of 400 seconds, then the addition of relatively small doses of aprotinin (plasma concentrations >2 μM) will extend the ACT to >700 seconds.

A second confounding variable is related to the measurement of the ACT. Currently two methods are commonly used for measurement of the automatic clotting time. Both use different systems for activation of coagulation and monitoring of the time to clot formation. The Hemochron (International Techdyne Corporation, Edison, NJ) uses celite as the activator and a rotating magnet as the detector. The HemoTec system (HemoTec Inc., Englewood, CO) uses kaolin as the activator and a reciprocating daisy wheel as the sensor. A comparison of the two systems reveals significant differences between results when these instruments are used on the same blood sample drawn during clinical open-heart surgery.[42] The response of these systems to heparin and additional aprotinin are also significantly different. This difference is again due to the effect of the activator. Kaolin is a very powerful activator of the intrinsic coagulation system.[38] Because of this activity aprotinin has little effect

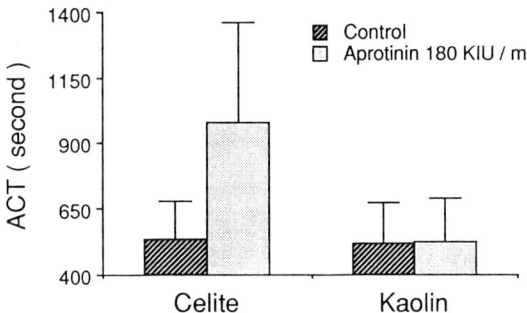

FIGURE 6. Results (mean ± SD) for the ACT when stimulated with celite or kaolin. Control samples are from the blood of patients heparinized, using clinical criteria, before surgery. After aprotinin was added to these samples to give a final concentration of 180 KIU/ml, the assay was repeated. The celite system is more affected by the added aprotinin. From data in reference 58.

on activation due to kaolin,[58] whereas clotting induced by contact with other surfaces is inhibited by aprotinin.[38]

The difference in the response of the two activation systems to blood from patients with the addition of heparin and heparin plus aprotinin is thus not surprising (Fig. 6).[58] The ACT with the celite (the activator in the Hemochron system) was more affected by the addition of aprotinin (180 KIU/ml) than the samples stimulated with kaolin (the activator in the HemoTec system). This difference, as well as the variability in response to heparin alone and in combination with aprotinin, has also been shown for the APTT (essentially the ACT in a cell-free system).[18]

What strategies can be adopted in clinical practice to ensure adequate heparin dosing?

(1) Suggest an Empirical Number Such as 750–800 Seconds.

Based on the understanding of the actions of aprotinin on the ACT (Fig. 4), many centers have adopted a policy of maintaining the ACT at >750–1000 seconds by the administration of additional heparin, if required.[43] Obviously this is a totally empirical suggestion and relies on a measurement that is essentially outside the range of the machine. Nonetheless, adopting this policy has resulted thus far in no major problems. Particularly when aprotinin is used, maintaining this ACT does not lead to the requirement of more protamine at the end of the procedure, nor does an ACT of 750 seconds throughout bypass lead to excessive postoperative bleeding.[45] This is similar to data from studies in which prostacyclin was used. Fish and colleagues reported that the ACT was about 700 seconds in patients receiving prostacyclin. However, the treated patients did not receive additional protamine and had significantly less postoperative bleeding.[17]

(2) Use Heparin Concentrations.

The principle of this technique is that it is possible to perform a functional heparin assay with the HemoTec Heparin Management System (HMS). This machine uses a multiple-chamber cartridge to plot a heparin titration curve. The cartridge contains various quantities of protamine, and the stimulus is tissue thromboplastin. The use of tissue thromboplastin should overcome the effects of aprotinin with contact activation. Potential drawbacks relate to (1) the cost of the apparatus and the assay systems; (2) the relationship between the heparin dose and plasma concentrations, which are known to be poorly correlated[60]; and (3) the fact that the heparin concentration is not related easily to ACT, which has been recognized since the earlier days of cardiac surgery.[51] A decreased sensitivity to heparin is seen in children, patients who have had preoperative infusions of heparin, and patients requiring preoperative intraaortic balloon counterpulsation. These are the patients most likely to benefit substantially from the use of aprotinin therapy. The lack of sensitivity to heparin appears not to be related to AT III activity, clotting factors, fibrinogen concentration, or platelet count.[15] It would therefore be extremely difficult to predict which patients may not be adequately anticoagulated, despite adequate concentrations of heparin, throughout bypass. In these circumstances it is easy to predict that clot formation may be more likely.

(3) Perform a Heparin Dose/ACT Response Before the Administration of Aprotinin.

Unless a dose/response study can be performed in the hours before surgery, a delay in the administration of aprotinin is inevitable. This in turn may lead to a reduction in the efficacy of therapy. This approach removes, for example, the advantage of the absence of bleeding before CPB in cases in which it may be significant, such as reoperations. Measuring the amount of heparin to administer to patients after the initial bolus of aprotinin may lead to difficulties in calculation, depending on the system used. The slope of the heparin dose/response curve in the presence of aprotinin is less steep when kaolin is used as activator compared with celite. For the same ACT value this means that a greater dose of heparin is suggested when the HemoTec system is used. Whether this is a theoretical or practical problem remains to be established.

(4) Neutralize the Aprotinin Prior to Performing the ACT.

It is easy to raise both IgM and IgG antibodies to aprotinin; plasma concentrations are measured with an ELISA technique. It may therefore be possible to add an antibody that neutralizes aprotinin to the ACT tube before measurement. This approach has not been studied.

(5) Measure Some Aspect of the Final Common Pathway of the Coagulation System.

In principle it is possible to define the action of heparin alone on the coagulation system by measuring factors Xa and IIa in the final common pathway (Fig. 4). Currently measurements of factor Xa rely on chromogenic assays of plasma samples. This technology is therefore too cumbersome for routine clinical use. The alternative is to measure the thrombin time. Addition of thrombin to plasma and/or blood induces clot formation. The time for clot formation is prolonged in the presence of heparin. Some centers routinely use the thrombin time as opposed to the ACT to assess the adequacy of heparinization.[27] Both Hemochron and HemoTec manufacture automatic systems for measuring the thrombin time. However, to obtain a degree of reproducibility, the test tube has been modified to include not only thrombin but also protamine and snake venom. This so called HiTT system, manufactured by Hemochron, is currently under evaluation both in normal practice and in combination with aprotinin therapy. The current system has four major problems: (1) The relationship of the HiTT value to the ACT and concentration of heparin is currently unknown. (2) A normal value cannot be measured because non-anticoagulated blood clots within about 30 seconds after stimulus. Blood which is weakly anticoagulated also clots too rapidly to measure the effect accurately. (3) Because the contents of the tubes are unstable once they are reconstituted, results of the test cannot be precisely reproduced. (4) The cost of the assay is high.

CONCLUSIONS

The current high-dose regimen of aprotinin was not originally intended to represent an optimal means of reducing blood loss and preventing transfusion. Therefore, the scope to develop the optimal dose regimen for specific procedures and patients is considerable. Indeed, the concept of high-dose aprotinin has led to more questions than answers, especially as use of the drug increases, encompassing other types of surgery and extending into other countries of the world.

The use of lower-dose regimens has met with some success. However, the effectiveness of lower doses relies on the reported endpoint. The observation that a lower dose of aprotinin delivered to the oxygenator has benefit is tempered by the fact that 75% of all patients in reported studies still receive donor blood products during primary myocardial revascularization. In addition, lower dosages have not shown absolute benefits equal to the higher-dose protocols in any at-risk group. Furthermore, no studies have yet reported an increase in the incidence of specific complications with the high-dose regimen. In particular, no current evidence suggests an increase in thrombotic complications when anticoagulation has been controlled to provide what is currently perceived as adequate heparinization.

There seems to be little rationale for modifying the total dose of aprotinin in the current regimen—except to determine if a *higher* dose results in increased benefit. The appropriate dose for a certain situation and the criteria and methods for measuring adequate and appropriate anticoagulation still require substantial studies to determine the safest and most effective use of this remarkable therapy.

REFERENCES

1. Angelini GD, Cooper GJ, Lamarra M, Bryan AJ: Unorthodox use of aprotinin to control life-threatening bleeding after cardiopulmonary bypass. Lancet i:799-800, 1990.
2. Aoki N, Yoshida N: Inhibition of platelet aggregation by protease inhibitors. Possible involvement of proteases in platelet aggregation. Blood 52:1-12, 1978.
3. Bidstrup BP, Harrison J, Royston D, et al: Aprotinin therapy in cardiac surgery: A report on use in 42 UK cardiac centres. Ann Thorac Surg, 1993 (in press).
4. Bidstrup BP, Royston D, McGuiness C, Sapsford RN: Aprotinin in aspirin treated patients. Perfusion 5:77-81, 1990.
5. Bidstrup BP, Royston D, Sapsford RN, Taylor KM: Effect of aprotinin on need for blood transfusions in patients with endocarditis having open heart surgery. Lancet i:366-367, 1988.
6. Bidstrup BP, Royston D, Taylor KM, Sapsford RN: Reduction in blood loss and blood use after cardiopulmonary bypass with high dose aprotinin (Trasylol). J Thorac Cardiovasc Surg 97:364-372, 1989.

7. Blauhut B, Gross C, Necek S, et al: Effects of high-dose aprotinin on blood loss, platelet function, fibrinolysis, complement and renal function after cardiopulmonary bypass. J Thorac Cardiovasc Surg 101:958-967, 1991.
8. Braude S, Nolop KB, Fleming JB, et al: Increased pulmonary transvascular protein flux after canine cardiopulmonary bypass: Association with lung neutrophil sequestration and tissue peroxidation. Am Rev Respir Dis 134:867-872, 1986.
9. Carrel T, Bauer E, Garcia E, et al: Reduktion des postoperativen Blutverlustes und des Fremblutverbrauches in der herzchirurgie mit Aprotinin: Erfahrrungen mit untersciederlicher Dosierung. Helv Chir Acta 58:365-378, 1991.
10. Clasen C, Jochum M, Mueller-Esterl W: Feasibility study of very high dose aprotinin in polytrauma patients. In Schlag G, Redl H (eds): First Vienna Shock Forum: Pathophysiological role of mediators and mediator inhibitors in shock. New York, Alan R. Liss, 1987, pp 175-183.
11. Culliford AT, Gitel SN, Starr N, et al: Lack of correlation between activated clotting time and plasma heparin during cardiopulmonary bypass. Ann Surg 193:105-111, 1981.
12. de Smet AAEA, Joen MCN, van Oeveren W, et al: Increased anticoagulation during cardiopulmonary bypass by aprotinin. J Thorac Cardiovasc Surg 100:520-527, 1990.
13. Dietrich W, Barankay A, Hähnel CH, Richter JA: High-dose aprotinin in cardiac surgery: Three years experience in 1,784 patients. J Cardiothorac Vasc Anesth 6:324-327, 1992.
14. Dietrich W, Spannagl M, Jochum M, et al: Influence of high-dose aprotinin treatment on blood loss and coagulation pattern in patients undergoing myocardial revascularization. Anesthesiology 73:1119-1126, 1990.
15. Esposito RA, Culliford AT, Colvin SB, et al: Heparin resistance during cardiopulmonary bypass: The role of heparin pretreatment. J Thorac Cardiovasc Surg 85:346-353, 1983.
16. Esposito RA, Culliford AT, Colvin SB, et al: The role of the activated clotting time in heparin administration and neutralization for cardiopulmonary bypass. J Thorac Cardiovasc Surg 85:174-185, 1983.
17. Fish KJ, Sarnquist FH, van Steenis C, et al: A prospective, randomised study of the effects of prostacyclin on platelets and blood loss during coronary bypass operations. J Thorac Cardiovasc Surg 91:436-442, 1986.
18. Francis J, Howard C: The effects of aprotinin on the response of the activated partial thromboplastin time (APTT) to heparin. Blood Coagul Fibrinolysis 4:35-40, 1993.
19. Freise J, Schmidt FW, Magerstedt P, et al: Gabexate mesilate and camostat: New inhibitors of Phospholipase A_2 and their influence on the alpha-amylase activity in serum from patients with acute pancreatitis. Clin Biochem 18:224-229, 1985.
20. Fritz H, Wunderer G: Biochemistry and applications of aprotinin, the kallikrein inhibitor from bovine organs. Arzneimittelforsch 33:4:479-494, 1983.
21. Goodenough LT, Johnson MF, Toy PTCY: The variability of transfusion practice in coronary artery bypass surgery. JAMA 265:86-90, 1991.
22. Gravelee GP, Haddon WS, Rothberger HK, et al: Heparin dosing and monitoring for cardiopulmonary bypass. J Thorac Cardiovasc Surg 99:518-523, 1990.
23. Hannekum A, Reuter HD, Dalichau H, et al: Anlage und zussammenfassendes Ergebnis einer Klinischen Doppelblindstudie bei Operationen am offenen Herzen. Einfluss von Aprotinin auf Thrombozytenzahl und-funktion. In Dudziak R, Kirchhoff PG, Reuter HD, Schumann F (eds): Proteolyse und Proteinaseninhibition in der Herz-und Gefasschirurgie. Stuttgart, Schattauer, 1985, pp 222-233.
24. Harder MP, Eijsman L, Roozendaal KJ, et al: Aprotinin reduces intraoperative and postoperative blood loss in membrane oxygenator cardiopulmonary bypass. Ann Thorac Surg 51:936-941, 1991.
25. Harke H, Gennrich M: Aprotinin-ACD Blut. 1. Experimentelle Untersuchungen über den Einfluss von Aprotinin auf die plasmatische und thrombozytäre Gerinnun. Anaesthetist 29:266-276, 1980.
26. Harke H, Steinen G, Rahman S, et al: Aprotinin ACD Blut II: Der Einfluss von Aprotinin auf die Freisetzung zellulärere Medioraten un Enzyme im Konservenblut. Anaesthetist 31:165-171, 1982.
27. Heller W, Fuhrer G, Gallimore MJ, et al: Changes in the kallikrein-kinin-system after different dose regime of aprotinin during cardiopulmonary bypass operations. Adv Exp Med Biol 247B:43-48, 1989.
28. Kallis P, Tooze JA, Talbot S, et al: Aprotinin treatment rather than prophylaxis for excessive bleeding following cardiac surgery. Blood (in press).
29. Ketterl R, Haas S, Heiss A, et al: Zur Wirkung des natürlichen Proteinaseninhibitors Aprotinin auf die Plättchenfunktion beim alloarthroplastischen Hüftgelenkersatz. Med Welt 33:480-486, 1982.

30. Ketterl R, Haas S, Lechner F, et al: Wirkung von Aprotinin auf die Thrombozytenfunktion während Hüft-Totalendoprosthesenoperation. Med Welt 31:1239–1240, 1980.
31. Kirklin JK, Westaby S, Blackstone EH, et al: Complement and the damaging effects of cardiopulmonary bypass. J Thorac Cardiovasc Surg 86:845–852, 1983.
32. Koestering H, Kirchoff PG, Voelker P, et al: Untersuchungen der Blutgerinnungsveraenderungen während und nach Operationen mit Hilfe der Herz-Lungen–Maschine. Thoraxchirurge 21:534–543, 1978.
33. Kraut E, Frey EK, Werle E: Über die Inaktivierung des Kallikreins. Hoppe-Seyler's Zeitschrift für Physiologische Chemie 192:1–21, 1930.
34. Kunitz M, Northrop JH: Isolation from beef pancreas of crystalline trypsinogen, trypsin, a trypsin inhibitor and an inhibitor trypsin compound. J Gen Physiol 19:991–1007, 1936.
35. Kurusz M, Schneide B, Brown BP, et al: Filtration during open heart surgery: Devices, techniques, opinions and complications. Proc Am Acad Cardiovasc Perfusion 4:123–129, 1983.
36. Laskowski M, Kato I: Protein inhibitors of proteinases. Ann Rev Biochem 49:593–626, 1980.
37. Lu H, Soria C, Commin P-L, et al: Hemostasis in patients undergoing extracorporeal circulation: The effect of aprotinin (Trasylol). Thromb Haemos 66:633–637, 1991.
38. Maria-Teresa PL, Ratnoff OD, Everson B: Inhibition of the activation of hageman factor (factor XII) by aprotinin (Trasylol). J Lab Clin Med 119:580–585, 1992.
39. Moorehead MT, Westenguard JC, Bull BS: Platelet involvement in the activated clotting time of heparinized blood. Anesth Analg 63:394–398, 1984.
40. Mössinger J, Dietrich W, Spanngel M, et al: Influence of aprotinin on coagulation patterns and blood loss in infants undergoing surgery for congenital heart defects. Anesthesiology 75(3A):A77, 1991.
41. Pratt CW, Church FC: Antithrombin: Structure and function. Semin Hematol 28:3–9, 1991.
42. Reich DL, Zahl K, Perucho MH, Thys DM: An evaluation of two activated clotting time monitors during cardiac surgery. J Clin Monit 8:33–36, 1992.
43. Royston D: High-dose aprotinin therapy: A review of the first five years experience. J Cardiothorac Vasc Anaesth 6:76–100, 1992.
44. Royston D: The serine antiprotease aprotinin (Trasylol): A novel approach to reduce postoperative bleeding. Blood Coag Fibrinol 1:55–69, 1990.
45. Royston D, Bidstrup BP, Sapsford RN, Taylor KM: Reduced blood loss after open heart surgery with aprotinin is associated with an increase in the activated clotting time (ACT). J Cardiothorac Anesth 3:80, 1989.
46. Royston D, Bidstrup BP, Taylor KM, Sapsford RN: Effect of aprotinin on the need for blood transfusion after repeat open heart surgery. Lancet ii:1289–1291, 1987.
47. Royston D, Braude S, Nolop KB, Hughes JMB: 113m Indium protein flux does not reflect degree or outcome in respiratory failure. Am Rev Respir Dis 139:A380, 1989.
48. Royston D, Fleming JS, Desai JB, et al: Increased peroxide product generation associated with open heart surgery: Evidence for free radical generation. J Thorac Cardiovasc Surg 91:759–766, 1986.
49. Royston D, Minty BD, Wallwork J, et al: The effects of surgery with cardiopulmonary bypass on alveolar-capillary barrier function in man. Ann Thorac Surg 40:133–142, 1985.
50. Scott D, Au J: The Edinburgh experience—low dose Trasylol. In Freidel N, Hetzer R, Royston D (eds): Blood Use in Cardiac Surgery. New York, Springer Verlag, 1991, pp 263–265.
51. Senning A: Plasma heparin concentrations in extracorporeal circulation. Acta Chir Scand 117:55–59, 1959.
52. Spiess BD, Tuman KJ, McCarthy RJ, et al: Thrombelastography as an indicator of postcardiopulmonary bypass coagulopathy. J Clin Monit 3:25–30, 1987.
53. Tabuchi N, van Oeveren W, Eijsman L, et al: Preserved hemostasis during the combined use of aprotinin and aspirin in CABG operations. In Freidel N, Hetzer R, Royston D (eds): Blood Use in Cardiac Surgery. New York, Springer Verlag, 1991, pp 245–251.
54. van Oeveren W, Harder MP, Roozendaal KJ, et al: Aprotinin protects platelets against the initial effect of cardiopulmonary bypass. J Thorac Cardiovasc Surg 99:788–797, 1990.
55. van Oeveren W, Jansen NJ, Bidstrup BP, et al: Effects of aprotinin on haemostatic mechanisms during cardiopulmonary bypass. Ann Thorac Surg 44:640–645, 1987.
56. Vandevelde C, Fondu P, DuBois-Primo J: Low-dose aprotinin for reduction of blood loss after cardiopulmonary bypass. Lancet i:1157–1158, 1991.
57. Von der Emde J, Mahmoud FO, Esperer HD: Retransfusion of postoperative drainage blood. In Freidel N, Hetzer R, Royston D (eds): Blood Use in Cardiac Surgery. New York, Springer Verlag, 1991, pp 129–132.

58. Wang J-S, Lin C-Y, Hung W-T, et al: In vitro effects of aprotinin on activated clotting time measured with different activators. J Thorac Cardiovasc Surg 104:1135-1140, 1992.
59. Wildevuur CHRH, Eijsman L, Roozendaal KJ, et al: Platelet preservation during cardiopulmonary bypass with aprotinin. Eur J Cardiothorac Surg 3:533-538, 1989.
60. Zimmerli W, Huber I, Bouma BN, Lämmle B: Purified human plasma kallikrein does not stimulate but primes neutrophils for superoxide production. Thromb Haemst 62:1121-1125, 1989.

Chapter 11

The Use of Desmopressin in Cardiopulmonary Bypass Surgery

G. Mariani, M.D., P. Arcieri, M.D., and F. Pizzo, M.D.

Patients who undergo cardiopulmonary bypass (CPB) for open-heart surgery are often susceptible to intraoperative and postoperative bleeding.[11,53,54,56] Life-threatening hemorrhage may require blood component therapy and/or reoperation, which occurs in about 3% of patients.[60] Bleeding from surgical wounds, which occurs in many patients, can be ascribed either to surgical damage to blood vessels or to inaccurate surgical hemostasis.

HEMOSTATIC CHANGES IN CPB

Systemic bleeding may be the consequence of an acquired defect of hemostatic function.[7,10,11,22,27,41,47,48] Because of the numerous variables associated with CPB, the causes of hemostatic derangement can be many and complex, including (1) drugs administered before surgery, (2) anesthesia, (3) complexity and duration of the surgical procedure, (4) artificial surfaces (oxygenators), (5) hypothermia, (6) hemodilution, (7) heparinization and heparin neutralization, and (8) transfused blood products. These factors may bring about a number of hemostatic changes that eventually lead to bleeding. Abnormalities most frequently diagnosed include prolongation of clotting tests related to anticoagulant treatment (heparin); low platelet count and/or altered platelet function; low fibrinogen titers; complex changes of clotting tests due to hemodilution or disseminated intravascular coagulation; and enhanced fibrinolytic activity. Strong evidence, however, suggests that the major contributors to hemostatic derangement in CPB are alterations of platelet function and/or number.[7,9,10,11,18,21-23,27,28,41,47-49,62,64]

Immediately after the initiation of extracorporeal circulation, platelet count decreases,[27] partly because of the dilution of blood with nonblood priming agents for the oxygenator apparatus. Bleeding time is most often prolonged, even if the platelet count is >80–90,000, indicating a functional defect as well. A number of functional abnormalities, associated with impaired platelet adhesion and aggregation[4,9,10,21,22,47] and a prolongation of bleeding time, have been documented in platelets from patients undergoing CPB. Some studies[20,27] have demonstrated that immediately after the onset of bypass, a depletion of alpha-granules is accompanied by an increase in the plasma of proteins released from platelet alpha-granules (beta-thromboglobulin [BTG] and platelet factor 4 [PF4]) as well as thromboxane B_2. These data indicate a transient activation of platelets; bleeding time and platelet count gradually return to normal after discontinuation of bypass.

Although the exact mechanism responsible for this platelet dysfunction remains unknown, the most probable cause seems related to a reversible membrane abnormality, as demonstrated by the reduced platelet aggregation induced by various agonists (adenosine diphosphate [ADP], epinephrine, collagen, ristocetin)[41] and the reduced expression of membrane glycoproteins Ib, IIb, and IIIa, which function as receptors for the adhesive proteins (von Willebrand's factor, fibrinogen).[23] Platelet defects are more pronounced when a bubble oxygenator rather than a membrane oxygenator is used.[11,21] Coating of the oxygenator with albumin or low-molecular-weight dextran helps to minimize the activation of platelets.[1,11]

PHARMACOLOGIC APPROACHES EMPLOYED TO COUNTERACT PLATELET DYSFUNCTION IN CPB

Attempts have been made to reduce platelet activation during CPB. Antiplatelet agents such as aspirin,[18] dipyridamole,[50] and prostaglandin EI (PGE1)[2,3,62] have been used without success. Despite early optimism, administration of prostacyclin (PGI2)[1,3,15] does not obviate the need for heparin,[15] even though PGI2 has been shown to reduce platelet degranulation and plasma levels of BTG and PF4.[6,21,61] Clinical studies demonstrate that PGI2 reduces, although not to a statistically significant degree, blood loss during CPB.[6,61]

The pathophysiology and clinical features of the bleeding diathesis subsequent to CPB share characteristics that are amenable to treatment with desmopressin acetate (DDAVP). In fact, DDAVP, a synthetic analog of the hormone vasopressin, induces a broad spectrum of pharmacologic reactions with hematologic consequences, including release from endogenous storage sites of (1) tissue plasminogen activator (TPA),[35,39,42] which causes a mild activation of the fibrinolytic system, and (2) the factor VIII/von Willebrand's factor (FVIII/vWF) complex.[25,42,43,46] The second effect forms the basis of the widespread therapeutic use of desmopressin in the treatment of mild hemophilia A and von Willebrand's disease.[8,13,24,38,43,45,57] DDAVP also improves hemostasis by unknown mechanisms in many hematologic and nonhematologic syndromes, including congenital and acquired platelet defects[12,19,32,44] and surgical bleeding,[31,33] in which the FVIII/vWF complex is within the normal range. A possible explanation for this improvement is provided by the studies of Sloand et al.,[59,60] who demonstrated that in vitro DDAVP increases the expression on the platelet membrane of GPIb, the receptor for vWF. If this occurs in vivo as well, DDAVP may act on the whole mechanism of platelet adhesion, which is of paramount importance for so-called primary hemostasis.

CLINICAL STUDIES

With this clinical and biologic background, a number of trials have been carried out to ascertain the clinical usefulness of DDAVP in reducing blood loss after complex cardiac surgery with CPB. Characteristics of the published trials[4,5,16,26,29,30,34,36,51,53,54,56,63] are outlined in Table 1.

Czer et al.[16] pioneered the studies of DDAVP by demonstrating that patients with excessive bleeding after open-heart surgery required less blood component therapy (red cells and platelets) and had to undergo reoperation much less frequently if treated with DDAVP (Table 2). A year later Salzman et al.[54] performed the first prospective, randomized, double-blind trial in unselected patients who required open-heart surgery with CPB. This study confirmed the indications provided by Czer's study, showing that blood loss during the 24-hour postoperative period was 40% less and transfusion requirements 34% less in the group receiving DDAVP. Details of Salzman's study are given in Table 3.

The beneficial effect of DDAVP shown by Salzman's study appeared to be correlated to the elevation of vWF and possibly to its high-molecular-weight multimers. Involvement of the multimers was not confirmed by Weinstein et al.,[63] who ascribed the hemostatic improvement to the rise of factor VIII or to the exposure of new binding sites on endothelial cells.

In 1988 and 1989, however, two important prospective, randomized, double-blind trials[26,51] failed to demonstrate any efficacy on the part of DDAVP in reducing the total blood loss in cardiac surgery with CPB in adults (Table 4). These negative findings were confirmed by a similar study carried out in children.[56]

In the early trials, patients who had to undergo coronary artery bypass grafting (CABG) were excluded because of the concern that the rise in vWF (and, above all, the high-molecular-weight multimers) may cause an early graft occlusion with thrombosis. Since Hackman's study, which included a number

TABLE 1. Characteristics of the Trials on Desmopressin in Open-Heart Surgery

Author (1st)	Year	Ref. No.	Patients	Treated	Controls
Czer	1985	16	Bleeding patients	23	16*
Salzman	1986	54	Complex cardiac surgery	35	35
Rocha	1988	51	Valvular heart disease + septal defects	50	50
Hackman	1989	26	Elective cardiac surgery + CABG	76	76
Sears	1990	56	Cardiac surgery (children)	30	30
Anderson	1990	4	CABG	10	9
Lazenby	1990	34	CABG	30	30
Hedderich	1990	29	CABG	31	31
Lo Cicero	1991	36	CABG	74	91
Rocha	1992	53	Various cardiac surgical procedures	30+30	30
Ansell	in press	63	Valvular heart surgery	41	42

* Not randomized, not double-blinded.
CABG = coronary artery bypass grafting.

TABLE 2. Blood Component Requirements (Units) and Reoperation Rates in Czer's Study

Blood Components	Desmopressin (n = 23)	Controls (n = 16)	Significance (p)
Red blood cells	4.5 ± 3.0	7.0 ± 4.7	.015
Platelets	4.0 ± 6.7	11.8 ± 9.1	.004
Plasma	2.7 ± 2.8	4.2 ± 2.6	n.s.
Total	15.3 ± 13.4	29.2 ± 19.3	.02
Reoperation	2 (9%)	12 (75%)	.001

TABLE 3. Detailed Results of Salzman's Study

	Desmopressin (n = 35)	Placebo (n = 35)	Significance (p)
Type of surgery			
Valve replacement	19	21	–
CABG	10	6	–
Valve + CABG	5	7	–
Other	1	1	–
Duration of surgery (min)	373	392	n.s.
Duration of bypass (min)	144	159	n.s.
Blood loss (ml)			
Intraoperative	592 ± 358	993 ± 858	.015
0–12 hr	512 ± 289	803 ± 471	.003
12–24 hr	215 ± 113	414 ± 429	.013
0–24 hr	1,317 ± 487	2,210 ± 1,415	.001
RBC transfused (units)	2.6 ± 2.1	3.7 ± 3.3	.079
vWF (u/dl)			
Before operation	185 ± 76	179 ± 78	n.s.
After treatment	180 ± 53	146 ± 55	.02

TABLE 4. Principal Results in Rocha's and Hackman's Studies

	Blood Loss		
	Intraoperative	Total	
			Red blood cells used
Rocha et al., 1988			
Desmopressin	131 ± 106*	458 ± 206*	1,642 ± 705[†]
Placebo	193 ± 137	536 ± 304	1,574 ± 645
p	.02	NS	NS
			Patients transfused (%)
Hackman et al., 1989			
Desmopressin	200[†]	1,138[†]	96
Placebo	200	1,010	91
p	NS	NS	NS

* = ml/m².
[†] = ml.
NS = not significant.

TABLE 5. Trials Including CABG Only: Desmopressin vs. Placebo with Regard to Blood Loss and Transfusion Requirements

	Desmopressin	Placebo	Significance (p)
Anderson et al.			
No. of patients	10	9	
Total blood loss (ml)	852 ± 223	1,020 ± 422	NS
Lazenby et al.			
No. of patients	30	30	
Blood loss 0–12 h	465 ± 207	511 ± 221	NS
Blood loss 12–24 h	236 ± 127	260 ± 112	NS
RBC transfused (unit)	2.8 ± 2.1	2.2 ± 1.8	NS
Hedderich et al.			
No. of patients	31	31	
Total blood loss (ml)	1,716 ± 688	1,826 ± 849	NS
RBC transfused (unit)	3.6 ± .8	3.4 ± 1.3	NS
LoCicero et al.			
No. of patients	74	91	
Total blood loss (ml)	1,306 ± 688	896 ± 33	.001
RBC transfused (unit)	1.23 ± .8	.35 ± .8	.005

RBC = red blood cells, NS = not significant.

of patients undergoing CABG, four trials involving this frequent open-heart operation have been published[4,29,34,36]; in none did treatment with desmopressin demonstrate reduced blood loss during or after CPB (Table 5). In one trial,[36] moreover, controls bled significantly less than the treatment group (Table 5).

In 1992 two significant trials[5,53] provided definitive evidence that desmopressin does not reduce either blood loss or transfusion requirements in unselected open-heart surgical patients (Table 6). Moreover, in one of the two studies,[53] the timing of desmopressin administration was also considered; the drug was given twice, first on completion of CPB and then 6 hours later. This schedule modification yielded no improvement compared either with controls or with patients who received the drug only once (Table 6). However,

TABLE 6. The Most Recent Trials of Desmopressin in Open Heart Surgery

	Desmopressin		Placebo or Controls	p
Ansell et al.				
No. of patients	41		42	
Total blood loss	1,065		830	NS
Rocha et al.				
No. of patients	30*	30†	30	
Total blood loss‡	515 ± 310	465 ± 228	432 ± 236	NS
RBC transfused§	1.26 ± 89	1.20 ± 1.1	1.22 ± 1.1	NS

* Patients treated with one DDAVP administration.
† Patients treated with two DDAVP administrations.
‡ ml/m^2
§ ml × 10^3
RBC = red blood cells, NS = not significant.

desmopressin was reported as causing side effects in none of the published studies, except in one child with cyanotic heart disease.[53] Specifically, increased frequency of thrombotic episodes such as myocardial infarction, stroke, or deep venous thrombosis has not been documented.

CONCLUSION

The results of the studies reviewed in this chapter demonstrate that desmopressin reduces neither blood loss nor transfusion requirements in the typical patient who undergoes an open-heart surgical procedure with CPB. In fact, the majority of such patients have only moderate blood loss, and in this setting desmopressin seems to be useless.

However, in a subset of patients at higher risk for bleeding, who so far have not been clearly categorized, desmopressin may be of substantial advantage. This subset could include reoperations[52,55]; pretreatment with aspirin or other strong inhibitors of platelet cyclooxygenase[14,17]; severe platelet dysfunction and excessive bleeding >2 hours after termination of CPB; and chronic renal or liver failure. Accurate screening of hemostatic function, including bleeding time, before and after surgery may help to identify patients who can benefit from desmopressin.

Recent reports indicate that intraoperative administration of aprotinin significantly reduces blood loss in patients undergoing open-heart surgery. This agent seems to be a better alternative than DDAVP: it is hoped that definitive evidence of its usefulness will soon be available.

REFERENCES

1. Addonizio PV, Macarak EJ, Nicolaou KC, et al: Effects of prostacyclin and albumin on platelet loss during in vitro simulation of extracorporeal circulation. Blood 53:1033, 1979.
2. Addonizio PV, Makarak EJ, Niewiarowski S, et al: Preservation of human platelets with prostaglandin E during in vitro simulation of cardiopulmonary bypass. Circ Res 44:350, 1979.
3. Addonizio PV, Strauss JF, Macarak EJ, et al: Preservation of platelet number and function with prostaglandin E during total cardiopulmonary bypass in rhesus monkey. Surgery 83:619, 1978.
4. Anderson TLG, Solem JO, Tengborn L, et al: Effects of desmopressin acetate on platelet aggregation, von Willebrand factor and blood loss after cardiac surgery with extracorporeal circulation. Circulation 81:872, 1990.
5. Ansell J, Klassen V, Lew SB, et al: Does desmopressin acetate prophylaxis reduce blood loss after valvular heart surgery? A randomized, double-blind study. J Thorac Cardiovasc Surg 104:117, 1992.
6. Aren C, Feddersen K, Radegran K: Effects of prostacyclin infusion on platelet activation and postoperative blood loss in coronary bypass. Ann Thorac Surg 36:49, 1983.
7. Bachmann F, McKenna R, Cole ER, et al: The hemostatic mechanism after open-heart surgery. I. Studies on plasma coagulation factors and fibrinolysis in 512 patients after extracorporeal circulation. J Thorac Cardiovasc Surg 70:76, 1975.
8. Berry EW: DDAVP—clinical use and therapeutic limitations in patients with congenital bleeding disorders. The Auckland experience. In Mariani G, Mannucci PM, Cattaneo M (eds): Desmopressin in Bleeding Disorders. London, Plenum Publishing, 1993, in press.
9. Beurling-Harbury C, Galvan CA: Acquired decrease in platelet secretory ADP associated with increased postoperative bleeding in post-cardiopulmonary bypass patients and in patients with severe valvular heart disease. Blood 52:13, 1978.
10. Bick RL: Alterations of hemostasis associated with cardiopulmonary bypass: Pathophysiology, prevention, diagnosis and management. Semin Thromb Hemost 3:59, 1976.

11. Bick RL: Hemostasis defects associated with cardiac surgery, prosthetic devices, and other extracorporeal circuits. Semin Thromb Hemost 11:249, 1985.
12. Cattaneo M, Mannucci PM: Desmopressin in the treatment of congenital and acquired defects of platelet function. In Mariani G, Mannucci PM, Cattaneo M (eds): Desmopressin in Bleeding Disorders. London, Plenum Publishing, 1993, in press.
13. Castaman G, Ruggeri M, Di Bona E, et al: Management of spontaneous bleedings and prevention of bleeding after dental extractions and other surgical procedures in mild hemophilia A and von Willebrand's disease: Ten years of experience at the Vicenza hemophilia and thrombosis center. In Mariani G, Mannucci PM, Cattaneo M (eds): Desmopressin in Bleeding Disorders. London, Plenum Publishing, 1993, in press.
14. Chard RB, Kam CA, Nunn GR, et al: Use of desmopressin in the management of aspirin-related and intractable hemorrhage after cardiopulmonary bypass. Aust NZ J Surg 60:125, 1990.
15. Coppe D, Sobel M, Seamans L, et al: Preservation of platelet function and number by prostacyclin during cardiopulmonary bypass. J Thorac Cardiovasc Surg 81:274, 1981.
16. Czer L, Bateman T, Gray RJ, et al: Prospective trial of DDAVP in treatment of severe platelet dysfunction and hemorrhage after cardiopulmonary bypass. Circulation 72(Suppl III):111, 1985.
17. Czer LSC, Capon SM: Clinical experience in disorders of haemostasis. Drug Invest 2(Suppl 5):32, 1990.
18. DeLaval ME, Hill JD, Mielke CH, et al: Blood platelets and extracorporeal circulation. J Thorac Cardiovasc Surg 69:144, 1975.
19. DiMichele DM, Hathaway WE: Use of DDAVP in inherited and acquired platelet dysfunction. Am J Hematol 33:39, 1990.
20. Ditter H, Heinrich D, Matthias FR, et al: Effects of prostacyclin during cardiopulmonary bypass in men on plasma levels of beta-thromboglobulin, platelet factor 4, thromboxane B_2, 6-keto prostaglandin F_1 alpha and heparin. Thromb Res 32:393, 1983.
21. Edmunds LH, Ellison N, Colman RW, et al: Platelet function during cardiac operation: Comparison of membrane and bubble oxygenators. J Thorac Cardiovasc Surg 83:805, 1982.
22. Friedenberg WR, Myers WO, Plotke ED, et al: Platelet dysfunction associated with cardiopulmonary bypass. Ann Thorac Surg 25:298, 1978.
23. George JN, Pickett EB, Saucerman S, et al: Platelet surface glycoproteins: Studies on resting and activated platelets and platelet membrane microparticles in normal subjects and observations in patients during adult respiratory distress syndrome and cardiac surgery. J Clin Invest 78:340, 1986.
24. Ghirardini A, Chistolini A, Tirindelli MC, et al: Clinical evaluation of subcutaneously administered DDAVP. Thromb Res 49:363, 1988.
25. Grant PJ: Regulation of haemostasis: The role of arginine vasopressin. In Mariani G, Mannucci PM, Cattaneo M (eds): Desmopressin in Bleeding Disorders. London, Plenum Publishing, 1993, in press.
26. Hackmann T, Gascoyne RD, Naiman SC, et al: A trial of desmopressin (1-deamino-8-D-arginine vasopressin) to reduce blood loss in uncomplicated cardiac surgery. N Engl J Med 321:1437, 1989.
27. Harker LA, Malpass TW, Branson HE, et al: Mechanism of abnormal bleeding in patients undergoing cardiopulmonary bypass: Acquired transient platelet dysfunction associated with selective alpha-granule release. Blood 56:824, 1980.
28. Harker LA: Bleeding after cardiopulmonary bypass. N Engl J Med 314:1446, 1986.
29. Hedderich GS, Petsikas DJ, Cooper BA, et al: Desmopressin acetate in uncomplicated coronary artery bypass surgery: A prospective randomized clinical trial. Can J Surg 33:33, 1990.
30. Israels SJ, Kobrinski NL: Serious reaction to desmopressin in a child with cyanotic heart disease. N Engl J Med 32:1563, 1989 [letter].
31. Johnson RG, Murphy JM: The role of desmopressin in reducing blood loss during lumbar fusion. Surgery 171:223, 1990.
32. Kobrinski NL, Israel ED, Gerrard JM, et al: Shortening of bleeding time by 1-deamino-8-D-arginine vasopressin in various bleeding disorders. Lancet 1:1145, 1984.
33. Kobrinski NL, Letts M, Patel LR, et al: 1-desamino-8-D-arginine vasopressin (Desmopressin) decreases operative blood loss in patients having Harrington rod spinal fusion surgery. Ann Intern Med 107:446, 1987.
34. Lazenby WD, Russo I, Zadeh BJ, et al: Treatment with desmopressin acetate in routine coronary artery bypass surgery to improve hemostasis. Circulation 82(Suppl IV):413, 1990.

35. Levi M, de Boer JP, Roem D, et al: Plasminogen activation in vivo upon intravenous infusion of DDAVP: Quantitative assessment of plasmin-2-antiplasmin complex with a novel monoclonal antibody based radioimmunoassay. Thromb Haemost 67:111, 1992.
36. LoCicero J, Massad M, Matano J: Effect of desmopressin acetate on hemorrhage without identifiable cause in coronary bypass patients. Am J Surg 57:165, 1991.
37. Longmore DS, Bennett G, Gueirra D, et al: Prostacyclin: A solution to the problems of extracorporeal circulation. Lancet 1:1002, 1979.
38. Lusher JM, Miller E, Wiseman CH, et al: Use of highly concentrated intranasal spray formulation of desmopressin in persons with congenital bleeding disorders. In Mariani G, Mannucci PM, Cattaneo M (eds): Desmopressin in Bleeding Disorders. London, Plenum Publishing, 1993, in press.
39. MacGregor IR, Roberts E, Prowse CV, et al: Changes in plasma t-PA, PAI and factor VIII following I.V. and S.C. injection of DDAVP in healthy volunteers. Thromb Haemost 58:366, 1987 [abstract].
40. Malpass TW, Hanson SR, Savage B, et al: Prevention of acquired transient defect in platelet plug formation by infused prostacyclin. Blood 57:736, 1981.
41. Mammen EF, Koets MH, Washington BC, et al: Hemostatic changes during cardiopulmonary by-pass surgery. Semin Thromb Hemost 11:727, 1985.
42. Mannucci PM, Aberg M, Nilsson IM, et al: Mechanism of plasminogen activator and factor VIII increase after vasoactive drugs. Br J Haematol 30:81, 1975.
43. Mannucci PM, Canciani MT, Rota L, et al: Response of factor VIII/vWF to DDAVP in healthy subjects and patients with hemophilia A and von Willebrand disease. Br J Haematol 47:283, 1981.
44. Mannucci PM, Vicente V, Vianello L, et al: Controlled trial of desmopressin (DDAVP) in liver cirrhosis and other conditions associated with a prolonged bleeding time. Blood 67:1148, 1986.
45. Mariani G, Ciavarella N, Mazzucconi MG, et al: Evaluation of the effectiveness of DDAVP in surgery and in bleeding episodes in haemophilia and von Willebrand's disease. A study on 43 patients. Clin Lab Haematol 229, 1984.
46. Mayadas TN: Von Willebrand factor and P-selectin targeting to and release from endothelial cell-specific storage granules. In Mariani G, Mannucci PM, Cattaneo M (eds): Desmopressin in Bleeding Disorders. London, Plenum Publishing, 1993, in press.
47. McKenna R, Bachmann F, Whittaker B, et al: The hemostatic mechanism after open heart surgery. II. Frequency of abnormal platelet functions during and after extracorporeal circulation. Thorac Cardiovasc Surg 70:298, 1975.
48. Mohr R, Golan M, Martinowitz U, et al: Effect of cardiac operation on platelets. J Thorac Cardiovasc Surg 92:434, 1986.
49. Musial J, Niewiarowski S, Dershosk D, et al: Loss of fibrinogen receptors from the platelet surface during simulated extracorporeal circulation. J Lab Clin Med 105:514, 1985.
50. Nuutinen LS, Mononen P: Dipyridamole and thrombocyte count in open heart surgery. J Thorac Cardiovasc Surg 70:707, 1975.
51. Rocha E, Llorens R, Paramo JA, et al: Does desmopressin acetate reduce blood loss after surgery in patients on cardiopulmonary bypass? Circulation 77:1319, 1988.
52. Rocha E, Llorens R, Paramo JA: Desmopressin and surgical hemostasis. N Engl J Med 322:1563, 1990 [letter].
53. Rocha E, Paramo JA, Llorens R, et al: Desmopressin in cardiac surgery with extracorporeal circulation. In Mariani G, Mannucci PM, Cattaneo M (eds): Desmopressin in Bleeding Disorders. London, Plenum Publishing, 1993, in press.
54. Salzman EW, Weinstein MJ, Weintraub RM, et al: Treatment with desmopressin acetate to reduce blood loss after cardiac surgery: A double-blind randomized trial. N Engl J Med 314:140, 1986.
55. Salzman EW: Desmopressin and surgical hemostasis. N Engl J Med 322:1085, 1990 [letter].
56. Sears MD, Wadsworth LD, Rogers PC, et al: The effect of desmopressin acetate (DDAVP) on postoperative blood loss after cardiac operations in children. J Thorac Cardiovasc Surg 98:217, 1990.
57. Seremitis SV, Aledort LM: Nasal spray desmopressin: Laboratory and clinical implications. In Mariani G, Mannucci PM, Cattaneo M (eds): Desmopressin in Bleeding Disorders. London, Plenum Publishing, 1993, in press.
58. Shulman S: The effectiveness of desmopressin in patients with disorders of primary haemostasis. In Mariani G, Mannucci PM, Cattaneo M (eds): Desmopressin in Bleeding Disorders. London, Plenum Publishing, 1993, in press.

59. Sloand EM, Sloand J, Kessler C, et al: Loss of glycoprotein Ib from platelets on hemodialysis (HD) or cardiopulmonary bypass (CABG) is followed by its re-expression on the platelet membrane. Blood 78:388a, 1991.
60. Sloand EM, Kessler CM, Sloand J, et al: DDAVP corrects the platelet dysfunction produced by cardiopulmonary by-pass, hemodialysis and prolonged storage: Re-expression of glycoprotein Ib on the platelet membrane. In Mariani G, Mannucci PM, Cattaneo M (eds): Desmopressin in Bleeding Disorders. London, Plenum Publishing, 1993, in press.
61. Walker ID, Davidson JF, Faichney A, et al: A double blind study of prostacyclin in cardiopulmonary bypass surgery. Br J Haematol 49:415, 1981.
62. Wachtfogel YT, Musial J, Jenkin S, et al: Loss of platelet $alpha_2$-adrenergic receptors during simulated extracorporeal circulation prevention with prostaglandin E1. J Lab Clin Med 105:119, 1985.
63. Weinstein M, Ware JA, Troll J, et al: Changes in von Willebrand factor during cardiac surgery: Effect of desmopressin acetate. Blood 71:1648, 1988.
64. Wenger RK, Lukasicwicz H, Mikuta BS, et al: Loss of platelet fibrinogen receptors during clinical cardiopulmonary bypass. J Thorac Cardiovasc Surg 97:235, 1989.

Chapter 12

Management of Patients with Acute Myocardial Infarction Who Require Cardiac Surgery after Failed Thrombolysis

Alan W. Heldman, M.D., and William R. Bell, Jr., M.D.

Thrombolytic drug therapy has become established in the past decade as standard treatment for acute transmural myocardial infarction (MI) and is also used to treat thrombotic coronary and graft occlusion in patients without acute MI. Some patients require emergency cardiac surgery in these settings; their management is detailed herein. Patients in the thrombolytic state are at increased risk for bleeding complications, in addition to the other risks of emergency surgery. The need for transfusion of blood products (with the potential for complications from transmissable disease), prolonged or difficult surgery, and morbidity or mortality may result from the drug-induced coagulopathy. Selection of patients for emergency operation should integrate a knowledge of these risks with the potential for reducing infarct size, stabilizing hemodynamic compromise, and providing definitive therapy for severe multi-vessel coronary disease. For the cardiologist, anesthesiologist, and cardiothoracic surgeon, an understanding of the mechanisms of drug-induced changes in coagulation and of their correction is indispensable.

A number of large clinical trials have demonstrated the value of appropriately administered thrombolytic treatment for acute MI. Most commonly, these drugs are given intravenously to patients with transmural infarction who present within 4-6 hours of the onset of ischemia. Benefit of thrombolytic treatment is not clearly established for nontransmural infarcts or for patients presenting after many hours or days of ischemia.

MECHANICAL REVASCULARIZATION FOLLOWING THROMBOLYTIC THERAPY

Clinical trials of mechanical revascularization as a complement to thrombolytic therapy for acute MI or after attempted thrombolysis has failed have demonstrated limited application for percutaneous transluminal coronary angioplasty (PTCA) and for coronary artery bypass grafting (CABG). Mathey[22] reported additional benefit from early surgical revascularization after thrombolysis with the use of intracoronary streptokinase. In the current era, with intravenous thrombolytic therapy the norm, the strategy of immediate PTCA after administration of recombinant tissue plasminogen activator (r-TPA) has been examined in three trials.[28,31-33] In each, immediate angioplasty did not improve left ventricular (LV) function but did increase complications, notably blood transfusion and emergency CABG, which was required in 3-7% of patients treated with r-TPA and immediate PTCA. Angioplasty revascularization may be beneficial for patients with a persistently occluded vessel after failed thrombolysis. Emergency CAGB, used for failed sequential thrombolytic therapy and PTCA in the Thrombolysis and Angioplasty in Acute MI (TAMI) trial, was associated with significant improvement in LV function.[17,18]

Most patients with acute MI can be managed conservatively. Urgent catheterization and revascularization with PTCA or CABG were tested as strategies for recurrent ischemia or hemodynamic instability after thrombolytic therapy in the TAMI-V study.[23] A small number of patients initially assigned to a conservative strategy required early catheterization, and a small number of those required emergency CABG.

In our experience, consultation for emergency coronary operation despite recent thrombolytic therapy is requested for patients in whom (1) thrombolytic therapy for acute MI has failed, and multivessel coronary disease is known or suspected; (2) thrombolytic therapy and PTCA for acute MI have failed; or (3) PTCA, with adjunctive intracoronary thrombolytic therapy for angiographically visualized coronary thrombus, has failed. In each situation, surgical risk is increased over that for elective operation. In one study,[6] emergency coronary surgery (defined by its use for refractory ongoing ischemia) carried a 15% operative mortality; the subgroup taken directly to the operating room from the catheterization laboratory suffered only a 4% mortality rate, whereas patients brought from the ward or intensive care unit suffered a significantly higher mortality rate of 22.4%.

In another study,[21] patients undergoing emergency operation within 12 hours of receiving 1.5 million units of intravenous streptokinase had a mean blood loss 2½ times greater than patients undergoing emergency operation without thrombolytic therapy for acute MI. Bleeding and the need for reexploration decreased in patients whose surgery was deferred for more than 12 hours. In a metaanalysis, the operative mortality after thrombolysis (2.8%) was similar to that for emergency operation after failed angioplasty (3.6%) and to that for emergency operation in acute MI (4.9%).[1]

THROMBOLYTIC DRUGS

The thrombolytic drugs in current clinical use are streptokinase (SK), urokinase (UK), anisoylated plasminogen-streptokinase activator complex (APSAC), and recombinant tissue plasminogen activator (r-TPA). These drugs are quite similar in their effect on the coagulation system. The initially hoped-for fibrin clot specificity of r-TPA has not been realized. All coagulation proteins are affected; the depletion of fibrinogen may persist longer with SK and

APSAC than with r-TPA and UK,[25] but bleeding complicates treatment with all drugs of this class.[30] Most bleeding occurs at sites of vascular puncture, and until coagulation is restored, invasive procedures should be avoided if possible. Because streptokinase and APSAC are antigenic, neither should be given to a patient who has been previously treated with either in the previous 6 months.

Intracranial hemorrhage, the most feared complication of thrombolytic therapy, is often devastating. If suspected, all thrombolytic, anticoagulant, and antiplatelet drugs must be stopped, and coagulation should be restored. A computerized tomographic scan of the brain and neurosurgical consultation are needed; surgical decompression has also been used.[8]

ANTICOAGULANT AND ANTIPLATELET DRUGS

Adjunctive anticoagulant and antiplatelet therapy is an important part of coronary care, and patients needing emergency CABG can be expected to have received, besides thrombolytics, a number of other medications affecting coagulation. Aspirin was shown to reduce mortality in acute MI in the ISIS-2 study.[15] Aspirin irreversibly acetylates platelet cyclooxygenase, inhibiting platelet aggregation and thus impairing a normal mechanism of rapid hemostasis. This effect can last for up to 2 weeks after aspirin is stopped. Aspirin and other causes of platelet dysfunction prolong the bleeding time.

Studies have shown that aspirin does[2] or does not[26] cause increased surgical bleeding complications. Aspirin has been shown to improve survival after CABG,[16] probably by a beneficial effect on graft patency.[10] However, in the special case of emergency surgery soon after thrombolytic therapy, discontinuing or withholding aspirin seems prudent once the decision is made to operate.

Intravenous heparin is also given to patients with unstable angina and acute MI. Potential benefits of heparin anticoagulation include the stabilization of coronary thrombi and the prevention of mural thrombi, systemic embolism, venous thrombi, and pulmonary embolism. The activated partial thromboplastin time (aPTT) is the usual test for monitoring heparin therapy; the activated clotting time (ACT) is also used. Heparin therapy should not complicate emergency cardiac surgery; its anticoagulant effects significantly diminish within 90 minutes of discontinuation. However, ongoing heparin therapy can make more difficult the laboratory assay of the degree of thrombolytic drug-induced fibrinolysis. Fortunately, there are ways to solve this problem, as discussed below.

Some patients with acute MI receive oral anticoagulant therapy with warfarin, including patients with chronic atrial fibrillation, mechanical prosthetic valves, recent prior transmural anterior MI, and a history of thromboembolic disease. The prothrombin time (PT) is prolonged by warfarin. Prolongation of the PT can be corrected with fresh frozen plasma transfusion or with aquamephyton (vitamin K_1), as detailed below.

EVALUATION BEFORE OPERATION

When emergency surgery is to be undertaken in a patient who has recently received a thrombolytic drug, the coagulation system must be carefully and completely evaluated. The PT and aPTT are measured. These tests are prolonged by thrombolytic agents; however, when heparin is present, it is impossible to distinguish whether heparin or the thrombolytic is responsible for prolongation of the aPTT. Heparin can be continued until shortly before operation; in this setting, the concentration of fibrinogen is the most important measure of the persistence of thrombolytic effect. A number of assays for fibrinogen are available[24]; however, we favor using a kit with antibody directed against human fibrinogen, which accurately quantifies plasma fibrinogen in the presence of heparin (American Biogenetic Sciences, Inc., Copiague, NY). The reptilase time and the Arvin time are also tests that can identify persistent depletion of fibrinogen in a heparinized patient. The Arvin time, which uses ancrod as the in vitro coagulant, is unaffected by heparin therapy.[3] The ACT is used to monitor heparin therapy in many catheterization laboratories and operating rooms; like the aPTT, the ACT is prolonged by thrombolytic therapy as well as by heparin.

The PT may be prolonged by thrombolytic drugs; however, oral anticoagulant therapy, vitamin K deficiency, and liver disease with synthetic failure also prolong the PT. If any of these conditions is known or suspected, specific therapy should be given, as detailed below.

The thrombin time (TT) is used to monitor thrombolytic therapy when long courses of treatment (12–72 hours) are planned (e.g., vascular thrombosis or pulmonary embolism). For the brief therapy used in acute MI, TT monitoring is not required and may delay therapy.

Platelet number should be evaluated wth an automated complete blood count, and thrombocytopenia should be confirmed by visual inspection of the blood smear to distinguish spuriously low values caused by platelet clumping. Thrombolytic drugs can cause thrombocytopenia.[25] In the clinical setting, platelet function is usually evaluated with the bleeding time. Because the bleeding time is also prolonged by the fibrinolytic state,[11] however, it is best measured after adequate replacement therapy, as determined by the fibrinogen assay. Aspirin prolongs the bleeding time; platelet transfusion may be required if the bleeding time remains dramatically prolonged after repletion of fibrinogen. Other drugs used in acute coronary care, including nitroglycerin[5] and calcium channel blockers,[34] may also have antiplatelet effects.

A complete blood count also includes the hematocrit value, which is useful as a baseline in case of bleeding. Appropriate specimens of blood should also be sent to the blood bank so that crossmatching can be performed before surgery.

RESTORING COAGULATION

Once a decision is made for emergency surgery, no further thrombolytic drugs should be given. The duration of the drug-induced coagulopathy varies, depending on the type and amount of drug given. As noted, small doses of intracoronary thrombolytics may produce only a modest coagulopathy, as demonstrated by mild prolongation of the aPTT and TT and by a normal concentration of fibrinogen.

Large doses of thrombolytics, systemically administered, produce a more spectacular derangement of the coagulation studies, and the concentration of fibrinogen is decreased. If the fibrinogen is <75-100 mg/dl, cryoprecipitate should be given for replacement. One bag of cryoprecipitate (defined as the amount that contains 80-100 units of factor VIII) raises the concentration of fibrinogen by 5-7 mg/dl in a 70-kg patient. Cryoprecipitate should be rapidly available from the blood bank. After transfusion, the concentration of fibrinogen should again be determined, with the goal of attaining a level >100 mg/dl. In addition to fibrinogen, factors VIII and XIII and plasminogen are supplied by cryoprecipitate.

If antiplatelet drugs have been given, a template bleeding time should be measured after repletion of fibrinogen. If the bleeding time is markedly prolonged (>10-12 minutes), then platelet transfusion may be advisable. Similarly, if thrombocytopenia is present, platelets should be given. One bag of platelet concentrate typically produces a 10,000/ml rise in the platelet count. In aspirin treated patients who have a prolonged bleeding time, 25% of the total platelet mass should be replaced with fresh platelets obtained from aspirin-free donors (approximately 6 bags of platelet concentrate) to restore near-normal function.

In a dog model, prolongation of the bleeding time by r-TPA was potentiated by aspirin; this effect, along with the bleeding tendency, was inhibited by aprotinin, a serine protease inhibitor and antifibrinolytic agent.[9] Aprotinin has been found to reduce blood loss in routine coronary surgery[4] and has been used for emergency operation after intracoronary streptokinase with apparently good results.[7] In early clinical trials, the drug has been well tolerated, although a serious allergic reaction is reported in at least 1 patient who had been previously exposed to the drug. Aprotinin appears to be a promising drug for reducing blood loss in high-risk cardiac surgery, including surgery after thrombolytic therapy. However, the risks of graft thrombosis or of reocclusion of the infarct vessel may be increased; this possibility bears careful evaluation.

The other antifibrinolytic drugs in use are tranexamic acid[12] and epsilon-aminocaproic acid (EACA). We use EACA, which has the shorter half-life, in settings of severe hypofibrinogenemia, in cases in which there is a platelet problem as well as an active fibrinolytic state or when there is no time to confirm adequate replacement therapy before surgery. EACA is given intravenously or orally; for adult patients, the initial dose of 5 g is followed by 2 g every 4 hours. The doses of EACA and tranexamic acid are reduced in the presence of renal or hepatic dysfunction. In critically ill patients, disseminated intravascular coagulopathy (DIC) contraindicates treatment with antifibrinolytic drugs, which may result in vascular thrombosis.

When warfarin anticoagulation has been given or when vitamin K deficiency is present, aquamephyton (vitamin K_1), administered intravenously (10 mg over 2 minutes or more), can usually reverse vitamin K-dependent anticoagulation within 24-48 hours if liver function is normal. Reinstitution of warfarin anticoagulation may be more difficult afterwards; transmural anterior infarction, ventricular aneurysm, atrial fibrillation, and valve replacement may mandate postoperative anticoagulation. Patients with a strong need for anticoagulation (for example, those with recurrent thromboembolism) should receive intravenous heparin while waiting for reversal or restoration of oral anticoagulation.

When the PT is prolonged because of liver disease, vitamin K may not normalize coagulation. Infusion of fresh frozen plasma (FFP) rapidly corrects the defects caused by depletion of vitamin K-dependent factor and by liver disease, but its effect lasts only a few hours; repeated infusions are required. FFP is also used when a PT prolonged by warfarin must be corrected immediately, as for truly emergent surgery.

Besides clotting factors, it may also be necessary to transfuse red blood cells before, during, or after surgery. The intravascular volume load applied by these measures can easily cause or worsen pulmonary edema, especially in patients with LV dysfunction. Careful attention to fluid management is mandatory, and pulmonary artery catheterization should be considered for patients with LV dysfunction. As with the arterial puncture site for coronary angiography and angioplasty, the site for central venous catheterization must be selected with care in patients with coagulopathy; a compressible site is always preferable. For the central venous catheter, a brachial venous approach is best, and the jugular vein is preferred over the noncompressible subclavian vein.

Unanticipated problems with hemostasis during and after cardiac surgery are not infrequent, even with elective surgery. Platelet dysfunction, possibly caused by contact with the membrane oxygenator and roller pumps during cardiopulmonary bypass, is a well-described phenomenon.[19] Desmopressin acetate (DDAVP) was found to reduce blood loss after cardiac surgery[29]; its value remains unclear, however, for routine surgery.[27] DDAVP may be useful for patients pretreated with aspirin.[20] In cases in which thrombolytics have been given and coagulation factors have been repleted with cryoprecipitate and plasma, we treat persistent bleeding with EACA and platelet transfusion. Aprotinin has also been recommended for preventing the platelet dysfunction (and possibly fibrinolysis) that follows cardiopulmonary bypass.[14] Aprotinin artifactually prolongs the ACT, complicating the intraoperative monitoring of heparin while on cardiopulmonary bypass.[34]

With rational analysis of the mechanisms of coagulation and hemostasis and with therapy directed at specific defects, most problems can be solved. The application of these techniques allows preoperative assessment of the risk of bleeding and guides pre-, intra-, and postoperative management of the patient with heart disease.

ACKNOWLEDGMENT

The authors thank R. Scott Stuart, M.D., and Steven P. Schulman, M.D., for helpful reviews of this manuscript.

Supported in part by NIH research grant HL 36260 from the NHLBI of the National Institutes of Health, Bethesda, MD.

REFERENCES

1. Barner HB, Lea JW, Naunheim KS, Stoney WS: Emergency coronary bypass not associated with preoperative cardiogenic shock in failed angioplasty, after thrombolysis, and for acute myocardial infarction. Circulation 79(Suppl I):I-152-159, 1989.
2. Bashein G, Nessly ML, Rice AL, et al: Preoperative aspirin therapy and reoperation for bleeding after coronary artery bypass surgery. Arch Intern Med 151:89-93, 1991.
3. Bell WR, Tomasulo PA, Alving BM, Duffy TP: Thrombocytopenia occurring during the administration of heparin. Ann Intern Med 85:155-160, 1976.

4. Dietrich W, Barankay A, Dilthey G, et al: Reduction of homologous blood requirement in cardiac surgery by intraoperative aprotinin application—clinical experience in 152 cardiac surgical patients. Thorac Cardiovasc Surg 37:92-98, 1989.
5. Diodati J, Theroux P, Latour JG, et al: Nitroglycerin at therapeutic doses inhibits platelet aggregation in man. J Am Coll Cardiol 11:54A, 1988 [abstract].
6. Edwards FH, Bellamy RF, Burge JR, et al: True emergency coronary artery bypass surgery. Ann Thorac Surg 49:603-611, 1990.
7. Efstratiadis T, Munsch C, Crossman D, Taylor K: Aprotinin used in emergency coronary operation after streptokinase treatment. Ann Thorac Surg 52:1320-1321, 1991.
8. Eleff SM, Borel C, Bell WR, Long DM: Acute management of intracranial hemorrhage in patients receiving thrombolytic therapy: Case reports. Neurosurgery 26:867-869, 1990.
9. Garabedian HD, Gold HK, Leinbach RC, et al: Bleeding time prolongation and bleeding during infusion of recombinant tissue-type plasminogen activator in dogs: Potentiation by aspirin and reversal with aprotinin. J Am Coll Cardiol 17:1213-1222, 1991.
10. Gaveghan TP, Gebski V, Baron DW: Immediate post-operative aspirin improves vein graft patency early and late after coronary bypass surgery. A placebo controlled, randomized study. Circulation 83:1526-1533, 1991.
11. Hirsch DR, Goldhaber SZ: Bleeding time and other laboratory tests to monitor the safety and efficacy of thrombolytic therapy. Chest 97(Suppl 4):124S-131S, 1990.
12. Horrow JC, Van Riper DF, Strong MD, et al: Hemostatic effects of tranexamic acid and desmopressin during cardiac surgery. Circulation 84:2063-2070, 1991.
13. Hunt BJ, Segal H, Yacoub M: Monitoring heparin by the activated clotting time when aprotinin is used during cardiopulmonary bypass. Thromb Haemost 65:1025, 1991.
14. Hunt BJ, Yacoub M: Aprotinin and cardiac surgery. Br Med J 303:660-661, 1991.
15. ISIS collaborative group: Randomised trial of intravenous streptokinase, oral aspirin, both, or neither among 17,187 cases of suspected acute myocardial infarction: ISIS-2. Lancet 2(8607):349-360, 1988.
16. Johnson WD, Kayser KL, Hartz AJ, Saedi SF: Aspirin use and survival after coronary bypass surgery. Am Heart J 123:603-608, 1992.
17. Kereiakes DJ, Califf RM, George BS, et al: Coronary bypass surgery improves global and regional left ventricular function following thrombolytic therapy for acute myocardial infarction. TAMI study group. Am Heart J 122:390-399, 1991.
18. Kereiakes DJ, Topol EJ, George BS, et al: Emergency coronary artery bypass surgery preserves global and regional left ventricular function after intravenous tissue plasminogen activator therapy for acute myocardial infarction. J Am Coll Cardiol 11:899-907, 1988.
19. Kirklin JK, Westaby S, Blackstone EH, et al: Complement and the damaging effects of cardiopulmonary bypass. J Thorac Cardiovasc Surg 86:845-857, 1983.
20. Lazenby WD, Russo I, Zadeh BJ, et al: Treatment with desmopressin acetate in routine coronary artery bypass surgery to improve postoperative hemostasis. Circulation 82(Suppl 5):V413-419, 1990.
21. Lee KF, Mandell J, Rankin JS, et al: Immediate versus delayed coronary grafting after streptokinase treatment: Postoperative blood loss and clinical results. J Thorac Cardiovasc Surg 95:216-221, 1988.
22. Mathey DG, Rodewald G, Rentrop P, et al: Intracoronary streptokinase, thrombolytic recanalization and subsequent surgical bypass of remaining atherosclerotic stenosis in acute myocardial infarction: Complementary combined approach affecting reduced infarct size, preventing reinfarction and improving left ventricular function. Am Heart J 102:1194-1202, 1981.
23. Muller DW, Topol EJ, Ellis SG, et al: Determinants of the need for early acute intervention in patients treated conservatively after thrombolytic therapy for acute myocardial infarction. TAMI-5 study group. J Am Coll Cardiol 18:1594-1601, 1991.
24. Palareti G, Maccaferri M, Manotti C, et al: Fibrinogen assays: A collaborative study of six different methods. Clin Chem 37:714-719, 1991.
25. Rao AK, Pratt C, Berke A, et al: Thrombolysis in myocardial infarction (TIMI) trial—phase I: Hemorrhagic manifestations and changes in plasma fibrinogen and the fibrinolytic system in patients treated with recombinant tissue-type plasminogen activator and streptokinase. J Am Coll Cardiol 11:1-11, 1988.
26. Rawitscher RE, Jones JW, McCoy TA, Lindley DA: A prospective study of aspirin's effect on red blood cell loss in cardiac surgery. J Cardiovasc Surg 32:1-7, 1991.
27. Rocha E, Llorens R, Paramo JA, et al: Does desmopressin acetate reduce blood loss after surgery in patients on cardiopulmonary bypass? Circulation 77:1319-1323, 1988.

28. Rogers WJ, Baim DS, Gore JM, et al: Comparison of immediate invasive, delayed invasive, and conservative strategies after tissue-type plasminogen activator. Results of the Thrombolysis in Myocardial Infarction (TIMI) phase II-A trial. Circulation 81:1457–1476, 1990.
29. Salzman EW, Weinstein MJ, Weintraub RM, et al: Treatment with desmopressin acetate to reduce blood loss after cardiac surgery—a double blind randomized trial. N Engl J Med 314:1402–1406, 1986.
30. Sane DC, Califf RM, Topol EJ, et al: Bleeding during thrombolytic therapy for acute myocardial infarction: Mechanisms and management. Ann Intern Med 111:1010–1022, 1989.
31. Simoons ML, Arnold AE, Betriu A, et al: Thrombolysis with tissue plasminogen activator in acute myocardial infarction: No additional benefit from immediate percutaneous coronary angioplasty. Lancet 1(8579):197–202, 1988.
32. The Thrombolysis in Myocardial Infarction (TIMI) research group: Immediate versus delayed catheterization and angioplasty following thrombolytic therapy for acute myocardial infarction. TIMI II-A results. JAMA 260:2849–2858, 1988.
33. Topol EJ, Califf RM, George BS, et al: A randomized trial of immediate versus delayed angioplasty after intravenous tissue plasminogen activator in acute myocardial infarction. N Engl J Med 317:581–588, 1987.
34. Yamada Y, Furui H, Furumichi T, et al: Inhibitory effects of endothelial cells and calcium channel blockers on platelet aggregation. Jpn Heart J 31:201–215, 1990.

Chapter 13

Heparin-induced Thrombocytopenia and Platelet Activation in Cardiovascular Surgery

Harry L. Messmore, M.D., Sucha Nand, M.D., and John Godwin, M.D.

Heparin-induced thrombocytopenia (HIT) is a disorder seen in approximately 5% of all patients receiving heparin. It may be mild and clinically inapparent, or it may be severe and accompanied by serious hemorrhage or thrombosis. Thrombosis frequently involves arteries of medium and large size, results in ischemia of extremities or organs (coronary thrombosis, cerebral artery thrombosis), and occurs in about 0.5% of patients (10% of patients who develop HIT).[39] HIT is immune-mediated and should be distinguished from platelet activation as a nonspecific complication of cardiopulmonary bypass (CPB) surgery in terms of pathogenesis and clinical manifestations.

HIT should also be distinguished from the transient decrease in platelet counts seen in some patients immediately after administration of heparin. Such a reaction is of little or no clinical consequence; no antibody is involved. The mechanism is unclear, but it is likely to result from nonspecific binding of higher-molecular-weight molecules of heparin to platelets and platelet sequestration or removal. Thrombosis does not occur, but bleeding may occur on rare occasions. This acute reversible phenomenon was first described in animals in the 1940s and in humans in 1962.[6,19]

This chapter discusses the clinical features, diagnosis, pathophysiology, treatment, and strategies for prevention of HIT. Although the acute reversible phenomenon was previously called heparin-induced thrombocytopenia, this diagnosis now properly applies only to the delayed-onset, immune-mediated disorder.[37] The pathophysiology and clinical manifestations of nonimmune platelet activation associated with CPB is also discussed below.

HIT was not recognized with any regularity by clinicians until about 1975, 35 years after heparin came into clinical use. In an important study published in 1958 Weissman and Tobin pointed out that heparin therapy could be associated with arterial thromboembolism. They did not note thrombocytopenia, but they observed that the thrombi (most frequently in the aorta) were composed predominantly of platelets and fibrin—so-called white clots. The 10 patients in their study had emboli from the aorta into peripheral arteries with total occlusion of many major vessels.[72] In 1974 Klein and Bell reported disseminated intravascular coagulopathy (DIC) during heparin therapy,[40] and in 1976 Bell reported on 52 patients who were prospectively studied for thrombocytopenia (platelet <100,000) during heparin therapy. Sixteen of the 52 developed thrombocytopenia while receiving bovine lung heparin by continuous infusion. Two patients experienced hemorrhage. No thrombotic complications were reported.[7]

In 1973 Rhodes et al. reported thrombocytopenia and thrombosis in patients receiving heparin. An antibody to platelets, demonstrated by a complement lysis method, persisted for several weeks after heparin was stopped.[6] By 1981 the antibody was known to be IgG.[11,52]

A number of studies demonstrated that the problem was more frequently observed with bovine lung heparin than with porcine heparin, but the frequency was at least 3-5% with porcine mucosal (gut) heparin.[39] The dose and route of administration were not significant factors in development of HIT, but the frequency may be less with the subcutaneous route.[36,39]

Several critical reviews of this syndrome by Ansell and Deykin,[4] Kelton,[37] and Bell[6] during the 1980s helped to bring together results of a number of studies of diagnostic methods for detecting the antibody and management of the patient. A number of substitute drugs were proposed and tested, including low-molecular-weight heparin and heparinoids, snake venom (ancrod), and fibrinolytic agents.[12,18,20,44,46,71]

No complication of drug therapy is more hazardous and dramatic than HIT. At this time, however, we lack effective, readily available substitutes for clinical conditions that require acute or readily reversible anticoagulation.

DIAGNOSIS OF HEPARIN-INDUCED THROMBOCYTOPENIA

The diagnosis of HIT is based on the finding of a platelet count that has decreased by 50% from the pretreatment level or has fallen below $100,000/\mu l$ with no apparent cause other than heparin therapy and has persisted for 2 days or more.[6] The platelet count should be monitored at least every 2 days during therapy. In the majority of cases, the platelet count does not fall before the fifth day. The simultaneous occurrence of venous or arterial thrombosis with thrombocytopenia increases the likelihood that the thrombocytopenia is due to heparin.

When the diagnosis is suspected, heparin should be stopped and blood should be drawn for in vitro testing, preferably after 4-6 hours, when, as a rule, heparin is gone from the blood. If blood is drawn while the patient is heparinized, the laboratory should be made aware of this fact. Heparin can be removed from plasma or serum in the laboratory before testing.[73] Platelet aggregation[36] and serotonin release are the most commonly used tests. The former is easy to perform and avoids radioactive materials. It is highly specific but insensitive, with a high percentage (40-50%) of false negatives. The serotonin-release test is more sensitive but uses radioactive serotonin. In most laboratories a result can be reported within 3 hours of request.[38,65]

Several other methods have been recently reported (Table 1). One or more of these may replace currently used tests. One of the tests (Amiral et al.[1]) is

TABLE 1. Laboratory Testing for Heparin-Induced Thrombocytopenia

Test Method	Authors	Reference
Platelet aggregation	Fratantoni et al.	24
Platelet aggregation	Kelton et al.	36
Serotonin release	Sheridan et al.	65
Elisa (platelet IgG)	Howe et al.	34
Elisa (PF-4 heparin)	Amiral et al.	1
Platelet activation	Greinacher et al.	29

based on the author's finding that platelet factor 4 is the antigen from platelets that binds to heparin to form the antigenic stimulus for antibody production in HIT. This point is of special interest to the discussion of pathophysiology (see below).

Testing the patient's serum or plasma in vitro for antiplatelet activity (aggregation or release reaction) is not essential for diagnosis, but a positive result increases the probability that the thrombocytopenia is heparin-related. A negative test does not exclude the diagnosis, but a positive test confirms the diagnosis with 90–95% certainty. A return of the platelet count to pretreatment levels within 10 days is confirmatory. In some cases the platelet count returns to normal while the patient continues to receive heparin.[6]

False-positive tests may occur if the patient has alloantibodies to platelet antigens or HLA antigens. Testing for platelet aggregation or release reaction when heparin is added to the patient's own platelet-rich plasma (PRP) allows exclusion of alloantibodies as the cause of the aggregation. HLA-matched donor platelets may be used in testing if they are available. False-positive reactions may occur when the donor platelets are aggregated with heparin and normal serum or plasma. In such cases PRP from a different donor must be used for testing.

PATHOPHYSIOLOGY

Much about the pathophysiology of HIT is incompletely understood and controversial despite nearly 20 years of research. The immune nature of the disorder is not in question. HIT is caused by the development in susceptible patients of an antibody that interacts with platelets in the presence of heparin. The nature of the antibody seems unique among drug-induced antiplatelet antibodies because it activates the platelets as well as causes thrombocytopenia. But the nature of the antigenic stimulus for production of HIT antibody, the site(s) of platelet interaction with the antibody, the role of heparin or heparinoids in triggering the interaction of the antibody with platelets, and the mechanism(s) of thrombosis are still an enigma.

HIT Serum Factor-Immunoglobulin

Natelson first called attention to the association of heparin therapy with a severe, persistent thrombocytopenia and demonstrated in vitro reduction of the platelet count after incubation of the patient's PRP with heparin.[58] Not long thereafter, Rhodes demonstrated that the factor responsible for HIT was present in the serum of two patients and that it caused in vitro platelet aggregation in the presence of heparin. He proposed that the factor was an immunoglobulin.[62] Rhodes' method of in vitro platelet aggregation testing with heparin (1 U/ml), patient serum, and control platelets is used, with minor modifications, in many studies of the mechanism of heparin-dependent platelet activation and in diagnostic testing to the present day. Rhodes also observed that higher amounts of heparin (8 U/ml) reduced the heparin-dependent platelet aggregation response. In a series of elegant studies exploring the nature of the interaction of the heparin-dependent serum factor with platelets, Green demonstrated that the factor was stable at 56°C and labile at 100°C; that it was precipitated from plasma by 50% ammonium sulfate; and that it was nondialyzable.[28] These findings are consistent with the chemical properties of an immunoglobulin. Further studies strengthened the concept that the HIT-serum factor was an immunoglobulin,[5,24,69] and direct evidence was provided by repeated isolation of the factor from the IgG fraction of the plasma of patients with HIT by column chromatography and immunopurification methods.[14,15,38]

The Antigen and the Antibody

Heparin is weakly immunogenic, and immunologic reactions are unusual.[24] The nature of the antigen(s) with which HIT-dependent antibodies react is of considerable interest; it has been difficult, however, to determine if HIT-dependent antibodies react with free heparin, heparin-platelet complexes, or platelet membrane proteins that are neoantigens. Heparin interacts by an electrostatic mechanism with several proteins and has been reported to associate with immunoglobulin.[25,49] Most studies have not detected a specific immune interaction of HIT-dependent antibodies with free heparin. Green was unable to demonstrate the binding of radiolabeled heparin to the immunoglobulin fraction of HIT plasma.[28] However, Cines found a two- to threefold increase over control IgG in radiolabeled heparin bound to partially purified IgG from patients with HIT.[15] He could not eliminate the possibility that the reaction was nonspecific, resulting from ionic interaction of a highly charged heparin component and unspecified HIT IgG components.

Several investigators have proposed that HIT-dependent antibodies bind directly to platelets or to platelet-heparin complexes. Lynch and Howe showed that HIT sera incubated with fixed platelets produced mildly elevated platelet surface-bound immunoglobulin; immunoglobulin binding was markedly enhanced by coincubation of sera with heparin.[47] In addition, they studied the platelet antigens that interacted with HIT-dependent antibodies. Solubilized platelet proteins were separated by SDS-PAGE, then transferred to nitrocellulose strips (Western blot). HIT sera in the presence of heparin showed binding to platelet proteins of 180, 124, and 82 kd. These platelet antigens were determined to be surface membrane components by iodination studies of intact platelets,[47] but none is the platelet Fc receptor (40 kd).[44] The level of immunoglobulin from HIT sera bound to these antigens in the absence of heparin was low, but normal sera did not bind to the antigens with or without heparin. Heparin has been shown to bind to unactivated normal platelets,[64] to gel-filtered and activated platelets,[33] and to Bernard-Soulier and Glanzmann's platelets.[33] Using the Western Blot technique, Lynch and Howe showed that radiolabeled heparin bound to the same 180, 124, and 82 kd proteins as HIT sera.[47] These platelet membrane sites may not be specific for heparin, for Horne has shown that highly charged polysaccharides inhibit the binding of heparin to platelets.[32] These observations are also consistent with data from Green, who was able to remove the heparin-dependent platelet aggregation reaction by preincubation of HIT sera with washed platelets exposed to heparin but not with washed platelets alone.[28]

Role of the Platelet in the HIT Immune Reaction

The antibodies associated with quinidine-induced thrombocytopenia do not lyse platelets from patients with Bernard-Soulier syndrome (BSS) (lack of platelet membrane glycoproteins Ib-IX and V).[43] These antibodies react with the GPIb complex of human platelets. On the other hand, HIT-dependent antibodies react with both BSS platelets and Glanzmann platelets.[12,38] Several lines of evidence support the role of the platelet Fc receptor in the HIT-dependent antibody interaction. Kelton demonstrated that normal human and goat IgG Fc fragments inhibit the platelet release reaction of HIT-dependent antibodies. The platelet release reaction can also be inhibited by F(ab')$_2$ from HIT sera but not from normal sera.[38] Castaldi demonstrated that rabbit IgG and its purified Fc fragments strongly inhibit platelet aggregation induced by HIT-dependent antibody.[9] Rabbit IgG interacts strongly with the human platelet Fc receptor. Several investigators have shown that the interaction of HIT-dependent antibodies and platelets can be blocked by a monoclonal antibody, IV.3, to the FcγRII receptor.[2,13,38]

The role of the GPIb complex in the receptor in HIT-dependent antibody platelet interaction appears to be indirect. Messmore and colleagues have shown that a monoclonal antibody to GPIb blocks platelet aggregation (MOAB SZ2) induced by HIT-dependent antibody and that heparin inhibits the binding of asialo von Willebrand's factor (vWF) to platelets.[53] Yet BSS platelets demonstrate platelet release induced by HIT-dependent antibody. Chong showed that a monoclonal antibody to GPIb inhibited the HIT-dependent platelet release reaction of normal platelets but not BSS platelets.[13] He also suggested an explanation for this paradox: the close proximity of GPIb to the Fc receptor[55] results in stearic hindrance by anti-GPIb antibodies to the Fc receptor interaction of HIT-dependent antibodies.

The nature of platelet activation by HIT-dependent antibodies is still incompletely understood. The role of complement in platelet activation has not been studied frequently, but complement appears to be necessary for the reaction. Cines has shown that partially purified HIT-IgG did not induce platelet release reaction in the absence of plasma or in C4-deficient plasma.[15] Similarly Chong has shown complement dependence for platelet aggregation induced by HIT-dependent antibody.[10] Heparin's role in triggering the reaction may be nonspecific. Heparin potentiates the interaction of HIT-IgG with the FcII receptor, but so may other substances, including dextran sulfate (but not dextran) and salmon sperm DNA[2] as well as epinephrine.[60] Greinacher studied the reaction of HIT sera with different heparins, polysaccharides, and heparinoids.[29] He demonstrated platelet release reaction induced by HIT-dependent antibody with the low-molecular-weight heparins (KABI 2165, Enoxaparin, CY216) and with dextran sulfate and pentosan sulfate. No reaction occurred with ORG 10172, De-n-sulfated heparin, dermatan sulfate, or dextran. Heparin or dextran sulfate bound to beads did not adsorb the HIT-dependent antibodies and prevented heparin-induced platelet release.

Thus the exact nature of the heparin–antibody–platelet interaction is still unknown. Heparin and other charged substances bind to platelets. This initial binding of heparin may trigger a neoantigen on the platelet surface responsible for the production of HIT-dependent antiplatelet antibodies; the antibodies may be directed to a heparin-platelet antigen; or they may react with circulating heparin, as an immune complex. The weight of the evidence supports triggering of platelet aggregation and release by platelet-FcγRII interaction. It is likely that the Fc portion of the HIT-dependent antibodies combines with the FcγRII. Complement is involved in the process of platelet activation by an undefined mechanism.

Heparin also has a role in potentiating or triggering the platelet activation reaction, which appears to be a nonspecific property of many charged substances that bind to platelets. It is unclear whether true heparin–antiheparin antibody immune complexes are circulating or binding to the platelet Fc receptor. Heparin clearly binds to platelets independent of the Fc receptor, and no circulating immune complexes have been demonstrated.[44] A more plausible explanation of the Fc-dependent nature of platelet activation induced by HIT-dependent antibody has been suggested by Anderson,[3] who demonstrated that a platelet's FcγRII can be activated by the Fc portion of antibodies bound to another platelet. He showed that an anti-GPIIb/IIIa monoclonal antibody bound the GPIIb/IIIa of one platelet and the antibody's Fc portion bound to the FcγRII of another platelet in a cell–cell interaction. His model corresponds with many of the features known about platelet activation induced by the HIT-dependent antibody. Thus the circulating immune complex in HIT may be a HIT-dependent antibody bound to platelets by specific F(ab')$_2$ interaction with a heparin-platelet antigen or platelet neoantigen. This platelet–antibody complex then triggers platelet activation by interaction of the Fc portion of the antibody with the FcγRII of another platelet (Fig. 1).

The thrombocytopenia in this disorder is quite variable and does not correlate with the dose of heparin. It is of considerable interest that the time to recovery after discontinuing heparin varies from 2–10 days. Delayed recovery may be due to several factors. The antibody may interact with sulfated glycosaminoglycans (heparan sulfate) on the endothelium, with consumption of platelets at the site of interaction or with partially activated platelets that have a platelet neoantigen on their surface. Recent reports demonstrate that sulfated polysaccharides of certain types can induce an immune reaction to platelets, just like heparin, and that the antibody aggregates platelets in the presence of heparin. Conversely, the heparin-induced antibody causes platelets to be aggregated by sulfated polysaccharides.[23,29] It may be speculated that all highly sulfated polysaccharides can induce a change in the platelet surface that exposes a neoantigen, giving rise to an antibody and an immune reaction.

Thromboembolic Component

Thrombotic and thromboembolic complications are the most devastating injuries produced by heparin. About 25% of the thromboses are venous and 75% are arterial. Mortality is approximately 30%; amputation is necessary in 20% or

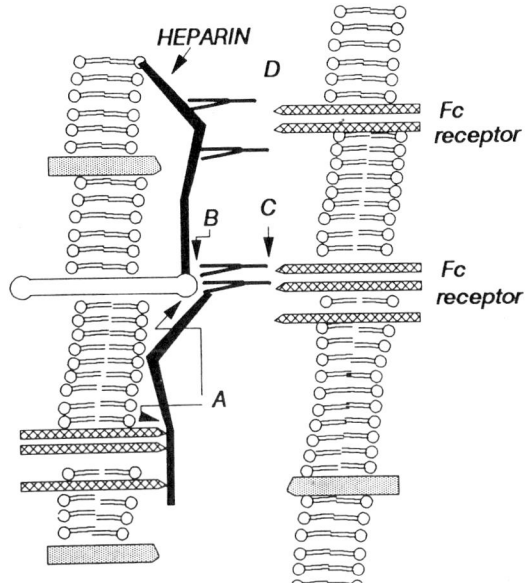

FIGURE 1. HIT-dependent antibody platelet activation. A, Heparin binds to platelets by adherence to specific membrane proteins. B, Heparin binding exposes neoantigens. C, HIT-dependent antibodies bind to heparin-membrane protein or neoantigen complex via specific F (ab')$_2$ interaction. D, The Fc portion of HIT-dependent antibodies interacts with the FcγRII of another platelet, triggering platelet release. The mechanism of activation depends on this cell-cell interaction. Alternatively the binding of HIT-dependent antibodies may be to heparin bound to platelets; this complex interacts with FcγRII receptor of another platelet.

more.[37] Continuation of heparin therapy after the development of thrombosis probably results in even more thromboembolic episodes.

The reason for the predominance of arterial thromboembolism and the predilection of the aorta as the site of the initial thrombus formation in the arterial system is unknown.[33] Some investigators, who routinely examined the aorta with imaging techniques, have shown the development of thrombi in situ in affected patients.[68] We evaluated a similar case that embolized both legs and possibly the coronary arteries (Fig. 2). The patient died from acute MI while the platelet count was still $<50,000/\mu l$. At autopsy the aorta was studded with 1–2-cm sessile thrombi (Fig. 3), which on histologic examination were found to be predominantly platelets and fibrin (Fig. 4).

One might speculate that the thrombi form at sites of atherosclerotic plaques where platelets are already adherent and that the immune reaction at that site induces rapid build-up of a platelet-fibrin thrombus. Alternatively, when platelets are bound to atherosclerotic plaques, they undergo a release reaction, making platelet factor 4 or release-related neoantigens on the platelet surface available to the antibody and heparin simultaneously. This results in an immune reaction with further release of platelet products such as thromboxane A$_2$ and ADP, which recruit more platelets to the site. Therapeutic use of protamine sulfate to interrupt this reaction has not been reported, but it does interrupt the HIT-serum-dependent aggregation of platelets by heparin in vitro[51] and may be useful therapeutically, particularly when thrombosis is occurring.[68]

HIT may recur when heparin is given on subsequent occasions. With repeat courses it frequently occurs earlier than 5 days.[37] The severity of clinical reactions in terms of platelet count or thrombotic complications has been found to be no worse in patients receiving heparin on subsequent occasions than in patients receiving an initial course. An interesting phenomenon is the lack of an immune reaction in some patients who are rechallenged with the

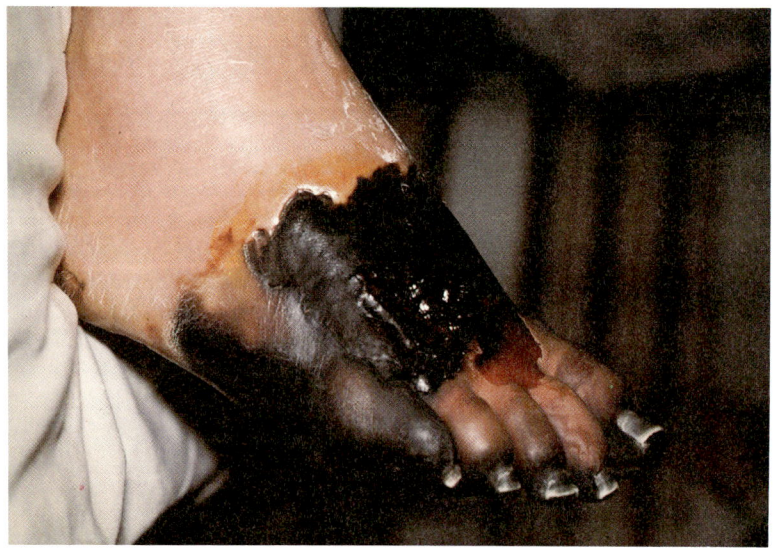

FIGURE 2. Ischemic necrosis of the foot.

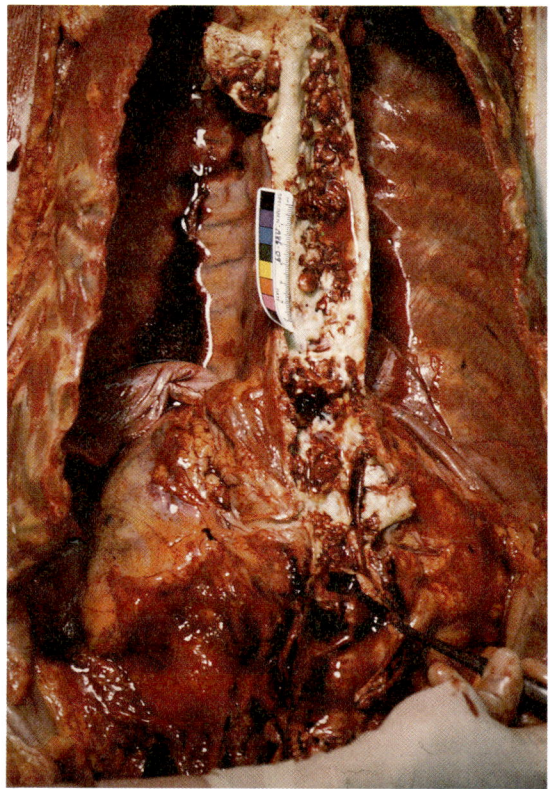

FIGURE 3. Abdominal aorta filled with thrombi.

drug.[37] As mentioned above, the resolution of thrombocytopenia may occur while heparin therapy is being continued.[6]

MANAGEMENT

The decisions to be made after the diagnosis of HIT are complex and may require consultation with a variety of experts. The seriousness of the complications requires immediate cessation of all heparin. A number of pitfalls must be avoided when discontinuation of heparin is ordered. Some patients may have an arterial line that is kept open with heparin. Special effort should be made to see that heparin is stopped in lines and flushes, in addition to stopping the parenteral infusions. Heparin-coated catheters should be avoided.[54] If a patient must have an angiogram or is placed on a balloon pump or hemodialysis, measures to avoid heparin are necessary. A number of clinical approaches may be helpful in avoiding heparin in these circumstances (see below).

The initial question to be answered is whether all anticoagulation can be safely stopped. If so, the solution is easy if no serious bleeding or thrombotic complications have occurred. If anticoagulation must be continued, Coumadin should be substituted if thrombocytopenia is of modest degree and thrombosis is absent. In the presence of hemorrhage or thrombosis, the heparin must be stopped.[6,37] If anticoagulation must be continued for a particular reason, a substitute drug may be advised. Much of the literature in this regard is necessarily anecdotal, and substitute drugs must be used with caution because of the uncertainty of effectiveness and side effects. Several of the more common indications for anticoagulation are listed below, along with possible substitute agents.

Massive Deep Vein Thrombosis With or Without Pulmonary Embolism. Thrombolytic agents such as streptokinase or urokinase may be followed by warfarin.[18,42] If thrombolytic therapy is contraindicated, a heparinoid such as Lomoparan,[12] a snake venom (ancrod),[20] or hirudin is effective.[57] Dextran has been used for deep vein thrombosis,[6] but when the thrombosis is massive or associated with pulmonary embolism, dextran may fail to block the growth of the thrombus. Each of these agents should be accompanied by warfarin therapy and stopped as soon as the prothrombin time is therapeutic. Low-molecular-weight heparins may also be substituted, provided they are negative in the HIT test.[37,46]

Arterial Thrombosis. Intraarterial thrombolytic agents with or without mechanical probing of the thrombus have been useful when given by infusion for hours or days.[17,22,41] Antiplatelet drugs or warfarin may be useful to prevent rethrombosis.[48] The antiplatelet agents most commonly used in this setting are combinations of aspirin and dipyridamole, Iloprost (an analog of prostacyclin), or all three.[30]

Cardiopulmonary Bypass Surgery. Anticoagulation is mandatory to perform CPB safely. If a patient has a life-threatening problem requiring emergency surgery and has a past diagnosis of HIT, a test for the HIT antibody should be carried out. The patient's own PRP should be tested by the addition of heparin and the results interpreted in comparison with suitable controls. If the test is negative, the patient can probably be placed on bypass long enough for surgery without significant hazard.[59] Postoperative use of heparin is

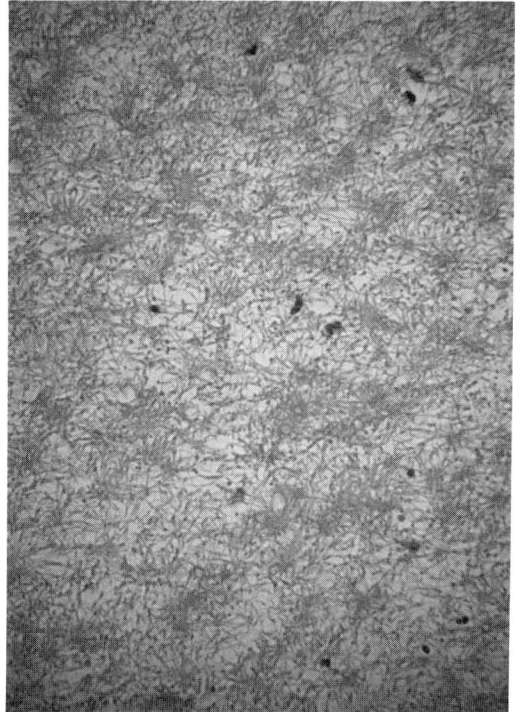

FIGURE 4. Platelet-fibrin thrombus (white clot) from the aorta.

hazardous and should be avoided. The patient does not always respond to a second heparin treatment with antibody formation; in vitro testing is recommended if more heparin therapy is needed.

If the heparin antibody test is positive or if the patient has thrombocytopenia while on heparin (a strong indication that HIT is present), CPB may be performed with a substitute drug. Bypass has been successfully carried out with low-molecular-weight heparin, but the HIT test must be performed first with low-molecular-weight heparin and the patient's serum or by adding the drug to the patient's PRP. If the test is negative, the procedure can probably be performed safely.[71] The drug should not be continued in the postoperative period because of possible antibody formation. Most low-molecular-weight heparins cross-react with the heparin-induced antibody because they contain some molecules of standard heparin. The heparinoid ORG 10172 (Lomoparan) apparently contains little or no heparin. It has been used safely a number of times, but postoperative bleeding has been a problem in some patients. Lomoparan contains heparan sulfate, dermatan sulfate, and a small amount of low-molecular-weight heparin.[67] Interaction with the heparin antibody is much less likely to occur with this drug than with other low-molecular-weight heparins that are commercially produced.[12] One of the problems with ORG 10172 is that it has a relatively long half-life and cannot be completely neutralized with protamine sulfate. Dermatan sulfate was effective in a dog model[8]; the investigators suggested that it may be the ideal agent for this purpose.

Hirudin has been studied in dogs in our laboratories and found to be safe and effective for CPB in this setting.[70] In the near future one of these drugs may be made available for human trial.

Hemodialysis. A number of available drugs permit hemodialysis while circumventing the heparin antibody. Prostacyclin analogs,[45,66] dermatan sulfate,[63] and Lomoparan[31] have been used with good results in the patient with renal failure requiring dialysis. Whenever a glycosaminoglycan is used, the drug should first be tested to make sure it does not aggregate platelets in the presence of the patient's serum or plasma.

Intraaortic Balloon Pumping. We have successfully substituted a low-molecular-weight heparin (CY 216) for heparin in a patient with HIT who needed an IABP for 10 days. During that time the platelet count rose from 70,000/μl to more than 300,000/μl. However, low-molecular-weight heparins cross-react with the HIT antibody. For that reason Lomoparan may be safe, but no trials of the drug for this indication have yet been reported.

NEWER THERAPIES FOR HEPARIN-ASSOCIATED THROMBOCYTOPENIA

Ancrod, derived from the venom of Malayan pit viper, is a rapidly acting defibrinogenating agent. It has been reported to be useful in patients developing HIT.[20] Of 11 treated patients, all had recovery of platelet counts in 2-10 days. Ancrod was started at 1-2 U/kg every 24 hours, and the dose was titrated to keep the fibrinogen level between 0.5-1 g/L. Only 1 patient developed a soft-tissue bleed. These results are promising, but further trials are necessary.

Recombinant hirudin is currently under trial for numerous thrombotic and hypercoagulable states.[21,50] This rapid and specific inhibitor of thrombin acts by forming with thrombin a tight stoichiometric complex. It also inhibits platelet function and prolongs the bleeding time. Initial reports indicate that hirudin may be a safe and effective anticoagulant. No published reports, however, focus on use of hirudin in patients with HIT. A single patient with HIT and bilateral venous thrombosis was treated successfully with hirudin at Loyola University Medical Center.[57]

The use of plasmapheresis and intravenous gammaglobulins in patients with HIT is anecdotal.[27,56] In a patient with thrombosis, these therapies can be used only to reverse the immune mechanism of HIT; anticoagulant or thrombolytic agents are still required.

PREVENTIVE MEASURES

Because HIT is such a devastating problem, it would be wise to avoid heparin, when at all possible, for any purpose. The development of substitute drugs is, therefore, an important priority. Fortunately, a number of substitutes are under investigation, including low-molecular-weight heparin, dermatan sulfate, synthetic thrombin inhibitors, hirudin and hirulogs, natural factor Xa inhibitors, and antiplatelet agents. Until these are available, it would be wise to monitor platelet counts closely in patients on heparin and to avoid its use for more than 5 consecutive days. Patients should be made aware of the fact that they have received heparin therapy, and this information should be included in their medical history.

Nonspecific Platelet Activation During Cardiopulmonary Bypass

In patients placed on CPB, the platelet count is routinely lowered to about 50% because of hemodilution. Further lowering may occur because of binding of platelets to foreign surfaces and activation of platelets with aggregation and release reaction or partial release reaction.[74] When anticoagulation is inadequate, thrombin generation occurs, followed by thrombin-mediated platelet aggregation. Release of ADP from damaged red cells and platelets also causes aggregation and release.

Functionally impaired platelets in the circulation during CPB result in a prolonged bleeding time independent of the lowered platelet count. The causes of this dysfunction are believed to be hypothermia and contact of the platelet with synthetic surfaces.[74] Plasma or urine contain platelet release products such as thromboxane B_2 and platelet factor 4.[74] Platelet alpha granules are depleted, but dense granules are intact in most platelets. The platelet defect can be prevented by infusion of PGE-1 or prostacyclin.

Several possible mechanisms may underlie development of platelet dysfunction, but this phenomenon appears to be of little clinical impact; no correlation of the defect and bleeding has been improved. Prophylactic transfusions of platelets are not indicated. Platelet defects induced by preoperative drugs such as aspirin are an important cause of bleeding and may be remedied by transfusions of intact platelets.[74] Platelet transfusions are a rational approach to bleeding in the presence of thrombocytopenia and/or a defective platelet function.

Desmopressin (des arginine vasopressin) causes release of von Willebrand's factor from the endothelium. It has not been shown to reduce bleeding when used prophylactically in CPB patients. However, it may be useful in patients who bleed postoperatively and have not responded to other measures, particularly if the bleeding time is prolonged.[74]

REFERENCES

1. Amiral J, Bridley F, Dreyfus M, et al: Platelet factor 4 complexed to heparin is the target for antibodies generated in heparin induced thrombocytopenia. Thromb Haemost 68:95-96, 1992.
2. Anderson GP: Insights into heparin-induced thrombocytopenia. Br J Haematol 80:504-508, 1992.
3. Anderson GP, van de Winkel JGJ, Clark L: Anti-GPIIb-IIIa (CD41) monoclonal antibody induced platelet activation requires Fc receptor-dependent cell-cell interaction. Br J Haematol 79:75-83, 1991.
4. Ansell J, Deykin D: Heparin induced thrombocytopenia and recurrent thromboembolism. Am J Hematol 8:325-332, 1980.
5. Babcock RB, Dumper CW, Scharfman WB: Heparin-induced immune thrombocytopenia. N Engl J Med 295:237-241, 1976.
6. Bell WR: Heparin associated thrombocytopenia and thrombosis. J Lab Clin Med 111:600-605, 1988.
7. Bell WR, Tomasulo PA, Alving BM, et al: Thrombocytopenia occurring during the administration of heparin: A prospective study in 52 patients. Ann Intern Med 85:155-160, 1976.

8. Brister SJ, Heigenhauser GJF, Austin J, et al: Dermatan sulfate anticoagulation during cardiopulmonary bypass reduces bleeding and eliminates the need of protamine neutralization. Thromb Haemost 65:863, 1991 [abstract 593].
9. Castaldi PA, Davies PH, Berndt MC: Antiplatelet heparin-dependent antibody interacts with the platelet Fc-receptor. Thromb Haemost 43:61, 1985 [abstract].
10. Chong BH, Grace CS, Rozenberg MC: Heparin induced thrombocytopenia: Effect of heparin platelet antibody on platelet. Br J Haematol 49:531-540, 1981.
11. Chong BH, Pitney WR, Castaldi PA: Heparin-induced thrombocytopenia: Association of thrombotic complications with heparin-dependent IgG antibody that induces thromboxane synthesis and platelet aggregation. Lancet 2:1246-1249, 1982.
12. Chong BH, Ismail F, Cade J, et al: Heparin induced thrombocytopenia: Studies with a new low molecular weight heparinoid, Org 10172. Blood 73:1592-1596, 1989.
13. Chong PL, Fawaz I, Chesterman CN, et al: Heparin-induced thrombocytopenia: Mechanism of interaction of the heparin-dependent antibody with platelets. Br J Haematol 73:235-240, 1989.
14. Cimo PL, Moake JL, Weinger RS, et al: Heparin-induced thrombocytopenia: Association with a platelet aggregating factor and arterial thrombosis. Am J Hematol 6:125-133, 1979.
15. Cines DB, Kaywin P, Bina M, et al: Heparin-associated thrombocytopenia. N Engl J Med 303:788-795, 1980.
16. Cines DB, Tomaski A, Tannenbaum S: Immune endothelial-cell injury in heparin-associated thrombocytopenia. N Engl J Med 316:581-589, 1987.
17. Clifton GD, Smith MD: Thrombolytic therapy in heparin associated thrombocytopenia with thrombosis. Clin Pharmacol 5:597-601, 1986.
18. Cohen JI, Cooper MR, Greenberg CS: Streptokinase therapy of pulmonary emboli with heparin associated thrombocytopenia. Arch Intern Med 145:1725-1726, 1985.
19. Copley AL, Robb TP: Studies on platelets. III. The effect of heparin in vivo on the platelet count in mice and dogs. Am J Clin Pathol 12:563-570, 1942.
20. Demers C, Ginsberg J, Brill-Edwards P, et al: Rapid anticoagulation using ancrod for heparin associated thrombocytopenia. Blood 78:2194-2197, 1991.
21. Editorial. Hirudin: Return of the leech. Lancet 340:579-580, 1992.
22. Fiessinger JN, Aiach M, Roncato M, et al: Critical ischemia during heparin induced thrombocytopenia. Treatment by intraarterial streptokinase. Thromb Res 33:235-238, 1984.
23. Follea G, Hamandjian I, Trzeciak MC, et al: Pentosan polysulphate associated thrombocytopenia. Thromb Res 42:413-418, 1986.
24. Frantantoni JC, Pollet R, Gralnick HR: Heparin-induced thrombocytopenia: Confirmation of diagnosis with in vitro methods. Blood 45:395-401, 1975.
25. Glueck GJ, Kaplan AP, Levy RI, et al: A new mechanism of exogenous hyperglyceridemia. Ann Intern Med 71:1051-1062, 1969.
26. Gollub S, Ulin AW: Heparin-induced thrombocytopenia in man. J Lab Clin Med 59:433-435, 1962.
27. Grau E, Linares M, Angels Alaso M: Heparin induced thrombocytopenia response to intravenous immunoglobulin in vivi and in vitro. Am J Hematol 39:312-313, 1992.
28. Green D, Harris K, Reynolds N, et al: Heparin immune thrombocytopenia: Evidence for a heparin-platelet complex as the antigenic determinant. J Lab Clin Med 91:167-175, 1978.
29. Greinacher A, Michels I, Mueller-Eckhardt C: Heparin associated thrombocytopenia: The antibody is not heparin specific. Thromb Haemost 67:547-549, 1992.
30. Gruel Y, Lermusiaux P, Lang M, et al: Usefulness of antiplatelet drugs in management of heparin associated thrombocytopenia and thrombosis. Ann Vasc Surg 5:552-555, 1991.
31. Henney CHP, ten Cate JW, ten Cate H, et al: Use of a new heparinoid as anticoagulant during acute hemodialysis of patients with bleeding complications. Lancet 1:890-893, 1983.
32. Horne MK: Heparin binding to normal and abnormal platelets. Thromb Res 51:135-144, 1988.
33. Horne MK, Chao ES: Heparin binding to resting and activated platelets. Blood 74:238-243, 1989.
34. Howe SE, Lynch DM: An enzyme-linked immunosorbant assay for the evaluation of thrombocytopenia induced by heparin. J Lab Clin Med 105:554-559, 1985.
35. Hrushesky W: Thrombocytopenia induced by low dose subcutaneous heparin. Lancet ii:1286, 1977.
36. Kelton JG, Sheridan D, Brain H, et al: Clinical usefulness of testing for a heparin-dependent platelet-aggregating factor in patients with suspected heparin-associated thrombocytopenia. J Lab Clin Med 103:606-612, 1984.
37. Kelton JG: Heparin induced thrombocytopenia. Haemostasis 16:173-186, 1986.

38. Kelton JG, Sheridan D, Santos A, et al: Heparin induced thrombocytopenia: Laboratory studies. Blood 72:925-930, 1988.
39. King DJ, Kelton JG: Heparin associated thrombocytopenia. Ann Intern Med 100:535-540, 1984.
40. Klein HG, Bell WR: Disseminated intravascular coagulopathy during heparin therapy. Ann Intern Med 80:477-481, 1974.
41. Koltun WA, Gardiner GA, Harrington DP, et al: Thrombolysis in the treatment of peripheral arterial vascular occlusions. Arch Surg 122:901-905, 1987.
42. Krueger SK, Andres E, Weenand E: Thrombolysis in heparin induced thrombocytopenia with thrombosis. Ann Intern Med 103:159, 1985.
43. Kunicki TJ, Aster RH: Absence of the platelet receptor for drug dependent antibodies in the Bernard-Soulier Syndrome. J Clin Invest 62:716-719, 1978.
44. Kunicki TJ, Newman PJ: The molecular immunology of human platelet proteins. Blood 80:1386-1404, 1992.
45. Leehy DJ, Kanak RJ, Messmore HL, et al: Heparin associated thrombocytopenia in maintenance hemodialysis patients. Int J Artif Organs 10:390-392, 1987.
46. Leroy J, Leclerc MH, Delahousse B, et al: Treatment of heparin-associated thrombocytopenia and thrombosis with low molecular weight heparin (CY216). Semin Thromb Hemost 11:326-329, 1985.
47. Lynch DM, Howe SE: Heparin-associated thrombocytopenia: Antibody binding specificity to platelet antigens. Blood 66:1176-1181, 1985.
48. Makhoul RG, McCann RL, Austin EH, et al: Management of patients with heparin associated thrombocytopenia and thrombosis requiring cardiac surgery. Ann Thorac Surg 43:617-621, 1987.
49. Marciniak E: Binding of heparin in vitro and in vivo to plasma proteins. J Lab Clin Med 84:344-356, 1974.
50. Markwardt F: Hirudin and its derivatives as anticoagulants. Thromb Haemost 66:141-152, 1991.
51. Messmore HL, unpublished observation.
52. Messmore HL, Fareed J, Parvez Z, et al: Studies on the mechanism of heparin-induced thrombocytopenia. Thromb Haemost 46:215, 1981 [abstract 0679].
53. Messmore HL, Griffin B, Koza M, et al: Interaction of heparinoids with platelets: Comparison with heparin and low molecular weight heparins. Semin Thromb Hemost 17(Suppl):57-59, 1991.
54. Moberg PQ, Geary VM, Shiekl FM: Heparin induced thrombocytopenia: A possible complication of heparin-coated pulmonary artery catheters. J Cardiothorac Anesth 4:226-228, 1990.
55. Moore A, Ross GD, Nachman RL: Interaction of platelet membrane receptor with von Willebrand factor, ristocetin, and the Fc region of immunoglobulin G. J Clin Invest 62:1053-1060, 1978.
56. Nand S, Robinson J: Plasmapheresis in the management of heparin associated thrombocytopenia with thrombosis. Am J Hematol 28:204-206, 1988.
57. Nand S, unpublished case, 1992.
58. Natelson EA, Lynch EC, Alfrey CP, et al: Heparin-induced thrombocytopenia: An unexpected response to treatment of consumption coagulopathy. Ann Intern Med 71:1121-1125, 1969.
59. Olinger GN, Hussey CV, Olive JA, et al: Cardiopulmonary bypass for patients with previously documented heparin induced platelet aggregation. J Thorac Cardiovasc Surg 87:673-677, 1984.
60. Pfueller S, David R: Different platelet specifications of heparin-dependent platelet aggregating factors in heparin-associated immune thrombocytopenia. Br J Haematol 64:149-159, 1986.
61. Quick AJ, Shanberge JN, Stefanini M: The effect of heparin on platelets in vivo. J Lab Clin Med 33:1424-1430, 1948.
62. Rhodes GR, Dixon RH, Silver D: Heparin induced thrombocytopenia with thrombotic and hemorrhagic manifestations. Surg Gynecol Obstet 136:409-416, 1973.
63. Ryan FE, Lane DA, Flynn A, et al: Dermatan sulfate (MF 701) in hemodialysis for chronic renal failure. Thromb Haemost 65(Suppl 1):S116, 1991.
64. Shanberge JN, Kambayashi J, Nakagawa M: The interaction of platelets with a tritium-labeled heparin. Thromb Res 9:595-609, 1976.
65. Sheridan D, Carter C, Kelton JG: A diagnostic test in heparin induced thrombocytopenia. Blood 67:27-30, 1986.
66. Smith MC, Kowit D, Crow JW, et al: Prostacyclin substitution for heparin in long-term hemodialysis. Am J Med 73:669-678, 1982.

67. Stiekema JCJ, Wynand HP, Van Dinther TG, et al: Safety and pharmacokinetics of the low molecular weight heparinoid ORG 10172 administered to healthy elderly volunteers. Br J Clin Pharmacol 27:39-48, 1989.
68. Towne JB, Bernhard VM, Hussey C, et al: White clot syndrome: Peripheral vascular complications of heparin therapy. Arch Surg 114:372-377, 1979.
69. Wahl TO, Lipschitz DA, Stechschulte DJ: Thrombocytopenia associated with antiheparin antibody. JAMA 240:2560-2562, 1978.
70. Walenga J, Bakhos M, Messmore HL, et al: Potential use of recombinant hirudin as an anticoagulant in a cardiopulmonary bypass model. Ann Thorac Surg 51:271-277, 1991.
71. Warkentin TE, Kelton JG: Heparin induced thrombocytopenia. Annu Rev Med 40:31-44, 1989.
72. Weismann RE, Tobin RW: Arterial embolism occurring during systemic heparin therapy. Arch Surg 76:219-227, 1958.
73. White MM, Siders L, Jennings LK, et al: The effect of residual heparin on the interpretation of heparin induced platelet aggregation in the diagnosis of heparin associated thrombocytopenia. Thromb Haemost 68:88, 1992.
74. Woodman RC, Harker LA: Bleeding complications associated with cardiopulmonary bypass. Blood 76:1680-1687, 1990.

Chapter 14

Monitoring of Platelet Function in the Cardiovascular Surgery Patient

Ricardo Manrique, M.D.

From the hemostatic point of view, cardiovascular surgery with extracorporeal circulation (ECC) has a different postoperative outcome from similar surgery without ECC. For example, implantation of a coronary bypass graft without ECC seldom has significant bleeding in the postoperative period. However, the same type of surgery with ECC produces a larger loss of blood and the risk of serious bleeding is higher. The implication is clear: artificial heart-and-lung circulation causes the hemostatic changes and the bleeding tendency. In these hemostatic changes platelets play an important role.

Over the past years we have been concerned about how best to monitor hemostatic changes that occur during open-heart surgery with ECC. The specific intent is to detect changes in platelet function, number, or both that could lead to intra- or postoperative hemostatic problems. Moreover, a practical means of monitoring must detect disorders within a short time frame, before they lead to deleterious consequences. Testing must provide early diagnosis, which allows early decision-making and thus avoids complications.

Since 1967 we have been involved with open-heart surgery and hemostatic abnormalities. We have studied open-heart surgery from different standpoints, including preoperative homeostatic diagnosis, type of surgery, type of oxygenator, priming, use of roller pump, dosage of heparin and protamine, and results of laboratory tests. The ultimate objective is to reduce the incidence of bleeding and thrombotic complications.

In the early years of open-heart surgery we mainly studied patients undergoing valve replacement or correction of congenital cardiovascular defects.[9] Our goals were (1) testing of different technical set-ups during open-heart surgery to create a perfusion routine with minimal disruption of hemostasis; (2) prophylaxis of intra- and postoperative bleeding; and (3) with the incorporation of coronary patients, prophylaxis of thrombosis to avoid intraoperative myocardial infarction (MI) and postoperative thromboembolic complications.

Very early we learned that platelets, both number and function, are important parameters in maintaining an optimal ECC procedure. A poorly controlled

ECC induces severe hemostatic alterations with subsequent bleeding. Moreover, the use of large amounts of procoagulant proteins, antifibrinolytic drugs, and platelet concentrates predisposes to thrombosis or disseminated intravascular coagulation (DIC).

HEMOSTATIC ACTIVATION IN EXTRACORPOREAL CIRCULATION

Platelets

Platelets are blood corpuscles adapted to circulate in contact with normal endothelial surfaces. Impelling platelets through nonendothelial, artificial channels modifies their behavior. Physiologically activated platelets become sticky, form aggregates, and adhere to endothelium-free surfaces. During ECC the activation of platelets results from their circulation through nonendothelial, artifical surfaces of the oxygenator, tubing lines, and reservoirs. The nonpulsatile flow of the roller pump and the presence of mechanical and chemical aggression in the circulation are other important factors.[4]

All studies of platelets after cardiopulmonary bypass (CPB) agree that ECC induces changes in platelet number and function.[3,9,13] Well-documented data indicate that activated platelets release their granular content and become exhausted thrombocytes or ghost particles (Fig. 1). These ghost particles become involved in abnormal aggregation phenomena, mainly in the artificial device.[7,25] We have found thrombocyte aggregates in the blood reservoir after CPB or in the blood filter of the arterial line (Fig. 2). When the thrombocytes are hyperreactive, this phenomenon is amplified.[24]

Many observations reveal activation of platelets during ECC, such as increased release of endogenous proteins, platelet factor 4, and β-thromboglobulin.[15] Stable products from activation of the arachidonic acid pathway, thromboxane B_2 are also increased. Electronmicroscopy shows change in platelet shape and degranulation.[14] Platelet functions are also modified, with abnormal responses to activators. This abnormality is related to changes in the structure of the platelet membrane. Glycoproteins (GP) play an important role

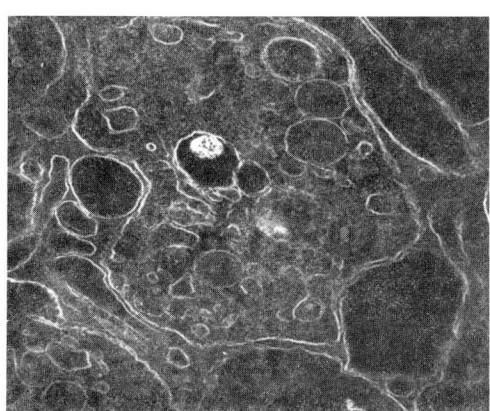

FIGURE 1. Electronmicroscopy of a totally degranulated and exhausted platelet after an 85-minute perfusion time during coronary bypass surgery. Platelet reactivity index before surgery was 301.

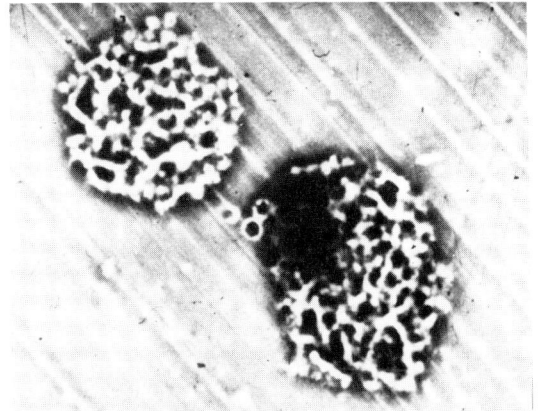

FIGURE 2. Platelet aggregates taken from the oxygenator reservoir after an 82-minute bypass time during coronary bypass surgery. Platelet reactivity index before surgery was 230.

as platelet membrane receptors for specific stimuli. GPs are modified through chemical or physical mechanisms. Decreased activity of GPIb (receptor for von Willebrand's factor) and GPIIb/GPIIIa (receptor for fibrinogen) have been documented, whereas GPIV (receptor for collagen) shows a minimal reduction and can often be hyperactive.[6,17,19,20] This complex pattern of inactivation/activation results from the presence of circulating proteases during ECC.

Vasoactive Substances

Reports indicate that thrombin can reduce the surface expression of GPIb.[8] Plasmin, another protease activated during ECC, has the capacity to modify GPs in platelet membrane.[1,16] Complement fragment C5B-9, which significantly increases during ECC, is also an activator of platelets.[22] High concentrations of bradykinin and kallikrein can damage the vessel wall. All these elements belong to the contact activating system of coagulation. In our opinion such reactions are inherent to the use of large artificial surfaces.

To understand the reason for high levels of these vasoactive substances, one needs to remember that CPB in heart surgery has special characteristics not shared with other applications of ECC. In hemodialysis, artificial hepatic devices, infusion of antitumor drugs, or certain types of cardiovascular support, the amount of blood flowing into the extracorporeal device is a fraction of the total blood volume. In open-heart surgery the entire blood volume is circulated through the pump. Moreover, in heart surgery blood is in contact with open tissues, thus increasing the likelihood of contamination with tissue thromboplastin.

Contact System

The contact of blood with nonendothelial surfaces activates the contact system, a common meeting point of many life-preserving reactions. The activation of factor XII puts into motion a complicated system rich in interactions of the coagulant, inflammatory, fibrinolytic, and immunologic systems, with increased vasodilation and stimulation of permeability-pain mediators. In this complex reaction kininogen is transformed into bradykinin and prekallikrein

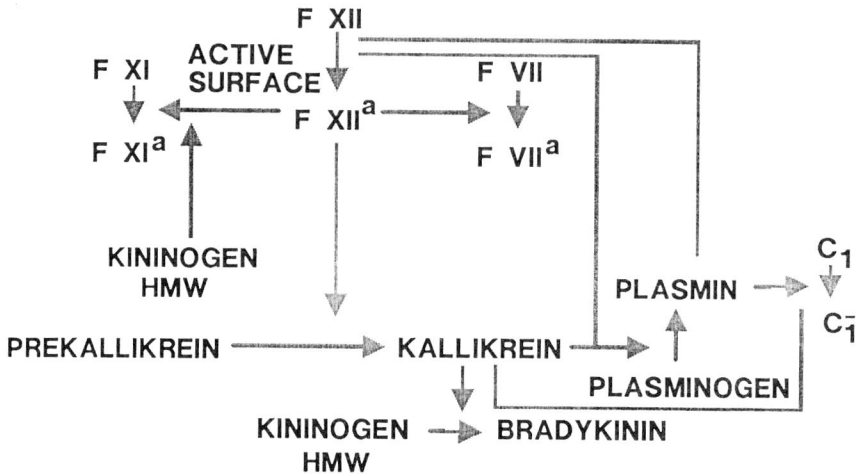

FIGURE 3. The contact activation complex and its integration with many vital systems.

into kallikrein (Fig. 3). Normally these substances are neutralized by the lung. For instance, if they are injected into the venous system of an animal, no activity is found in the left atrium; the lung passage is sufficient to neutralize completely these activities. In open-heart surgery the pulmonary circuit is left out of the circulation. This translates into a large production of vascular active substances (because of the contact with nonendothelial surfaces) but no neutralization (because lung contact is removed). The inevitable consequence is an increase in production and life span of vasoactive polypeptides.[10]

Environmental Factors

The involvement of platelets in reactions with synthetic material in ECC depends on environmental factors and platelet reactivity. Environmental factors are inherent to ECC; they are exogenous to the patient, generic to any heart surgery with ECC, and impossible to remove totally. It is desirable, however, to minimize their effects, thus controlling the determinant factors. Variables such as duration of CPB and presence of hemolysis are important additional elements. Platelet reactivity is a functional, endogenous, individual parameter that determines the consequences of the environmental factors on platelet number and function.

MONITORING PLATELETS IN ECC

The ideal test for monitoring platelet function is a global, real-time test. Many methodologies to study platelets exist. In general, however, they are time-consuming, and the relatively short time of ECC allows no real window to run a test and to obtain the results in time to modify a dangerous situation.

From the practical viewpoint, not many tests can satisfy the given prerequisites. Few studies in the literature address this issue. On the other hand, many studies have focused on blood samples taken during the ECC period and processed later. The results of these tests did not help to make any corrective decision. Therefore, they did not constitute true monitoring.

We counted platelets and ran a platelet retention test using a collagen chamber. The platelet retention test was chosen because it is a global test that can be executed using whole blood and in a few minutes, if possible in the operating room. Platelets were counted with the help of an electronic counter, and the retention test was completed in 5 minutes. We worked with heparinized blood taken directly from the oxygenator during ECC. Normal values for the platelet retention test are 30–50%. In the laboratory we ran parallel tests for platelet aggregation, platelet factor 4, clot retraction, fibrinogen, prothrombin time (PT), partial thromboplastin time (PTT, after ECC), thrombin time, protamine titration, euglobulin lysis and levels of fibrin degradation products (FDPs), free plasma hemoglobin and hematocrit as well as a thromboelastogram. This protocol required from 20–30 minutes during ECC. This study protocol is not our standard procedure now.

Platelet Count

The first task was to evaluate thrombocytopenia. We observed that patients with a similar platelet count during ECC did not have the same postoperative course. The correlation with platelet function was more important than the thrombocyte number alone. Thrombocytopenia may result from environmental factors, such as anticoagulant strength, priming of the oxygenator, physical and chemical aggressions, perfusion time, and protamine dose, to name the most evident.

Effect of Anticoagulation

We studied 220 consecutive patients divided into 2 subgroups. Patients received either 3 or 5 mg heparin/kg body weight. All were controlled with the protamine titration test and activated clotting time (ACT). Patients receiving 3 mg heparin/kg did not receive reinforcement doses. Patients with 5 mg heparin/kg received reinforcement doses to maintain an ACT similar to that at the beginning of perfusion. The number and function of platelets were better in patients who received 5 mg/kg heparin and were reinforced to maintain full anticoagulation during ECC (ACT around 600 sec) (Tables 1 and 2).

TABLE 1. Effect of Heparin Dose on the Platelet Count

	Heparin Dose		
Time	5 mg/kg	3 mg/kg	p
0 minutes	286 ± 42*	294 ± 48*	0.19
30 minutes	250 ± 52	232 ± 48	0.01
60 minutes	225 ± 58	198 ± 41	0.0004
90 minutes	195 ± 47	151 ± 53	0.000004
120 minutes	172 ± 44†	125 ± 38‡	0.00002

The group using the higher heparin dose has better platelet count preservation. Results are given as platelet number × $10^3/\mu l$.
* (n = 110)
† (n = 49)
‡ (n = 47)

TABLE 2. Effect of Heparin Dose on the Platelet Retention Test

Time	Heparin Dose 5 mg/kg	Heparin Dose 3 mg/kg	p
0 minutes	40 ± 3.7*	39 ± 4.1*	0.13
30 minutes	42 ± 3.8	37 ± 4.1	0.001
60 minutes	41 ± 4.4	34 ± 4.6	0.0006
90 minutes	42 ± 4.8	33 ± 4.8	0.0004
120 minutes	39 ± 5.2†	33 ± 5.4‡	0.002

The lower heparin dose is not as effective at preserving platelet function. Results are given as % for platelet retention.
* (n = 110)
† (n = 49)
‡ (n = 47)

Effect of Hemodilution

We studied the influence of oxygenator priming in 102 patients: 50 patients with mitral disorders, 20 with aortic disorders, 27 with mitral and aortic disorders, and 5 with mitral, aortic, and tricuspid valve disease, all rheumatic in origin. Forty-four patients were operated with full blood and 58 with hemodilution. All patients had a normal platelet count before surgery (286,000 and 294,000/µl).

The thrombocyte number decreased during ECC, with the reduction proportional to time if anticoagulant strength was maintained. During the first 20 minutes, an important functional difference was observed between patients receiving full blood priming and patients receiving hemodilution. Although the difference in platelet number was not significant, the thrombocyte function was better preserved with hemodilution (Tables 3 and 4). The reasons are related to rheologic factors. The hematologic trauma during ECC is reduced by lower blood viscosity and decreased shear force. Therefore, we set limits to hemodilution and consider a hematocrit of 25% as acceptable. Hematocrits below this level are used only in special cases.

TABLE 3. Effect of Hemodilution vs. Full Blood Priming on the Platelet Count

Time	Priming Hemodilution	Priming Full Blood	p
0 minutes	325 ± 40*	317 ± 35†	0.18
20 minutes	308 ± 32	286 ± 32	0.06
40 minutes	291 ± 33	265 ± 32	0.01
60 minutes	276 ± 31	224 ± 28	0.001
90 minutes	254 ± 29‡	201 ± 27§	0.0001
120 minutes	233 ± 26∥	189 ± 32∥∥	
Hematocrit	30 ± 5%	46 ± 3%	

A lower hematocrit offers better hemorrheologic conditions and preserves platelet. Results are given as platelet number × $10^3/\mu l$.
* (n = 58) § (n = 16)
† (n = 44) ∥ (n = 3)
‡ (n = 12) ∥∥ (n = 2)

TABLE 4. Effect of Hemodilution vs. Full Blood Priming on the Platelet Retention Test

Time	Priming		p
	Hemodilution	Full Blood	
0 minutes	42 ± 3.4*	43 ± 3.6†	0.23
20 minutes	45 ± 3.8	39 ± 4.2	0.002
40 minutes	44 ± 3.9	34 ± 4.6	0.0003
60 minutes	42 ± 4.4	34 ± 4.2	0.001
90 minutes	40 ± 4.6‡	33 ± 4.4§	0.001
120 minutes	40 ± 4.8∥	30 ± 5.3¶	
Hematocrit	30 ± 5%	46 ± 3%	

Hemodilution reduces platelet function damage. Results are given as % for platelet retention.
* (n = 58)   § (n = 16)
† (n = 44)   ∥ (n = 3)
‡ (n = 12)   ¶ (n = 2)

The importance of rheologic factors can be better understood if the consequences of high hematocrits are analyzed. In children with cyanotic congenital heart defects and hematocrit values >56%, the platelets drop more than 30% in the first 20 minutes on ECC and maintain a faster reduction rate than in patients with previous hemodilution and preoperative hematocrit values between 46–50%. In cases with high hematocrit values, acute intraoperative hemodilution did not compensate hemostatically to the same degree as preoperative hemodilution.

The reason for these differences is that hemodilution sets new hemodynamic rules. From the hemostatic point of view hemodilution should be performed with oncotic positive solutions to increase the plasma volume. In cases of preoperative hemodilution, we observe a better performance of plasma coagulation factors, a reduction in the reactive fibrinolytic plasma activity, and a rise in platelet number with release of new platelets from the bone marrow. These reactions are not present in the acutely hemodiluted patient. In other words, preoperative hemodilution improves the patient's postoperative status. We use blood for priming only under special indications, as in children with low body weight, to avoid an aggressive dilution (when the total blood volume is less than the priming volume) during surgery.

In our opinion, patients with hematocrit values >56% should be hemodiluted before surgery because the hemorrheologic conditions increase blood trauma during ECC. Blood trauma is characterized by high levels of free plasma hemoglobin, increased platelet destruction, fall in fibrinogen, and rise in levels of FDPs.

The thrombocyte changes in patient groups were typical. At first both groups showed platelet activation, but only in the group with preoperative hemodilution did the platelets reduce to normal and become slowly hypoactive. In the group with high hematocrit values and acute hemodilution, an increase in platelet function was accompanied by a reduction in number; but after 40 minutes a faster and more pronounced dysfunction was observed, with a higher rate of dysfunction in the last period of perfusion.

Effect of Erythrocyte Damage

Physical hemotrauma, resulting in high levels of plasma free hemoglobin, can be related to several factors. For example, in old banked blood the mechanical resistance of the erythrocytes is reduced during the storage period because of altered pH, release of cytolytic products from leukocytes, packing of red cells, and metabolic changes. Mechanical factors can also challenge the vitality of the red cells. High hemolysis results when aspiration is performed with intense suction.[2,9] The high vacuum produces erythrocyte deformation in the aspiration lines. But this negative force disappears when the blood arrives at the reservoirs, and the erythrocyte returns to its previous form. These rapid and intense changes in shape create a cavitation phenomenon. Consequently, the erythrocyte breaks, releasing hemoglobin into the plasma. Schistocytes and circulating erythrocyte ghosts appear.[11] The collapse of the aspiration tubes is a danger signal indicating excessive suction.

Erythrocyte lysis induces changes in platelet function, in relation to release of adenosine diphosphate (ADP) and the membrane itself. We have found a large amount of platelets trapped in the arterial line blood filter when hemolysis is excessive. When the level of free hemoglobin is >50 mg/dl and increases more than 10 mg/30 minutes, there is a risk of platelet dysfunction (Table 5). The best solution is to reduce the suction force, to check for free plasma hemoglobin, and to increase diuresis and alkalinization (sharp control of hydration and serum levels of sodium and potassium) if necessary.

Effect of Oxygenation

Chemical hemotrauma, mainly related to the use of high oxygen concentration during perfusion, induces a significant modification of platelet shape. The most impressive number of exhausted platelets after massive release was found in patients with high pO_2 levels. Values >500 mmHg that last longer than 30 minutes produce major changes.

Effect of Time

The time factor determines the formation of vasoactive substances, which affects the extent of deleterious effects on the hemostatic system and also explains the effect of ECC on the immune system. Major alterations induced in the complement system, initially with activation, lead eventually to depletion of complement factors.

TABLE 5. Effect of Hemolysis on Platelet Function

Time	Platelet Retention Test	Plasma Hemoglobin
0 minutes	37 ± 4.4	7
20 minutes	30 ± 3.9	24
40 minutes	28 ± 5.2	35
60 minutes	26 ± 5.8	50
90 minutes	26 ± 6.0	70

Hemolysis decreases platelet number and function. Results are given as % for platelet retention and mg/dl for plasma free hemoglobin (n = 2).

Effect of Protamine

The most dramatic changes in platelet number and function are observed after the use of protamine. Protamine produces side effects dependent on the amount administered, speed of infusion, and route of application. Because protamine is not without risk to the hemostatic system, it should be given only in the amount needed to neutralize circulating heparin. During ECC heparin acts as a protector against thrombin formation and inhibits the thrombin that is eventually formed. Neutralization of heparin may release an activated factor that produces enough thrombin to threaten the stability of the hemostatic system.

A second important factor relevant to the modification induced by protamine is the time at which the drug is used. By the end of the ECC environmental factors have induced such important changes in homeostasis that any accessory agent can prompt alterations that break the unstable equilibrium and produce massive bleeding or thrombosis that began in the operating room. Protamine can be the perfect trigger.

At the time of a fast venous injection of protamine the FDP levels increased, platelet number dropped, and fibrinogen levels were reduced. Sometimes these phenomena were correlated with a decrease of lung complacency and cardiac arrhythmia. We calculate the amount of the protamine dose by titration. If the titration assay is not available or if time is too limited, we calculate the dose of protamine in milligrams on the basis of the initial dose of heparin. In the operating room we prefer to use the arterial tree to inject protamine. Initially we inject only half of the calculated dose, and we run an ACT 5 minutes later. The rest is injected in small doses if the coagulation time does not return to the preperfusion value and consumptive coagulopathy is ruled out. If an additional dose of protamine is required later, we use the intravenous route, dilute the calculated amount of protamine 1:1 with glucose 5% in water, and inject slowly over 5-15 minutes.

We particularly warn against the dangerous combination of low doses of heparin with high doses of protamine. This combination leads to the most severe alterations in platelets and plasma factors.[11]

THE PLATELET REACTIVITY TEST

The platelet reactivity test is performed in vitro and measures platelet maximal response to a standard stimulus within a fixed period. The platelet reactivity test does not assess the relation between thromboxane and prostacyclin. It depends on maximal production of thromboxane in a platelet suspension induced by pig aorta collagen. The reaction follows a linear regression; thus it is a quantitative phenomenon. The upper borderline of the normal range is achieved at 35% of the scale; the remaining 65% of the scale permits recognition of hyperreactive platelets. These two characteristics of the test make it quite adequate for detection of hyperreactivity.

Four reactions with different conditions are run; addition of the four endpoints of the reactions gives the platelet reactivity index (PRI). The normal range for the PRI is 90-140. In relationship to aspirin and coronary bypass surgery, we found that most of the patients who bled after heart surgery with ECC had a PRI below 100 on the day of surgery (Table 6). We run a PRI for

TABLE 6. Aspirin and Myocardial Revascularization Surgery

Patients taking aspirin with a PRI <100
Number of patients: 22
Mean PRI: 84.6 ± 8.2
Mean transfusion volume: 2580 ± 400 ml
Mean bleeding volume (48 h): 2820 ± 736 ml

PRI = platelet reactivity index.

all patients on aspirin who are candidates for aortocoronary bypass surgery. If the index is below 100, the occlusion risk is low, but the risk of surgery-related bleeding is high. We recommend deferment of surgery, allowing 3–5 days for recovery of normal platelet function.

In general, aspirin can increase intra- and postoperative bleeding.[23] We complete this statement by saying, "Aspirin can induce bleeding if platelet reactivity is below the minimal hemostatic borderline." In our opinion the normalization of platelet hyperreactivity by an antiplatelet drug (for surgical patients we recommend a PRI between 100–150) cannot increase bleeding after cardiac surgery (Figs. 4 and 5). The consequences of ECC are quite different in patients with hyperreactive platelets and in patients with normal or hyporeactive platelets (Fig. 6).

The most important group with hyperreactive platelets are coronary patients. This cohort of atherosclerotic patients frequently has abnormalities in blood coagulation. The easiest to demonstrate is the increased fibrinogen level associated with hyperreactive platelets and resulting in a higher incidence of vascular occlusions in the postoperative period. Aortocoronary bypass occlusion may be as high as 11% during the first 2 weeks after surgery. The use of antiplatelet drugs significantly reduces this figure.[5]

Thromboembolic complications also occur more frequently in aortocoronary graft patients than in other open-heart surgery groups, such as valvular or congenital cases.[18,21] The high rate of coronary bypass occlusion detected in many studies may be related to operative use of procoagulant plasma factors, platelet infusions, and large amounts of antifibrinolytic drugs. Patients with

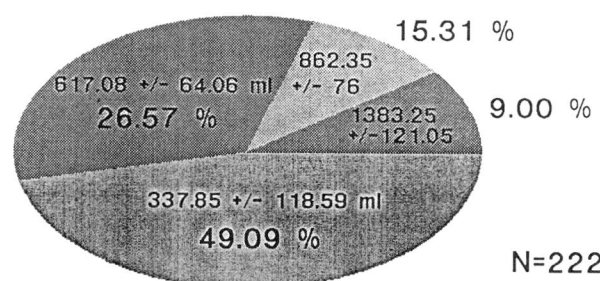

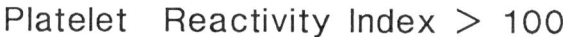

FIGURE 4. Distribution of the drainage volume in patients with normal platelet reactivity index (without aspirin) and normal blood coagulation tests.

Platelet Reactivity Index > 100

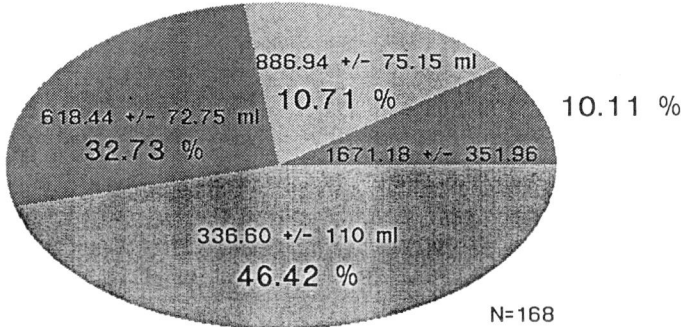

FIGURE 5. Distribution of the drainage volume in patients taking aspirin with PRI >100 and normal blood coagulation tests.

hyperreactive platelets should be treated before surgery to avoid intraoperative acute vascular occlusion or risk of bleeding immediately after surgery, with a secondary thrombotic phase during the 7th–18th postoperative day. The normalization of platelet function correlates with reduction in thrombogenesis and hemostatic problems.

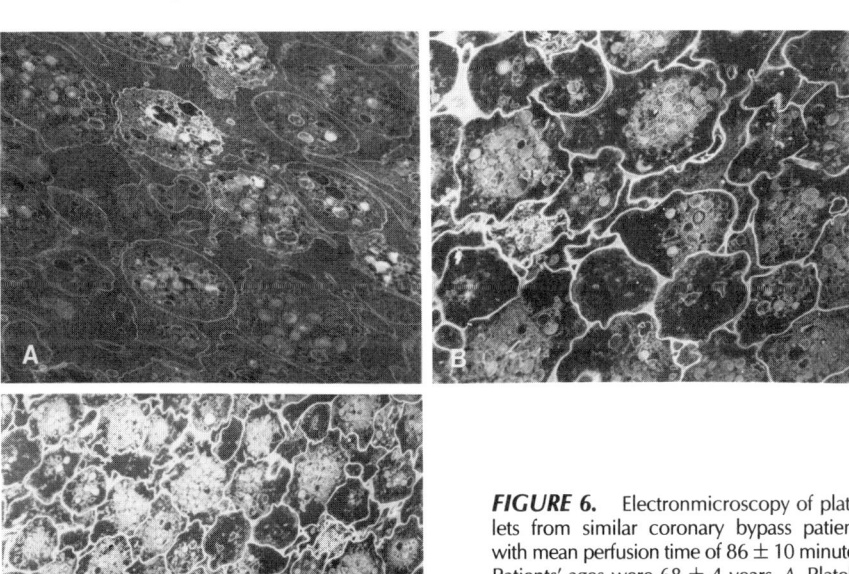

FIGURE 6. Electronmicroscopy of platelets from similar coronary bypass patients with mean perfusion time of 86 ± 10 minutes. Patients' ages were 68 ± 4 years. A, Platelet Reactivity Index (PRI) before surgery was 301; B, PRI before surgery was 200; C, PRI before surgery was 124.

Just as we are committed to prophylaxis of bleeding, so we are also concerned with prophylaxis of thromboembolism. This point needs to be stressed because recent discussions of prophylactic measures against bleeding have disregarded the risk of thromboembolism. Commitment to prevention of bleeding should not compromise homeostasis. We must remember that the hemostatic equilibrium is easy to break in the postperfusion period.

Large amounts of procoagulant proteins, platelet concentrates, or hemostatic drugs increase the risk of thrombosis and transform cardiovascular surgery into an unacceptable, expensive medical procedure. Antifibrinolytic drugs are helpful in relatively small doses. We began the use of aprotinin 25 years ago.[10,12] From our experience the large doses reported by Royston and coworkers are too high because they are antiphysiologic.[21] We believe that fibrinolysis protects against thrombosis. A massive inhibition of the system may induce intravascular fibrin deposit with ischemic consequences.

CONCLUSION

Since 1967 our aim has been to prevent bleeding without increasing the risk of thrombosis. In thousands of cardiovascular operations with CPB, not once have we used platelet concentrates, and only in 3 cases have we used blood factors. For coronary bypass surgery the mean thoracic drainage in the first 48 hours has been 589.6 ± 341.8 ml. The patients in our surgical group are categorized by severity of illness, need for multiple surgical procedures, and advanced age.

Hemostatic prophylaxis should always begin with a preoperative hemostatic evaluation. Patients with thrombocytopenia, thrombocytopathy, or blood coagulation disorders need to be compensated before surgery. Emergent patients should have close hemostatic control to increase their chance of survival. Patients in a critical situation do not have a second chance.

We know that platelet number and function alone do not explain all cases of bleeding, which generally is caused by the interactions of multiple factors.

For all these reasons our effort should be directed to prophylaxis and not to treatment of bleeding. Prophylaxis is a relatively simple approach, whereas treatment of bleeding after CPB is always a complicated issue. Prevention is facilitated by a full sense of the platelet reactivity test, which provides objective data from which to make decisions.

REFERENCES

1. Adelman B, Michelson AD, Loscalzo J, et al: Plasmin effect on platelet glycoprotein IB-von Willebrand factor interaction. Blood 65:32-37, 1985
2. Boonstra PW, Van Imhoff GW, Eysman L, et al: Reduced platelet activation and improved hemostasis after controlled cardiotomy suction during clinical membrane oxygenator perfusions. J Thorac Cardiovasc Surg 89:900-906, 1985.
3. Davies GC, Sobel M, Salzman EW: Elevated plasma fibrinopeptide A and thromboxane B2 levels during cardiopulmonary bypass. Circulation 61:808-814, 1980.
4. Faymonville ME, Deby-Dupont G, Larbuisson R, et al: Prostaglandin E2, prostacyclin, and thromboxane changes during nonpulsatile cardiopulmonary bypass in humans. J Thorac Cardiovasc Surg 91:858-866, 1986.
5. Fuster V, Chesebro JH: Role of platelets and platelet inhibitors in aortocoronary vein-graft disease. Circulation 73:227-232, 1986.

6. George JN, Pickett EB, Saucerman S, et al: Platelet surface glycoproteins. J Clin Invest 78:340-348, 1986.
7. Harker LA, Malpass TW, Branson HE, et al: Mechanism of abnormal bleeding in patients undergoing cardiopulmonary bypass: Acquired transient platelet disfunction associated with selective alpha granule release. Blood 56:824-834, 1980.
8. Hourdille P, Heilman I, Combire R, et al: Thrombin induce a rapid redistribution of platelet glycoprotein Ib-IX complex within the membrane systems of activated human platelets. Blood 76:1503-1513, 1990.
9. Manrique R: Blood Coagulation and Heart Surgery. São Paulo, Brazil, IDPC, 1968.
10. Manrique R: Protease Inhibitors and Heart Surgery. São Paulo, Brazil, IDPC, 1983.
11. Manrique R: Hemostasia and Open Heart Surgery. Doctoral Dissertation. Lima, Peru, San Marcos University, 1973.
12. Manrique R: Thromboembolic-prophylaxis in Cardiovascular Surgery. CLAHT XII International Congress on Hemostasis and Thrombosis. Bueños Aires, Argentina, November 1991.
13. Martin JF, Daniel TD, Towbridge EA: Acute and chronic changes in platelet volume and count after cardiopulmonary bypass induced thrombocytopenia in man. Thromb Haemost 57:55-58, 1987.
14. Martin JF, Towbridge EA, Salmon G, Plumb J: The biological significance of platelet volume: Its relationship to bleeding time, platelet thromboxane B2 production and megakaryocyte nuclear DNA concentrations. Thromb Res 32:443-460, 1983.
15. Mezzano D, Aranda E, Urzua J, et al: Changes in platelet beta-thromboglobulin, fibrinogen, albumin, 5-hydroxytryptamine, ATP, and ADP during and after surgery with extracorporeal circulation in man. Am J Hematol 22:133-142, 1986.
16. Michelson AD, Barnard MR: Plasmin induced redistribution of platelet glycoprotein Ib. Blood 76:2005-2010, 1990.
17. Musial J, Niewiarowski S, Hershock D, et al: Loss of fibrinogen receptors from the platelet surface during simulated extracorporeal circulation. J Lab Clin Med 105:514-521, 1985.
18. Reis S, Polack J, Hirsh DR, et al: Frequency of deep venous thrombosis in asymptomatic patients with coronary artery bypass grafts. America Heart J 122:478-482, 1991.
19. Rinder CS, Bonnert J, Rinder HM, et al: Platelet activation and aggregation during cardiopulmonary bypass. Anesthesiology 74:388-393, 1991.
20. Rinder CS, Mathew JP, Rinder HM, et al: Modulation of platelet surface adhesion receptors during cardiopulmonary bypass. Anesthesiology 75:563-570, 1991.
21. Royston D, Taylor KM, Bidstrup BP, Sapsford RN: Effect of aprotinin on need for blood transfusion after repeat open-heart surgery. Lancet 2:1289-1291, 1987.
22. Salama I, Hugo F, Heinrich K, et al: Deposit of terminal C5b-9 complement complexes on erythrocytes and leukocytes during cardiopulmonary bypass. N Engl J Med 318:408-414, 1988.
23. Sethi GS, Copeland JG, Goldman S, et al: Implications of preoperative administration of aspirin in patients undergoing coronary artery bypass grafting. J Am Coll Cardiol 15:15-20, 1990.
24. Solis T, Kennedy PS, Beall A, et al: Cardiopulmonary bypass: Microembolization and platelet aggregation. Circulation 52:103-106, 1975.
25. Zilla P, Fasol R, Groscurth P, et al: Blood platelets in cardiopulmonary bypass operations. J Thorac Cardiovasc Surg 97:379-388, 1989.

Chapter 15

Blood Utilization and the Role of the Transfusion Medicine Specialist in Cardiac Surgery

David B. Calandra, M.D., and Roland E. Lonser, M.D.

The development of cardiopulmonary bypass (CPB) in the 1950s and 1960s has allowed more complex and diversified surgical procedures to be successfully performed. The theoretic, technical, and mechanical refinements of CPB have resulted in a much safer and systematic approach to this type of surgery. Much attention has been directed toward decreasing the mechanical damage and functional alterations to blood. In addition, the recent focus on the risks of allogeneic blood transfusion has resulted in a renewed effort to improve further the safety of blood transfusion for open-heart surgery. This chapter focuses on a community hospital's approach to managing, as safely as possible, the use of blood components in open-heart surgery. Particular attention is directed to the use of autologous blood components, the evaluation of the plasma saver (Haemonetics Plasma System, Haemonetics Corporation, Braintree, MA) as a potential tool to reduce use of allogeneic blood, and the involvement of the specialist in transfusion medicine as a member of the cardiac surgery team.

The impact of this topic is clear when one reviews the number of operative procedures requiring CPB and the number of allogeneic blood transfusions. In the United States approximately 300,000 operative procedures are performed annually with CPB.[1] The majority of these procedures are primary and reoperative aortocoronary bypass, valve replacement (aortic, mitral, and tricuspid), correction and/or palliation of congenital heart disease, and cardiac transplantation, along with many rarely performed operations. The frequency of transfusion is high and represents some 10% of all the red blood cells transfused in the U.S. annually.[13]

While the nation's supply of blood has never been safer, the risks of receiving allogeneic blood components are still significant. The best information available indicates that immediate or delayed adverse effects occur in 10–15% of transfusion recipients.[22] The most common serious effects are acute hemolytic transfusion reactions (1/25,000/U),[22] viral hepatitis-C (1/3000/U),[10] and transfusion-associated acquired immunodeficiency syndrome (AIDS) (1/300,000/U).[9,22] One additional category of adverse effects is the immunologic consequences of blood components. This category includes graft versus host disease,[14] decreased resistance to postoperative infection,[20,24] and increased incidence of remote tumor metastasis.[3] The exact incidence of these problems is not known, but their serious nature is of concern.

A major complication of open-heart surgery requiring CPB is bleeding. Approximately 3 in 100 patients require a second operation for evaluation of excessive postoperative mediastinal drainage. Until recent years, essentially 100% of all CPB patients received allogeneic blood transfusions. Although CPB has significantly improved, disruption of the normal blood coagulation system is still severe.

The altered coagulation is due to many factors, including hypothermia, hemodilution, pharmacologic agents, hypotension, and thrombogenic surfaces.[6] Hypothermia is thought to increase the risk for hemorrhage by interfering with platelet function.[11,18] The exact mechanism is not clear. Hemodilution results in increased bleeding mainly because of platelet dilution. Numerous pharmacologic agents have clear and predictable effects on hemostasis, including common medications such as Coumadin, heparin, streptokinase, tissue plasminogen activator (TPA), urokinase, aspirin, dipyridamole, ticlopidine (Ticlid), and other platelet inhibitors. A detailed discussion of all medications known to affect hemostasis is beyond the scope of this chapter. One particular agent that in our experience repeatedly gives problems is Coumadin. One must keep in mind that the prothrombin time (PT) measures the vitamin K-dependent clotting factors II, VII, IX and X. The PT is most sensitive to levels of factor VII. After a dose of vitamin K the doubling time for regeneration of factor VII is 6 hours, after which the PT normalizes. Because factors II, IX, and X require a longer time to normalize, the patient may experience increased bleeding as a result of decreased levels of factors II, IX, and X, even with a normal PT. Hypotension is usually a problem only when severe and associated with hypoxemia. In this case the risk of developing disseminated intravascular coagulation (DIC) is increased. The mechanism for this association is not entirely clear. Finally, contact of the patient's blood with the plastic surfaces in the CPB circuit can lead to platelet activation as well as initiation of both coagulation and fibrinolysis pathways and activation of complement.[2,18] The above factors and many other potential alterations of normal hemostasis in an individual patient may lead to significant coagulopathy and thus result in bleeding.

The specialist in transfusion medicine is in a unique position to participate effectively in the management of the patient undergoing open-heart surgery. With a knowledge of coagulation and blood components, rapid assessment can be facilitated and appropriate therapy instituted in a timely manner. The goal of transfusion medicine is to limit the patient's exposure to allogeneic blood products. Among the ways to accomplish this goal are use of autologous blood products obtained pre-, intra-, and postoperatively; the lowering of the transfusion trigger (accepting lower hemoglobin levels); use of nonblood pharmacologic agents (e.g., Fluosol; see other chapters in this volume for discussion); the initiation of biologic response modifiers (e.g., erythropoietin); and, probably foremost, strict adherence to criteria for use of allogeneic blood components (Table 1).[1,12,13,17,26]

The hematologic parameters in Table 1 are used to help determine the need for blood components in patients with persistent postsurgical bleeding after reversal of the standard heparin dose with protamine.

TABLE 1. Transfusion Threshold

Hemoglobin (Hgb)	Less than 7.0 gm/dl
Hematocrit (Hct)	Less than 21%
Platelet count (Plts)	Less than $50–100 \times 10^9$/L
Protime (PT)	Greater than 20 sec
Activated partial thromboplastin time (APTT)	Greater than 55 sec
Fibrinogen	Less than 200 mg/dl

ALLOGENEIC BLOOD COMPONENTS

Hinsdale Hospital is a 440-bed acute care facility. The open-heart program is designed to treat emergent and elective cardiac conditions. The majority of operations are myocardial revascularizations (primary and reoperative), valve replacement, valve reconstruction, resection and reconstruction of ventricular aneurysm, and adult intracardiac defects, such as atrial septal defects. The data to be reviewed and discussed result from a complete study of 608 consecutive patients undergoing open-heart procedures from January 1, 1989–June 30, 1992. The distribution of patients is 167 women and 441 men.

The use of allogeneic red cells is presented in Table 2. These data have been compiled to encompass the entire hospitalization period from admission to discharge. All patients are evaluated before surgery as potential candidates for preoperative collection of autologous whole blood (see below). In addition, intraoperative techniques minimize extraneous and excessive use of allogeneic red cells, including acute normovolemic hemodilution and red cell salvage with the Haemonetics Cell Saver IV (Haemonetic Corporation, Braintree, MA). During the immediate postcardiotomy period all shed mediastinal blood is salvaged. If >400 ml is collected, it is readministered to the patient. All these pre-, intra-, and postoperative methods have been used in all patients who meet the established criteria.

The result of this multimodality approach to minimize use of allogeneic red cells has been excellent. The data in Table 2 indicate that 70% of all men and 30% of all women required no transfusion of red cells during their entire hospital stay. Overall, over 50% of all patients operated required no transfusion of allogeneic red cells. Patients who received <2 units of allogeneic red cells had critically low hematocrits while on CPB (16–18% or less). The need for red cell infusion with low hematocrit is well established.

TABLE 2. Allogeneic Red Cells*

	Males	Females
0 unit	305	52
1 unit	11	18
2 units	59	37
3 units	20	17
4 units	15	19
5 or more units	31	24

* Red cells given during the time from admission to discharge.

TABLE 3. Blood Component Use (Allogeneic) Other Than Red Cells*

Fresh Frozen Plasma	Cryoprecipitate	Platelet Concentrate+
52 (3 units)	7 (14 bags)	116 (1.6 units)
(8.6%)	(1.2%)	(19%)

* Number of patients receiving product with average per patient in parentheses; percent in parentheses is total patients in study receiving product.

Table 3 demonstrates the use of blood components other than red cells during the study period. When possible, all of these allogeneic products are single-donor products to further reduce exposure to multiple donors.

The use of fresh frozen plasma (FFP) was generally based on documented parameters of abnormal clotting and excess postcardiotomy loss of blood. In 52 patients (8.6% of total), FFP was administered (Table 3). The mean number of units of FFP per patient was 3. The FFP units were prepared as single donor units of 500 ml of plasma each, which is roughly equivalent to 2 units of standard FFP prepared from 2 separate donors.

The use of cryoprecipitate was based on documented abnormal levels of fibrinogen, excess mediastinal blood loss, or recent exposure to thrombolytic agents such as urokinase, streptokinase, and TPA. In 7 patients (1.2% of total) cryoprecipitate was administered (Table 3). The mean number of units of cryoprecipitate per patient was 14 bags. A cryoprecipitate bag is a standard bag of approximately 10-15 ml, prepared from a unit of whole blood in the usual fashion.

The use of platelet concentrate was based on documented low platelet counts ($50-100 \times 10^9$/L or less), excessive mediastinal blood loss, and/or recent exposure to standard antiplatelet agents such as aspirin or persantine. In 116 patients (19% of total), platelet concentrate was administered (Table 3). A unit of platelet concentrate, prepared by apheresis techniques from single donors, is equivalent to 6-10 standard randomly pooled donor units. The volume ranged from 200-400 ml of plasma with 3×10^{11} to 5×10^{11} platelets/unit.

Most patients used allogeneic red cells and no other blood components. The patients who required red cells alone weighed <60 kg and/or had preoperative hematocrits of <33%. This subset of patients was predominantly female—an observation made by others.[5] The smaller patients (<60 kg) have less intravascular volume, and with the standard method of hemodilution used for CPB the hematocrit of these patients frequently reaches critical levels (<16-18%). The volume of prime solution, which is approximately 1500 ml of solute, and the oxygenator are potential sources for altering the overall dilution effect. Thus, with smaller prime volume and smaller oxygenator size, this effect could be minimized. Such techniques would be most appropriate for smaller patients (<60 kg), who are most frequently women.

The patients needing cryoprecipitate generally had serious bleeding during the immediate postoperative period. All patients receiving cryoprecipitate use allogeneic red cells, FFP, and platelet concentrate. The hematologic parameters of clotting in these patients were markedly affected with thrombocytopenia (<$50-100 \times 10^9$/L), abnormal PTs (>20 seconds, n = 10-14 sec), and abnormal activated partial thromboplastin times (APTTs >55 seconds, n = 20-31 sec). The subset of patients who received only platelet concentrate was quite remarkable. These 16 patients received no other blood component

Chapter 15

Blood Utilization and the Role of the Transfusion Medicine Specialist in Cardiac Surgery

David B. Calandra, M.D., and Roland E. Lonser, M.D.

The development of cardiopulmonary bypass (CPB) in the 1950s and 1960s has allowed more complex and diversified surgical procedures to be successfully performed. The theoretic, technical, and mechanical refinements of CPB have resulted in a much safer and systematic approach to this type of surgery. Much attention has been directed toward decreasing the mechanical damage and functional alterations to blood. In addition, the recent focus on the risks of allogeneic blood transfusion has resulted in a renewed effort to improve further the safety of blood transfusion for open-heart surgery. This chapter focuses on a community hospital's approach to managing, as safely as possible, the use of blood components in open-heart surgery. Particular attention is directed to the use of autologous blood components, the evaluation of the plasma saver (Haemonetics Plasma System, Haemonetics Corporation, Braintree, MA) as a potential tool to reduce use of allogeneic blood, and the involvement of the specialist in transfusion medicine as a member of the cardiac surgery team.

The impact of this topic is clear when one reviews the number of operative procedures requiring CPB and the number of allogeneic blood transfusions. In the United States approximately 300,000 operative procedures are performed annually with CPB.[1] The majority of these procedures are primary and reoperative aortocoronary bypass, valve replacement (aortic, mitral, and tricuspid), correction and/or palliation of congenital heart disease, and cardiac transplantation, along with many rarely performed operations. The frequency of transfusion is high and represents some 10% of all the red blood cells transfused in the U.S. annually.[13]

While the nation's supply of blood has never been safer, the risks of receiving allogeneic blood components are still significant. The best information available indicates that immediate or delayed adverse effects occur in 10–15% of transfusion recipients.[22] The most common serious effects are acute hemolytic transfusion reactions (1/25,000/U),[22] viral hepatitis-C (1/3000/U),[10] and transfusion-associated acquired immunodeficiency syndrome (AIDS) (1/300,000/U).[9,22] One additional category of adverse effects is the immunologic consequences of blood components. This category includes graft versus host disease,[14] decreased resistance to postoperative infection,[20,24] and increased incidence of remote tumor metastasis.[3] The exact incidence of these problems is not known, but their serious nature is of concern.

A major complication of open-heart surgery requiring CPB is bleeding. Approximately 3 in 100 patients require a second operation for evaluation of excessive postoperative mediastinal drainage. Until recent years, essentially 100% of all CPB patients received allogeneic blood transfusions. Although CPB has significantly improved, disruption of the normal blood coagulation system is still severe.

The altered coagulation is due to many factors, including hypothermia, hemodilution, pharmacologic agents, hypotension, and thrombogenic surfaces.[6] Hypothermia is thought to increase the risk for hemorrhage by interfering with platelet function.[11,18] The exact mechanism is not clear. Hemodilution results in increased bleeding mainly because of platelet dilution. Numerous pharmacologic agents have clear and predictable effects on hemostasis, including common medications such as Coumadin, heparin, streptokinase, tissue plasminogen activator (TPA), urokinase, aspirin, dipyridamole, ticlopidine (Ticlid), and other platelet inhibitors. A detailed discussion of all medications known to affect hemostasis is beyond the scope of this chapter. One particular agent that in our experience repeatedly gives problems is Coumadin. One must keep in mind that the prothrombin time (PT) measures the vitamin K-dependent clotting factors II, VII, IX and X. The PT is most sensitive to levels of factor VII. After a dose of vitamin K the doubling time for regeneration of factor VII is 6 hours, after which the PT normalizes. Because factors II, IX, and X require a longer time to normalize, the patient may experience increased bleeding as a result of decreased levels of factors II, IX, and X, even with a normal PT. Hypotension is usually a problem only when severe and associated with hypoxemia. In this case the risk of developing disseminated intravascular coagulation (DIC) is increased. The mechanism for this association is not entirely clear. Finally, contact of the patient's blood with the plastic surfaces in the CPB circuit can lead to platelet activation as well as initiation of both coagulation and fibrinolysis pathways and activation of complement.[2,18] The above factors and many other potential alterations of normal hemostasis in an individual patient may lead to significant coagulopathy and thus result in bleeding.

The specialist in transfusion medicine is in a unique position to participate effectively in the management of the patient undergoing open-heart surgery. With a knowledge of coagulation and blood components, rapid assessment can be facilitated and appropriate therapy instituted in a timely manner. The goal of transfusion medicine is to limit the patient's exposure to allogeneic blood products. Among the ways to accomplish this goal are use of autologous blood products obtained pre-, intra-, and postoperatively; the lowering of the transfusion trigger (accepting lower hemoglobin levels); use of nonblood pharmacologic agents (e.g., Fluosol; see other chapters in this volume for discussion); the initiation of biologic response modifiers (e.g., erythropoietin); and, probably foremost, strict adherence to criteria for use of allogeneic blood components (Table 1).[1,12,13,17,26]

The hematologic parameters in Table 1 are used to help determine the need for blood components in patients with persistent postsurgical bleeding after reversal of the standard heparin dose with protamine.

therapy. All had significant postoperative bleeding with >200 ml/hour of mediastinal drainage and platelet counts ranging from <50-100 × 10^9/L. Dramatic control of bleeding was achieved rapidly with the administration of platelet concentrate. In our opinion, excessive blood loss can many times be averted by timely and adequate correction of platelet dysfunction with platelet concentrates. The 100 other patients requiring platelet concentrate received transfusion of other blood components.

AUTOLOGOUS BLOOD COMPONENTS

Because autologous blood components are obviously a superior blood product, every attempt should be made to obtain them when indications are clear. The following techniques of autologous blood salvage (with criteria for each) were used:

1. Preoperative whole blood collection. Criteria: If a delay of 3 or more days before surgery is anticipated, all patients meeting the American Association of Blood Banks donor criteria donated autologous blood at the rate of 1 unit every 3-4 days. These criteria are predonation hematocrit of 33% or more; absence of infection that may cause bacteremia; and removal of no more than 10-15% of total blood volume per donation episode.

2. Acute normovolemic hemodilution. Criteria: All patients with a hematocrit of 35% or more had between 300-600 ml (average: 1 unit) removed and held until the end of the procedure, then returned to the patient while the surgical wound was closed.

3. Intraoperative red cell salvage. Criteria: In all patients undergoing open-heart surgery the Haemonetics Cell Saver IV technology (Haemonetics Corporation, Braintree, MA) was used.

4. Postoperative shed blood salvage. Criteria: All patients undergoing open-heart surgery had a Deknatel Pleur-Evac Autotransfusion (Pfizer Hospital Products Group, Inc., Fall River, MA) salvage device hooked up in line with the chest-tube drainage. If 400 ml or more of blood was collected into the device at the end of 4 hours, the blood was sent to the transfusion service for appropriate washing and immediately returned to the patient for transfusion. NOTE: Washing of the salvaged blood is accomplished with the COBE 2991 Blood Cell Processor (Cobe Laboratories, Inc., Lakewood, CO), using 1000 ml normal saline (Abbott Laboratories, 0.9% sodium chloride injectable SP) per unit or salvage collection bag.

Table 4 shows the number of patients using the described autologous blood salvage techniques and the average amount of product used.

Eleven patients used autologous blood components only. Each was able to donate from 1-3 units of red cells preoperatively. Nine patients used all the donated blood; 1 used none of the 2 donated units. In several instances, the

TABLE 4. Red Blood Cells (Autologous)

Intraoperative Salvage	Acute Normovolemia Hemodilution	Postoperative Shed Blood	Preoperative Whole Blood
541 (5.5 units)	179 (1 unit)	84 (0.5 unit)	20 (1 unit)
(89%)	(29%)	(14%)	(3.3%)

blood was used several days after surgery according to the same transfusion criteria used for allogeneic products (Table 1). The risks of allogeneic blood transfusion have been well documented (e.g., hepatitis C, human immunodeficiency virus (HIV), acute hemolytic reaction).[22] Minimizing these risks is an important goal. Use of autologous blood components is one means of reducing the risks. Although these techniques are generally safe and without serious complications, caution must be exercised with each modality. The more serious of these potential problems have been described.

Some of the concerns in presurgical autologous donation of whole blood have been recently outlined.[23,27] Even though autologous donation is safe, a subgroup of high-risk patients may demand special monitoring while they donate because of significant hypotensive episodes. Infusion of crystalloid volume rapidly corrects these hypotensive episodes. This subgroup is characterized when one or more of the following criteria are met: history of angina, myocardial infarction, cardiac dysrhythmia, hypertension requiring two or more medications for control, congestive heart failure, valvular heart disease, congenital heart disease, seizure disorder, previous cerebral vascular accident, or demonstrated cerebral vascular insufficiency. The special monitoring for these donor patients includes automated blood pressure monitor, pulse oximeter and modified lead II electrocardiogram. An intravenous line with normal saline is also started before donation, and equal volumes are given after donation for partial replacement of the volume of blood removed during donation.[23]

With regard to intraoperative salvage a recently described problem called the salvaged blood syndrome should be considered.[4,7,19,21] The clinical findings are adult respiratory distress syndrome, anasarca, and/or DIC. The mechanism involved is hypothesized to be activation of the oxidative burst enzymatic pathway in exposed phagocytic cells in the salvaged blood, which leads to increased vascular permeability. In the case of DIC the infusion of platelet phospholipid and cellular debris is also thought to play a key role. Some evidence suggests that activation of complement plays an important role in triggering this sequence of events.

In our opinion, complement activation may be the key factor. In 12 years of experience with intraoperative salvage (over 3,000 cases involving all types of surgical procedures, including cardiovascular cases), we have not encountered this problem. Our hypothesis is that the anticoagulant used in collecting the shed blood for the cell salvage may be a key factor in whether or not one is likely to experience the salvaged blood syndrome. We use ACD-A Baxter Fenwal (Deerfield, IL) in a ratio of 1:5-1:8 (citrate to whole blood salvaged). Because citrate inactivates complement, it is likely that activation of factors leading to the salvaged blood syndrome is blocked, thus preventing clinical manifestation of the syndrome. (Citrate solutions may be used alone or in combination with heparin.)

Potential problems with the use of postsurgical shed mediastinal blood are also documented, including fever, DIC, and spurious elevation of cardiac enzymes.[16,25] We experienced one such nearly catastrophic complication: the development of profound acute hypotension with cardiac arrest within minutes of starting an infusion of 400 ml of shed mediastinal blood. The patient, who received approximately 25-50 ml of the postsurgical shed blood, was successfully resuscitated without long-term problems and discharged from the hospital. This hypotensive episode occurred in an otherwise stable, noncomplicated patient after coronary artery bypass. This type of reaction is typically seen with infusion of residual ethylene-oxide (an agent used to sterilize collection devices). Although we were unable to prove conclusively that ethylene-oxide was administered via the postsurgical mediastinal shed blood, we have begun washing all blood products obtained in this manner with 1000 ml of 0.9% sodium chloride solution/400 ml blood salvaged. Since initiating this protocol, we have had no similar episodes or other potential problems that may be seen with the infusion of activated clotting factors, cellular debris, or other materials.

PREOPERATIVE PLATELET-RICH PLASMA (PRP) STUDY

The use of PRP has been reported by some investigators to decrease perioperative transfusion requirements.[8] The following study was designed to evaluate this technique. The immediate preoperative autologous PRP study involved 31 consecutive patients undergoing coronary bypass surgery. The Haemonetics Plasma Saving System (Haemonetics Corporation, Braintree, MA) was used in accordance with the following criteria. Patients were subjected to harvesting of PRP immediately before or immediately after induction of anesthesia prior to placement on CPB. The product was returned to the patient at the end of surgery after heparin reversal. All other modalities of blood conservation and salvage discussed previously were employed in these patients.

The patient populations (study vs. control) were matched for age, sex, size, and severity of disease. Ten (30%) of the 31 study patients and 56 (30%) of the 185 control patients were women. Use of blood components by study patients was compared with use by control patients. The average volume of salvaged PRP was 552 ml/patient. The average platelet count in the salvaged product was 1.4×10^{11}. (This is the equivalent of 3 units of standard random donor platelet concentrate.)

Table 5 shows that 30% of the plasma salvage patients had increased mediastinal drainage vs. 14% of patients not using the plasma saver. The significance of this observed increase in postoperative mediastinal drainage in the plasma saver patients is not apparent from this study. No other findings of significance were seen.

The data comparing patients with PRP salvage versus patients without PRP salvage (our standard technique) do not support the routine use of this technique to minimize loss of blood and transfusion of allogeneic blood components (Table 5). The differences in the mean volume of packed red blood cells, FFP, cryoprecipitate, and platelet concentrate did not reach statistical significance. The shed mediastinal blood was slightly greater with PRP, but the difference was not statistically significant. This study shows no advantage or disadvantage in regard to use of allogeneic blood components between the two groups of patients.

This conclusion may be due to our patient population, who are not the types to require blood component support. In our opinion, centers reporting reduced use of blood components with this technique are experiencing more

TABLE 5. Comparison of Blood Components With and Without Platelet-rich Plasma Salvage

	Packed RBC	Fresh Frozen Plasma	Cryo-precipitate	Apheresis Platelet Concentrate (Single Donor)	Intra-operative Cell Salvage	Shed Mediastinal Blood*	Average Discharge Hct (%)
Patients with plasma salvage (31 pts.)	1.2 units per pt.	0.16 units per pt.	0.2 units per pt. (1 pt. used 8 units)	0.06 units per pt. (2 units total)	1147 ml/pt. or 5.1 units per pt.	1.4 units per pt. (10 pts.)	31
Patients without plasma salvage (185 pts.)	1.3 units per pt.	0.14 units per pt.	0	0.17 per pt. (31 units total)	1231 ml/pt. or 5.5 units per patient	1.0 unit per pt. (26 pts.)	33

* The shed mediastinal blood was tabulated only when the drainage was greater than 400 ml in the first 4 hours postoperatively.

conservation in blood components as a result of greater awareness and care in use of blood products; i.e., adherence to transfusion criteria may be stricter.

The study raises a number of questions that need answers:
1. Can a high-risk candidate for blood component use be defined?
2. When should autologous blood components be obtained from the patient?
3. Which products and in what quantities should products be obtained?
4. When should autologous products be returned to the patient?
5. Should autologous blood products always be returned to the patient?

ROLE OF THE SPECIALIST IN TRANSFUSION MEDICINE

The role of the specialist in transfusion medicine in open-heart surgery can be a critical one. The increased awareness and sensitivity of patients and families to transfusion-related diseases has resulted in a greater need for precise and timely use of allogeneic blood components. Specialists in transfusion medicine are in a unique position because of their knowledge and potential to act as an important liaison between the blood bank and the operating room. These physicians have specialized training in all aspects of coagulation, blood components, and red cell antibody identification (including cold agglutinins) as well as the infectious and immunologic consequences of blood transfusion. Specialists in transfusion medicine can provide guidance in the appropriate use of blood products before, during, and after open-heart surgery. They can also facilitate early recognition of heparin-induced platelet antibodies (HIPA) and potentially minimize the life-threatening aspects of this increasingly recognized syndrome. The specialist can also facilitate the early identification and verification of new, potentially useful modifiers from the fields of hematology and blood banking, including the biologic response modifiers such as erythropoietin and granulocyte colony stimulating factor. This area of basic research is ever expanding and may provide new and safer modulators that further minimize the need for allogeneic exposures.

The development and maintenance of responsible, strict criteria for use of blood components are important aspects of the role of the specialist in transfusion medicine on the cardiovascular surgery team. Timeliness, quality, and specific blood component used for individual patients are improved. In addition, the specialist is available to discuss and educate patient and family about issues surrounding blood transfusions.

SUMMARY

Overall, at least 50% of patients undergoing coronary bypass procedures do not need support with allogeneic blood products. This figure is much better for men (70%) than women (30%). The plasma saver did not affect the use of blood products either favorably or unfavorably.

With judicious use of autologous blood products, most patients requiring open-heart surgery can avoid exposure to allogeneic blood products. When possible, the use of single-donor blood components also reduces the exposure to allogeneic blood products. The specialist in transfusion medicine should be included as a member of the team caring for the open-heart surgery candidate. This involvement often begins presurgically.

REFERENCES

1. Audet A, Goodnough LT: Practice strategies for elective red blood cell transfusion. Ann Intern Med 116:403, 1992.
2. Bick RL: Platelet function defects: A clinical review. Semin Thromb Hemost 18:167-185, 1992.
3. Blumberg N, Triulzi DJ, Heal JM: Transfusion-induced immunomodulation and its clinical consequences. Trans Med Rev 4:24-35, 1990.
4. Bull BS, Bull MH: The salvaged blood syndrome: A sequel to mechanochemical activation of platelets and leukocytes. Blood Cells 16:5-23, 1990.
5. Cosgrove DM, Loop FD, Lytle BW, et al: Determinants of blood utilization during myocardial revascularization. Ann Thorac Surg 40:380-384, 1985.
6. Counts RB: Causes of bleeding in open heart surgery. In Baldwin ML, Kurtz SR (eds): Transfusion Practice in Cardiac Surgery. Arlington, VA, American Association of Blood Banks, 1991, pp 1-11.
7. DeLeuze PH, Intrator L, Liou A, et al: Complement activation and use of a cell saver in cardiopulmonary bypass. ASAIO Trans 36:M179-M181, 1990.
8. Del Rossi AJ, Cernaianu AC, Vertrees RA, et al: Platelet-rich plasma reduces postoperative blood loss after cardiopulmonary bypass. J Thorac Cardiovasc Surg 100:281-286, 1990.
9. Dodd RY: The risk of transfusion-transmitted infection. N Engl J Med 327:419-420, 1992.
10. Donahue JG, Muñoz A, Ness PM, et al: The declining risk of post-transfusion hepatitis C virus infection. N Engl J Med 327:369-383, 1992.
11. Edmunds LH, Addonzio VP Jr: Massive transfusion. In Colman RW, Hirsh J, Marder VJ, Salzman EW (eds): Hemostasis and Thrombosis, 2nd ed. Philadelphia, J.B. Lippincott, 1987, p 916.
12. Ellison N, Campbell FW, Jobes DR: Postoperative hemostasis. Semin Thorac Cardiovasc Surg 3:33-38, 1991.
13. Goodnough LT, Johnston MF, Ramsey G, et al: Guidelines for transfusion support in patients undergoing coronary artery bypass grafting. Ann Thorac Surg 50:675-683, 1990.
14. Greenbaum BH: Transfusion-associated graft-versus-host disease: Historical perspectives, incidence, and current use of irradiated blood products. J Clin Oncol 9:1889-1902, 1991.

15. [deleted]
16. Griffith LD, Billman GF, Daily PO, Lane TA: Apparent coagulopathy caused by infusion of shed mediastinal blood and it prevention by washing of the infusate. Ann Thorac Surg 47:400-406, 1989.
17. Jones JW, Rawitscher RE, McLean TR, et al: Benefit from combining blood conservation measures in cardiac operations. Ann Thorac Surg 51:541-546, 1991.
18. Khuri SF, Wolfe JA, Josa M, et al: Hematologic changes during and after cardiopulmonary bypass and their relationship to the bleeding time and nonsurgical blood loss. J Thorac Cardiovasc Surg 104:94-107, 1992.
19. Maggart M, Stewart S: The mechanisms and management of noncardiogenic pulmonary edema following cardiopulmonary bypass. Ann Thorac Surg 43:231-236, 1987.
20. Murphy P, Connery C, Hicks G, Blumberg N: Homologous transfusion is associated with post-operative infection in coronary bypass surgery patients. Ann Clin Lab Sci 22:260, 1992.
21. Murray DJ, Gress K, Weinstein SL: Coagulopathy after reinfusion of autologous scavenged red blood cells. Anesth Analg 75:125-129, 1992.
22. Smith DM Jr, Dodd RY: Transfusions-Transmitted Infections. Chicago, IL, American Society of Clinical Pathologists, 1991, pp 9-10.
23. Spiess BD, Sassetti R, McCarthy RJ, et al: Autologous blood donation: Hemodynamics in a high-risk patient population. Transfusion 32:17-22, 1992.
24. Triulzi DJ, Vanek K, Ryan DH, Blumberg N: A clinical and immunologic study of blood transfusion and postoperative bacterial infection in spinal surgery. 32:517-524, 1992.
25. Wahl GW, Feins RH, Alfieres G, Bixby K: Reinfusion of shed blood after coronary operation causes elevation of cardiac enzyme levels. Ann Thorac Surg 53:625-627, 1992.
26. Welch HG, Meehan KR, Goodnough LT: Prudent strategies for elective red blood cell transfusion. Ann Intern Med 116:393-402, 1992.
27. Zussa C, Polesel E, Salvador L, et al: Efficacy and safety of predeposit blood autodonation in 500 cases of myocardial revascularization. Scand J Thorac Cardiovasc Surg 24:171-175, 1990.

Chapter 16

The Use of Apheresis in Cardiac Surgery

John A. Robinson, M.D.

The therapeutic concept of apheresis is based on the ability to process whole blood into component parts and subsequently to return the modified product to the patient. Primitive apheresis could be achieved only by manual withdrawal of whole blood that was anticoagulated and then allowed to separate into fluid and cell phases, either by offline centrifugation or simple gravity techniques; the clinical situation determined whether the cells or plasma was then returned to the patient. Evaluation of the therapeutic efficacy of apheresis was hampered at this point in time by the technical impossibility of modifying large volumes of whole blood and safely returning it to the patient. This impasse was resolved after the development of safe, online blood processing by cell separators that could process up to 20 L (or more) of whole blood during a single treatment.

Current methodology of cell/plasma separation is based on treatment of ex vivo anticoagulated whole blood by either centrifugation that separates fluid from formed elements by density/flotation or membrane filtration that generates cellfree plasma by flux under pressure across membranes or hollow fibers that exclude the formed elements. Techniques of centrifugation can employ either discontinuous or continuous flow systems; discontinuous systems can be used with a single venipuncture site, but they can be time-consuming and often require extracorporeal volumes during separation that may pose risk to patients with borderline cardiac function. Under most circumstances, continuous flow systems require either two antecubital venipunctures or access by a dual-lumen pheresis/dialysis catheter in a central vein. A single-needle adaptation to the COBE Spectra continuous system is available for plasmapheresis and platelet collection.

Centrifuge cell separators can be used for erythrocyte exchange, lymphocytapheresis, plateletpheresis, leukopheresis, and plasma exchange, but membrane filtration is limited to treatment of diseases that benefit from alteration or removal of plasma only and currently cannot be used for effective separation of cell populations.

Volume replacement appropriate to the whole blood component being removed is provided to maintain normovolemia. An additional therapeutic benefit available in most apheresis machines is the ability to increase or decrease fluid balance within a narrow range during treatment. The standard colloid used for volume replacement during plasmapheresis and cellular pheresis procedures is 5% human serum albumin spiked with 8.0 mEq/L of calcium gluconate. Transfusionists, cardiac surgeons, anesthesiologists, and apheresis personnel differ as to whether albumin or low-molecular-weight hydroxyethyl starch should be used for maintenance of adequate plasma volume during cardiopulmonary bypass (CPB). We use 5% albumin exclusively, but other groups have used 6% hydroxyethyl starch without complication. Nonetheless, most investigators agree that a colloid rather than a crystalloid is the optimal replacement fluid for autologous plasma.[3] In most patients, acid citrate dextrose A provides adequate anticoagulation. Because whole blood, processed by either method, comes in contact with plasticware, complement activation can occur, as ample in vitro evidence demonstrates. As a general rule, centrifugal separation generates less C3a than filtration.[9] Significant clinical sequelae of complement activation are almost nonexistent during therapeutic apheresis; however, the superimposition and possibly additive effect of CPB complement activation has not been carefully studied.

Almost all current apheresis equipment is at least semiautomated and has appropriate safety/alarm systems that prevent development of inappropriate fluid imbalances during the procedure. Monitors of access and return pressure as well as air in the tubing are standard on automated systems.

In general, complications during or after therapeutic or donor apheresis are rare.[1] The most common complication of any significance is a vasovagal reaction with transient hypotension, which may be more pronounced in patients with autonomic neuropathies; however, simple postural changes and volume expansion usually suffice to control it. Hypotension can also occur if apheresis equipment with relatively high extracorporeal volume is used in patients who are volume-depleted or taking drugs that blunt pressure-regulating mechanisms. In the rare circumstance in which homologous fresh frozen plasma is used for replacement, serious transfusion reactions may occur, but they are infrequent. The most serious morbidity relates not to the procedure itself, but to the frequent need, especially in critically ill patients, for central line access and its attendant complications. Patients with extensive liver disease or low ionized calcium for any reason, patients receiving superimposed citrate in fresh frozen plasma, and children are somewhat more susceptible to citrate toxicity. Most equipment, however, has the flexibility to alter the ratio of citrate anticoagulant flow to whole blood and thus to prevent bothersome tingling and symptomatic hypocalcemia.

Continuing improvements in the technology of fluid and cell separation have fostered creative uses of apheresis in cardiovascular surgery (Table 1). The availability of equipment and plasticware that minimize extracorporeal whole blood volume (200 ml or less) during processing allows rapid and efficient treatment of patients even with severe hemodynamic compromise. On the horizon are two-step blood filtration methods that hold great promise for even more selective removal of cellular and protein components from processed whole blood and less need for nonautologous replacement of albumin.

TABLE 1. Apheresis in Cardiac Surgery

Plasmapheresis	Platelet collection
Preoperative prophylactic strategy	Postoperative use of autologous
Hyperviscosity diseases	platelets for hemostasis
Waldenstrom's macroglobulin	
Multiple myeloma	**Automated erythrocyte exchange**
Cryoglobulinemia	Sickle-cell hemoglobinopathies
Cold agglutinin disease	
Postoperative strategy	
Reinfusion of autologous plasma for hemostasis	
Complication related to therapy	
Heparin-induced thrombosis	

THERAPEUTIC PLASMA EXCHANGE

The first successful use of apheresis was the removal of serum proteins by plasmapheresis. Although the rationale of pathogenic antibody depletion appears straightforward, it may be too simplistic because plasma removal also depletes circulating cytokines and soluble antigens as well as enhances mechanisms of splenic clearance, presumably by decreasing the level of circulating antigen-antibody complexes. The latter may also be crucial for maintenance and regulation of idiotypic-antiidiotypic networks. Thus the therapeutic effects of plasmapheresis are most likely multifactorial.

Current apheresis technology with either centrifugation or membrane separation of plasma is efficient and rapid. Under normal circumstances and appropriate vascular access, 1–1.5 plasma volumes can be removed in a 2-hour period. Because the entire plasma fraction is removed, global depletion (63–86%) of all plasma components occurs, not just the putative or potentially pathogenic antibody molecules. The reduction of serum level of antibody varies with the immunoglobulin isotype. Immunoglobulin M, a large molecule with a molecular weight in the range of one million daltons, circulates predominantly within the intravascular space; its removal by plasma exchange is highly efficient (at times approaching 85%). The reappearance of IgM molecules in the patient's plasma depends basically on the rate of synthesis by the B-cell lymphoid system. Because IgG is not as large (approximately 160,000 daltons), it is not confined to the intravascular space; thus attempts to deplete substantially this class of antibody molecules are much more difficult. Usually, for example, removal of a volume of plasma equal to the patient's plasma volume depletes only about 60% of circulating IgG. If the amount of plasma depletion is increased during apheresis to 1.5 times the patient's plasma volume, removal of IgG increases only to about 80%. Further increases in volume of plasma removal result in only small additional increments of removal and are usually associated with increased side effects from the procedure itself, especially citrate toxicity. Because IgG, in contrast to IgM, has a wide distribution throughout both intra- and extravascular spaces, reequilibration of IgG into the intravascular space after initial depletion of the molecule by plasma exchange is rapid. This usually dictates more frequent apheresis when the treated disease is caused by IgG antibody.

Unfortunately, calculation of the appropriate plasma volume for removal during plasmapheresis is usually not achievable by scientific calculation and remains largely a clinical art shaped by previous experience with the disease in question. A standard plasma exchange is usually 1-1.5 plasma volumes. Need for rapid removal of IgM can justify 2.0-2.5 plasma volume exchanges. A crude assessment of a patient's plasma volume can be calculated by using 40 ml/kg as a common standard. However, hematocrit, body surface area, and gender are important variables in determining plasma volume; therefore, widely available normograms should be used for precise determination. Some modern cell separators calculate plasma volume by keyboard entry of appropriate variables during the procedure set-up.

The frequency of therapeutic plasma exchange treatments also remains unknown in almost all diseases in which it is shown to have efficacy; thus it too is dictated by individual clinical situations.

Plasmapheresis has predictable effects on plasma hemostatic factors. Factor VIII, antithrombin III, and several other clotting factors are decreased 30-40% immediately after a standard 1.5 volume exchange. The rate of fibrinogen depletion may be somewhat greater and, in some instances, may approach 75%. Just as the rates of depletion are variable, so are the rates of synthetic recovery. Up to 72-96 hours may elapse in some patients before return of fibrinogen and other clotting factors to accepted normal levels. However, extensive use of plasmapheresis in various clinical situations has not been associated with significant bleeding, and depletion of clotting factors is apparently more of a cosmetic than a functional aberration. Severe bleeding is more likely to occur in situations with concomitant impairment of factor synthesis, especially in patients with advanced liver disease. The risk of a potentially dangerous hemostasis deficiency can be averted by substituting fresh frozen plasma products for other colloid replacement during plasmapheresis.

Symptomatic hypocalcemia secondary to the citrate required for anticoagulation during plasmapheresis is common. In the nonsurgical setting, symptoms are limited usually to circumoral paresthesias or ill-defined myalgias. Severe reactions occur rarely. In many circumstances in cardiac surgery, the patient is unable to describe the beginning of hypocalcemic symptoms, and the usual warning mechanism that activates reduction of the proportion of citrate to plasma by changing the rate of infusion is not present. Thus, during anesthesia and surgery, the electrocardiogram as well as serum calcium should be carefully monitored, and the lowest possible ratios of citrate to whole blood should be used.

A very rare complication that is nonetheless highly relevant to cardiac surgery may result from a significant reduction of plasma cholinesterase by plasmapheresis. Some patients have retarded resynthesis of the enzyme, and prolonged apnea during induction of anesthesia has been reported.[7]

The significant depletion of antibody proteins during plasmapheresis may also lead to a temporary decrease in a patient's ability to respond to bacterial infection. Synthesis of antibodies to new antigens in the normal host is usually extremely rapid, and most clinical situations require little antibody replacement. But in the severely debilitated host, in the patient undergoing cardiac or lung transplantation, in other artificially immunocompromised patients, and in patients requiring placement of a ventricular assist device, intravenous immunoglobulin fractions (100 mg/kg) should be given after plasmapheresis.

SPECIFIC INDICATIONS FOR PLASMAPHEREIS

The common clinical setting that prompts use of therapeutic plasma exchange (TPE) in cardiac surgery is the perceived need to remove pathogenic antibodies that have the potential to cause hemolysis, impaired microcirculation, or thrombosis.

Hyperviscosity Syndrome

In the rare instance when a patient with a hyperviscosity syndrome related to multiple myeloma, Waldenstrom's macroglobulinemia, or abnormal cryoproteins requires cardiac surgery, TPE is the primary method for rapid reduction of high viscosity values caused by abnormal plasma proteins and thus for normalization of intra- and postoperative capillary rheology.[14] A concomitant salutary effect of plasmapheresis during removal of abnormal serum proteins in most hyperviscosity syndromes is reversal of the commonly associated platelet defect; this effect further decreases the risk of serious postoperative bleeding.

Heparin-Associated Thrombocytopenia with Thrombosis

Approximately 5–15% of patients treated with heparin develop thrombocytopenia. A minority of these develop a somewhat paradoxical and potentially catastrophic complication of venous or arterial thrombosis (or both). Heparin-induced thrombosis has a high mortality rate and has necessitated amputation in approximately 20% of survivors. Because the heparin-induced syndromes are widely thought to be antibody-mediated, they become suitable candidates for remediation by plasmapheresis. We have previously reported the usefulness of plasmapheresis in a patient with heparin-induced thrombosis.[11] She had undergone successful aortofemoral bypass surgery but on the fourth postoperative day developed a painful, cold right foot that rapidly became ischemic and required amputation on day 7. Three days later the patient complained of similar pain in the left foot but did not respond to infusion of Dextran 40. She had received heparin prior to bypass surgery, and the heparin-associated aggregation test was strongly positive. Heparin was stopped; therapy with Dextran 40 and aspirin was begun.

In the face of no improvement, we elected to begin plasmapheresis; a 1.5 plasma volume exchange led to an immediate decrease in pain and significantly improved results from the platelet aggregation test. Her platelet count rose to 90,000 and, after the second plasma exchange, normalized (Fig. 1). Although the distal phalanges, which had become completely gangrenous, were lost, the foot became warm and arterial pulses returned. The patient was able to ambulate with assistance shortly thereafter. Subsequent reports have confirmed the efficacy of plasmapheresis in this devastating syndrome; our continuing experience leads us to believe that aggressive, early intervention with plasmapheresis can be life-saving.

Conversely, the temptation to use TPE to reduce heparin-associated platelet antibody without thrombosis should be resisted. No reliable evidence suggests that plasmapheresis is efficacious in accelerating the reversal of heparin-induced thrombocytopenia; in fact, theoretical concepts suggest that it

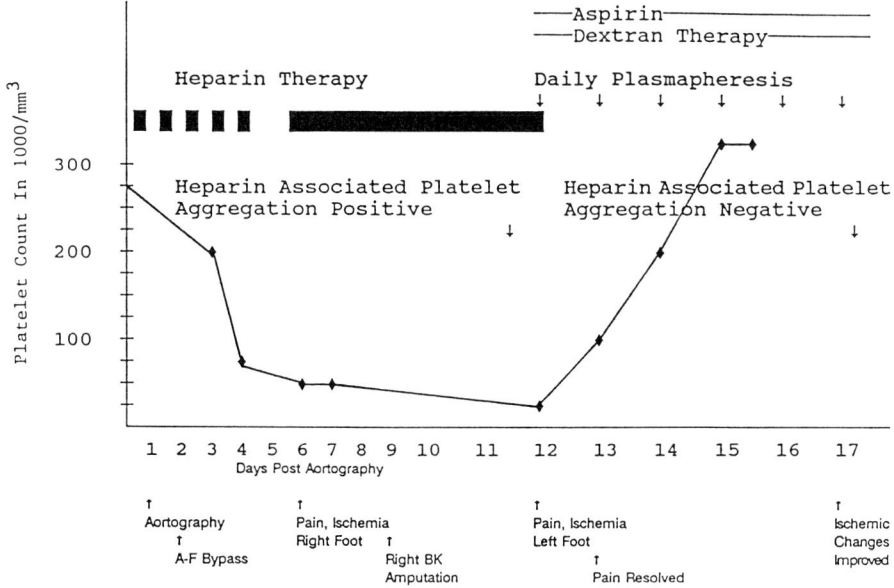

FIGURE 1. Clinical course of a patient with heparin-induced thrombosis treated with plasmapheresis.

may even extend the syndrome by prompting antibody rebound after treatment is stopped. The identification of platelet crystallizable fragment receptors as the binding site of heparin-immunoglobulin complexes[16] may stimulate the development of specific columns to remove only the pathogenic complexes during double filtration pheresis. Fortunately, the impending availability of low-molecular-weight heparin may decrease the incidence of heparin-induced thrombosis and thrombocytopenia, thus removing the need for pheresis.

Cold Agglutinin Disease

Cold agglutinin disease is a relatively rare cause of autoimmune hemolytic anemia. Significant hemolysis may occur after binding of a temperature-dependent IgM autoantibody to I-erythrocyte antigens. The thermal amplitude and activation of the antibody varies widely from patient to patient, and antibody coating of cells usually occurs as they traverse cool body areas such as skin and digits. Once the IgM binds to an erythrocyte, intravascular agglutination occurs; the complement system may also be activated as antibody-coated cells and recirculate to areas of warmer temperature. The resultant hemolysis is usually mild to moderate but in rare situations can be acute and fulminant.

Systemic and myocardial hypothermia during CPB may activate autoantibody-induced agglutination and lead to massive hemolysis, myocardial ischemia, or maldistribution of cardioplegia. Low titers of cold agglutinin antibodies are common in many patients and may be viewed as normally occurring autoantibodies. Although the threat that cold agglutinins pose to both surgeon and patient has been overemphasized, the detection of cold agglutinin in a patient scheduled for CPB can pose a vexing problem for the cardiac surgeon.[13] If a patient has exceptionally high titers of cold agglutinins as well as evidence of hemolysis and anemia, the surgeon should suspect an underlying lymphoproliferative disease. Elective procedures should be postponed until malignancy or autoimmune disease is ruled out. In most circumstances a cold agglutinin is detected in an otherwise normal patient scheduled for surgery.

Unfortunately, the in vitro detection and quantitation of cold agglutinin correlates loosely with its ability to cause in vivo hemolysis; thus simple measurement of cold agglutinin titer during the preoperative work-up may well be of little help in predicting which patients will develop significant agglutination and hemolysis during and after cooling. Determination of thermal amplitude—that is, the critical temperature at which the autoantibody begins to bind to erythrocytes—may be most helpful in the preoperative work-up of a patient with cold agglutinin. In most institutions, however, precise determination of the temperature is not routinely available. When it is, the most direct solution is to perform the surgical procedure at a temperature higher than the thermal amplitude of the autoantibody. In many situations, the thermal amplitude is reported as 4, 20, or 37°C. Cold agglutinins active only at 4°C are not dangerous; only those with amplitudes between 20-37°C are problematic. In such a situation, with cold agglutinin titers >1:200, it may be prudent to be safe rather than sorry and to use plasmapheresis before surgery. Fortunately, a 2.0 plasma volume exchange is usually quite effective in acutely reducing cold agglutinins because the antibody is an IgM isotype distributed mainly in the intravascular space. The plasmapheresis procedure can be technically difficult, especially with high thermal amplitude antibodies, because erythrocyte agglutination at ambient temperatures of the extracorporeal circuit may occur without meticulous care to maintain plasticware, machines, and replacement fluid at higher temperatures than usual. The timing of plasmapheresis is also critical because the half-life of IgM, especially if the antibody is produced by monoclonal B-lymphocyte disease, may be <2-4 days; thus the procedure should be performed immediately (within 24 hr) before CPB.

In addition to performing the procedure at temperatures >32°C, the surgeon should use warm cardioplegia and warmed replacement fluids and blood components. A practical note is that erroneous low hematocrits may be reported during CPB if blood samples are allowed to cool before centrifugation.[15]

SPECIFIC INDICATIONS FOR CELLULAR APHERESIS

Although plasmapheresis has been widely used for several decades in a wide variety of diseases as well as in normal donors for production of homologous fresh frozen plasma, only recently has interest in removal of specific cell components from native blood increased. Burgeoning interest in the use of modified immune effector cells for cancer treatment, collection of hematopoietic stem cells for reconstitution of bone marrow after chemotherapy, and the urgent need for maximal restriction of allogenic blood component transfusions have been the driving forces behind the development of new cell separators capable of harvesting immense numbers of specific cell populations rapidly and efficiently. The need for enhancing blood conservation and autologous reuse seems not only intuitively obvious, but also imperative in the face of the continuing threat of blood-borne disease transmission. Even though sensitive and specific methods are now available to screen blood donors for the presence of lethal retroviruses and hepatitis, the specter of antibody negative-virus positive donors is still quite real. The probability of an infectious homologous blood component in the United States is extremely low, but even minimal risk of transmitting a potentially fatal infectious component mandates maximal use of autologous blood products in cardiac surgery. Reduced exposure to allogenic blood components and cytomegalovirus is very important for recipients of thoracic organ transplants. A third, equally important reason for exploiting apheresis for autologous component harvesting is that the troublesome aberrations in hemostasis after CPB persist as clinically important morbidities in spite of refinements in surgical technique and procedure.

Cardiovascular and orthopedic surgeons, in collaboration with transfusionists, have responded with innovative schemes to use autologous blood components. Not only have surgeons salvaged intraoperative erythrocytes, but they are now beginning to use apheresis for autologous, preoperative collection of platelet-rich plasma components for eventual postoperative reinfusion.

The window of opportunity for using cell separators for rapid collection of platelets or platelet-rich plasma is the 24 hours before surgery. Because harvested platelets maintain at least 50% function for periods up to 5 days, earlier harvesting of platelet-rich plasma is theoretically possible, but usually not practical in most cardiac surgery settings. Fortunately, the efficiency of mobile cell separators does not impinge on other mandatory preoperative procedures; thus platelets can be collected in the anesthesia holding area or the actual surgical suite up to the moment the patient is placed on pump. Suitable candidates for preoperative platelet collection should have peripheral platelet counts above 150,000 mm^3; lower counts may result in surgery in a patient with a platelet count <100,000 mm^3. The major plasma-cell component collected preoperatively and used in postoperative infusion to improve hemostasis is autologous plasma with varying amounts of platelets; the number depends on procedure, duration of collection, and availability of platelets in the peripheral blood.

Forty-five patients scheduled for aortocoronary bypass surgery underwent pheresis after induction of anesthesia.[4] The apheresis procedure was completed before onset of surgery. Patients excluded from the study were those with ejection fractions <50% or left ventricular end-diastolic pressures >20 mmHg. We have successfully performed 1.5 plasma volume exchanges in patients with much more severe hemodynamic compromise and do not believe moderately severe ventricular dysfunction is a contraindication to preoperative harvesting of autologous components if the pheresis equipment has low extracorporeal whole blood volumes (<200 ml) and uses continuous flow collections. In any event, apheresis in this study protocol was performed by two different methods: plasmapheresis, which generated platelet-poor plasma, and platelet collection, which generated platelet-rich plasma. Averages of platelet counts/product were not provided.

Patients were randomly divided into two treatment groups and a control group; the autologous plasma products were returned after termination of extracorporeal circulation. Blood loss over the next 24 hours was significantly greater in the control group that received no autologous plasma product. Two patients in the control group also required transfusion of homologous packed red cells, whereas neither group receiving autologous reinfusion required homologous products. Sequential measurement of laboratory hemostatic variables consistently showed that concentrations of antithrombin III and fibrinogen were higher in the groups that received plasma components.

Giordano and colleagues compared 57 patients who underwent CPB surgery without reinfusion of autologous platelet-rich plasma with 30 patients who underwent similar surgery with reinfusion of preoperative, apheresis-generated autologous platelet-rich plasma.[8] Both patient groups received intraoperative autotransfusion cell salvage, and the study group received the autologous platelet product immediately after CPB when heparin neutralization had been completed. The study group that received platelets harvested by apheresis of approximately 1 whole-blood volume immediately before surgery required less postoperative plasma and platelet transfusion. The total postoperative platelet requirement in the treatment group was significantly reduced by 3.53 random donor units/case. During the 2 months when the infusion of autologous platelet-rich plasma was available at the medical center, no postoperative platelets were required in saphenous vein grafting procedures or in a small number of reoperative bypass procedures. Overall, after the institution of this program, homologous blood exposures per case fell from 14 to 6 component units; in addition, the cost benefit was significant.[6]

A third group of investigators also used apheresis to generate platelet-rich plasma from 15 patients during a 24-hour period before scheduled surgery.[12] The harvested product per patient ranged from 8-17 platelet units (5×10^{10} platelet/unit) in 300-350 ml plasma and was reinfused after protamine neutralization of heparin on termination of CPB. The study and control groups were stratified by risk factors that included past history of sternotomy, prior history of myocardial infarction, and history of bleeding tendency. The pheresis-treated group were higher-risk patients. The results mirror the previously discussed studies in reduced use of all homologous blood products and significant cost benefit in the group reinfused with autologous components. The conclusion appears to be that relatively simple techniques of blood component harvesting in the immediate preoperative period can generate hemostatically functional products that are useful for reducing the need for postoperative use of homologous blood components.

An additional benefit to preoperative apheresis has been postulated by Davis and associates,[5] who studied 32 patients who received autologous platelet- and leukocyte-enriched plasma after aortocoronary grafting. As in previous studies, comparison with historical controls documented a decrease in postoperative bleeding and need for homologous blood products as well as a significant reduction in cost. Additional observations of interest were that patients reinfused with platelet-leukocyte-rich autologous plasma had higher PaO_2 and higher PaO_2/FiO_2 at the time of extubation. The investigators implied that an 11% reduction in circulating leukocytes as well as platelets immediately before surgery minimized the toxic sequelae of CPB-driven, complement-activated sequestration of neutrophils in pulmonary capillaries. One should be skeptical of this implication. If indeed the improved PaO_2 is a genuine finding, it is more likely that postoperative return of plasma withdrawn during the preoperative collection of enriched plasma product protected pulmonary function from neutrophil adhesion to alveolar capillaries by making available complement, chemotaxis, and regulators of adhesion molecules. This possible additional benefit of apheresis to the cardiac surgeon, however, could be a deciding factor in the postoperative course of a debilitated patient and deserves to be documented in a randomized trial with appropriate controls.

At this point a caveat must be evoked. The use of small 1-1.5 whole-blood volume apheresis to generate such platelet-rich plasma does not yield the number of platelets necessary to regain hemostasis in cardiac surgical procedures that result in severe, multifactorial bleeding diathesis. The amount of blood that would have to be processed in the immediate preoperative setting is not feasible with current technology and may also result in reducing the count of circulating platelets to dangerous levels during surgery. The next logical step to define further the benefit of preoperative collection of autologous product is proper organization of a multicenter trial to identify which cardiac surgery patients will benefit most from such technology and which do not require it.

ERYTHROCYTE EXCHANGE

Little attention has been devoted to improving the technology of red blood cell exchange. The exception is the COBE Spectra, a continuous-flow centrifugal system that provides automated exchange of erythrocytes. Specific patient data are provided to the system, along with physician-determined goals that include desired hematocrit and a target percentage of hemoglobin reduction. The system then calculates the exchange necessary to reach the goals. A frequent complication of discontinuous-flow exchange of erythrocytes is extracorporeal clotting, which does not occur in the continuous system. The optimal range of timing for a red cell exchange is not known, but most clinicians recommend 24 hours before surgery.

Furthermore, although surgical folklore suggests a high frequency of postoperative complications in sickle-cell hemoglobinopathies, no definite consensus requires preoperative transfusion of erythrocytes or exchange transfusion in these patients. A group of 66 patients with sickle-cell hemoglobinopathies were retrospectively analyzed for the incidence of postoperative complications related to preoperative transfusions. No advantage accrued to the transfused patients.[2] Adverse clinical sequelae may simply be less frequent than expected with the use of contemporary, improved preoperative preparation of the patient and management of anesthesia. Although none of the patients in the study had undergone cardiac surgery, the theoretical complications are clear: reduced capillary blood flow and tissue hypoxia secondary to stasis caused by sickle erythrocytes during unavoidable changes in pH, PaO_2, and temperature during CPB. In this setting, it seems prudent to increase oxygen-carrying capacity and to reduce the potential for sickle-cell capillary stasis by preoperative red cell exchange. The in vitro rheology of blood approaches normal when it contains <40% hemoglobin-containing cells.[10] This finding has prompted the widespread adoption of 50% or less hemoglobin as a requirement before cardiac surgery in a patient with sickle-cell hemoglobinopathy.

ACKNOWLEDGMENT

The author thanks Brenda J. Smith for expert manuscript and graphic preparation.

REFERENCES

1. Barnes A: Untoward effects of plasmapheresis. In Nosé PS, Malchesky PS, Smith JW (eds): Therapeutic Apheresis: A Critical Look. Cleveland, ISAO Press, 1984, pp 11-14.
2. Bischoff RJ, Williamson A III, Dalali MJ, et al: Assessment of the use of transfusion therapy perioperatively in patients with sickle cell hemoglobinopathies. Ann Surg 207:434-438, 1988.
3. Boldt J, Kling D, Zickman B, et al: Acute plasmapheresis during cardiac surgery: Volume replacement by crystalloids versus colloids. J Cardiothorac Anesth 5:564-570, 1990.
4. Boldt J, von Bormann B, Kling D, et al: Preoperative plasmapheresis in patients undergoing cardiac surgery procedures. J Cardiothorac Anesth 72:282-288, 1990.
5. Davies GG, Wells DG, Mabee TM, et al: Platelet-leukocyte plasmapheresis attenuates the deleterious effects of cardiopulmonary bypass. Ann Thorac Surg 53:274-277, 1992.
6. Davies GG, Wells DG, Mabee TM, et al: Plateletpheresis and the cost of heart operations. Ann Thorac Surg 53:940-945, 1992.
7. Evans RT, MacDonald R, Robinson EAE: Suxamethonium apnea associated with plasmapheresis. Anesthesia 35:198-201, 1980.
8. Giordano GF, Rivers SL, Chung GKT, et al: Autologous platelet-rich plasma in cardiac surgery: Effect on intraoperative and postoperative transfusion requirements. Ann Thorac Surg 46:416-419, 1988.
9. Konstantin P, Neumann HJ: The advantages of centrifugation in therapeutic plasmapheresis. In Smit CT, Kater L (eds): Advances in Haemapheresis. Kluwer Academic Publications 25:5-11, 1991.
10. Lessins LS, Kurant Sin-Mills J, Klug PP, et al: Determination of rheologically optimal mixtures of AA and SS erythrocytes. Blood 50(Suppl):111-114, 1977.
11. Nand S, Robinson JA: Plasmapheresis in the management of heparin-associated thrombocytopenia with thrombosis. Am J Hematol 28:204-206, 1988.
12. Noon GP, Jones J, Fehir K, Yawn DH: Use of preoperatively obtained platelets and plasma in patients undergoing cardiopulmonary bypass. J Clin Apheresis 5:91-96, 1990.
13. Park JV, Weiss CI: Cardiopulmonary bypass and myocardial protection: Management problems in cardiac surgical patients with cold autoimmune disease. Anesth Analg 67:75-78, 1988.
14. Reinhart WH, Lutolf O, Nydegger U, et al: Plasmapheresis for hyperviscosity syndrome in macroglobulinemia Waldenstrom and multiple myeloma: Influence on blood rheology and the microcirculation. J Lab Clin Med 119:69-76, 1992.
15. Rowbottom SJ: Hypothermia, myocardial protection, and cold agglutinin disease. Anesth Analg 67:1192-1193, 1988.
16. Warkentin TE, Kelton JG: Heparin-induced thrombocytopenia. Prog Hemost Thromb 10:1-34, 1991.

Chapter 17

Control and Treatment of Hemostasis in Patients with a Total Artificial Heart: The Experience of La Pitié

Jacques Szefner, M.D., and Christian Cabrol, M.D.

The rapid development of cardiovascular surgery in general and of heart transplantation in particular has highlighted the increasing needs for different orthotopic and heterotopic circulatory assist devices and for research directed toward the permanent and independent total artificial heart (TAH). Furthermore, the gap between the patient population that could benefit from a heart transplant and the number of potential donors (which has almost reached a plateau of stability throughout the world) is constantly widening. Support therapy that serves as a bridge to heart transplantation, therefore, has become even more important.

When the recovery of the heart appears difficult or impossible, a circulatory assist device becomes necessary, either to restore normal function or to enable the patient to wait for transplantation. The optimal conditions therefore require (1) careful choice of the appropriate type of assistance to ensure correct hemodynamics and recovery of various functions (e.g., renal, hepatic); (2) absence of infection; and (3) control of hemostasis.

This chapter summarizes the control and treatment of hemostasis in patients implanted with a Symbion Jarvik-7 TAH. Implantation, performed in an orthotopic position, requires cardiopulmonary bypass (CPB). Because the common denominator among postoperative complications with all forms of circulatory assistance is deviation from adequate coagulation that leads to thrombosis, bleeding, or both, we can extrapolate the application of follow-up and treatment protocols. The general principles are not restrictive and can be adapted to other clinical conditions in which the various systems of hemostasis are activated. In the last few years at La Pitié Hospital, we have established a follow-up of hemostasis that carefully correlates the global study of platelet function and coagulolytic balance with the clinical state of the patient in the pre- and postoperative (both immediate and remote) periods.

The topics covered in this chapter include (1) presentation and outcome of cases; (2) approach to hemostasis, including specific methods and tests, control of fibrinolysis, stabilization of platelet function, and balanced coagulation; (3) brief account of the longest implantation; and (4) conclusions drawn from the experience at La Pitié.

PRESENTATION OF SYMBION JARVIK-7 TAH CASES

From April 1986 to December 1991, 60 patients received a Jarvik-7, including 52 men and 8 women between the ages of 15 and 57 (mean ± SD = 39.22 ± 11.41). The indications for surgery were primary dilated cardiomyopathy (22 patients), ischemic cardiomyopathy (21), acute late graft rejection (5), primary graft failure (4), postpartum cardiomyopathy (4), valvular cardiomyopathy (1), and miscellaneous (3). The total duration of CPB ranged from 95–427 minutes (mean ± SD = 158.5 ± 61.52, and the total implantation time was 1589 days, ranging from 1–603 days (mean ± SD = 26.48 ± 78.47).

Patients suffered strong and permanent aggression (continuous injury) at every level of each coagulation system. Disturbances were caused in the perioperative period by global heart failure, different anticoagulant treatments, and CPB of long duration. In the postoperative period they were caused first by implantation of four mechanical valves and two pneumatic ventricles with extensive blood contact that resulted in turbulent flow and somewhat later by infection. For patients with either a Jarvik-7 TAH or other types of circulatory assist devices, the effects on hemostasis are ultimately the same.

RESULTS

The results obtained for all patients include (1) control of biologic bleeding, which enabled us to detect other causes of bleeding and permitted rational use of blood products; (2) absence of thromboembolic accidents; (3) absence of thrombi at high-risk sites after explantation, as confirmed by microscopic analysis by the manufacturer (Score SOP-035); and (4) absence of iatrogenic bleeding.

APPROACH TO HEMOSTASIS

Because problems are posed at every level of hemostasis, control of all systems involved is imperative, including (1) the platelet system; (2) the procoagulant system and its regulation (the inhibitory system); and (3) the fibrinolytic system. The fundamental role of hemorrheology must also be taken into account, for all systems are tightly interwoven. The changes detected in the various systems do not appear as isolated phenomena but as a unit; thus they require a multiple therapeutic strategy. The specific modalities determine the follow-up protocol (coagulolytic assessment). Treatment must be adapted to the individual patient, and four major objectives should be attained:

1. Strict normocoagulability must be achieved and maintained by respecting, on the one hand, the potential of the inhibitory system and, on the other, thrombin formation compatible with normal hemostasis but incompatible with an excessive hemostatic capacity.

2. The first objective must be associated with platelet stabilization to enable the platelet to respond effectively when it is needed (primary hemostasis) but with a high-sensitivity threshold that allows it be be indifferent to the effects of CPB, to changes in laminar flow, to implantation of prostheses, and to foreign material.

3. At the same time the fibrinolytic system must be left intact, with constant surveillance to ensure that physiologic triggering of this system maintains hemostatic balance of the whole.

4. Clearly this whole must always be adapted to the changing clinical and surgical status of the patient.

Methods of Assessment

Blood samples are drawn for (1) preoperative assessment (day-1); (2) assessment 30 minutes after neutralization of heparin by protamine (day-0) when CPB is terminated; (3) daily assessment while the patient is in intensive care; and (4) assessment 2 or 3 times a week in cases of long-term implantation without complications. Evaluations are carried out more frequently when complications arise.

Specific Tests

To achieve an effective appraisal of hemostasis and thereby protect against accidents, routine screening must be supplemented with a variety of tests aimed at specific targets.

Platelet Activation. The first test necessary for control of platelet activation is the **platelet count**, a decrease in which may be the first sign of consumption coagulopathy. The **hematocrit value** is also important because of its influence on global coagulability and on the sludge phenomenon. **Platelet aggregation** may be assessed with four inductors: adenosine diphosphate (ADP), adrenalin, collagen, and arachidonic acid. We concentrate essentially on deduction of existing relations between in vitro reactivity curves (or rather their absence) and in vivo reactivity curves. In assessing **platelet factor 4** (PF4) and **beta-thromboglobulin** (βTG), it is important to remember that in vivo concentrations are inversely proportional to in vitro activity. The systemic determination of PF4 and βTG in plasma helps to detect in vivo platelet hyperactivity and thus constitutes a reliable measurement of the efficiency of the stabilizing and antiaggregant treatment. PF4 is fixed to the endothelium after being released by platelets into plasma, has a short half-life (5 min), and helps to prevent the combination of heparin with antithrombin III (AT III). βTG, together with other compounds, is responsible for platelet adhesion and for the interactions between platelets and between vessels and platelets. It also has a different metabolism and renal elimination (half-life: 100 min).

Procoagulant System and Its Inhibitory Regulation. Analysis of the procoagulant system begins with assessment of the **prothrombin time** (PT) and **activated partial thromboplastin time** (APTT) in order to appreciate the deficit created with or without anticoagulant treatment. The second test focuses on **fibrinogen**, the raw material of the clot structure. **Thromboelastography** (TEG) on recalcified whole blood is the only test sensitive to global coagulability and enables study of the different phases of coagulation. It can reveal the kinetics, dynamics, and syneresis of clot formation as well as the structural quality of the clot. From the TEG is obtained the **thrombodynamic potential index** (TPI), which permits labeling of global coagulation as normo-, hyper-, or hypocoagulable. **Raby's Transfer Test** on plasma allows control of heparin therapy and detects circulating thromboplastinic material. We maintain a test value >1, which indicates adequate anticoagulant activity.

The determination of **AT III in plasma** (AT IIIp), the main inhibitor and regulator of thrombin formation, and **in serum** (AT IIIs) allows calculation of the **antithrombinic potential index** (API) by subtraction of AT IIIs from AT IIIp. In turn, the API indicates adaptation of inhibition to global coagulability. In cases of serious clinical deterioration (i.e., disseminated intravascular coagulation [DIC] of any origin), the appearance of the **pinching phenomenon** provides a more precise indication of prognosis and treatment. The pinching phenomenon is characterized by the decrease of AT IIIp and the increase of AT IIIs (which reflects the exhaustion of AT III), both of which are associated with hypocoagulability. Finally, the determination of **activated factor X in plasma** (FXa p) and **in serum** (FXa s) indicates the speed of thrombin formation.

Fibrinolytic System. Analysis of the fibrinolytic system relies on three tests: (1) The **reptilase time** indicates the antithrombinic action of fibrinogen/fibrin degradation products (FDPs), even under anticoagulant therapy. (2) Assessment of **Alpha-2-antiplasmin**, the most powerful inhibitor of fibrinolysis, which shows the degree of activation of the fibrinolytic system. (3) An increase in **FDPs** is a clear sign of greater deposit of fibrin.

Other Targets. The following tests are used as needed:

Ivy bleeding time, as modified by Borchgrevink, for study of platelet adhesiveness

Wu-Hoak test for detection of circulating platelet aggregates

Platelet aggregation with other inductors

Raby's K test, a safety test with use of oral anticoagulants (inhibitors of vitamin K)

Counts of protein C and protein S, vitamin K-dependent inhibitors of coagulation

Assessment of heparin cofactor II, another inhibitor of coagulation

Assessment of fibrinopeptide A for detection in outpatients of traces of thrombin formation

D-dimer screening test of the activation of coagulation (if $<$ 500 ng/ml, further testing is unnecessary)

Tissue-type plasminogen activator (t-PA), plasminogen activator inhibitor (PAI), plasminogen, and venous occlusion test for verifying the failure of the profibrinolytic system

These tests allow optimal surveillance of hemostasis and institution of appropriate therapy. Although in appearance extensive, the series can be performed in any moderately equipped hemostasis laboratory, either manually or, in most cases, automatically or semiautomatically. Time and cost depend on resources of the laboratory. The cost, however, is justified by the clinical results. In patients who have undergone heart surgery, these tests help to avoid empirical administration of antifibrinolytic, anticoagulant, or antiaggregant treatments.

OBJECTIVES OF THERAPY

A brief description of the basic objectives for effective control of hemostasis in all patients contributes to a clearer understanding of the rationale for the different treatments. The objectives of therapy are (1) to stop fibrinolysis; (2) to stabilize platelet function; and (3) to balance coagulation.

Stopping Fibrinolysis

Fibrinolysis is due to the activation of plasminogen after it has overcome the effect of its inhibitors. Active plasmin protease formed is physiologically inhibited mainly by alpha-2-antiplasmin. This inhibition can lead to exhaustion if the activation of the fibrinolytic system has been too great or of too long duration. Disseminated intravascular coagulation (DIC) results, mainly in the microcirculation.

The follow-up of DIC is of the utmost importance. Our protocol distinguishes four distinct phases of DIC, each with a different biologic profile and a different therapeutic approach: (1) compensated thrombophilia; (2) clot kinetic-structure dissociation; (3) generalized hypocoagulability, with the pinching phenomenon; and (4) secondary fibrinolysis.

Phase 1. Compensated Thrombophilia

Factors	Conserved	Platelet count	Normal
Fibrinogen	Normal	Platelet aggregation	Slightly ↓
Reptilase time	Moderately ↑	Platelet proteins (PF4-βTG)	Slightly ↑
Plasma AT III	Normal or ↑	Plasminogen	Normal
Serum AT III	↓	Alpha-2-antiplasmin	Normal
API	↑	FDP	(-) or (+)
TEG r	5		
k	2		
MA	60		
TPI	75		

Treatment: Abstain from treating, but closely survey the evolution of the process.

Phase 2. Clot Kinetic-structure Dissociation

Factors	Moderately ↓	Platelet count	↓
Fibrinogen	↑ or ↓	Platelet aggregation	↓
Reptilase time	↑	Platelet proteins (PF4-βTG)	↑
Plasma AT III	↓	Plasminogen	↓
Serum AT III	↓	Alpha-2-antiplasmin	Normal or ↓
API	Normal or ↓	FDP	(+) or (++)
TEG r	6-10		
k	±20		
MA	30-35		
TPI	2.7		

Treatment: Heparin, 10-20 IU/kg/day; dipyridamole, 150-200 mg every 6 hours.

Phase 3. Generalized Hypocoagulability with Pinching Phenomenon

Factors	↓ ↓	Raby's transfer test	(+) (<1)
Fibrinogen	↑ or ↓	Platelet count	↓ ↓
Reptilase time	↑ ↑	Platelet aggregation	↓ ↓ or (−)
Plasma AT III	↓ ↓	Platelet proteins (PF4-βTG)	↑ ↑
Serum AT III	↑	Plasminogen	↓ ↓
API	↓ or ↓ ↓	Alpha-2-antiplasmin	↓ ↓
TEG r	30–40	FDP	(++)
k	∞		
MA	∞		
TPI	0		

Treatment: Heparin, 5–10 IU/kg/day; dipyridamole, 200–300 mg every 6 hours; fresh frozen plasma or fresh whole blood to replace missing factors.

Phase 4. Secondary Fibrinolysis

Factors	↓ ↓ ↓	Raby's transfer test	(−) (>1)
Fibrinogen	↑ or ↓ ↓	Platelet count	↓ ↓
Reptilase time	↑ ↑ ↑	Platelet aggregation	(−)
Plasma AT III	↓ ↓ ↓	Platelet proteins (PF4-βTG)	↑ ↑ ↑
Serum AT III	↓ ↓	Plasminogen	↓ ↓
API	↓ or ↓ ↓	Alpha-2-antiplasmin	↓ ↓ ↓ or (−)
TEG r	40	FDP	(+++)
k	∞		
MA	∞		
TPI	0		

Treatment: Aprotinin, 125,000 KIU intravenously, followed by a drip of 500 KIU/min; heparin, 5–10 IU/kg/day; dipyridamole, 200–300 mg every 6 hours; fresh frozen plasma, fresh whole blood, cryoprecipitates, fibrinogen, and AT III concentrates, when needed.

DIC in its diverse phases is a frequent phenomenon, and its diagnosis is extremely important for the evolution and prognosis of the patient. Of our first 40 patients to undergo implantation of a TAH, 31 were diagnosed with DIC, and only 8 of this total could receive a transplant. On the other hand, all of the patients without DIC (n = 9) were given a transplant. Patients in whom DIC occurred only in the immediate postoperative period (n = 23) had a greater probability of undergoing transplantation (30% vs. 59% of patients without immediate postoperative DIC) compared with patients with later-onset septic DIC (n = 19) (5% vs. 77% in patients without later-onset DIC) or with patients with DIC in both the immediate postoperative period and later, who had absolutely no chance of undergoing transplantation (0% vs. 100% without DIC).

Immediate postoperative DIC reflects the severe clinical condition of the patient before intervention, which is aggravated by surgical trauma. Early-onset DIC is, however, easier to treat because its etiology is frequently resolved by implantation of the artificial heart and improved cardiac output. DIC due to infection is not easily resolved, because sepsis created a situation that is only partially corrected by appropriate hemostatic treatment. This serious condition considerably hampers later implantation of a donor heart and, if not reversed by antibiotic therapy, precludes transplantation. When DIC occurs both in the immediate postoperative and in later periods, it effectively rules out heart transplantation.

In 85% of patients with immediate postoperative bleeding (32% of the total), tests showed that diffuse bleeding was closely related to DIC in its late phases. However, our diagnostic protocol detected DIC in 45% of patients with no postoperative bleeding (68% of the total), allowing early and frequently life-saving treatment. Immediate postoperative DIC may reflect direct passage into one of the phases of DIC, even if overt bleeding does not occur. DIC can then become severely complicated without early diagnosis and treatment.

Bleeding occurred in 12% of patients without postoperative DIC (42% of the total). On the other hand, among patients with immediate postoperative DIC (58% of the total), 48% presented with immediate overt bleeding, because they had passed directly into the late phases of DIC. With appropriate early treatment, in spite of the high risk, we were able to avoid hemorrhage in all of the remaining 52% who had no overt bleeding but biologically proved DIC.

Fibrinolysis, therefore, must be detected and then stopped, because fibrinolysis and prefibrinolysis are frequent phenomena. DIC must be closely monitored (especially for decrease of alpha-2-antiplasmin and plasminogen, increase of FDPs, and presence of the pinching phenomenon) and treated as early as possible (aprotinin, 125,000 KIU intravenously, followed by a drip of 500 KIU/min) until biologic data are normalized.

Close analysis of the different phases of DIC demonstrates that although biologic hypocoagulability is manifested as hemorrhage, in fact it is a simple translation of a state of overt and decompensated hypercoagulability. The assertion that hypercoagulability does not always lead to thrombosis may confuse the clinician, because no distinct parameter or precise marker can predict both situations. Because hemostatic functions take place in whole blood, thereby forming the thrombi, any assessment limited to plasma alone is necessarily incomplete, especially when the patient is in disequilibrium due to hemodilution (CPB). The best available indicator of the overall situation is a single, inexpensive, and rapid test: thromboelastography (TEG) on recalcified whole blood.

The thromboelastogram (Fig. 1) has different parameters: reaction time (r) up to a deflection of 1 mm (normal value: 12-15 mm); coagulation time (k) up to a deflection of 20 mm (normal value: 9-13 mm); and maximal amplitude

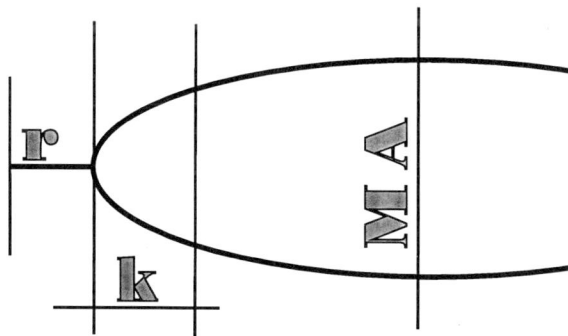

FIGURE 1. Parameters of the thromboelastogram.

(MA), corresponding to the clot's dynamics and its final structure. A conversion table reveals the elasticity constant (ϵ), or it can be calculated as follows:

$$\epsilon = \frac{100 \times MA}{100 - MA}$$

The thrombodynamic potential index (TPI) is obtained by the formula:

$$\frac{\epsilon}{k}$$

The TPI allows qualification of global coagulation as normocoagulable (TPI of 6-15), hypocoagulable (TPI <6), or hypercoagulable (TPI >15).

Hypercoagulability detected by the TEG has no sequelae if it is compensated by the main inhibitor and regulator of thrombin formation, AT III. However, measurement of plasma AT III alone does not supply a true appreciation of its inhibitory and regulatory activity. This compensation is more clearly shown by the measurement of AT III in serum, which allows determination of the effect of AT III in impeding thrombus formation, its availability for combination, and its remaining potential for combination. Calculation of the antithrombinic potential index (API) by subtracting serum AT III from plasma AT III (normal values: 35-45) makes possible an appreciation of the adaptive capacity of inhibition to global coagulability.

Confronted with violent acceleration of thrombin formation (of any origin), AT III makes an effort to adapt to increased solicitation, as demonstrated by an increased—or at least normal—API. As mentioned above, the exhaustion of the inhibitor and its failure to adapt, reflected by a decrease in plasma AT III and an increase in serum AT III (thus giving a greatly reduced, or even absent, API) is what we call the **pinching phenomenon**. This phenomenon manifests biologically as hypocoagulability (with, of course, underlying hypercoagulability) and clinically as overt bleeding.

In our first 56 patients, after analysis of the correlation between the pinching phenomenon and DIC in the same clinical periods described above (Fig. 2), we confirmed that the pinching phenomenon is a reliable indicator of the thrombophilic state that accompanies DIC in its final phases. In the immediate postoperative period, the pinching phenomenon is parallel to the last phases of DIC (initial phases do not present this phenomenon). However, the presence of the pinching phenomenon in patients without DIC reflects the gravity of the multiple organ failure that preceded surgical intervention and that was corrected by the TAH. In sepsis, the correlation is more significant: of 27 patients with septic DIC, the pinching phenomenon was present in 26, whereas it occurred in no patient without septic DIC (n = 29). Similar ratios are found in patients with both postoperative and later-onset septic DIC.

At the same time we analyzed the relationship between the pinching phenomenon and the probability of transplantation (Fig. 3). Data in the immediate postoperative period, although at the limit of statistical significance because of the small number of cases, the varying etiologies of multiple organ failure before intervention, and the intervention itself, show a tendency that may be confirmed later. In contrast, of patients with late-onset sepsis and the pinching phenomenon only 1 (4%) of 26 could undergo transplantation; the same ratio was observed among patients with both immediate postoperative and late-onset sepsis (n = 17), none of whom could undergo transplantation.

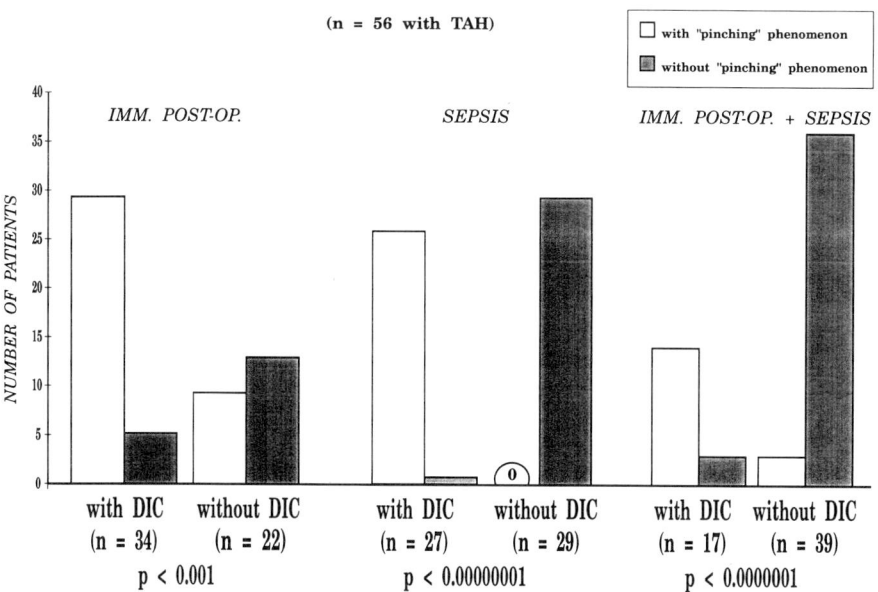

FIGURE 2. Pinching phenomenon and DIC.

In addition, the pinching phenomenon is closely correlated with renal failure; the presence of both greatly diminishes the probability of transplantation ($p < 0.00005$).

Sepsis can also be suspected in the presence of the pinching phenomenon (which reflects a severe and frequently ominous evolution) and may be later

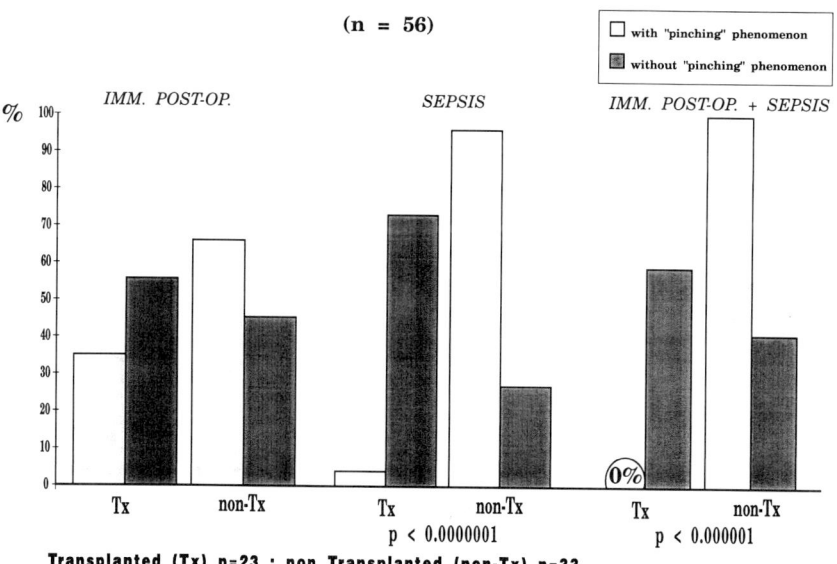

FIGURE 3. Pinching phenomenon evolution in patients with TAH.

confirmed by systematic blood cultures and by other signs of infection. This suspicion allows initiation of an appropriate antibiotic treatment or at least constitutes an alarm signal showing change from the previously normal state. In all such cases, patients were treated as if they were in phase 3 or 4 of DIC. In many cases, unfortunately, a fatal outcome could not be avoided; hemorrhage, however, was never the main cause of death.

In current practice, the pinching phenomenon can contribute greatly to the study of hypercoagulability, although it still requires further investigation.

Stabilizing Platelet Function

The behavior of platelets is conditioned by a special metabolism based on prostaglandin synthesis; it can be either beneficial by ensuring primary hemostasis or harmful by triggering in vivo activation with strong and permanent aggression (continuous injury). Harmful behavior occurs with valvular prostheses, bypasses, grafts, and circulatory assist devices. The platelet plays an important role in triggering and maintaining a thrombophilic state that can degenerate into thrombosis. This state must be controlled and corrected according to clinical and surgical conditions. Among the various platelet functions, we have therefore reconsidered the basic aspects of platelet aggregability.

After analysis of >20,000 aggregation curves, performed by turbidimetry, we have observed a basic discrepancy between these curves and those resulting from the determination of PF4 and βTG. We therefore conclude that, just as the hypocoagulability demonstrated during progressive consumption coagulopathy is only the clinical reflection of decompensated hypercoagulability, so the hypoaggregability that often appears in high-risk situations is only the visible reflection of a decompensated hyperaggregability. In cases of strong and permanent aggression, such as CPB and implantation of a prosthesis, platelet hyperactivation occurs (Fig. 4). On the one hand, it interferes with the platelets'

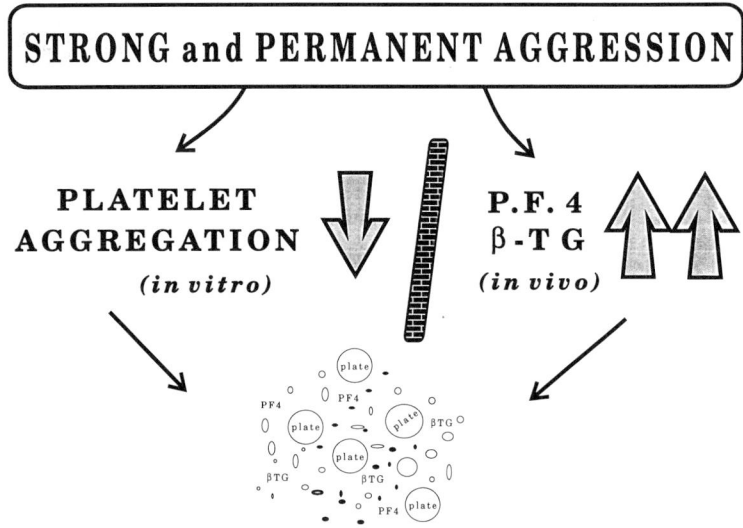

FIGURE 4. Platelet function during strong and permanent aggression.

primary hemostatic functions because few platelets remain unscathed; this explains the hypoaggregability and possible hemorrhage. On the other hand, the platelets have been depleted of their granule content (e.g., PF4, βTG, thrombin, thromboxane A_2) which are released into plasma and activate other platelets. Thus the formation of circulating aggregates is increased, and adequate heparinization is prevented. By in vitro aggregation, therefore, the platelets may be judged hypoaggregable, but in vivo, because they are strongly stimulated, they may aggregate. This seeming paradox explains the many thromboembolic accidents that have no apparent cause: conventional and simple aggregation tests disguise this phenomenon, which occurs even in the absence of thrombocytopenia.

Degranulation (release of PF4, βTG, and other metabolites) is not always associated with thrombocytopenia, but it is closely related to change in the intraplatelet level of cyclic adenosine monophosphate (cAMP), which regulates the sensitivity threshold of the platelet to external inductors of aggregation (Fig. 5). This threshold is modified in many cases of strong and permanent aggression (e.g., CPB, valves, bypasses, grafts, assist devices), thus leading to harmful exocytosis. Increases in cAMP lead to the phosphorylation of several platelet proteins. The inhibitory effects of cAMP on activation of protein kinase C, mobilization of calcium ions, fibrinogen-receptor exposure, myosin light-chain phosphorylation, actin polymerization, and cytoskeletal assembly result from inhibition of receptor-mediated phospholipase C activation. Recent studies also indicate that cAMP inhibits platelet aggregation at steps distal to activation of protein kinase C and calcium-dependent protein kinase.

How have we managed to avoid the phenomenon of degranulation and to stabilize the metabolic pool of the platelet? Abundant evidence supports the theory that an increase in intraplatelet cAMP, while stabilizing several enzymatic reactions, depresses platelet aggregation and secretion (degranulation) and thereby mediates many of the effects of inhibitory agonists. We have tried to increase the amount of beneficial intraplatelet cAMP by inhibition of phosphodiesterase (Fig. 6) with high doses of dipyridamole. High-dose dipyridamole inhibits phosphodiesterase, thus reducing breakdown of cAMP,

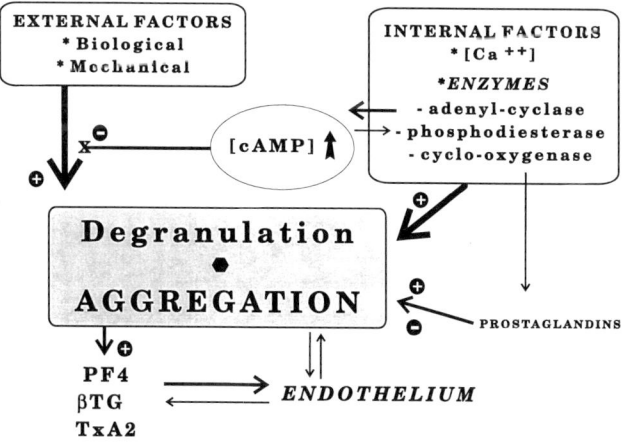

FIGURE 5. Mechanism of degranulation-aggregation.

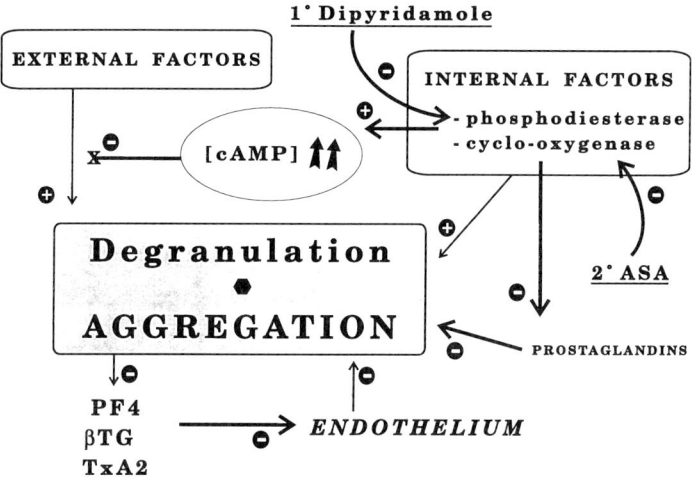

FIGURE 6. Action of dipyridamole and aspirin.

and also activates adenylate cyclase by a prostacyclin-mediated effect on the platelet membrane. In addition, dipyridamole increases plasma levels of adenosine by inhibiting its uptake by vascular endothelium and red blood cells, thus enhancing the activity of platelet adenylate cyclase. Because dipyridamole prolongs the shortened platelet survival time, platelet activation is reduced both with prostheses and with CPB, thus diminishing immediate postoperative blood loss. Consequently, we strongly recommend the administration of high doses of dipyridamole a few days before any invasive procedure.

For us, the fundamental role of dipyridamole is not as an antiaggregant, but rather as a stabilizer of the platelet's metabolic pool, allowing the platelet to adapt to the new situation (such as various prostheses and grafts or changes in blood flow). Because the platelet then becomes less receptive to the usual inductors, secretion of platelet products (e.g., PF4, βTG, thromboxane, thrombospondin, permeability factor) is inhibited. These products are all able to generate endothelial changes and thus activate other platelets, further amplifying the phenomenon.

When stabilization has been attained, low-dose aspirin is given to control the release reaction; it inhibits cyclooxygenase but leaves the PGI2 system intact. (Prostacyclin synthesized in the endothelium is a powerful vasodilator and antiaggregant.) Aspirin irreversibly acetylates the serine residue at the active site of cyclooxygenase both in the platelet (which is unable to generate new enzymes) and in the endothelium (which can resynthesize cyclooxygenase). This suggests a differential effect in regard to duration of the synthetic capacity of thromboxane A_2 and PGI2. Because aspirin is rapidly absorbed in the stomach and upper small intestine, it reaches significant levels in plasma in 20 minutes, and platelet inhibition occurs in 50-70 minutes. Although the drug itself is rapidly cleared from circulation, its effect on platelet secretion lasts for the life of the platelet (7-10 days), even at low doses.

The administration of aspirin alone, regardless of dose, does not take into account the physiologic attitude of the platelet toward strong and permanent aggression (Fig. 4). Aspirin displays an antiplatelet attitude because it can act only against platelets able to resist the aggression; that is, those responsible for primary hemostasis. Such intervention encourages bleeding. The removal of the thromboembolic risk still remains uncertain because the platelets have already released their contents and are capable of forming aggregates, with little or no sensitivity to aspirin.

If platelet adhesiveness is not controlled (Ivy test <18 minutes and/or abnormally low Wu-Hoak coefficient), we add ticlopidine to the above treatment in a very low dose (250 mg on alternate days or even every 3 days) in order not to exceed a bleeding time >23 minutes. Thus other side effects are avoided. The strong antiadhesive activity of ticlopidine is due to interference in fixation of fibrinogen to the platelet through interaction with glycoproteins on the platelet membrane.

Our goal in regard to platelet function is to obtain a satisfactory balance with (1) control of platelet aggregation (i.e., no appearance of a second wave with ADP and adrenalin; no response with arachidonic acid; and normal response with collagen); (2) maintenance of the plasma levels of PF4 and βTG within normal limits (accepted variation: <10 ng/ml for each); and (3), depending on the case, maintenance of the bleeding time (Ivy test modified by Borchgrevink) between 11-13 minutes (with the Jarvik-7, >18 min). Platelet function must be stabilized because of exaggerated in vivo platelet activation. Stabilization is appreciated by a significant increase in the plasma level of platelet proteins (PF4 and βTG) and a consequent decrease in platelet aggregation.

The normal level of βTG is always higher than that of PF4, and the determination of both, in spite of technical problems, makes possible a better understanding of the efficacy of stabilizing treatment. Unfortunately, as yet few biologic tests at the clinician's disposal are able to detect platelet activity. It is necessary, however, to consider renal function when interpreting the results because βTG is eliminated by the kidneys. In cases of acute renal failure, lowered clearance of βTG results in an increase in plasma levels that bears no relation to platelet hyperactivity. (In these frequent cases, the results from determination of urinary βTG, sometimes rendered impossible by lack of urine, were aleatoric and unreliable). This fact, which can conceal the stabilizing effect of treatment, constrains us to study the changes in the levels of PF4, even though its rate of liberation and its route of elimination are quite different.

The exaggerated in vivo activation of platelets, as shown in cases of strong and permanent aggression (e.g., TAH), is normalized by high doses of dipyridamole (150-300 mg every 6 hours) as a platelet stabilizer that induces a fundamental change in platelet metabolism. Dipyridamole is administered immediately during the postoperative period.

Once platelet stabilization is achieved and platelet aggregation (as measured by turbidimetry) indicates that reactivity has recovered, we then add small doses of aspirin (100 mg/day or every other day) as a platelet antiaggregant to control degranulation, which can then occur only after greatly increased activity of the agonists (as with a vascular breach). Numerous clinical trials have demonstrated that the combination of dipyridamole and aspirin clearly prevents or significantly reduces thromboembolic accidents; this effect is highly dose-dependent. Indeed, several major trials based on low doses of dipyridamole and high doses of aspirin have provided inconsistent and questionable results, also producing bleeding as well as gastrointestinal and other well-known complications.

The platelet treated with high-dose dipyridamole becomes less sensitive to proaggregant factors (thus resulting in decreased thromboembolic risk) but recovers its hemostatic capacities (thus resulting in decreased risk of bleeding). This dual effect allows the performance of invasive procedures, such as endomyocardial, transbronchial, hepatic, and renal biopsies, and even major surgery without stopping the stabilizing treatment and without bleeding complications. In fact, among all patients who underwent transplantation after an implanted TAH (which requires another CPB), no significant bleeding was present in the postoperative period.

Balancing Coagulation

Control of coagulation involves a balance between the different pathways of thrombin formation and the activity of the most powerful inhibitor, AT III (Fig. 7). We depart from the conventional model of thrombin formation (with intrinsic and extrinsic pathways) because it does not take into account the determinant factor of kinetics—that is, the speed of the enzymatic reactions. Our model is a little different (Fig. 8). At the onset of activation, the intrinsic and extrinsic pathways should no longer be considered as independent, but as interacting; this interaction involves several elements common to both pathways (e.g., factor VII). Furthermore, a rapid pathway (including a feedback mechanism) and a slow pathway for thrombin formation should be taken into account.

The rapid—or hemostatic—pathway requires the presence of four essential elements in addition to factors IXa, VIII, and VIIa: factor Xa, factor Va, ionized calcium, and factor III (phospholipids). These four elements (called prothrombinase) activate prothrombin (factor II) into intermediate II, which, in a second phase, is transformed into thrombin (factor IIa); this thrombin then transforms fibrinogen into fibrin. This process requires the addition of the concept of feedback: a small quantity of thrombin formed by the different pathways (or coming from the degranulation of platelets) is used to transform prothrombin into intermediate I. In the presence of factors Xa, Va, III, and ionized calcium, intermediate I gives rise to intermediate II, which, in the presence of the same

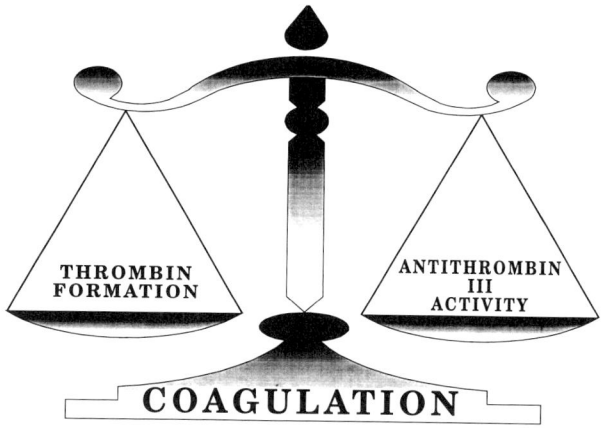

FIGURE 7. Coagulation balance.

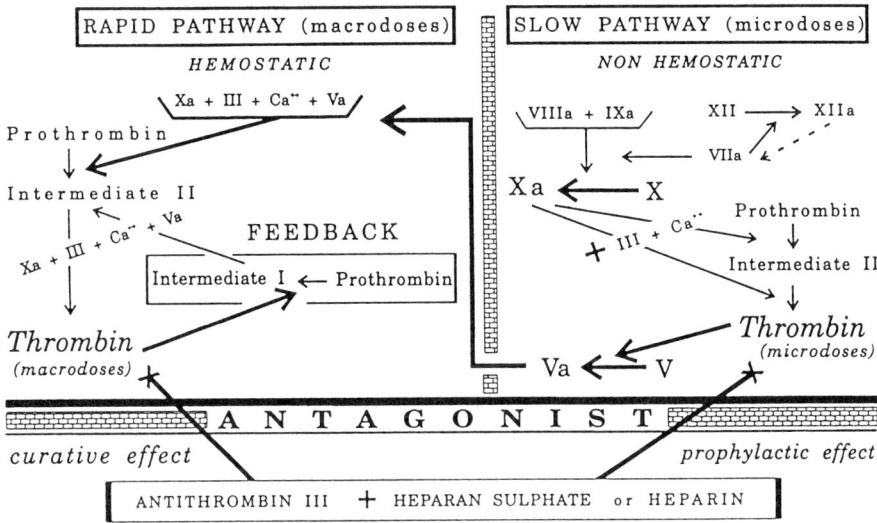

FIGURE 8. Thrombin formation and its regulation (according to Bellon and Szefner).

elements, forms active thrombin. Thus, thrombin formation provides positive feedback for additional thrombin formation.

The slow—or nonhemostatic—pathway implies the presence of factors VIIIa and IXa, which, in the presence of factor VIIa, activate factor X into factor Xa. Factor Xa, in the presence of factor III and ionized calcium, activates prothrombin into intermediate II, which in the presence of factor Xa, ionized calcium, and factor III, gives rise to factor IIa, a microdose of slowly formed thrombin. All these reactions are carried out in the absence of factor V, which is activated into factor Va via the microdose of thrombin. Factor Va, in the presence of ionized calcium, and factors Xa and III, transforms intermediate II into factor IIa, a macrodose of thrombin in the accelerated pathway. The activation of factor V is essential to complete the rapid formation, because it acts as a receptor of factors II and Xa.

The fibrin formation system is permanently thwarted by an inhibitory system that regulates thrombin formation, ensuring the equilibrium and normal modulation of coagulation. The principal inhibitors of thrombin are AT III (the most important), proteins C and S (the synthesis of which depends on vitamin K), heparin cofactor II, and lipoprotein-associated coagulation inhibitor (LACI), which has a sequence homology with Künitz-type trypsin inhibitors but no well-known function. The action of AT III is considerably enhanced physiologically by heparan sulfate (normally present in the blood) and therapeutically by heparin. When heparin and AT III combine, the low-molecular-weight fraction of heparin acts prophylactically against the microdose of thrombin; in the slow formation pathway, this action prevents the activation of factor V into factor Va as well as the association of factor Va with factor Xa, factor III, and ionized calcium, which in high doses transforms intermediate II into macrodoses of rapidly forming thrombin. On the other hand, the high-molecular-weight fraction of heparin acts against macrodoses and therefore has a direct antithrombinic effect.

The inhibitory system of thrombin is therefore in permanent equilibirum with the procoagulant system, and the state of this equilibrium can be evaluated at any moment by the following tests: (1) determination of AT III; (2) calculation of the API; (3) calculation of the TPI; (4) measurement of factor Xa; and (5) Raby's transfer test.

Determination of Antithrombin III

AT III—or rather its rate of activity expressed as a percentage (that is, its capacity to combine with thrombin)—is determined both in plasma and serum. Determination of AT III in plasma indicates its total capacity to combine and therefore reflects its level in the blood, that is, its combination potential. Because the serum represents the remainder of the blood after formation of a clot, determination of AT III in serum indicates the quantity of antithrombin remaining in the blood after coagulation.

Calculation of the Antithrombin Potential Index

If we subtract AT III in serum from AT III in plasma, we can evaluate the percentage of antithrombin that has been used in the formation of the clot—that is, the quantity that combined with thrombin—and consequently the fraction still capable of combining with thrombin. The result is the antithrombin potential index (API). The study of variations in the API provides valuable information on the state of coagulation when it is compared with the TPI (see below).

Determinations of AT III in plasma and in serum and calculation of the API also make it possible to understand the effect of anticoagulant treatments. Heparin, for example, does not fundamentally modify thrombin formation; it simply diminishes the quantity by reinforcing the antithrombin inhibitory system that neutralizes the microdose of thrombin formed in the slow pathway (low-molecular-weight fraction). Thus it prevents the activation of factor V and noticeably diminishes the activity of the rapid pathway and consequently of macrodoses of thrombin (high-molecular-weight fraction). These macrodoses of thrombin, which are nevertheless formed in small quantities, are neutralized by heparin's direct opposition to thrombin. However, to counteract the decrease in factor V, hyperactivity of factor X gives rise to a certain amount of thrombin by the rapid pathway.

Treatment by oral anticoagulants (inhibitors of vitamin K) thwarts the formation of factors II (prothrombin), VII, IX, and X as well as formation of proteins C and S, which is normally carried out in the liver and is vitamin K-dependent. The manner in which thrombin is produced is thus profoundly disturbed. Because the slow pathway is not modified, microdoses of thrombin are available to activate factor V. The resultant quantity of factor Va does not find 100% of the coagulation factors necessary for the rapid pathway, but only, for example, 30%. Factor Va, therefore, is able to transform this 30% into thrombin—totally and rapidly. This thrombin is only minimally neutralized, if at all, by AT III for two main reasons: (1) antithrombin activity that is not enhanced by heparin is less efficient, and (2) antithrombin usually arrives too late to neutralize the thrombin that has already transformed fibrinogen into fibrin and has settled at this level. This low level of activity for antithrombin seems quite obvious when AT III is determined in serum; it is, as a matter of fact, only slightly lower than or even equal to the level of AT III in plasma; consequently, the API is greatly diminished.

In patients receiving inhibitors of vitamins K, a state of normo- or even hypercoagulability can persist, in spite of the deficit in coagulation factors, because the inhibitory system is inefficient (AT III is not activated, as mentioned above, and production of proteins C and S is diminished.) Thus thrombin is not neutralized, and the risks of thrombosis are increased. Treatment with oral anticoagulants is usually monitored exclusively through determination of the prothrombin rate or Quick's time. If this test shows an increase in prothrombin rate, the usual practice is to increase the dosage of vitamin K inhibitors, thus further lowering the production of coagulation factors without diminishing hypercoagulability. Inhibitors of coagulation are thus deprived of efficient action, and the patient is at risk for both bleeding and thrombosis.

The measurement of AT III in plasma with a specific chromogenic substrate shows only the combination of AT III with high-molecular-weight heparin. In fact, this measurement is performed with an excess of thrombin over a short period of time: moreover, the totality of AT III cannot be mobilized, and only the part of the protein that corresponds to rapid movement is shown. This test cannot explore the prophylactic effect of AT III, which acts on factor Xa and corresponds to slow movement.

Calculation of the Thrombodynamic Potential Index

The TPI, derived from the TEG performed on recalcified whole blood, makes it possible to determine if the patient's status is normo-, hyper-, or hypocoagulable. Three examples illustrate the value of the TPI in combination with the API.

1. If, in a biologic state of hypercoagulability characterized by a TPI of 40, the activity of AT III in plasma is normal, but the API is high (60-70), then the state of hypercoagulability is offset by a greater consumption of antithrombin. Therefore, less antithrombin remains in the serum, and the plasma-serum difference (the API) is increased. Hypercoagulability is then compensated.

2. If the biologic state of hypercoagulability, before any alteration in the plasma activity of AT III, demonstrates a marked decrease in the API, then hypercoagulability does not bring about a greater consumption of antithrombin, which is not properly activated. A significant amount of antithrombin remains in the serum, and the plasma-serum difference (the API) is small. In this case, hypercoagulability is not compensated by greater inhibition; this decompensated hypercoagulability, called the thrombophilic state, is propitious to thrombosis.

3. If we observe hypocoagulability (TPI <6) in the thromboelastogram, associated on the one hand with decreased AT III activity in plasma (because of either insufficient production or excessive consumption) and on the other hand with increased activity in serum, the significant reduction in the API can be explained by the reversal of activities, with plasma activity diminishing and serum activity increasing. This pinching phenomenon arises from a serious disturbance in coagulation because (1) hypocoagulability corresponds

to greatly enhanced consumption of the coagulation factors that is not compensated and can therefore lead to bleeding and (2) the decrease in API corresponds to a serious decrease in antithrombinic activity that can therefore lead to thrombosis.

Measurement of Factor Xa

The systematic measurement of factor Xa in serum has led to the following observations:

1. In patients treated with heparin, we have noted a significant increase in factor Xa in serum, which seems to indicate that a hyperactive system comes into play to compensate for the total or partial absence of factor Va. The low-molecular-weight fraction of heparin has neutralized the microdose of thrombin necessary to activate factor Va.

2. On the other hand, in patients treated with oral anticoagulants, in whom factor V fully conserves its activation properties, only a few molecules of factor Xa are activated. But they are activated totally, because they do not have to compensate for any deficit of factor Va. In this case the determination of activated factor X in serum is clearly independent of the determination of the residual activation in plasma; thus the quantity and the quality of thrombin become relevant concerns. In other words, complete but rather weak activity of factor Xa provokes a thrombin activity that is sufficient to maintain a state of normo- or hypercoagulability in spite of the deficit created.

The magnitude of the problem described above can be appreciated when the activity of AT III in serum is determined, because it can sometimes be slightly less than, equal to, or greater than that in plasma. (In the last case, the negative difference in API corresponds to the part that, for technical reasons related to the speed of the reaction, cannot be measured in plasma.) This risk factor must be taken into account, because the inhibitory system of the patient is inefficient and thrombin is not neutralized. Thus the risk of thrombosis is increased. If this phenomenon coincides with a decrease in the prothrombin time—that is, an increase in the prothrombin rate—and if this is the only information available to the doctor, he or she may increase the dose of oral anticoagulants, putting the patient at risk for bleeding and thrombosis simultaneously. Therefore, for efficient inhibition of vitamin K, it is necessary to obtain a TPI of 6-8, an API of 9-15, and a serum level of factor Xa not less than 10%.

In practice, our goal is to achieve a satisfactory balance in coagulation. This balance can be verified by the application of specific tests with specific indices. We have been able to reduce the immediate or long-term risk of thromboembolism by establishing reproducible limits for these indices within which we can maintain a satisfactory balance: (1) a normal API value between 35-45; (2) a TPI as measured by TEG between 6-15; and (3) a serum level of factor Xa between 10-20%.

In the cases reported in this study, we have applied these parameters throughout the duration of the implant to maintain values compatible with what we consider to be the most adequate coagulation balance possible. It must nevertheless be taken into account that the API can be reduced as a function of global coagulability (as measured by TEG), which can itself be more or less weak.

Raby's Transfer Test

To give an idea of the heparinization achieved in relation to the dose, we use Raby's transfer test on plasma, which was devised in 1969. Indeed, the postoperative phase of a Jarvik-7 TAH implant is characterized by thromboplastinic activity that generates real and potential hypercoagulability. This hypercoagulant activity is created and maintained by the introduction of a complex device that interrupts the laminar flow, resulting in turbulence and eddies. This thromboplastinic activity can also be detected by the transfer test on plasma.

The reaction time (r) of plasma rich in platelets is determined by TEG for the patient and for a control, as well as for a mixture of the two. The quotient should be calculated as follows:

$$\frac{r\ mixture}{r\ control}$$

(The r for the mixture is not the sum of r for the patient and r for the control, because the two plasmas are mutually corrected and yield a specific r for the mixture.) A quotient <1 indicates a nonneutralized hypercoagulability, and the test is said to be positive. A quotient >1 indicates a sufficient anticoagulant activity, and the test is said to be negative.

In fact, the calculation of this quotient, together with the study of the variations in TPI, API, and serum factor Xa, constitutes an indispensable reference for the efficient control of heparin therapy. When the test result is >1, the API tends to decrease (thus indicating reduced consumption of AT III and greater residual AT III in serum) because the preexisting thromboplastinic capacity is reduced or has disappeared, bringing about reduced production of thrombin.

Clinical Application

Taking the techniques and values discussed above into account, how are we going to treat thromboembolism and the different phases of DIC to maintain a satisfactory balance?

In our experience, the most appropriate anticoagulant to date is doubtlessly heparin, which can act both on factor Xa generation of thrombin and on consumption of excessive thrombin through adaptation of the natural inhibitor (AT III). Its mode of action is therefore physiologic. Heparin therapy is used on two occasions: (1) during CPB and (2) for maintenance of appropriate anticoagulation for each patient.

For CPB we recommend an efficient anticoagulation adjusted to preexisting imbalances. The basic dose of 120 IU/kg of heparin is adjusted during the operation to maintain a Hemochron value of 450 ± 50. We also neutralize this anticoagulation with a dose of protamine equivalent to two-thirds (60%) of the total dose of heparin injected during the operation. This avoids any overdosage of protamine that can lead to heparinlike rebound after about 30 minutes. This effect is the cause of frequent, uncontrolled bleeding after CPB (without the participation of the fibrinolytic system). Indeed, heparin injected at the beginning of CPB follows one of two directions: it combines, or it remains free. Only free heparin has to be neutralized.

One must take into account, among other factors, the elimination of heparin during CPB and the fact that surgery produces an accelerated turnover of heparin. Thus, when protamine is injected in the usual way (dose for dose, or sometimes more), it has an excessive effect that leads to the dissociation of the AT III–heparin–thrombin complex. As a result of this dissociation, free molecules (AT III–heparin) are returned to the circulation, where they are once more ready to combine with hemostatic thrombin. Thus, our experience demonstrates that only those patients in whom the total dose of injected protamine is less than the total dose of injected heparin do not show the phenomenon of rebound bleeding.

To maintain appropriate anticoagulation apart from CPB, imbalances are corrected first by intravenous low-dose heparin and then by modulated subcutaneous doses. Heparin therapy is monitored by Raby's transfer test on plasma. The following goals are to be achieved: (1) a constantly negative transfer test; (2) a satisfactory function of the inhibitory system in relation to the availability of AT III in plasma and to the quantity of thrombin to be neutralized; and (3) a quantity of factor Xa in serum that corresponds to thrombin formation in harmony with the two parameters above.

More importance is thus given to the transfer test than to TEG on whole blood, because the goal is balance between the procoagulant capacity and the inhibitory capacity, regardless of the biologic potential of coagulation. For these reason the doses that we use vary between 10–50 mg/day (∼1,000–5,000 IU/day), beginning in the immediate postoperative period. We later adapt these doses to different clinical situations. Massive doses of anticoagulants are therefore unnecessary.

This heparin therapy provides efficient antithrombinic and prophylactic effects, while retaining adequate function of the inhibitory system and thrombin formation sufficient for satisfactory hemostasis but insufficient for a state of hypercoagulability.

BRIEF ACCOUNT OF THE LONGEST IMPLANTATION

A brief account of our longest implantation shows the practical aspect of the objectives stated above. Normally the Jarvik-7 TAH is used as a temporary bridge to heart transplantation. In one patient, however, a permanent heart was practically impossible to transplant because of an extremely high antibody titer, which almost certainly would have resulted in rejection of the graft.

On July 21, 1988, a 37-year-old woman was admitted for postpartum dilated cardiomyopathy of 10 years' duration. Her history indicated regular consumption of alcohol and two episodes of ventricular tachycardia. A phlebography in 1980 had demonstrated thrombophlebitis of the left leg. Anti-HLA antibodies demonstrated a positive titer to 4 of the 25 determinants. In spite of these factors as well as multiple organ failure, we decided to implant a TAH.

Complications included preoperative renal and hepatic failure as well as DIC in phase 2, which was exacerbated after CPB. Duration of CPB was 142 minutes; in this case, the total dose of heparin was 150 mg and of protamine, 90 mg. After CPB the patient presented with phase-3 DIC, which was treated with aprotinin, heparin, dipyridamole at high doses, packed red blood cells, and AT III concentrates. The moderate bleeding was therefore controlled. She then presented with anuria and difficulties in awakening, but on the third postoperative day her status returned to normal and she was extubated.

When lymphocytotoxicity worsened (17/18 antibodies present), different procedures (plasmapheresis, prescription of intravenous immunoglobulins) were undertaken to allow transplantation of a compatible donor heart. Unfortunately, the procedures did not produce the expected results.

During the 10 sessions of plasmapheresis, performed on alternate days, another problem in the control of hemostasis appeared. Each session entailed the exchange of 3 times the patient's plasma volume, bringing about a profound change in coagulolytic and platelet equilibrium. This change had to be corrected carefully and rapidly to avoid hemorrhage or thrombosis at the end of each plasma exchange. Transesophageal echocardiography was performed on the 200th and 300th days after implantation to monitor and verify correct functioning of the four valves and to demonstrate patency of the circuit. The only infectious incident was a superficial abscess around one of the cutaneous openings of the activation lines; this abscess was drained and healed with no important effect on hemostasis.

The patient also experienced depression, which was treated with antidepressant drugs and psychotherapy. This condition led to immobilization for extended periods of time, which necessitated constant increase and adjustment in anticoagulant and antiaggregant treatment.

The hemodynamic state was almost always satisfactory, in spite of two transient ischemic attacks (scotomas, monoplegia) that left no sequelae. They were explained by the accidental interruption (for 2 and 3 days, respectively) of the administration of aspirin and identified in the laboratory by modifications noted in the equilibrium of hemostatic function. The patient presented no thomboembolic signs, no focal neurologic signs, and no neurologic deficit. This was confirmed by two computerized axial tomograms of the head and by her capacity to walk around with the portable console and to carry out simple manual tasks.

Unfortunately, in spite of a biologic profile of normocoagulability and normoaggregability, the patient suffered a massive acute brain hemorrhage due to rupture of a previously undetected mycotic aneurysm. She died on the 603rd day after implantation of the TAH. At explantation the Jarvik-7 had no evidence of macroscopic thrombus or fibrin at high-risk sites.

The therapeutic protocol, which was modulated according to diverse clinical situations and results of laboratory tests, can be briefly described as follows:

1. Because the patient had phase 3-4 DIC, aprotinin was administered in the immediate postoperative period at an intravenous dose of 125,000 KIU, followed by a constant drip of 500 KIU/min for 6 days.

2. Blood derivatives were limited to a strict minimum, according to our usual practice. However, the patient's course necessitated transfusion and compensation for certain deficits with fresh frozen plasma, AT III, fibrinogen concentrates, and packed red blood cells, notably in the immediate postoperative period, during sessions of plasma exchange, and in cases of deglobulization or mechanical hemolysis.

3. Heparin, first administered intravenously, then subcutaneously after normalization of all systems, was used at doses ranging from 1,000-22,500 IU/day.

4. Because the patient had a bad combination of heparin with its cofactor, AT III, pentosan polysulfate was necessary to mobilize heparin cofactor II, at doses of 100 mg/day or on alternate days.

5. Dipyridamole was given at doses ranging from 900-1,500 mg/day as a platelet stabilizer.

6. Aspirin was given at doses between 50-200 mg/day as a platelet antiaggregant.

7. Ticlopidine had to be administered sporadically, at a dose of 250 mg on alternate days.

8. Pentoxifylline was given at doses ranging from 400-800 mg/day to ameliorate the hemorrheology through enhancement of the flexibility of red blood cells and modulation of both the fibrinogen level and leukocyte-platelet interactions.

This case is unique among the other 59 implantations that we performed because of numerous problems at the level of hemostasis with potentially fatal complications; these problems were linked to characteristics of the patient and to the exceptional duration of implantation (the longest, to date, in the world).

CONCLUSION

The development of new inotropic agents and new circulatory assist devices has enabled us to envision the ultimate (and forthcoming) system: the permanent and independent total artificial heart. This is particularly important because the demand for donor hearts is increasing, although the supply remains limited. Adequate support strategies are imperative; optimal conditions imply a good choice of circulatory assistance to ensure stable hemodynamic function as well as recovery of adequate renal, hepatic, and other organ functions, absence of infection, and control of hemostasis.

Thus far we have described how the protocol for control of platelet function and coagulolytic balance can be adapted to each situation and to each patient. The results are encouraging. Control of hemostasis with its three main objectives—to stop fibrinolysis, to stabilize platelet function, and to balance coagulation—requires complex and innovative approaches. Certain of our points of view and explanations may be considered disquieting because they clash with conventional wisdom and acquired habits of thinking.

We hope that the nonspecialist gains a clearer understanding—if not of the elimination, then at least of the considerable reduction—of the ever-present nightmare of incessant bleeding and unexpected thrombosis. Certain conclusions can now be advanced:

1. The various alterations in platelet function and coagulolytic kinetics linked to TAH implant require permanent anticoagulation and permanent antiaggregation as well as suitable follow-up.

2. Follow-up must be carried out with a protocol capable of exploring all systems involved and of modulating treatment to individual needs.

3. Patients in the preoperative period are in a thrombophilic condition of varying degrees of severity and thus are much more prone to coagulolytic imbalances after surgical trauma. The protocol must take this factor into account.

4. Postoperative modifications require multidisciplinary treatment to control any decompensations; for instance, fibrinolytic bleeding, a relatively frequent phenomenon that demands a specific emergent strategy.

5. In the presence of single or multiple organ failure, the evolution of parameters is particularly reproducible, giving a perfect indication of the patient's subsequent clinical course.

6. Variations in the parameters provide an indispensable guide for modulation of treatment, making it possible to reduce thromboembolic accidents and to control the various postoperative and infectious states of DIC.

The use of the Jarvik-7 TAH in association with a strict protocol for control and treatment of coagulation disorders has been encouraging in our experience. This experience enables us, when the need arises, to perform with confidence long-term implantations of artificial hearts. Indeed, we think that the Jarvik-7 TAH is reliable and easy to use, offering a high level of safety for carefully selected patients. Patients should be young (<45 years), with no contraindication for transplantation and with acute heart failure of recent onset and no associated irreversible failure of other organs. For such critically ill patients, if no donor heart is immediately available, this technique seems to be the only possibility to reestablish a stable and satisfactory clinical condition during bridge to transplantation, which can then be carried out without urgency.

At the same time, in our experience, the progress attained with our protocol for control and treatment of hemostasis makes it possible (1) to avoid immediate bleeding (a frequent source of high mortality in early implants in other series) and (2) to avoid the formation of thromboses responsible for serious thromboembolic accidents.

We can extrapolate the application of our protocol to other clinical conditions, because the general principles are not restrictive and apply to different pathologic conditions in which the diverse systems of hemostasis are activated and to various types of circulatory assistance. We have had experience with almost all types of assist devices, applying the diagnostic and therapeutic protocol described above and obtaining the same results.

Cardiovascular surgery and cardiology have become increasingly efficient and complex, thanks to the diversity of the leading-edge techniques used for the diagnosis and treatment of previously untreatable pathologies. Advanced medical teams cannot content themselves with incomplete studies; they can and should have access to complete data.

Hemostasis has evolved in a similar fashion. Incomplete assessment and empirical therapy belong to the past. We must reconsider and restructure the control of coagulation to avoid oversimplifications that rarely reflect clinical reality.

Our study is certainly incomplete, but we have tried to share the fruit of several years' experience with the numerous problems presented by hemostasis in an advanced cardiovascular setting. We do not pretend to solve all the problems encountered, but to demonstrate that appropriate monitoring and treatment can significantly enhance the chances of success for a permanent heart transplant.

However, although certain aspects remain unclear and need further investigation, the protocol we have described permits us to reduce significantly thromboembolic accidents and to correct the disequilibriums that give rise to hemorrhage. We see a paradox between the considerable progress in cardiovascular surgery and complementary disciplines and the lethargy into which the criteria for control of hemostasis have fallen. An innovative spirit is necessary to address the totality of these methods as well as the interpretation and treatment that must follow. The need for teamwork seems clear and inevitable.

During great journeys the first step is always the longest.

Confucius

ACKNOWLEDGMENT

We appreciate the invaluable suggestions and criticism of Jack G. Copeland, M.D., Professor of Cardiovascular and Thoracic Surgery at the University of Arizona, Tucson, Arizona.

SELECTED BIBLIOGRAPHY

Al-Mondhiry H, Pae W, Miller C, Pierce WS: Platelet and fibrinogen survival in calves implanted with artificial heart and ventricular assist device—correlation with autopsy findings. Thromb Haemost 67:413-416, 1992.

Anderson LO, Barrowcliffe TW, Holmer E, et al: Molecular weight dependency of the heparin potentiated inhibition of thrombin and activated Factor X. Effect of heparin neutralization in plasma. Thromb Res 15:531-541, 1979.

Anido G, Freeman DJ: Heparin assay and protamine titration. Am J Clin Pathol 76:410-415, 1981.

Baille Y, Monties JR, Goudard A, et al: Le traitement par l'héparine des hémorragies per et postopératoires en chirurgie cardiaque. A propos de 121 observations. Ann Chir Thorac Card 9:79-87, 1970.

Barzu T, Molho P, Tobelem G, et al: Binding of heparin and low molecular weight heparin fragments to human vascular endothelial cells in culture. Nouv Rev Fr Hematol 26:243-247, 1984.

Batlle Fonrodona J, Lopez-Berges C: Proteínas plasmáticas en la relación pared vascular y plaquetas. XXVII Reunion de la Asociación Española de Hematología y Hemoterapia, Salamanca, October 23-25, 1986.

Beguin S, Kessels H, Dol F, Hemker HC: The consumption of antithrombin III during coagulation: Its consequences for the calculation of prothrombinase activity and the standardisation of heparin activity. Thromb Haemost 68:136-142, 1992.

Bellon JL, Castellanos CR, Arevalo JM: Estudio del comportamiento cinético de la Antitrombina III en contracepción y alcoholemia. Presse Medicale 2:325-328, 1983.

Bellon JL, Bores C, Puigvert A, et al: Dos casos de trombosis mortal de prótesis mitral (Bjork, Carpentier, Edwards). Estudio de los parámetros de la coagulación. Med Klin 211:30, 1979.

Bellon JL, Bores C, Miralles PJ, et al: Hemorragias graves por déficit del complejo protrombínico en portadoras et prótesis y cardíacas (Hepatopatías y AVK). Control y tratamiento. Med Klin 208:47, 1978.

Bellon JL, Camarasa M, Grifols E: Un caso grave de hematoma retroplacentario. Nueva pauta de tratamiento conservador. Anales Centro de Estudio, Clinica Nuestra Señora del Pilar 1:195-200, 1983.

Bellon JL, Castellanos CR, Arevalo JM: Potential hazards of thromboembolic accidents in people older than sixty five years in comparison with control groups. VIII International Congress of Thrombosis, Istanbul, Turkey, 1984.

Bellon JL, Garces J, Nolla M: Study of blood coagulation parameters of one hundred seriously ill patients admitted to the CCU unit of Ntra. Sra. del Mar Hospital in Barcelona during two years. Crit Care Med 9:2-12, 1981.

Bellon JL, Massot M, Bores C, et al: Accidentes vasculares cerebrales a repetición en una mujer joven hipertensa. Estudio de las alteraciones de la agregación plaquetar, FP4 y de los parámetros de la coagulación. Sangre 25:1082-1093, 1980.

Bellon JL, Miralles PJ, Nunez JL, et al: Results of coagulation controls made during seven years in sixty mechanical valve prostheses and during four years in eighty bioprosthesis carriers. Thoughts about antithrombin III and factor X behaviour. VIII International Congress on Thrombosis, Istanbul, Turkey, 380, 4-7, 1984.

Bellon JL, Szefner J, Cabrol A and C, Castellanos C: Protocole concernant l'exploration hémobiologique de patients soumis à C.E.C. et son évolution clinique. Variante proposée à la neutralisation classique de l'anticoagulation. Paris, France, C.E.C.E.C., 1987.
Bellon JL, Szefner J, Cabrol C: Coagulation et coeur artificiel. Paris, Masson, 1989.
Bjorklid E, Storm E, Osterud B, Prydz H: The interaction of the protein and phospholipid components of tissue thromboplastin (factor III) with the factor VII and X. Scand J Haematol 14:65-70, 1975.
Boyer C, Wolf M, Lavergne JM, Larrieu MJ: Thrombin generation and formation of thrombin-antithrombin III complexes in congenital antithrombin III deficiency. Thromb Res 20:207-218, 1980.
Cabrol C, Gandjbakhch I, Pavie A, et al: Transplantation coeur et coeur-poumons. Chirurgie (Mémoires de l'Académie) 114:284-295, 1988.
Cabrol C, Gandjbakhch I, Pavie A, et al: Current problems in cardiac transplantation. In Terasaki P (ed): Clinical Transplants. University of California at Los Angeles Press, 1987, pp 1-6.
Cabrol C, Gandjbakhch I, Pavie A, et al: Total artificial heart as a bridge for transplantation: La Pitié 1986 to 1987. J Heart Transplant 7:12-17, 1988.
Casu B: Structure of heparins and their fragments. Nouv Rev Fr Hematol 26:211-219, 1984.
Chan V, Chan TK: Heparin-antithrombin III binding. Haemostasis 8:373-389, 1979.
Choay J, Petitou M, Lormeau JC, et al: Structure-activity relationship in heparin: A synthetic pentasaccharide with high affinity for antithrombin III and eliciting high anti-factor Xa action. Biochem Biophys Res Comm 116:492-499, 1983.
Clarke R, Mayo G, Price P, Fitzgerald G: Suppression of thromboxane A_2 but not of systemic prostacyclin by controlled-release aspirin. N Engl J Med 325:1137-1141, 1991.
Collen D, Bounameaux H, Lunen H, Verstraete M: Analysis of coagulation and fibrinolysis during intravenous infusion of recombinant human tissue-type plasminogen activator in patients with acute myocardial infarction. Circulation 73:511-517, 1986.
Copeland J: Cardiac transplantation. Curr Probl Cardiol 13:157-224, 1988.
Copeland J, Smith R, Icenogle T, et al: Orthotopic total artificial heart bridge to transplantation: Preliminary results. J Heart Transpl 8:124-138, 1989.
De-Caterina R, Giannessi D, Boem A, et al: Equal antiplatelet effects of aspirin 50 or 324 mg/day in patients after acute myocardial infarction. Thromb Haemost 54:528-532, 1985.
De Vries WC: The total artificial heart. In Sabiston DC, Spencer FC (eds): Surgery of the Chest, 4th ed. Philadelphia, W.B. Saunders, 1983, pp 1629-1639.
De Vries W: The permanent artificial heart: Four case reports. JAMA 259:6, 1988.
Downing HR: The interaction of protease, antithrombin III and heparin. J Lab Clin Med 95:777-782, 1980.
Dunn FW, Soria J, Soria C, et al: Fibrinogen binding on human platelets: Influence of different heparins and of pentosan polysulphate. Thromb Res 29:141-148, 1983.
Dutch TIA Trial Study Group: A comparison of two doses of aspirin (30 mg vs 283 mg a day) in patients after a transient ischemic attack or minor ischemic stroke. N Engl J Med 325:1261-1266, 1991.
Engelberg H: Heparin and the prevention of atherosclerosis. In Wiley-Liss (ed): Basic Research and Clinical Application. New York, 1990.
Esposito R, Culliford A, Colvin S, et al: Heparin resistance during cardiopulmonary bypass. The role of heparin pretreatment. J Thorac Cardiovasc Surg 85:346-353, 1983.
Fareed J, Kumar A, Walenga JM, et al: Antithrombotic actions and pharmacokinetics of heparin fractions and fragments. Nouv Rev Fr Hematol 26:267-275, 1984.
Farrar D, Hill PD, Gray L, et al: Heterotopic prosthetic ventricles as a bridge to cardiac transplantation. N Engl J Med 318:333-340, 1988.
Fischer AM, Tapon-Bretaudiere J, Bros A, Josso F: Respective roles of antithrombin III and alpha-2-macroglobulin in thrombin inactivation. Thromb Haemost (Stutt) 45:51-54, 1981.
Fuster V, Chesebro J: Aortocoronary vein-graft disease: Experimental and clinical approach for the understanding of the role of platelets and platelet inhibitors. Circulation 72(Suppl V):V-65-70, 1985.
Griffith B, Hardesty R, Kormos R, et al: Temporary use of the Jarvik-7 TAH before transplantation. N Engl J Med 316:130-134, 1987.
Griffith B, Kormos R, Hardesty R, et al: The artificial heart: Infection-related morbidity and its effect on transplantation. Ann Thorac Surg 45:409-414, 1988.
Hemker HC: The mode of action of heparin in plasma. Thromb Hemost 17-36, 1987.
Hemker HC, Beguin S: Mechanisms of thrombin formation. Thrombosis Research Institute Inaugural Symposium, London, 1990.

Hemker HC, Lindhout TH: A clotting scheme for 1984. Nouv Rev Fr Hematol 26:227-231, 1984.
Hirsh J: Heparin-induced bleeding. Nouv Rev Fr Hematol 26:261-266, 1984.
Jarvik RK: The total artificial heart. Sci Am 244:74-80, 1981.
Johnson K, Prieto M, Joyce L, et al: Summary of the clinical use of the Symbion total artificial heart: A registry report. J Heart Lung Transplant 11:103-116, 1992.
Kakkar VV, Bentley PG, MacGregor IG, et al: Antithrombin III and heparin. Lancet 12:103-104, 1980.
Kang YG: Monitoring and treatment of coagulation. In Hepatic Transplantation. Praeger, 1986, pp 151-173.
Kawaguchi A, Gandjbakhch I, Pavie A, et al: Factors affecting survival in total artificial heart recipients before transplantation. Circulation 82(Suppl IV):IV-322-IV-327, 1990.
Kawaguchi A, Gandjbakhch I, Pavie A, et al: Liver and kidney function in patients undergoing mechanical circulatory support with Jarvik-7 artificial heart as a bridge to transplantation. J Heart Transplant 9:631-637, 1990.
Kinlouegh-Rathbone R, Packham M, Perry D, et al: Lack of stability of aggregates after thrombin induced reaggregation of thrombin-degranulated platelets. Thromb Haemost 67:453-457, 1992.
Kunin C, Dobbins J, Melo J, et al: Infectious complications in four long-term recipients of the Jarvik-7 artificial heart. JAMA 259:6, 1988.
Kwan-Gett CS, Wu Y, Collen R, et al: Total replacement artificial heart and driving-system with inherent regulation of cardiac output. ASAIO Trans 15:245-266, 1969.
Larcan A, Alexandre P, Lambert H, et al: Diagnostic, surveillance et traitements des coagulopathies de consommation par le test de transfert. Nouv Presse Med 15:2586, 1981.
Larcan A, Lambert H, Gerard A: Consumption coagulopathies. New York, Masson, 1987.
Larcan A, Stoltz JF, Stoltz M: Microcirculation et Hémorhéologie. Paris, Masson, 1970.
Lauri D, Zanetti A, Dejana E, Gaetano G: Effects of dipyridamole and low-dose aspirin therapy on platelet adhesion to vascular endothelium. Am J Cardiol 58:1261-1264, 1986.
Levine S, Sorenson R, Harris M, Knieriem L: The effect of platelet factor 4 (PF4) on assays of plasma heparin. Br J Haematol 57:585-596, 1984.
Levinson M, Smith R, Cork R, et al: Thromboembolic complications of the Jarvik-7 TAH: Case report. Artif Organs 10:236-244, 1986.
Lorenz R, Weber M, Kotzur J, et al: Improved aortocoronary bypass patency by low-dose aspirin (100 mg daily). Effects on platelet aggregation and thromboxane formation. Lancet 9:1261-1264, 1984.
Lundsgaard-Hansen P, Ehrengruber E, Frei E, et al: Antithrombin III and related parameters in surgical patients receiving blood components. Vox Sang 46:19-28, 1983.
Marciniak E, Gockerman JP: Kinetics of elimination of antithrombin III concentrate in heparinized patients. Br J Hematol 48:617-625, 1981.
Martin P, Horkay F, Rajah SM, Walker DR: Monitoring of coagulation status using thromboelastography during pediatric open heart surgery. Internat. J Clin Monit Comput 8:183-187, 1991.
Mehta J, Mehta P: Dipyridamole and aspirin in relation to platelet aggregation and vessel wall prostaglandin generation. J Cardiovasc Pharmacol 4:688-693, 1982.
Muggeo M, Calabro A, Businaro V, et al: Blood clotting, fibrinolytic and hemorrheological parameters in ischemic vascular disease: The effects of pentoxifylline in the treatment of acute cerebral vascular disease. Pharmatherapeutica 3:74-90, 1983.
Muneretto C, Pavie A, Gandjbakhch I, et al: Determinants of survival in the use of TAH as a bridge to transplantation. J Cardiovasc Surg 30:80, 1989.
Muneretto C, Rabago G Jr, Pavie A, et al: Mechanical circulatory support as a bridge to transplantation: Current status of total artificial heart in 1989 and determinants of survival. J Cardiovasc Surg 31:486-491, 1989.
Palinski W, Torsellini A, Doni L: Influence of platelet activation on erythrocyte deformability. Thromb Haemost (Stutt) 49:84-86, 1983.
Pifarre R, Sullivan HJ, Montoya A, et al: The use of the Jarvik-7 total artificial heart and the Symbion ventricular assist device as a bridge to transplantation. Surgery 108:681-685, 1990.
Poller L: Optimal therapeutic range for oral anticoagulation. In Poller L (ed): Recent Advances in Blood Coagulation, 5th ed. Edinburgh, Churchill Livingstone, 1991.
Raby C: Coagulations intravasculaires disséminées et localisées. Paris, Masson, 1974.
Ring M, Feinberg W, Levinson M, et al: Platelet and fibrin metabolism in recipients of the Jarvik-7 artificial heart. J Heart Transplant 8:225-232, 1989.
Schoen P, Lindhout T, Franssen J, Hemker HC: Low molecular weight heparin-catalized inactivation of factor Xa and thrombin by antithrombin III—effect of platelet factor 4. Thromb Haemost 66:435-441, 1991.

Scrutton M, Athayde CH: The biochemical basis for the regulation of platelet responsiveness. In Page C (ed): The Platelet in Health and Disease. Oxford, Blackwell Scientific Publications, 1991.

Siess W, Lapetina G: Functional relationship between cyclic AMP-dependent protein phosphorylation and platelet inhibiton. Biochem J 271:815–819, 1990.

Sinzinger H, Grady J, Fitscha P: Platelet deposition on human atherosclerotic lesions is decreased by low-dose aspirin in combination with dipyridamole. J Int Med Res 16:39–43, 1988.

Solis E, Leger P, Muneretto C, et al: Clinical application and patient selection in the use of a total artificial heart as a bridge for transplantation. Eur J Cardiothorac Surg 2:65–71, 1988.

Soloway HB, Christiansen TW: Heparin anticoagulation during cardiopulmonary bypass in an antithrombin III deficient patient. Am J Clin Pathol 73:723–725, 1980.

Soria C, Soria J, Diner H: Revue générale sur le mécanisme d'action du polysulfate de pentosan sur la coagulation et sur la fibrinolyse. Symposium Internationale Polysulfate de Pentosane. Paris, France, 1985.

Soria J, Soria C: Biologie du fibrinogène. Place de la pentoxifylline. J Mal Vasc 14:25–28, 1989.

Spero JA, Lewis JH, Hasiba U: Disseminated intravascular coagulation. Findings in 346 patients. Thromb Haemost 43:28–33, 1980.

Spiess B, Tuman K, McCarthy R, et al: Thromboelastography as an indicator of post-cardiopulmonary bypass coagulopathies. J Clin Monit 3:25–30, 1987.

Stewart ME, Douglas JT, Lowe GDO, et al: Prognostic value of beta-thromboglobulin in patients with transient cerebral ischemia. Lancet 27:2215, 1983.

Stratton JR, Ritchie JL: Reduction of indium-111 platelet deposition on Dacron vascular grafts in humans by aspirin plus dipyridamole. Circulation 73:325–330, 1986.

Szefner J: Apport de l'étude de la fontion plaquettiare et de la cinétique coagulo-lytique dan le contrôle et le traitement des transplantés cardiaques. In Sandoz (ed): Transplantation Cardiaque. Rueil-Malmaison, 1989, pp 80–87.

Szefner J: Le contrôle et la traitement de l'hémostase des malades sous le coeur artificiel total: L'experience de La Pitié. In Sandoz (ed): Transplantation Cardiaque et Pulmonaire. France, Rueil-Malmaison, 1991, pp 293–307.

Szefner J, Bellon JL, Cabrol C: Coagulation and Artificial Heart, 2nd ed. Paris, Masson, 1993.

Szefner J, Bellon JL, Castellanos C, et al: Méthode de surveillance et d'établissement d'un traitement anticoagulant chez les porteurs d'un coeur artificiel Jarvik 7. Paris, XII Journées d'Etudes du CECEC, 1987.

Szefner J, Desruennes M, Gandjbakhch I, et al: Heterotopic heart transplantation: Hemostasis well controlled in correlation with echocardiography. J Cardiovasc Surg 30:79, 1989.

Szefner J, Desruennes M, Gandjbakhch I, et al: Transplantation cardiaque hétértopique: Résultats encourageants à partir d'une nouvelle étude de l'hémostase et de l'échocardiographie. II Cuore Riv Cardiochir Cardiol (Suppl 3):266, 1988.

Szefner J, Miralles A, Bors V, et al: Disseminated intravascular coagulation: Our experience with 40 patients with a total artificial heart. J Heart Transplant 9:56, 1990.

Szefner J, Pavie A, Gandjbakhch I, et al: Apport de l'étude de la fonction plaquettaire et de la cinétique coagulolytique dans le contrôle et le traitement des malades sous coeur artificiel total Symbion type Jarvik 7. Deux années d'expérience. International Congress of Cardiology, American Heart Association, Marrakech, 1988.

Szefner J, Solis E, Pavie A, et al: The assessment of the supervision and treatment of hemostasis in 40 patients with a total artificial heart. Thromb Haemost 62:265, 1989.

Szefner J, Vaissier E, Arock M, et al: DIC in critically ill patients: Our experience with those having undergone TAH implants. Intensive Care Med 15:A-408, 1989.

Taylor KD, Gaykowski R, Keate KS, et al: Explant analysis of thirty-three bridges to transplant Jarvik-7 TAH devices. ASAIO Trans 33:738–743, 1987.

Teoh K, Christakis G, Weisel R, et al: Dipyridamole preserved platelets and reduced blood loss after cardiopulmonary bypass. J Thorac Cardiovasc Surg 96:332–341, 1988.

Teoh KH, Christakis GT, Weisel R, et al: Prevention of myocardial platelet deposition and thromboxane release with dipyridamole. Circulation 74(Suppl III):III-145–III-152, 1986.

Tidwell RR, Webster WP, Shaver SR, Geratz JD: Strategies for anticoagulation with synthetic protease inhibitors. Xa inhibitors versus thrombin inhibitors. Thromb Res 19:339–349, 1980.

Tollefsen DM: Activation of heparin cofactor II by heparin and dermatan sulfate. Nouv Rev Fr Hematol 26:233–237, 1984.

Unger F, et al: Assisted Circulation 3. Berlin, Springer Verlag, 1989.

Unger F, Olsen B, Oster H, Kolff WJ: Material and design factors in thromboembolization in TAH recipients living 100–2000 hours. Eur Surg Res 8:105–116, 1976.

Vairel EG, Bouty-Boye H, Toulemode F, et al: Heparin and a low molecular weight fraction enhances thrombolysis and by this pathway exercises a protective effect against thrombosis. Thromb Res 30:219–224, 1983.

Von Segesser L, Weiss B, Garcia A, et al: Reduced blood loss and transfusion requirements with low systemic heparinization: Preliminary clinical results in coronary artery revascularization. Eur J Cardiothorac Surg 4:639–643, 1990.

Yin ET, Giudice LC, Wessler S: Inhibiton of activated factor X-induced platelet aggregation: The role of heparin, the plasma inhibitor of activated factor X. J Lab Clin Med 82:390–398, 1973.

Zilla P, Fasol R, Groscurth P, et al: Blood platelets in cardiopulmonary bypass operations. J Thorac Cardiovasc Surg 97:379–388, 1989.

Chapter 18

Anticoagulation for Ventricular Assist Devices

A. Montoya, M.D., V.A. Lonchyna, M.D., and N. Moreno, M.D.

Ventricular assist devices (VADs) have been successfully applied for the hemodynamic stabilization of critically ill patients with profound cardiac failure that is unresponsive to inotropic and vasodilator support and intra-aortic balloon counterpulsation. Myocardial recovery has been reported to occur in up to 45% of patients with postcardiotomy cardiogenic shock who required mechanical assistance.[5,7,22,26,28,32,35] Patients with profound cardiogenic shock after acute myocardial infarction have a 100% mortality rate without the use of assist devices and a 23% survival rate with circulatory support.[24,33,42] Circulatory support with VADs has greatly improved survival in potential transplant recipients who deteriorate hemodynamically while waiting for a donor heart.[10,15,23,29,31] Mechanical assistance as a bridge to transplant was instituted in 534 patients reported in the Combined Registry for the Clinical Use of Mechanical Ventricular Assist Devices.[25] Sixty-seven percent underwent cardiac transplantation; 66% of patients with transplants were discharged.

Temporary circulatory support can be accomplished with left ventricular, right ventricular, and biventricular assist devices, which are of two types: nonpulsatile roller or centrifugal pumps (Biomedicus) and pulsatile pumps with a flexible blood sac enclosed in a rigid chamber. Pulsatile assist devices are connected to an external console and driven pneumatically via a percutaneous conduit.[34] Current pulsatile devices in clinical trials directed by the Food and Drug Administration (FDA) include the Thoratec (Pierce-Donachy), the Novacor, and the Thermocardiosystems HeartMate 1000.

The successful application of VADs involves accurate and timely selection of recipients who have severe myocardial failure without irreversible end-organ failure. Implantation of the device must improve secondary organ function with minimal complications. Hemorrhagic, thrombotic, and embolic complications are the major risk factors associated with mechanical circulatory assist devices. Equally as important as the desired improvement of hemodynamic performance is the minimization of complications that may jeopardize the successful outcome of circulatory assistance. Finally, discontinuance of circulatory support should be possible either because the myocardium has recovered or because the patient has received a transplant.

BLEEDING

Bleeding is the most common early complication related to the use of VADs. Fifty percent of patients requiring mechanical assistance and 40% of those who are bridged to transplant bleed in the immediate postoperative period.[25] This incidence can be related to insufficient hemostasis at the anastomotic sites. In addition, alterations in coagulation related to overheparinization, heparin rebound, inadequate heparin neutralization, and protamine excess can cause persistent bleeding. Other hemostatic defects causing hemorrhagic syndromes associated with VAD implantation are alteration of platelet function secondary to prolonged cardiopulmonary bypass (CPB) or related to a history of ingestion of aspirin or dipyridamole.[2,12,28]

The prolongation of bleeding time associated with CPB in excess of 2 hours is related to progressive platelet dysfunction. Under these circumstances, hemorrhage is present with abnormal bleeding times > 30 minutes that persist for hours after bypass despite platelet counts above 100,000/ml. Hypothermia is also a contributing factor to perioperative hemorrhage because it causes platelet dysfunction and sequestration.[3,12] Hemorrhage is directly proportional to the duration of CPB and the level of hypothermia.[12] Other hemostatic alterations accentuating CPB hemorrhage are primary fibrinolysis, thrombocytopenia, and disseminated intravascular coagulopathy (DIC).[2] A direct contributing factor to hemorrhage after the use of assist devices is a history of previous median sternotomy. Such patients require extensive lysis of adhesions and are at increased risk of severe postoperative bleeding.[11] Survival is significantly decreased when bleeding occurs as a complication after assisted circulation.[7,11,28] Therefore it is preferable to keep the patient in the operating room until hemostasis is accomplished, the chest is closed, heparin has been completely neutralized, and blood components are replaced.

THROMBOEMBOLISM

The therapeutic benefits of mechanical circulatory support have been overshadowed by the formation of clots within the assist devices that lead to long-term consequences related to strokes. Better device design with improvement in material and fabrication techniques, along with specific anticoagulation regimens and strict surgical protocols, has contributed to further decrease in the incidence of complications secondary to embolism. However, thrombus formation increases as the period of mechanical support is prolonged, and this complication is considered the primary drawback to its widespread long-term use.

Under normal circumstances blood remains fluid because of several factors. Living endothelial cells in the vessel wall actively synthesize antithrombotic agents such as prostacyclin and a heparinlike substance.[17] In addition, endogenous fibrinolytic activity, dispersion of procoagulant components of blood, and natural protease inhibitors such as antithrombin III and protein C help to prevent clotting within the vessel.[3]

Mechanical assistance requires contact between blood and synthetic material. This blood/surface interaction activates platelets that induce thrombus formation.[9,18] Anticoagulant and antiaggregatory therapy for patients with mechanical support does not fully prevent this thrombocyte activation.[41] Platelet aggregation and microembolism may occur as a result of abnormal flow conditions related to the configuration of the device, the biomaterial surfaces with which the blood interacts and fluid shear stress. Thrombi form in spite of large ratios of blood volume to synthetic surface, high flow rates, and smooth surfaces.[19] An additional means of preventing intravascular thrombus formation is the use of surface-bound heparin tubing and devices with an antithrombotic effect beyond that produced by the small amount of circulatory heparin that is washed from the surface. This technique retards the rate of thrombus formation rather than rendering the surfaces of the device nonthrombogenic.[19] Heparin coating improves the biocompatibility of existing VADs, thus decreasing the incidence of clot formation.[40]

Progress in device design, materials, and fabrication techniques have further improved hemodynamic performance and thus reduced thromboembolic complications. The result of these advances can be exemplified by calves with implanted total artificial hearts that survived for periods up to 210 days without anticoagulant therapy.[14] Nyilas attributes the absence of thromboembolism to deposition of a layer of plasma protein from the blood of the implanted host onto the smooth, nontextured surface of the device.[20] The blood interface must exhibit biologic stability, with the eventual formation of a cellular layer.[1,30] This pseudoneointima creates a passive blood-compatible lining that forms a selective barrier between blood and tissue and blocks contact-induced platelet activation. Synthetic polymer (Biomer) is an excellent material to fabricate smooth-contact surfaces. However, a microscopically smooth surface is extremely difficult to design,[4] and continuous stress forces caused by pump bladders that undergo constant flexing lead to failure of the pseudoneointima in long-term clinical applications.

An alternative design to circumvent this problem is the development of textured surfaces that provide the foundation for entrapment of cellular elements when the surface is initially exposed to blood. This innovation was incorporated into the HeartMate 1000 IP, a pneumatically driven LVAD designed by Poirier, which has been in clinical trials since 1986. Titanium microspheres are used in the pump housing and conduits and integrally textured polyurethane on the flexing pusher-plate diaphragm. When this textured surface comes in contact with blood, a well-adhered fibrin cellular coagulant develops, evolving into an extracellular matrix consisting of collagen, endothelial cells, and macrophages. A low incidence of thromboembolism on antiplatelet therapy alone results from long-term support with this device. Frazier reported the use of the HeartMate in 34 patients for up to 324 days. Anticoagulation was limited to 80 mg of aspirin and 225 mg of dipyridamole daily; no device-related thromboembolic events occurred.[10]

ANTICOAGULATION PROTOCOLS

In spite of progress in device design and fabrication, thrombus formation and embolization continue to be threats, and the optimal antithrombotic regimen for long-term clinical application remains a major challenge. Different anticoagulation protocols are recommended for the various VADs. However, protocols differ within the same institution, even for the same assist device.

Biomedicus Centrifugal Pump

The anticoagulant regimen is instituted 8–24 hours after implantation of the Biomedicus centrifugal pump when surgical bleeding is controlled and the chest-tube drainage is <50 cc/hr. Heparin is administered intravenously at 500–1000 U/hr. Its anticoagulant effect is monitored by the activating clotting time (ACT), which should range between 170–200 seconds. No bolus of heparin is given to initiate therapy or to adjust the ACT. In addition, antiplatelet aggregation therapy with dipyridamole is administered orally or via a nasogastric tube at a dose of 100 mg every 6 hours. This protocol, along with prophylactic antibiotics, is continued throughout the time the device is in place and until the patient is weaned from support or receives a transplant.

Pierce-Donachy (Thoratec)[6]

Several regimens of anticoagulation may be used with the Thoratec. Surgical bleeding is controlled by reversing heparin with protamine after CPB until chest-tube drainage is <25 cc/hr. Continuous infusion of heparin is then started at 400–1000 U/hr to maintain the ACT a 1.5 times normal. Alternatively, low-molecular-weight dextran is administered at 50 cc/hr for 24–36 hours, and then therapy is switched to heparin. A third protocol[38] uses intravenous dextran when the chest-tube drainage is <100 cc/hr for 3 consecutive hours. This protocol is continued until weaning from the device is begun, at which time heparin is administered. If the device is used as a bridge to transplantation, dextran is infused until oral dipyridamole and warfarin are given, and prothrombin time (PT) is maintained at 1.5 times control.[36]

Novacor

Anticoagulation for the Novacor is minimal and varies according to the clinical situation. Heparin is infused once postoperative bleeding has diminished to maintain a partial thromboplastin time (PTT) of 1.5 times normal. Low-molecular-weight dextran can be used alone or combined with low-dose heparin. With extended support, oral warfarin and dipyridamole have been used in place of dextran.

Thermocardiosystem Left Ventricular Assist Device (HeartMate)

The HeartMate has a well-defined anticoagulation protocol.[39] Heparin is reversed with protamine after implantation. Low-molecular-weight dextran is infused at a rate of 20 cc/hr postoperatively until the patient is able to take oral medication, at which time dipyridamole (75 mg 3 times daily) and aspirin (80 mg once daily) are initiated and continued for the duration of the implant. The pseudoneointimal biologic lining that forms within the device as a result of its unique surface composed of sintered titanium microphage (STM) has been very successful in limiting thrombin formation.[4] This, coupled with the use of bovine pericardial valves, has allowed safe use of the HeartMate without anticoagulation.

CONCLUSION

Considerable progress has been made in the development, indications, and application of VADs, which have led to improved survival in patients with refractory cardiogenic shock and are invaluable as a bridge to transplantation. Complications can be minimized with meticulous surgical technique and implementation of defined anticoagulant regimens. Advances in device design, material, and fabrication have greatly increased the scope of application of VADs.

REFERENCES

1. Berhard WF, LaFarge CG, Robinson TC, et al: An improved blood-pump interface for left ventricular bypass. Ann Surg 168:750-758, 1968.
2. Bick RL: Hemostasis defects associated with cardiac surgery, prosthetic devices and other extracorporeal circuits. Semin Thromb Hemost 11:249-280, 1985.
3. Bick RL, Bishop RC, Warren M, Stemmer E: Changes in fibrinolysis and fibrinolytic enzymes during extracorporeal circulation. Trans Am Soc Hematol 109, 1971 [abstract].
4. Dasse KA, Chipman SD, Sherman CN, et al: Clinical experience with textured contacting surfaces in ventricular assist devices. ASAIO Trans 10:418-425, 1987.
5. DeBakey ME: Left ventricular bypass pump for cardiac assistance. Am J Cardiol 27:3-11, 1971.
6. Farrar DJ: Thoratec Ventricular Assist Device System. Clinical Investigational Plan, 1988, p 25.
7. Farrar DJ, Hill D, Gray LA, et al: Heterotopic prosthetic ventricles as a bridge to cardiac transplantation. N Engl J Med 318:333-340, 1988.
8. Fasol R, Zilla P: Endothelialization of Artificial Heart Materials. Assisted Circulation 3. New York, Springer Verlag, 1989, pp 580-598.
9. Fasol R, Zilla P, Fishchlein T, Deutsch M: Surface morphology of circulating platelets: A suggested parameter for the monitoring of endothelial cell seeded grafts. J Cardiovasc Surg 30:398-401, 1989.
10. Frazier OH, Rose E, Macmanus Q, et al: Multicenter clinical evaluation of the HeartMate 1000 IP left ventricular assist device. Ann Thorac Surg 54:1019, 1992.
11. Gray LA, Ganzel BL, Mavroudis C, Slater D: The Pierce-Donachy ventricular assist device as a bridge to cardiac transplantation. Ann Thorac Surg 48:222-227, 1989.
12. Harker LA, Malpass TW, Branson HE, et al: Mechanism of abnormal bleeding in patients undergoing cardiopulmonary bypass: Acquired transient platelet dysfunction associated with selective and granule release. Blood 56:824-834, 1980.
13. Icenogle T, Copeland JG: Experience with the Total Artificial Heart as a Bridge to Transplantation. Assisted Circulation 3. New York, Springer Verlag, 1989, pp 260-268.
14. Jarvik RK, Lawson JH, Olsen DB, et al: Status of the artificial heart. Int J Artif Organs 1:21-29, 1978.
15. Kanter KR, McBride LR, Pennington DG, et al: Bridging to cardiac transplantation with pulsatile ventricular assist devices. Ann Thorac Surg 46:134-140, 1988.
16. Mansfield PB, Wechzak A: Tissue-cultured cells as an endothelial lining of prosthetic materials. In Norman JC (ed): Organ Perfusion and Preservation. New York, Appleton Century Crofts, 1986, pp 189-202.
17. Moncada S, Gryglewski R, Bunting S, Vane JR: An enzyme isolated from arteries transforms prostaglandin endoperoxides to an unstable substance that inhibits platelet aggregation. Nature 263:663-669, 1976.
18. Muller MM, Wholfahrt A, Nowak H, et al: Observations of human thrombocytes during total artificial heart replacement. Effects of aspirin on thromboembolism risk. Artif Organs (in press).

19. Musial J, Gluszko P, Edmunds H: Evaluation of surface-bound heparin and platelet inhibition in a centrifugal pump left ventricular assist system. World J Surg 9:72-77, 1985.
20. Nyilas E, Chiv T-H: Physiochemistry of blood/foreign surface interfacial phenomena. In Pierce WS (ed): Circulatory Assistance and the Artificial Heart. Washington, DC, U.S. Department of Health and Human Services, 1980, pp 81-134.
21. Nyilas E, Burnett P, Haag RM, Kupski EL: Surface microstructural factors and the blood compatibility of a silicone rubber. J Biomed Mater Res 4:368-374, 1970.
22. Pae WE, Miller CA, Matthews Y, Pierce WS: Ventricular assist devices for postcardiotomy cardiogenic shock. J Thorac Cardiovasc Surg 104:541-553, 1992.
23. Pae WE, Rosenberg G, Pierce WS: Ventricular Assistance: The Pennsylvania State University Experience. Assisted Circulation 3. New York, Springer Verlag, 1989, pp 115-131.
24. Pae WE, Pierce WS: Temporary left ventricular assistance in acute myocardial infarction and cardiogenic shock. Chest 79:629-695, 1981.
25. Pae WE: Combined Registry for the Clinical Use of Mechanical Ventricular Assist Devices. Personal communication, 1992.
26. Pennington DG, Samuels DL, Williams GW, et al: Experience with the Pierce-Donachy ventricular assist device in postcardiotomy patients with cardiogenic shock. World J Surg 9:37-46, 1985.
27. Pennington DG: Comment: Emergency management of cardiogenic shock. Circulation 79(Suppl I):I-149-I-151, 1989.
28. Pennock JL, Pierce WS, Wisman CB, et al: Survival and complications following ventricular assist pumping for cardiogenic shock. Ann Surg 198:469-478, 1983.
29. Pifarre R, Sullivan H, Montoya A, et al: Use of the total artificial heart and ventricular assist device as a bridge to transplantation. J Heart Transpl 9:638-642, 1990.
30. Poirier VK, Dasse KA: Clinical experience with the HeartMate 1000 IP blood pump. Woburn, MA, Thermocardiosystems, Inc., 1991.
31. Portner PM, Oyer PE, Pennington DG, et al: Implantable electrical left ventricular assist system: Bridge to transplantation and the future. Ann Thorac Surg 47:142-150, 1989.
32. Rose DM, Colvin SB, Culliford AT, et al: Long-term survival with partial left heart bypass following perioperative myocardial infarction and shock. J Thorac Cardiovasc Surg 83:483-492, 1982.
33. Schoen FJ, Palmer DC, Bernhard WF, et al: Clinical temporary ventricular assist. J Thorac Cardiovasc Surg 92:1071-1081, 1986.
34. Schoen FJ, Bernhard WF: Pathologic Considerations in Temporary Cardiac Assistance. Assisted Circulation 3. New York, Springer Verlag, 1989, pp 103-114.
35. Spencer FC, Eiseman B, Trinkle JK, Rossi NP: Assisted circulation for cardiac failure following intracardiac surgery with cardiopulmonary bypass. J Thorac Cardiovasc Surg 49:56-73, 1965.
36. Szukalski EA, Reedy JE, Pennington DG, et al: Oral anticoagulation in patients with ventricular assist devices. ASAIO Trans 36:M700-703, 1990.
37. Szycher M, Poirier VL, Tranzblauw C, et al: Biochemical, histological and ultrastructural assessments of pseudoneointimal linings derived from fibroblast-seeded integrally textured polymeric surfaces. J Biomed Mater Res 15:247-265, 1981.
38. Termuhlen DF, Swartz MT, Pennington DG, et al: Thromboembolic complication with the Pierce-Donachy ventricular assist device. ASAIO Trans 35:616-618, 1989.
39. Thermocardiosystems, Inc.: Investigational Plan for HeartMate 1000 IP LVAD System. 1991, p 30.
40. Von Segesser LK, Weiss BM, Bisang R, et al: Ventricular assist with heparin surface coated devices. ASAIO Trans 37:M278-M279, 1991.
41. Zilla P, Groscurth P, Varga G, et al: PGI and PGE induced morphological alterations in human platelets similar to those observed in the initial phase of activation. Exp Haematol 15:741-749, 1987.
42. Zumbro GL, Kitchens WR, Shearer G, et al: Mechanical assistance for cardiogenic shock following cardiac surgery, myocardial infarction and cardiac transplantation. Ann Thorac Surg 44:11-13, 1987.

Chapter 19

Surgical Considerations for Postoperative Bleeding

Bradford P. Blakeman, M.D., and Henry J. Sullivan, M.D.

Postoperative or perioperative bleeding is so much a part of open-heart surgery that it has its own code number in the American Medical Association Current Procedural Terminology (CPT).[60] Of greater importance are the potential problems that can occur with continued postoperative bleeding and reexploration, including wound infection; diseases transmitted by blood replacement (hepatitis and human immunodeficiency virus [HIV]); transfusion reactions; increased incidence of adult respiratory distress syndrome due to blood replacement; prolonged ventilation, greater potential for fluid overload; possible hemodynamic instability; increased risk of drop in systemic temperature because of prolonged operative procedures, with the possibility of arrhythmias and greater blood loss; and prolonged duration and increased cost of hospitalization for numerous reasons.[2,12,69]

The potential problems associated with postoperative bleeding have forced the cardiac surgeon to become compulsive about operative technique. However, as the cardiac surgeon knows, many sources of perioperative bleeding are uncontrollable, such as preoperative medications, liver disease, inherited coagulation defects, and thrombolytics. Even our so-called ally—the cardiopulmonary bypass (CPB) machine—can lead to coagulation disorders. This chapter organizes the many factors related to postoperative bleeding into a cohesive unit so that the cardiac surgeon can be better prepared to address bleeding problems. As expected, some overlap occurs with other chapters in this volume. However, whereas many of the other chapters were prepared by specialists in medicine, this chapter is written entirely from the viewpoint of the cardiac surgeon.

INCIDENCE

The percentage of patients who return to the operating room for bleeding after open-heart surgery ranges from 3-7% for routine procedures.[4,5,20,26,35,44,48,80] Similarly, the incidence in our experience of routine bypass surgery is 2.6% (Table 1). As predicted, certain procedures have a higher return rate for bleeding.

TABLE 1. Mediastinal Exploration for Postoperative Bleeding, Loyola University Medical Center, 1985-1992

Procedure	Total	Number Explored	%
Coronary artery bypass (CAB)	6430	171	2.6
Reoperative coronary artery bypass	882	106	12.0
Valve replacement with or without CAB	1391	123	8.8
Reoperative valve replacement	118	12	10.1
Cardiac transplant	209	25	11.9

Reoperative revascularization carries a 12% incidence in our institution. This rate no doubt results from the increased amount of dissection and longer pump runs. Other procedures with an increased incidence include valve replacement (primarily aortic and/or mitral), reoperative valve replacement, and cardiac transplant. The exceptionally high rate of reexploration for cardiac transplant is explained by the fact that many patients take Coumadin right up to the time of heart transplant. Commonly these patients are awaiting transplant on an outpatient basis. Moreover, because of chronic right-heart failure transplant patients often have insufficient amounts of clotting factors manufactured in the liver.

Other procedures in the literature that carry an increased risk for reexploration involve bypass with bilateral internal mammary arteries (IMAs).[48] As Lytle noted, in past years this particular procedure carried a risk of 17%. The incidence for reexploration, however, has decreased to 5% in recent years, with an incidence of 2% for single IMA bypass at the Cleveland Clinic. Use of the IMA for routine revascularization in chronic dialysis patients in our institution involved no increased bleeding problems.[7] In fact, in a small group of patients, none was returned for bleeding. Rich et al.[62] noted a 25% bleeding problem in patients over 75 years old. Reports also generally agree that patients with cyanotic heart disease have increased bleeding problems.[26] Clearly the incidence of reexploration is a universal problem for all cardiac surgeons.

PREOPERATIVE EVALUATION

Decreasing the incidence of postoperative bleeding should begin with preoperative evaluation of potential clotting problems. Management of a high-volume practice of heart surgery mandates a routine system to screen patients. The medical history should highlight any previous bleeding problems, such as epistaxis, hemoptysis, melena, or hematochezia. Family history should be explored to uncover possible inherited bleeding problems, such as hemophilia or von Willebrand's disease.[39,66,76]

Intake of medication should be carefully summarized, whether on a chronic or acute basis. Common drugs that may cause problems are aspirin (including aspirin-containing compounds such as cold medications), dipyridamole, heparin, Coumadin, and other antiinflammatory drugs. Table 2 lists other medications that can affect the normal clotting cascade. Aspirin, for example, can affect normal platelet aggregation for 5-7 days after ingestion.[23,43,54] Platelet abnormalities due to aspirin may result from inhibition of various factors, including thromboxane B_2, platelet function (by irreversible acetylation

TABLE 2. Common Drugs Interfering with Platelet Function in Surgical Patient Populations*

Ampicillin	Furosemide	Papaverine
Aspirin	Gentamicin	Penicillin
Carbenicillin	Glyceryl guaiacolate	Phenothiazines
Clofibrate	Ibuprofen	Propranolol
Diphenhydramine	Indomethacin	Sulfinpyrazone
Dipyridamole	Nitrofurantoin	Tricyclic amines

From Semin Thromb Hemost 11:253, 1985, with permission.
* Candidates for prosthetic devices.

of the active site of the platelet enzyme cyclooxygenase), production of prostaglandin by platelet and vessel walls, and platelet aggregation.[23,43,54] If possible, all aspirin should be discontinued for 7 days preoperatively because a single aspirin inhibits thromboxane B_2 for 5 days, which approximates the half-life of a platelet.[23,54] Unfortunately, the elevated bleeding time (as measured by Ivy or template) used to screen for platelet abnormalities does not correlate well with increased perioperative blood loss.[24] Kitcher, however, did note that bleeding was least in patients with a negative drug history and a normal bleeding time.[43]

The second aspect of screening for potential bleeding problems is a thorough physical examination. Particular notes should be made, for example, of excess bruising or any stigmata of liver abnormalities. The third part of screening includes preoperative laboratory work. The evaluation in our institution consists of a standard blood count with platelet count, prothrombin time (PT), partial thromboplastin time (PTT), Ivy bleeding time, and fibrinogen level. Screening for cryoglobulins is also appropriate when the patient has a routine type and cross-match performed in the blood bank. These tests should detect the majority of perioperative bleeding problems. If any significant problems are pinpointed, consultation with a hematologist is advised.

CAUSES OF POSTOPERATIVE BLEEDING

In addition to preoperative problems that may affect bleeding, many events at the time of surgery can contribute to blood loss and risk of reexploration. Engblom et al.[20] at reexploration found primarily minor bleeding due to coagulopathy, whereas Koshal[44] discovered that 78% of bleeding was due to surgical causes. The primary surgical sources were the bed of the IMA and the distal anastomosis of the obtuse marginal graft. Of importance, the majority of patients returning for bleeding had normal preoperative coagulation studies.[4]

Surgical bleeding can obviously be minimized by compulsive placement of sutures, appropriate reinforcement of suture lines and cannulation sites with Teflon, meticulous dissection of the IMA, and reinspection of all suture lines when the patient is weaned from CPB and normal blood pressure has been established. Control of blood pressure in the postoperative period, particularly when the heart is friable, is essential to minimize surgical bleeding.

The other significant cause of postoperative bleeding, as noted above, is a coagulation defect. Thrombocytopenia, which occurs simply from exposure to heparin,[21] can take two forms. The first, which occurs in 30–40% of patients, is due to a transient, reversible clumping, agglutination, and peripheral sequestration of platelets. The second, which occurs approximately 7-10 days after exposure to heparin, is due to heparin-induced antibodies. Despite this thrombocytopenia, as Pike noted,[61] quantitative platelet count has less to do with bleeding than does actual platelet function.

CPB contributes significantly to postoperative coagulation problems, as attested by multiple investigators.[6,8,11,17-19,25,27,29,31,37,42,49,50,52,55-57,59,72,74,75,83] Significant alterations by CPB in platelet count and function probably account for the majority of medically related bleeding problems. Between 60-70% of all platelets disappear in the first several minutes of bypass.[17] Both permanent destruction and reversible sequestration of platelets (often in the liver) occur.[17] The initial drop is the same with the bubbler and membrane oxygenators. However, return to a more normal platelet count is greater with the membrane than the bubbler oxygenator (70% for bubbler vs. 95% for membrane).[17]

This initial platelet drop is also much greater than can be explained by the hemodilution that occurs on CPB.[49,83] With membrane oxygenators, the platelet count decreases in the first few minutes and then stabilizes.[18] Presumably the platelets initially adhere to the surfaces of the oxygenator and other tubing, then no longer continue to do so. With the bubbler oxygenator, the platelet count continues to decrease gradually as long as the patient stays on CPB. The presumed damage to platelets with the bubble oxygenator results from the direct interface of blood and gas.[8,18] Continuance of this interface throughout the course of CPB explains the greater changes in platelet count with the bubbler oxygenator.

Cardiotomy or "inside" suction can also contribute to permanent platelet damage due to the interface because both air and blood are sent through the suction.[8] This problem can be lessened by decreasing the amount of suction. Differences in platelet function due to cardiotomy suction were noted only in unusual circumstances: after 3 hours on CPB and with cardiotomy suction exceeding 65 L.[8] The actual mechanism of damage is not fully understood.[6] The circulating platelets are uniformly activated during CPB through a process that involves release and partial degradation of alpha granules, but not of dense granules.[29] This platelet abnormality is confirmed by an increased bleeding time and a defect in normal platelet aggregation studies in vitro. The aggregability to adenosine diphosphate (ADP) and collagen is markedly impaired during CPB, but reaction to surface contact alone (ristocetin) is not altered.[49] However, both ADP and ristocetin are altered when protamine is used to reverse the heparin. Protamine probably further alters the membrane of the platelet and thereby affects its normal function.[49] ADP aggregation also slightly favors the membrane oxygenator versus the bubbler.[25]

Bleeding time, as measured by Harker,[29] showed that one group of patients had a bleeding time of 5 minutes preoperatively, 12 minutes after CPB started, and more than 30 minutes after 2 hours on bypass. Use of normothermia or hypothermia appears to make no significant difference in platelet aggregation.[29] In uncomplicated patients the bleeding time generally normalizes 1 hour after termination of CPB. Harker, however, identified a group of patients with significant bleeding in whom the platelet count was >100,000 but the bleeding time exceeded 20 minutes several hours after bypass. This obviously represents a group of patients at high risk of bleeding. As stated above, the majority of platelets are not destroyed but rather simply inhibited for a few hours.[18] It is not clear whether the return of platelet function is due to recovery or recruitment of new platelets. The postoperative platelet count rises to a maximum at 14–17 days and by 32 days postoperatively reaches a steady state of thrombopoiesis.[50]

The differences in membrane versus bubbler oxygenators should be highlighted. Although the membrane oxygenator accounts for less destruction and inhibition of platelets during bypass, the clinical significance is not as great as expected.[6,18,25,59] Using indium 111-labeled platelets, Peterson[59] demonstrated that the membrane compared with the bubbler preserved twice the number of platelets in circulation after 1 hour of bypass. As he pointed out, however, in shorter CPB runs (<2 hr) the positive effect of the membrane oxygenator is not noticeable. No clinical difference in semiporous or true membrane oxygenators has been observed.[72] Membrane oxygenators have also demonstrated less leukocyte sequestration, hemolysis, and complement activation.[72,75] Addition of steroids to the bubbler oxygenator can help to reduce leukocyte sequestration and complement activation.[11]

Multiple other coagulation factors have been evaluated to help to explain coagulopathy after CPB. Mammen monitored hematocrit (Hct); fibrinogen; factors II, V, X, VIII:C, and XI; antithrombin; plasminogen; alpha-2-antiplasmin; and platelets.[49] As CPB begins, the Hct drops because of hemodilution. All clotting factors decrease in parallel with hemodilution except for factors VIII:C and XI. By the end of CPB all clotting factors have returned to near normal levels except for factor V and, as previously noted, the platelet count. In the intensive care unit, Mammen noted a second drop in levels of fibrinogen, prothrombin, factor V, and antithrombin III. Moriau also noted that factor V was markedly decreased at the end of bypass, but by the end of 24 hours it had returned to normal.[57] Other investigators also corroborated that prolongation of PT due to a decrease of factor V is largely responsible for coagulopathy after CPB.[27,55,83] Wolk noted, as did Mammen, a continued drop in antithrombin in the intensive care unit.[83]

Increased fibrinolytic activity and secondary effects of fibrin-fibrinogen degradation products (FDPs) have been thought to increase bleeding because of their effects on coagulation. Milan[55] noted no increase in fibrin split products during bypass or for the next 2 days after CPB. Moriau[57] noted a transient rise in fibrinolysis but no increase in FDPs. Bick[6] points out that this possible explanation of disseminated intravascular coagulation (DIC) is unlikely because of adequate heparinization and the absence of uniform thrombocytopenia. Gralwick[27] also observed no increase in FDPs. Ulmas[74] noted an increase in fibrin split products in the bloodstream and chest-tube drainage. His findings demonstrated a large amount of fibrinolysis in the chest, but little or no fibrinolytic activity in the blood. In summary, hyperfibrinolytic activity is rarely responsible for excess bleeding.

Another occasionally quoted cause of excess bleeding is heparin rebound, which has been largely discounted by Harker,[29] Mammen,[49] and Bick.[6] Kirklin[42] also noted an increased risk of bleeding due to higher levels of C3a complement degradation products. The rate of complement activation does not differ between membrane and bubbler oxygenators.[75] It is doubtful, however, that complement activation plays a major role in postoperative bleeding. One other aspect of CPB that may affect bleeding as well as help to lower the hematocrit during surgery is damage to red blood cells. Deformability of red cells is a normal function to facilitate their passage through the microcirculation.

CPB decreases deformation by an average of 31%; this decrease continues for the next 3 days.[19] Lack of correlation with the length of time on CPB suggests that the injury occurs soon after CPB begins. The lack of deformability leads obviously to a shortened life span of the cell and the potential for anemia. Hirayama[31] noted that a 50% reduction in deformability is associated with more bleeding at 12 and 24 hours postoperatively. Deformability (or red cell filtration rate) normalizes at 6 weeks.

The cell-saver apparatus (CSA) has become routine in our practice. As noted above, when the cells are separated by the centrifuge system, all platelets are lost, and all protein, including the proteins in the clotting cascade, are removed.[28,51] Hall[28] also demonstrated that the CSA was associated with increased duration of CPB, operating time, and hospitalization. However, in a retrospective study the CSA unit appeared safe, caused no unusual risk of bleeding, and reduced transfusion of homologous blood.[28] Mayer[51] noted that patients in whom the CSA was used had comparable blood loss, no difference in postoperative coagulation cascades, and, most importantly, no increased bleeding. Although we use the CSA for all cases, we agree that it causes no increase in bleeding for the routine case. The amount of blood actually centrifuged amounts to only about 1 unit per patient. In situations involving greater blood loss, such as repair of aortic dissection, the amount of blood run through the CSA may cause sufficient loss of clotting factors and platelets to contribute to bleeding. Platelets, fresh frozen plasma, and cryoprecipitate may be necessary in prolonged cases with unusual blood loss. We concur that use of the CSA has dramatically reduced transfusions of homologous blood.

In conclusion, the devices used for surgery contribute to postoperative medical bleeding. The primary causes are qualitative defects of platelets, prolonged prothrombin time due to a decrease of factor V, and, to a minimal degree, decrease in red-cell deformability. Such knowledge can aid the physician in using platelets and fresh frozen plasma or cryoprecipitate to correct postoperative bleeding problems due to coagulopathy.

Medication-related Problems Causing Bleeding

The next significant cause of postoperative bleeding is preoperative medications. As noted above, because aspirin (ASA) and related drugs can affect platelet function for up to 5-7 days after ingestion, these medications should be stopped, if possible, before surgery. Ferraris noted that currently more patients take ASA because of previous coronary bypass; it is a commonly used drug that has been shown to decrease fatal and nonfatal cardiac events. Patients also take aspirin after angioplasty.[23] Though ASA does cause an increase in bleeding time, a strong correlation between amount of postoperative bleeding and bleeding time has not been found.[10,23,24,43,54]

Recent use of thrombolytics in the emergency room and cardiac catheterization laboratory for acute myocardial infarctions has also affected blood loss. The commonly used drugs include streptokinase, urokinase, tissue plasminogen activator (TPA), and anisoylated plasminogen streptokinase activator complex (APSAC).[14,38,40,41,45,46,70,71,73,78,81,82] Newer studies even combine the use of these drugs.[41] They are discussed in detail to aid the surgeon in counteracting their potentially great effect on perioperative blood loss.

Streptokinase is a potent thrombolytic agent that acts primarily by stimulation of plasminogen activator, thus leading to increased production of plasmin, which degrades many serum proteins, including polymerized fibrin meshwork.[46] It is not clot-specific and can initiate an overwhelming imbalance toward fibrinolysis. The half-life of streptokinase is 23 minutes, and the period of hyperplasminemia lasts for only a few hours; the resultant coagulopathy, however, lasts for up to 12-24 hours.[41,46] The group of patients with the most severe bleeding problems are those receiving systemic streptokinase, particularly in doses >1.5 million units.[46] As Lee noted, if patients receive systemic doses, blood loss and subsequent transfusion are increased in the first 12 hours. If, however, the streptokinase is given via an intracoronary approach in doses of 95,000-340,000 units, the incidence of perioperative bleeding is not excessive, even in patients taken immediately to the operating room.[38,81,82] Centers using either systemic or intracoronary streptokinase reported no excessive bleeding and no increased mortality if surgery was delayed for several days after discontinuance of the drug.[14,78,81,82] If the patient must go to the operating room within the first 24 hours after use of systemic streptokinase, then fibrinogen should be replaced with cryoprecipitate, which contains the highest concentration. Fibrinogen and antiplasmin levels as well as PT and PTT should be monitored in the postoperative period. E-aminocaproic acid might be helpful since it theoretically has the ability to cause dissociation of the streptokinase–plasminogen complex.[46]

The second most commonly used drug to lyse clots for acute myocardial infarction is urokinase, a naturally occurring enzyme with no antigenicity and no clot selectivity. Urokinase activates plasminogen directly by peptide bond cleavage.[41] Few catheterization laboratories presently use this drug alone; the approach is generally intracoronary. As with streptokinase, the intracoronary approach minimizes the risk of increased bleeding. The levels of antiplasmin as well as PT and PTT should be monitored in the postoperative period; cryoprecipitate is again the choice for source of fibrinogen.

Tissue plasminogen activator (TPA) is another of the popular drugs used for acute myocardial infarctions to lyse intracoronary blood clots. TPA is a serine protease produced in vascular endothelial cells by recombinant DNA.[41] TPA is different from streptokinase and urokinase in that it has more clot (fibrin) specificity, does not cause a systemic lytic state, and maintains relative preservation of the circulatory coagulation factors.[40,41,73] The breakdown of fibrinogen is generally 30-40%, which is less than with non–clot-specific agents; however, the clinical impression is that bleeding is as significant as with streptokinase or urokinase.[41] Kereiakes[40] operated on 24 patients within 7.3 hours after systemic administration of TPA, and 3 were reexplored for bleeding—2 because of diffuse oozing. Within the first 24 hours the 24 patients had received an average of 5.6 units of blood, 4 units of fresh frozen plasma, 3.9 units of cryoprecipitate, and 3 units of platelets. Obviously they required a significant amount of blood and blood-product replacement. Because fibrinogen is broken down, cryoprecipitate is again the obvious choice to reverse any coagulation problems.

The last thrombolytic agent in common use today is systemic anisoylated plasminogen streptokinase activator complex (anistreplase or APSAC). This chemically modified plasminogen streptokinase complex is associated with increased fibrin specificity.[41] Its half-life is 90-105 minutes. The fibrinolysis is concentrated at the site of the clot. If this agent is used before emergent surgery, cryoprecipitate most specifically reverses any coagulation problem.

PATTERNS OF BLEEDING AND INDICATIONS FOR REEXPLORATION

Strict indications for reexploration of the mediastinum for bleeding after open-heart surgery have not been well defined in the literature. The surgeon's pattern for reexploration is greatly influenced by individual training and opinions. The patterns of bleeding and indications for reexploration described below are general guidelines used in our institution.

The first pattern of bleeding is oozing that begins at the start of surgery and continues after weaning from CPB and administration of protamine. This pattern often occurs in reoperative patients who, even after meticulous control of surgical bleeding, drain >200 cc/hr from the chest tubes. If the patient continues to drain at this rate for more than 4-6 hours, reexploration is required. And if the patient becomes hemodynamically unstable with this degree of chest-tube drainage, reexploration is immediate. The logic of this approach is twofold: (1) the surgeon must prove by at least one reexploration that surgical bleeding is not involved, and (2) the evacuation of clot and blood may theoretically decrease consumption of coagulation factors within the mediastinum. During this 4-6 hour period, the coagulation profile is evaluated, and the patient is given platelet transfusions, fresh frozen plasma, cryoprecipitate, and blood as necessary. This group of postoperative bleeders probably accounts for the highest incidence of reexploration for bleeding. The surgeon must take care to avoid excessive time in the operating room with the chest open, because the patient's systemic temperature may drop below 35°C. If the temperature is falling, it is better to close the patient, with appropriate warming, and return for reexploration at a later time.

The second group of patients are "very dry" in terms of bleeding when the chest is initially closed. At some point postoperatively, active bleeding begins. This pattern is generally surgical bleeding and warrants immediate exploration. Common sources are a branch of the IMA, sternal wire through a chest wall vessel, a branch of an obtuse marginal vein graft, or occasionally an aortic suture line or cannulation site. If the aorta is involved, this bleeding can be catastrophic; however, if an operating room is available 24 hours a day and house staff are alert, the patient can be saved. The intensive care staff must also implement proper control of blood pressure. Abrupt rises in blood pressure can certainly lead to suture-line tears. Usually reimplementation of CPB is not necessary for these patients; however, quick access to CPB may salvage an occasional exception.

The third pattern of bleeding is the patient who has significant bleeding (>200 cc/hr) that suddenly stops. The clinical impression indicates no need for reexploration. Then the patient begins to have fluctuations in blood pressure, and inotropic support increases without a good explanation. Such a patient should always be reexplored, and the usual finding is a large clot on the right ventricle. Once this clot is evacuated, the patient stabilizes and has an uneventful postoperative course. This scenario is indicative of the acute tamponade, and many of the sequelae of the more chronic tamponade, such as neck vein distention, pulsus paradoxus, and low urine output, are not seen. Certainly return to the operating room should not be delayed until they appear.

The fourth pattern of bleeding is more subtle. The patient may have wide hemodynamic swings in the immediate postoperative period. Analysis of blood gases indicates that the hematocrit is dropping, but the chest-tube drainage remains well below 200 cc/hr. Suspicion of bleeding needs to be significant, and a chest x-ray can be helpful. A large fluid collection is visible in one pleura (Fig. 1). The patient needs to return to the operating room for exploration, evacuation of blood, and search for surgical bleeding.

PERIOPERATIVE METHODS TO REDUCE BLEEDING

In addition to administering blood and blood products to slow bleeding, two general methods may be used to reduce bleeding, one medical and one mechanical. The drugs most commonly discussed in the literature include desmopressin acetate (DDAVP), E-aminocaproic acid, tranexamic acid, and aprotinin. Because several of these drugs are discussed in other chapters, only a brief discussion is provided here.

DDAVP is a synthetic vasopressor analog that increases the plasma level of von Willebrand's factor.[30,67] It is known to improve hemostasis in mild hemophilia and in other conditions with defective platelet function.[30] In fact, de la Fuente[15] and Warrier[79] believe that the majority of patients with mild-to-moderate forms of hemophilia and von Willebrand's disease can be treated effectively with DDAVP instead of blood products. None of their patients, however, underwent open-heart surgery. The question remains whether routine use of DDAVP can reduce blood loss after open-heart surgery. Salzman[67] used the drug after CPB in 70 patients and noted improvement in blood loss and a decrease in the number of patients with blood loss > 2000 cc. Seear[68] and Rocha,[63] however, noted no reduction of blood loss in a combined group of over 160 children and adults when the drug was used routinely. Czer[13] used DDAVP selectively in patients with excess bleeding >100 cc/hr and

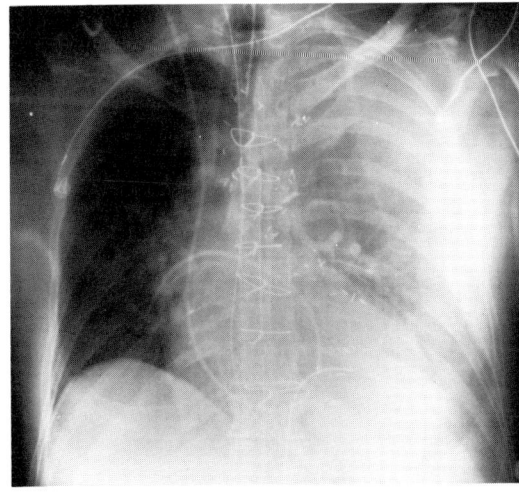

FIGURE 1. Chest x-ray taken 2 hours postoperatively demonstrates fluid collection in left chest in a patient with dropping hematocrit.

prolonged bleeding time >10 minutes. He noted a slowing of bleeding within 1 hour and an approximate 40% decrease in bleeding time. Twelve patients were subsequently explored, and 10 were found to have surgical bleeding. Although the verdict about DDAVP is still undecided, one can draw the following conclusions: (1) it plays a role in treatment of mild-to-moderate hemophilia or von Willebrand's disease; (2) routine use in all patients does not significantly alter blood loss; and (3) selective use in significant bleeders after CPB may reduce blood loss, but not if surgical bleeding is the cause.

Aminocaproic acid (EACA) is a 6-amino-hexanoic acid that effectively inhibits fibrinolysis. Although uncommon, primary hyperfibrinolysis may occur after CPB.[6] First, the other causes of surgical and medical bleeding should be ruled out. Next the surgeon should look for evidence of hypoplasminogenemia, circulating plasmin, and elevated FDPs. If these are found, then EACA is administered in a loading dose of 5 g over 1 hour, followed by 1 g/hr for the next 5 hours.[6]

The third drug sometimes used is tranexamic acid, a potent inhibitor of plasminogen. Theoretically it can be given as prophylaxis against fibrinolytic activity.[33,63] Tranexamic acid has a greater efficacy, longer half life, and stronger plasminogen-binding capability than EACA. Horrow[33] reported that patients receiving tranexamic acid demonstrated fewer fibrin split products and a marked decrease in plasminogen availability, whereas patients in the placebo group required more fresh frozen plasma.[33] More clinical studies are needed to determine whether the drug helps to reduce postoperative blood loss.

The final drug is aprotinin, which has recently created interest as a means of reducing bleeding. This drug is also discussed in greater detail elsewhere in this volume. Aprotinin is a serine proteinase inhibitor that probably has a platelet-sparing effect.[65] Although its exact mechanism of action is uncertain, it is thought to affect the von Willebrand-platelet interaction.[64,65] The drug is given from the start of surgery and in early studies has produced a significant decrease in blood loss.[1,64,65] Concern about a hypercoagulable state after surgery is not totally resolved, and a multicenter study that includes Loyola Medical Center is ongoing.

Cardiac surgeons have been particularly inventive in using mechanical means to slow perioperative bleeding. This discussion, although by no means exhaustive, demonstrates certain methods to slow bleeding, many of which certainly arose out of frustration. Topical glue has gained strong advocates among cardiac surgeons.[9,47,77] The usual method is to place cryoprecipitate in one syringe and topical thrombin in another. The syringes are then directed at the site of bleeding and squirted. The result is a gelatinous yellow substance that can help to control medical and even some minimal surgical bleeding.[9,47,77]

Another method (originally described by Cabrol[58]) to control bleeding when the ascending aorta is replaced is a fistula in the right atrial-to-periprosthetic space. This method is particularly useful if the sinuses of Valsalva are dilated. Presumably the majority of these fistulas close on their own soon after surgery.

Delayed sternal closure has been used by surgeons over the years to control bleeding.[16,22,53] Campo combined an open technique with packing of a friable aorta.[16] The obvious concern is the possibility of increased infection. Mestres[53] used delayed closure for 16 patients and reported no mediastinitis, but one late infection. Fanning[22] delayed closure in 57 patients (24 for bleeding) and subsequently reported 3 superficial infections and 1 fatality due to mediastinitis. Presumably the potential for infection is greater with this technique, and at least skin closure (with or without patch) should be achieved. Sterile technique for wound management should be used in conjunction with intravenous antibiotics. Delayed sternal closure was necessary on only two occasions in our own practice over the past 15 years.

Positive pressure ventilation with positive end-expiratory pressures (PEEPs) as high as 10–15 cm of H_2O has been used in several centers.[32,36,84] This method, which is appropriate only after coagulation problems are corrected, is thought to be successful because of overdistention of the lungs with tamponade bleeding.[36] Ilabaca[36] used this method in 15 patients (11 of whom bled an average of 330 cc/hr for 1–5 hr). Eleven were subsequently controlled with 10-15 cm of PEEP and 4 were reexplored. Zurick[84] randomized two groups of patients who had undergone routine heart surgery to either 10 cm or no PEEP. The result was no reduction in bleeding and no differences in the hematocrit, incidence of postoperative reexploration, or amount of blood administered. In all patients who returned for reexploration in Zurick's study,[84] the bleeding was due to surgical causes. Hoffman[32] noted that 5 cm of PEEP was not enough to be of help in reducing bleeding, but that 10 cm of PEEP was effective. These studies indicate that positive pressure ventilation may help to reduce medical bleeding but has no effect on surgical bleeding. This method should not be relied upon as a primary technique for reducing postoperative blood loss.

Of note, one surgeon actually clamped the chest tubes and created a controlled tamponade.[3] This technique is mentioned not to encourage use, but only to illustrate the frustration that surgeons experience when faced with the postoperative bleeder.

In conclusion, it should be firmly stated that mechanical methods must be viewed only as adjunctive techniques to control blood loss. Foremost is meticulous surgical technique, followed by correction of coagulation defects.

CONCLUSION

Although many experts have contributed to this volume on coagulation and blood preservation in cardiac surgery, it is the surgeon who is faced with sorting out the problems when a patient bleeds postoperatively. As mentioned previously, the surgeon must demonstrate that increased postoperative blood loss is not due to a surgical cause (even if the patient must be explored on more than one occasion). If coagulation disorders are present, meticulous surgical technique becomes increasingly important, along with appropriate replacement of blood products. Once surgical bleeding has been eliminated as a cause for blood loss, replacement of blood products, drugs such as DDAVP and aprotinin, or mechanical means can be used to slow bleeding. With the tools currently available to the surgeon, few if any patients should succumb to blood loss after routine cardiac surgery.

REFERENCES

1. Alajmo F, Calamai G, Perna AM, et al: High-dose aprotinin: Hemostatic effects in open heart operations. Ann Thorac Surg 48:536–539, 1989.

2. Angelini GD, Lamarra M, Azzu AA, Bryan AJ: Wound infection following early repeat sternotomy for postoperative bleeding: An experience utilizing intraoperative irrigation with povidone iodine. J Cardiovasc Surg 31:793-795, 1990.
3. Aravot DJ, Barak J, Vidne BA: Induction of controlled cardiac tamponade in the management of massive unexplained postcardiotomy bleeding: Case report and review of the literature. J Cardiovasc Surg 27:613-617, 1986.
4. Bachman F, McKenna R, Cole ER, Najafi H: The hemostatic mechanism after open-heart surgery: I. Studies on plasma coagulation factors and fibrinolysis in 512 patients after extracorporeal circulation. J Thorac Cardiovasc Surg 70:76-85, 1975.
5. Bahn CH, Annest LS, Miyamoto M: Pericardial closure. Am J Surg 151:612-615, 1986.
6. Bick RL: Hemostasis defects associated with cardiac surgery, prosthetic devices, and other extracorporeal circuits. Semin Thromb Hemost 11:249-280, 1985.
7. Blakeman BP, Sullivan HJ, Foy BK, et al: Internal mammary artery revascularization in the patient on long-term renal dialysis. Ann Thorac Surg 50:776-778, 1990.
8. Boonstra PW, van Imhoff GW, Eysman L, et al: Reduced platelet activation and improved hemostasis after controlled cardiotomy suction during clinical membrane oxygenator perfusions. J Thorac Cardiovasc Surg 89:900-906, 1985.
9. Borst HG, Haverich A, Walterbusch G, Maatz W: Fibrin adhesive: An important hemostatic adjunct in cardiovascular operations. J Thorac Cardiovasc Surg 84:548-553, 1982.
10. Burns ER, Billett HH, Frater RWM, Sisto DA: The preoperative bleeding time as a predictor of postoperative hemorrhage after cardiopulmonary bypass. J Thorac Cardiovasc Surg 92:310-312, 1986.
11. Cavarocchi NC, Pluth JR, Schaff HV, et al: Complement activation during cardiopulmonary bypass: Comparison of bubble and membrane oxygenators. J Thorac Cardiovasc Surg 91:252-258, 1986.
12. Culliford AT, Cunningham JN Jr, Zeff RH, et al: Sternal and costochondral infections following open-heart surgery: A review of 2,594 cases. J Thorac Cardiovasc Surg 72:714-726, 1976.
13. Czer LSC, Bateman TM, Gray RJ, et al: Treatment of severe platelet dysfunction and hemorrhage after cardiopulmonary bypass: Reduction in blood product usage with desmopressin. J Am Coll Cardiol 9:1139-1147, 1987.
14. Cook LS, Lucas SK, Cheatham JE, et al: Cardiovascular parameters after acute myocardial infarction and streptokinase administration in patients receiving coronary artery bypass grafts. Am J Surg 148:860-863, 1984.
15. de la Fuente B, Kasper CK, Rickles FR, Hoyer LW: Response of patients with mild and moderate hemophilia A and von Willebrand's disease to treatment with desmopressin. Ann Intern Med 103:6-14, 1985.
16. Del Campo C: Mediastinal packing for refractory nonsurgical bleeding after open-heart surgery. Can J Surg 28:55-56, 1985.
17. de Leval M, Hill JD, Mielke H, et al: Platelet kinetics during extracorporeal circulation ASAIO Trans 18:355-358, 1972.
18. Edmunds LH Jr, Ellison N, Colman RW, et al: Platelet function during cardiac operation: Comparison of membrane and bubble oxygenators. J Thorac Cardiovasc Surg 83:805-812, 1982.
19. Ekeström S, Koul BL, Sonnenfeld T: Decreased red cell deformability following open-heart surgery. Scand J Thorac Cardiovasc Surg 17:41-44, 1983.
20. Engblom E, Arstila M, Inberg MV, et al: Early results and complications of coronary artery bypass surgery: A consecutive series of 441 patients. Scand J Thorac Cardiovasc Surg 19:21-27, 1985.
21. Esposito RA, Culliford AT, Colvin SB, et al: Heparin resistance during cardiopulmonary bypass: The role of heparin pretreatment. J Thorac Cardiovasc Surg 85:346-353, 1983.
22. Fanning WJ, Vasko JS, Kilman JW: Delayed sternal closure after cardiac surgery. Ann Thorac Surg 44:169-172, 1987.
23. Ferraris VA, Ferraris SP, Lough FC, Berry WR: Preoperative aspirin ingestion increases operative blood loss after coronary artery bypass grafting. Ann Thorac Surg 45:71-74, 1988.
24. Ferraris VA, Swanson E: Aspirin usage and perioperative blood loss in patients undergoing unexpected operations. Surg Gynecol Obstet 156:439-442, 1983.
25. Friedenberg WR, Myers WO, Plotka ED, et al: Platelet dysfunction associated with cardiopulmonary bypass. Ann Thorac Surg 25:298-305, 1978.
26. Gomes MMR, McGoon DC: Bleeding patterns after open-heart surgery. J Thorac Cardiovasc Surg 60:87-97, 1970.

27. Gralnick HR, Fischer RD: The hemostatic response to open-heart operations. J Thorac Cardiovasc Surg 61:909-915, 1971.
28. Hall RI, Schweiger IM, Finlayson DC: The benefit of the Hemonetics cell saver apparatus during cardiac surgery. Can J Anaesth 37:618-622, 1990.
29. Harker LA, Malpass TW, Branson HE, et al: Mechanism of abnormal bleeding in patients undergoing cardiopulmonary bypass: Acquired transient platelet dysfunction associated with selective α-granule release. Blood 56:824-834, 1980.
30. Hedderich GS, Petsikas DJ, Cooper BA, et al: Desmopressin acetate in uncomplicated coronary artery bypass surgery: A prospective randomized clinical trial. Can J Surg 33:33-36, 1990.
31. Hirayama T, Roberts DG, Allers M, et al: Association between bleeding and reduced red cell deformability following cardiopulmonary bypass. Scand J Thorac Cardiovasc Surg 22:171-174, 1988.
32. Hoffman WS, Tomasello DN, MacVaugh H: Control of postcardiotomy bleeding with PEEP. Ann Thorac Surg 34:71-73, 1982.
33. Horrow JC, Hlavacek J, Strong MD, et al: Prophylactic tranexamic acid decreases bleeding after cardiac operations. J Thorac Cardiovasc Surg 99:70-74, 1990.
34. Hoylaerts M, Lijnen HR, Collen D: Studies on the mechanism of the antifibrinolytic action of tranexamic acid. Biochim Biophys Acta 673:75-85, 1981.
35. Hutter JA, Aps C, Hemsi D, Williams BT: The management of cardiac surgical patients in a general surgical recovery ward. J Cardiovasc Surg 30:273-276, 1989.
36. Ilabaca PA, Ochsner JL, Mills NL: Positive end-expiratory pressure in the management of the patient with a postoperative bleeding heart. Ann Thorac Surg 30:281-284, 1980.
37. Kalter RD, Saul CM, Wetstein L, et al: Cardiopulmonary bypass: Associated hemostatic abnormalities. J Thorac Cardiovasc Surg 77:427-435, 1979.
38. Kay P, Ahmad A, Floten S, Starr A: Emergency coronary artery bypass surgery after intracoronary thrombolysis for evolving myocardial infarction. Br Heart J 53:260-264, 1985.
39. Kelly JP, Thomas L, Moulder PV, Webb WR: Coronary bypass surgery in patients with circulating lupus anticoagulant. Ann Thorac Surg 40:261-263, 1985.
40. Kereiakes DJ, Topol EJ, George BS, et al: Emergency coronary artery bypass surgery preserves global and regional left ventricular function after intravenous tissue plasminogen activator therapy for acute myocardial infarction. J Am Coll Cardiol 11:899-907, 1988.
41. Killian DM, Scanlon PJ: Coronary thrombolysis and percutaneous transluminal coronary angioplasty in acute myocardial infarction. Card Surg: State Art Rev 6:113-132, 1992.
42. Kirklin JK, Westaby S, Blackstone EH, et al: Complement and the damaging effects of cardiopulmonary bypass. J Thorac Cardiovasc Surg 86:845-857, 1983.
43. Kitchen L, Erichson RB, Sideropoulos H: Effect of drug-induced platelet dysfunction on surgical bleeding. Am J Surg 143:215-217, 1982.
44. Koshal A, Murphy J, Keon WJ: Pros and cons of urgent exploratory sternotomy after open cardiac surgery. Can J Surg 29:186-189, 1986.
45. Krebber HJ, Mathey D, Kuck KJ, et al: Management of evolving myocardial infarction by intracoronary thrombolysis and subsequent aorta-coronary bypass. J Thorac Cardiovasc Surg 83:186-193, 1982.
46. Lee KF, Mandell J, Rankin JS, et al: Immediate versus delayed coronary grafting after streptokinase treatment: Postoperative blood loss and clinical results. J Thorac Cardiovasc Surg 95:216-222, 1988.
47. Lupinetti FM, Stoney WS, Alford WC Jr, et al: Cryoprecipitate-topical thrombin glue: Initial experience in patients undergoing cardiac operations. J Thorac Cardiovasc Surg 90:502-505, 1985.
48. Lytle BW, Cosgrove DM, Loop FD, et al: Perioperative risk of bilateral internal mammary artery grafting: Analysis of 500 cases from 1971 to 1984. Circulation 74(Suppl III):37-41, 1986.
49. Mammen EF, Koets MH, Washington BC, et al: Hemostasis changes during cardiopulmonary bypass surgery. Semin Thromb Hemost 11:281-292, 1985.
50. Martin JF, Daniel TD, Trowbridge EA: Acute and chronic changes in platelet volume and count after cardiopulmonary bypass induced thrombocytopenia in man. Thromb Haemost 57:55-58, 1987.
51. Mayer ED, Welsch M, Tanzeem A, et al: Reduction of postoperative donor blood requirement by use of the cell separator. Scand J Thorac Cardiovasc 19:165-171, 1985.
52. McKenna R, Bachmann F, Whittaker B, et al: The hemostatic mechanism after open-heart surgery: II. Frequency of abnormal platelet functions during and after extracorporeal circulation. J Thorac Cardiovasc Surg 70:298-308, 1975.

53. Mestres CA, Pomar JL, Acosta M, et al: Delayed sternal closure for life-threatening complications in cardiac operations: An update. Ann Thorac Surg 51:773-776, 1991.
54. Michelson EL, Morganroth J, Torosian M, MacVaugh H III: Relation of preoperative use of aspirin to increased mediastinal blood loss after coronary artery bypass graft surgery. J Thorac Cardiovasc Surg 76:694-697, 1978.
55. Milam JD, Austin SF, Martin RF, et al: Alteration of coagulation and selected clinical chemistry parameters in patients undergoing open heart surgery without transfusions. Am J Clin Pathol 76:155-162, 1981.
56. Mohr R, Golan M, Martinowitz U, et al: Effect of cardiac operation on platelets. J Thorac Cardiovasc Surg 92:434-441, 1986.
57. Moriau M, Masure R, Hurlet A, et al: Haemostasis disorders in open heart surgery with extracorporeal circulation: Importance of the platelet function and the heparin neutralization. Vox Sang 32:41-51, 1977.
58. Muehrcke DD, Szarnicki RJ: Use of pericardium to control bleeding after ascending aortic graft replacement. Ann Thorac Surg 48:706-708, 1989.
59. Peterson KA, Dewanjee MK, Kaye MP: Fate of indium 111-labeled platelets during cardiopulmonary bypass performed with membrane and bubble oxygenators. J Thorac Cardiovasc Surg 84:39-43, 1982.
60. Physician's Current Procedural Terminology 1992. Washington, DC, St. Anthony's Publishing, 1992.
61. Pike OM, Marquiss JE, Weiner RS, Breckenridge RT: A study of platelet counts during cardiopulmonary bypass. Transfusion 12:119-122, 1972.
62. Rich MW, Keller AJ, Schechtman KB, et al: Morbidity and mortality of coronary bypass surgery in patients 75 years of age or older. Ann Thorac Surg 46:638-644, 1988.
63. Rocha E, Llorens R, Paramo JA, et al: Does desmopressin acetate reduce blood loss after surgery in patients on cardiopulmonary bypass? Circulation 77:1319-1323, 1988.
64. Royston D, Bidstrup B: Reduction in postoperative blood loss in patients having open heart reoperations using high dose aprotinin (Trasylol). Anesthesiology 67:A23, 1987.
65. Royston D, Bidstrup BP, Taylor KM, Sapsford RN: Effect of aprotinin on need for blood transfusion after repeat open-heart surgery. Lancet December:1289-1291, 1987.
66. Ruggeri ZM, Mannucci PM, Lombardi R, et al: Multimeric composition of factor VIII/von Willebrand factor following administration of DDAVP: Implications for pathophysiology and therapy of von Willebrand's disease subtypes. Blood 59:1272-1278, 1982.
67. Salzman EW, Weinstein MJ, Weintraub RM, et al: Treatment with desmopressin acetate to reduce blood loss after cardiac surgery: A double-blind randomized trial. N Engl J Med 314:1402-1406, 1986.
68. Seear MD, Wadsworth LD, Rogers PC, et al: The effect of desmopressin acetate (DDAVP) on postoperative blood loss after cardiac operations in children. J Thorac Cardiovasc Surg 98:217-219, 1989.
69. Serry C, Bleck PC, Javid H, et al: Sternal wound complications: Management and results. J Thorac Cardiovasc Surg 80:861-867, 1980.
70. Skinner JR, Phillips SJ, Zeff RH, Kongtahworn C: Immediate coronary bypass following failed streptokinase infusion in evolving myocardial infarction. J Thorac Cardiovasc Surg 87:567-570, 1984.
71. Sterling RP, Walker WE, Weiland AP, et al: Early bypass grafting following intracoronary thrombolysis with streptokinase. J Thorac Cardiovasc Surg 87:487-492, 1984.
72. Teoh KH, Christakis GT, Weisel RD, et al: Blood conservation with membrane oxygenators and dipyridamole. Ann Thorac Surg 44:40-47, 1987.
73. Topol EJ, Nicklas JM, Kander NH, et al: Coronary revascularization after intravenous tissue plasminogen activator for unstable angina pectoris: Results of a randomized, double-blind, placebo-controlled trial. Am J Cardiol 62:368-371, 1988.
74. Umlas J: Fibrinolysis and disseminated intravascular coagulation in open heart surgery. Transfusion 16:460-463, 1976.
75. van Oeveren W, Kazatchkine MD, Descamps-Latscha B, et al: Deleterious effects of cardiopulmonary bypass: A prospective study of bubble versus membrane oxygenation. J Thorac Cardiovasc Surg 89:888-899, 1985.
76. Veltkamp JJ, Kerkhoven P, Loeliger EA: Circulating anticoagulant in disseminated lupus erythematosus: Proposed mode of action. Haemostasis 2:253-259, 1973/1974.
77. Vincente WVA, Lichtenstein SV, El-Dalati H, et al: Posterior wall disruption of the left ventricle after mitral valve replacement: Management of bleeding and cardiac enlargement. Can J Surg 30:249-251, 1987.

78. Walker WE, Smalling RW, Fuentes F, et al: Role of coronary artery bypass surgery after intracoronary streptokinase infusion for myocardial infarction. Am Heart J 107:826-829, 1984.
79. Warrier AI, Lusher JM: DDAVP: A useful alternative to blood components in moderate hemophilia A and von Willebrand disease. J Pediatr 102:228-233, 1983.
80. Wasser MNJM, Houbiers JGA, D'Amaro J, et al: The effect of fresh versus stored blood on post-operative bleeding after coronary bypass surgery: A prospective randomized study. Br J Haematol 72:81-84, 1989.
81. Wellons HA Jr, Schneider JA, Mikell FL, et al: Early operative intervention after thrombolytic therapy for acute myocardial infarction. J Vasc Surg 2:186-191, 1985.
82. Wilson JM, Held JS, Wright CB, et al: Coronary artery bypass surgery following thrombolytic therapy for acute coronary thrombosis. Ann Thorac Surg 37:212-217, 1984.
83. Wolk LA, Wilson RF, Burdick M, et al: Changes in antithrombin, antiplasmin, and plasminogen during and after cardiopulmonary bypass. Am Surg 51:309-313, 1985.
84. Zurick AM, Urzua J, Ghattas M, et al: Failure of positive end-expiratory pressure to decrease postoperative bleeding after cardiac surgery. Ann Thorac Surg 34:608-611, 1982.

Chapter 20

Cardiopulmonary Bypass in Children: Current Strategies in Anticoagulation and Hemostasis

Serafin Y. DeLeon, M.D., Jenny E. Freeman, M.D., Kalavathi P. Shenoy, M.D., and Carlos R. Suarez, M.D.

Anticoagulation and hemostasis differ in children and adults. This chapter presents the differences, along with pre-, intra-, and postoperative factors that influence anticoagulation and hemostasis in children undergoing cardiopulmonary bypass (CPB). The chapter also focuses on use of fresh whole blood versus blood components because of the smaller blood volume in children, in whom blood replacement therapy can have profound effects.

DEVELOPMENT OF THE HEMOSTATIC SYSTEM IN CHILDREN

Hemostasis refers to the maintenance of blood in a fluid state. The main determinant of blood fluidity is the balance between the coagulation and fibrinolytic pathways, the platelets and the vascular cell lining. In the neonate this hemostatic system is immature and remains so until 6 months of age.

Vascular-platelet Subsystem

Vascular contraction in response to injury is present in the fetus as early as 8 weeks of gestational age.[8] Furthermore, the vascular component is normal in full-term infants, along with capillary fragility and bleeding time.[6,23] Megakaryocytes are detected in the liver as early as the sixth gestational week, and platelets have been observed as early as 11 weeks of gestation. Most healthy term and preterm infants have platelet counts within the normal adult range.[27] The small percentage of term and preterm infants with platelet counts $<150 \times 10^9/L$,[1] are generally considered thrombocytopenic. Platelet function—and in particular platelet aggregation—is abnormal in the newborn; however, the underlying defect is not well understood.[58,59]

Humoral Subsystem

Before 10 or 11 weeks of gestation there is no evidence of fetal blood clotting or fibrinolytic activity.[70] Although it is difficult to establish a normal pattern, predictable patterns of hemostatic development have been proposed.[25] However, the newborn's hemostatic system is unique and different from that of the older child and adult.

Coagulation factors do not cross the placental barrier to any significant degree; the development of the hemostatic system is both gestational and postnatal age-dependent. Overall the coagulation factor levels are low at birth but quite variable (Table 1). However, fibrinogen, factor V, factor VIII procoagulant fraction (FVIII:C), and von Willebrand's factor (vWF) are within the normal adult range or higher at the time of birth. Factors XII and XI, prekallikrein (PK), and high-molecular-weight kininogen (HMWK) are low at birth, but postnatally they progressively increase and reach normal adult values by 6 months of age. Levels of factor XIII are also low at birth, but they rapidly increase to normal adult levels by 5 days of age.[5]

Levels of the vitamin K-dependent factors (II, VII, IX, and X) are significantly lower than in adults. Although individually they have different postnatal patterns of maturation, all four factors are in the adult range by 6 months of age.[5]

Levels for the most important and clinically significant inhibitors of coagulation—namely, AT III, protein C, and protein S—are low at birth and in the first week of life. AT III and protein S reach normal adult levels by 6 months of age; protein C levels, however, are still depressed by that age.[5]

Fibrinolytic activity is detectable at about 15 weeks of gestation, and fibrinolytic activity is increased in the newborn.[60] Although the system is activated at the time of birth, it is not fully developed.[4,21,60] Levels of plasminogen increase with advancing gestational age, achieving 50% of normal adult levels at term.

TABLE 1. Levels for Selected Coagulation Factors and Inhibitors in the Full-term Newborn

Test	Levels*
Fibrinogen	Normal
Factor II	Low
Factor V	Normal
Factor VII	Normal
Factor VIII	Normal
von Willebrand's factor	Normal
Factor IX	Low
Factor X	Low
Factor XI	Low
Factor XII	Low
Factor XIII	Low
Prekallikrein	Low
High-molecular-weight kininogen	Low
Antithrombin III	Low
Protein C	Low
Protein S	Low

* Compared with normal adult reference values.

MECHANISM OF NORMAL HEMOSTASIS

Although most hemorrhagic complications associated with surgery are due to traumatic or mechanical causes, occasionally they may be caused or aggravated by hemostatic disorders or deficiencies.

Primary Hemostatic System

The primary function of the platelet is preservation of vascular integrity and maintenance of normal hemostasis. Platelets provide the first line of defense against processes that may lead to blood loss after vascular injury. The process leading to formation of the platelet plug is known as primary hemostasis, which is achieved by platelet adherence to the vascular endothelial wall, followed by aggregation and the release reaction.

In order for platelets to adhere to the injured vessel wall, normal concentration and function of von Willebrand's factor is required. The activated adherent platelet normally releases several biochemical substances, such as thromboxane A_2 (a very potent vasoconstrictive and platelet aggregating agent), calcium, epinephrine, adenosine diphosphate (ADP), and serotonin. These mediators activate circulation platelets so that they bind to the initial platelet monolayer and facilitate further platelet aggregation and formation of the platelet plug.

Certain diseases and medications may interfere with normal platelet function. Von Willebrand's factor (vWF), a plasma protein composed of large multimers, supports platelet adhesion to the endothelial cell. Both quantitative and qualitative vWF protein abnormalities have been described. Quantitative deficiency of vWF (type I von Willebrand's disease) as well as deficiency of GPIb, the platelet membrane receptor site for vWF (Bernard-Soulier Syndrome), leads to impaired platelet adhesion to the endothelial wall and therefore a significant bleeding disorder. Qualitative abnormalities of vWF can also lead to significant hemorrhagic disorders. Changes affecting the pattern of vWF multimeric composition result in defective platelet adhesion and a clinically significant bleeding disorder (type II von Willebrand's disease).

Secondary Hemostatic System

The proteolytic enzymes that regulate the coagulation pathway exist in blood in their nonactive or zymogen form. As a defense to arrest bleeding or in response to a pathologic trigger, these zymogens are converted to their enzymatically active forms, usually through cleavage of a molecular fragment and therefore exposure of their active sites. A complex series of reactions, set into motion after endothelial damage, ultimately result in the generation of thrombin. Thrombin in turn catalyzes the generation of fibrin and further activates platelets. This process is also termed the secondary hemostatic system. Classically this system has been described as consisting of two different pathways, the intrinsic and extrinsic cascades (Fig. 1).

Disruption of the endothelial cell surface results in exposure of physiologic negatively charged surfaces, binding of factor XII to these surfaces, and consequently autoactivation of factor XII.[62,63] Factor XIIa and other smaller fragments of activated factor XII in turn activate factor XI, PK, HMWK, and plasminogen. Cleaved HMWK and kallikrein reciprocally activate factor XII,

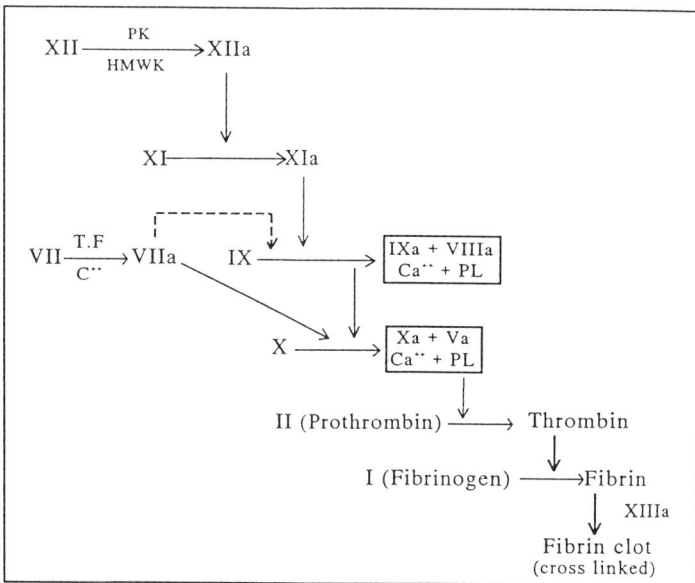

FIGURE 1. The coagulation pathway. The intrinsic pathway is initiated by exposure of plasma to a glasslike substance. Factor XII is then activated, and the intrinsic pathway is consequently activated. The extrinsic pathway activation is initiated when factor VII reads with tissue factor (TF), forming a complex that is capable of activating factors IX and X.

generating additional factor XIIa. Factor XIIa is then able to convert factor XI to factor XIa, which in turn interacts with factor IX and converts it to factor IXa. In the presence of activated factor VIII (FVIIIa) calcium and a phospholipid vesicle factor IXa convert factor X to its serine protease factor Xa.[33] Once factor Xa has been generated, this enzyme converts prothrombin to its serine protease thrombin. In vivo this process is catalyzed by a cofactor, factor Va, calcium, and a cell surface (namely, a phospholipid vesicle). The generation of thrombin leads to a stepwise degradation of fibrinogen and eventually to fibrin deposition.[56] The crosslinking of these fibrin polymers is then catalyzed by factor XIIIa. This crosslinking leads to formation of a more stable and mechanically stronger fibrin clot that is able to withstand the mechanical stress of the circulatory process.

Activation of the extrinsic pathway is initiated by the exposure of circulation plasma proteins to a membrane glycoprotein called tissue factor (TF). TF forms a stable complex with a plasma protein termed factor VII. The TF-factor VII complex is capable of activating factors X and IX and therefore merges with the intrinsic pathway.[51]

Fibrinolysis

Fibrinolysis is responsible for dissolution of the hemostatic clot. The fibrinolytic mechanism is activated at the start of the hemostatic process; as mentioned above, factor XIIa can activate plasminogen, thus initiating the transformation of plasminogen to plasmin. This process is part of the intrinsic plasminogen activation pathway, a process that involves biochemical substances normally present in plasma. The second plasminogen activator pathway is the extrinsic pathway, which depends on two major types of serine proteases—the tissue and urokinase types of plasminogen activator—as well as a second major group of plasminogen activators located within a variety of organs, such as the heart and lungs.

Plasmin is a proteolytic (trypsin-like) enzyme with broad specificity.[53] In addition to fibrin, other proteins—such as fibrinogen, factor V, factor VII, and components of the complement system—are susceptible to its proteolytic action. Plasmin leads to sequential fibrinogen-fibrin proteolysis and release of smaller fragments known as fibrin degradation products (FDPs).

PREOPERATIVE FACTORS

Cyanotic Congenital Heart Disease

Bleeding disorders and abnormalities in coagulation have been reported in patients with cyanotic congenital heart disease (CCHD). Hemostatic disorders, which most commonly are associated with thrombocytopenia and platelet dysfunction, appear related to the degree of hypoxemia and polycythemia.[22,29,31,38,42,46,67]

Other abnormal hemostasis parameters—such as prolonged prothrombin time (PT), partial thromboplastin time (PTT), and bleeding time (BT)—have also been reported in patients with CCHD. However, direct correlation between these abnormal tests and cyanosis cannot be made. Disseminated intravascular coagulation and increased fibrinolysis have been implicated but not proved.[45,49,67]

More recently, the use of molecular markers of hemostasis has more clearly defined the abnormalities of coagulation in cyanotic heart disease.[61] Using these molecular markers, we have found definite evidence of activation of the hemostatic system in children with CCHD as reflected by elevated levels of fibrinopeptide (FPA), which is one of the earliest products of fibrinogen degradation. This activation would not have been detected by routine screening tests such as PT, PTT, and factor levels. We also found marked activity of the platelet system in CCHD, as reflected by elevated levels of thromboxane B2 (TXB2), beta-thromboglobulin (βTG), and platelet factor (PF4). In addition to producing thrombocytopenia, this platelet activation could produce the qualitative platelet dysfunction previously reported in CCHD.

Currently, because patients with CCHD undergo early surgical intervention, extreme hypoxemia, cyanosis, and polycythemia are rarely seen. In the past, however, it was not uncommon to see patients with CCHD presenting with severe polycythemia and thrombocytopenia. In such patients preoperative plasmapheresis is indicated to reduce the hemoglobin level, to increase the platelet count, and to improve platelet aggregation, all of which decrease postoperative bleeding.[34] In our experience patients with CCHD (oxygen saturation of $\leq$80%) bled significantly more than patients with acyanotic heart disease (ACHD) in the first 48 hours postoperatively (649 $\pm$ 538 ml/m^2 vs. 274 $\pm$ 188 ml/m^2; p $<$.01). On reoperation, patients with CCHD bled 555 $\pm$ 531 ml/m^2 vs. 294 $\pm$ 203 ml/m^2, p $<$.05 for patients with ACHD.[17]

Acyanotic Congenital Heart Disease

Children with certain ACHDs have also been reported to have acquired hemostatic abnormalities. We and others have identified children with ventricular septal defect, atrial septal defect, and aortic stenosis who demonstrate qualitative abnormalities of vWF.[24] In particular, they have shown loss of the largest vWF multimers. The mechanism(s) responsible for the loss of these multimers in patients with congenital cardiac lesions is still unclear; however, theories include activation of platelet and/or endothelial cells from turbulent flows, which results in absorption of large multimers. In spite of this abnormality, patients have been able to undergo surgical correction of cardiac defects without excessive intra- or postoperative bleeding. In our experience, infusions of both cryoprecipitate and vasopressin (DDAVP) failed to correct the preexisting prolongation of the BT. Thus, acquired abnormalities of vWF can be present in some patients with ACHD.

In neonates with congenital heart disease who have been quite ill, abnormalities in the coagulation system may be related to hepatic dysfunction.[37] Kontras and colleagues[39] also found that 51% (65/111) of older children with ACHD showed laboratory evidence of a preexisting hemorrhagic diathesis, such as thrombocytopenia, prolonged BT, clot retraction, and capillary fragility. Hepatic dysfunction from heart failure has also been partially blamed for the hemorrhagic diathesis.

Preoperative Drugs

Unlike adults, children do not normally receive antiplatelet drug (acetylsalicylic acid) and Coumadin. In children we try to preserve the native cardiac valves to minimize long-term anticoagulation and reoperations.[15,17] We have been successful with preservation procedures involving the mitral, tricuspid, and pulmonary valves. For the aortic valve, new techniques are under development. In the event that valve replacement is necessary, biologic valves such as cryopreserved homograft and porcine valves are preferred to avoid the use of anticoagulants such as Coumadin, which are difficult to control in children.

In children with systemic pulmonary artery shunts and Fontan operations, we use antiplatelet drugs to minimize thrombosis of the shunt and formation of atrial thrombus due to sluggish blood flow in the Fontan patients.[13,19] The surgical considerations in children receiving antiplatelet drugs and anticoagulants are the same as in adults. Other medications with antiplatelet effects are listed in Table 2.

INTRAOPERATIVE TECHNIQUES

Prime and Hemodilution

Because of the small blood volume in infants and small children, the extracorporeal circuit for pediatric perfusion should use components that minimize surface area and hemodilution, yet provide adequate oxygenation and efficient heat exchange. The extent of hemodilution can significantly

TABLE 2. Medications with Antiplatelet Effects*

Drugs Inhibiting Platelet Function	Psychoactive drugs	Papaverine
Antiinflammatory drugs	Amitryptyline	Propranolol
Aspirin	Chlorpromazine	Sodium nitroprusside
Ibuprofen	Diazepam	Verapamil
Indomethacin	Doxepin	
Mefenamic acid	Imipramine	**Drugs Causing Thrombocytopenia**
Naproxen	Trifluoperazine	Antibiotics
Phenylbutazone	Anesthetic drugs	Cephalothin
Sulfinpyrazone	Halothane	Gentamicin
Antibiotics	Miscellaneous drugs	Sulfonamides
Carbenicillin	Alcohol	Diuretics
Nafcillin	Caffeine	Acetazolamide
Penicillin G	Diphenhydramine	Chlorothiazide
Ticarcillin	Cardiovascular drugs	Ethacrynic acid
Respiratory drugs	Adenosine	Furosemide
Aminophylline	Diltiazem	Cardiovascular drugs
Isoproterenol	Dipyridamole	Heparin
Theophylline	Hydralazine	Protamine
	Nitroglycerin	Quinidine

* This list is representative and not all-inclusive. From Campbell FW, Jobes DR, Ellison N: Coagulation management during and after cardiopulmonary bypass. In Hensley FA, Martin DE (eds): The Practice of Cardiac Anesthesia. Boston, Little, Brown, 1990, with permission.

affect the hematocrit and hemoglobin as well as coagulation factors and plasma oncotic pressure.

We prefer the membrane oxygenator (Cobe Cardiovascular Inc., Arvada, CO), which requires small priming volume. The smallest extracorporeal circuit requires 700 cc priming solution. The prime volume of the pediatric perfusion circuit generally varies from 700-1000 cc, depending on the size of the oxygenator and tubing. Balanced electrolyte solution is used, and depending on the weight of the patient, estimated blood volume, and hematocrit, blood is added to the prime to maintain a hematocrit of 18-22% during CPB. Generally, children whose weight is ≥10 kg have estimated blood volume of 700-800 cc (70-80 cc/kg). These children can have pure crystalloid prime, with an acceptable 50% dilution of the hematocrit and other blood components.

The safe limit of hemodilution in CPB is not clearly established.[52,57] Kawamura and colleagues[36] reported that in CCHD and ACHD hemodilution should be limited to 40% and 50%, respectively, because with high hemodilution, adequate oxygen transfer and stable hemodynamic conditions could not be maintained. In their study, however, mild hypothermia (33-35°C) was used. Milam and colleagues[46] reported that hemodilution up to 59% was well tolerated in cyanotic patients. The patients, however, were cooled to deep hypothermic temperatures (18-28°C). In spite of significant platelet reduction, postoperative reduction in values for fibrinogen, factors II, V, VIII, IX, and X, and slight prolongation of PT and PTT, no significant bleeding occurred compared with less hemodilution. At the other extreme Kawaguchi and colleagues[35] reported successful, totally bloodless open-heart surgery in children with hematocrit levels of ≥13%. Hetastarch was added for oncotic pressure, and moderate hypothermia was generally used (20-28°C).

Maintenance of oncotic pressure, which is also important to reduce fluid accumulation in the body, can be accomplished with whole blood, plasma, albumin, and less frequently hetastarch. Haneda and colleagues[26] reported less morbidity when the colloid osmotic pressure is maintained at 19 mmHg and total proteins at 5 g/100 cc.

Heparinization, Monitoring and Neutralization

Heparinization of children undergoing CPB has to take into consideration that children need larger heparin dose because of their higher rate of metabolism, which results in shorter heparin half-life.[29] Deep hypothermia that delays heparin decay is frequently used in surgery for complex congenital heart disease in children.[14,37]

In our current practice a baseline activated clotting time (ACT) is taken before instituting CPB with the Hemocron ACT timer (International Technidyne Corp., Edison, NJ). After heparin is administered at 3 mg/kg, another ACT is taken. We accept an ACT of ≥450 seconds. Thereafter, the ACT is checked every 30–45 minutes. Generally the ACT remains above the acceptable level and no further heparin dose is needed. One thousand units of heparin per unit of citrate-phosphate-dextrose blood is also added to the prime. After CPB the circulating free heparin is determined with the Hepcon HMS (Hemotec, Inc., Englewood, CO), and protamine is administered based on the heparin level.

The empirical dosing schedule for heparin during extracorporeal circulation should probably be reassessed because of known individual sensitivity to the drug. Akl and colleagues[3] reported ACTs ranging from 210 to >600 seconds in children after administration of 2 mg/kg of heparin. In addition to individual response, the biologic activity is known to vary among different batches of heparin (30–40%).[11]

Sensitivity or resistance to heparin can be tested with either the heparin dose curve/response (in vivo) or the heparin dose/response test (in vitro).[10,20,32,44] With the dose/response curve, the initial heparin is administered in 2–4 divided doses, with the ACT measured after each dose and plotted on linear coordinates. The heparin dose/response test measures clotting time in response to the addition of 1.5 and 2.5 units of heparin per cc of blood.[29]

Children generally require more heparin than adults. Akl and colleagues[3] reported that whereas most adults require a heparin dose equal to or lower than the conventional calculated dose to maintain the same ACT, most children (75%) require >110% of the conventional dose. Horkay and colleagues[29] reported that in vitro dose/response to heparin ranges from 2.2–4.9 mg/kg (mean: 3.3) in children compared with 2.1–4.5 mg/kg (mean: 3) in adults. In addition, they reported that the biologic half-life for heparin was shorter in children compared with adults (30 min vs. 60 min). Heparin requirement for children is not influenced by the presence of cyanosis, as reported by Babacan and colleagues.[7]

The acceptable and safe limits of ACT during CPB have not been clearly established. Young and colleagues[69] reported that fibrin monomers, indicating activation of the coagulation system, were detected with ACTs <400 seconds. They recommend that the lowest limits of ACT should be around 400–550 seconds. Akl and colleagues[3] recommended 450–550 seconds whereas Bull and colleagues[10] accepted ≥300 seconds. In an experimental study, Cardoso and colleagues[12] reported no difference in coagulation factors after CPB between

CURRENT CONFUSION

Certain well-established as well as other lesser known or newly emerging factors have helped, by their profusion and diversity, to produce what may be currently termed the confusion of reason and meanings as applied to understanding and recommending antithrombotic therapy. For this discussion, the terms warfarin and warfarin therapy are used interchangeably with anticoagulant and anticoagulant therapy, although other similarly acting anticoagulants could be substituted.[32]

Clearly adequate anticoagulation greatly reduces, but does not eliminate, the risk of thromboembolic events in patients with prosthetic heart valves.[4,17] The approximations of risk have been calculated by a number of means, and the estimates vary.[21] In fact, even the terms used to express incidence vary, ranging from events per 100 patient-years to simple percentages and actuarial computations. Such variations add further discongruities in comparing reports from different investigators.[21,63,65]

As a point of reference, the incidence of thromboembolic events in patients with mechanical heart valve replacements, expressed as episodes per 100 patient-years, has been reported to be 1.5-9.3 for ball valves; 0.7-4.6 for standard-disk Bjork-Shiley valves; 0.5-3.0 for the convexoconcave model; and 0.7-3.9 for St. Jude valves. An overall incidence of about 4 events per 100 patient-years has also been reported.[12,16,55] These estimations were derived from compilations of data pertaining to recipients of prosthetic heart valve(s) who received oral anticoagulant therapy.[58]

Even with the more modern, less thrombogenic mechanical valves, the estimated incidence of thromboembolic events is 2-5 per 100 patient-years. The risk is even higher in patients with atrial fibrillation, left atrial thrombus, left atrial enlargement, or prior thromboembolic events. It is probably also enhanced by factors such as hypertension, diabetes mellitus, carotid artery disease, smoking, and age >70 years, but such confounding variables have not been systematically studied. In the face of inadequate anticoagulation, the risk of thromboembolism has been reported to increase from two- to sixfold, whereas with excessive anticoagulation the risk of serious bleeding increases four- to eightfold.[21,57]

Although the risk for thromboembolism is generally acknowledged to be less with bioprosthetic valves than with mechanical valves, other operative factors, such as biases in patient selection (e.g., skewed toward inclusion of older patients with more advanced cardiac disease and associated effects such as atrial fibrillation) may act to vitiate direct comparisons.[58] Incidence of thromboemboli in recipients of bioprosthetic valves has been purported to be nearly nil, especially for patients with prosthetic tissue valves in the aortic position and without other overt risk factors (such as atrial fibrillation). Nevertheless, such complications have been reported at a rate as high as 2.9 per 100 patient-years in much the same patient cohort (i.e., recipients of bioprosthetic valves in the aortic position who were in sinus rhythm and received antithrombotic treatment for only the first 6-8 weeks after operation).[58] In recipients of tissue valves in the mitral position, who were in sinus rhythm and were treated with warfarin for only 8 weeks after operation, the rate of thromboembolic events was 1.9 per 100 patient-years.[58]

Major hemorrhagic complications during long-term therapy with oral anticoagulants after heart valve replacement have been reported (as absolute

Chapter 21

Antithrombotic Therapy in Patients with Substitute Heart Valves

*Sheldon M. Kahn, M.D., FACP,
and Rolf M. Gunnar, M.D., FACP, FRCP(E)*

Thrombus formation and arterial embolization remain the major complications following successful replacement of damaged heart valves and contribute adversely to both short- and long-term morbidity and mortality.[4,21,59] This holds true despite striking improvements in materials, structural and hemodynamic redesign of mechanical valves, and selective use of tissue (bioprosthetic) valves—advances that have significantly reduced thrombogenicity and consequently thromboembolic events.[4,21,57,63] Nonetheless, the devastating consequences of thromboembolism occur with sufficient frequency to warrant preventive measures, including antithrombotic therapy. Most often this is a life-long commitment, particularly for patients with mechanical heart valve replacements.[42,49,58,59] Such therapy, which has proved to be effective and increasingly safe, for the most part has depended on the use of an oral anticoagulant of the coumarin type, with or without the addition of one or more antiplatelet agents, primarily aspirin and dipyridamole.

Warfarin sodium, named after the Wisconsin Alumni Research Foundation, is the most widely used anticoagulant. Introduced into clinical usage over 50 years ago for treatment of various actual or predisposing thromboembolic conditions, it currently enjoys an upsurge in popularity.[28,32,64] The highly effective antithrombotic action of warfarin is mediated by the in-vivo reduction of the vitamin K-dependent clotting factors. However, when the anticoagulant intensity is excessive (i.e., International Normalized Ratio [INR] >5.0[42] or even >3.0), the risk of serious bleeding climbs steeply and alarmingly, at times from as small a dosage difference as 1 mg/day.[19,29,32,64] In the aggregate, this translates into an average dose of 4-5 mg/day for the therapeutic range deemed safer (less bleeding), yet still effective in reducing the risk for thromboembolism, as compared with the previous average dose of 5-6 mg/day.[29]

45. Maurer HM, McCue CM, Caul J, Still WJS: Impairment in platelet aggregation in congenital heart disease. Blood 40:207-216, 1972.
46. Milam JD, Austin SF, Nihill MR, et al: Use of sufficient hemodilution to prevent coagulopathies following surgical correction of cyanotic heart disease. J Thorac Cardiovasc Surg 89:623-629, 1985.
47. Morrell DF, Jaros GG, Thornington R: Calcium supplementation during cardiopulmonary bypass in paediatric surgery. S Afr Med J 66:367-368, 1984.
48. Naik SK, Knight A, Elliott M: A prospective randomized study of a modified technique of ultrafiltration during pediatric open-heart surgery. Circulation 84:III-422-III-431, 1991.
49. Naiman JL: Clotting and bleeding in cyanotic congenital heart disease. J Pediatr 76:333-335, 1970.
50. Neill CA: Postoperative hemolytic anemia in endocardial cushion defects. Circulation 30:801, 1964.
51. Nemerson Y: Tissue factor and hemostasis. Blood 71:1-8, 1988.
52. Ott DA, Cooley DA: Cardiovascular surgery in Jehovah's Witnesses. JAMA 238:1256-1258, 1977.
53. Robbins KC, Summaria L, Hsieh B, et al: The peptide chains of human plasmin: Mechanism of activation of human plasminogen. J Biol Chem 242:2333-2342, 1967.
54. Sayd HM, Dacie JV, Handley, et al: Hemolytic anemia of mechanical origin after open heart surgery. Thorax 16:356, 1961.
55.. Signori EE, Penner JA, Kahn DR: Coagulation defects and bleeding in open-heart surgery. Ann Thorac Surg 8:521-529, 1969.
56. Silver D, Hoch JR: Hemostasis in surgery. Resid Staff Phys 37:17-24, 1991.
57. Stein JI, Gombotz H, Rigler B, et al: Open heart surgery in children of Jehovah's Witnesses: Extreme hemodilution on cardiopulmonary bypass. Pediatr Cardiol 12:170-174, 1991.
58. Suarez CR, Fareed J, Tomich P: Neonatal hemostasis: Current concepts and relevance of molecular markers of hemostasis. In Stockman JA (ed): Developmental and Neonatal Hematology. New York, Raven Press, 1988.
59. Suarez CR, Gonzalez J, Menendez C, et al: Neonatal and maternal platelets: Activation at time of birth. Am J Hematol 29:18-21, 1988.
60. Suarez CR, Walenga J, Mangogna LC, Fareed J: Neonatal and maternal fibrinolysis: Activation at time of birth. Am J Hematol 19:365, 1985.
61. Suarez CR, Menendez CE, Griffin AJ, et al: Cyanotic congenital heart disease in children: Hemostatic disorders and relevance of molecular markers of hemostasis. Semin Thromb Hemost 10:285-289, 1984.
62. Tans G, Rosing J, Griffin JH: Sulfatide dependent autoactivation of human blood coagulation factor XII (Hageman factor). J Biol Chem 258:8215, 1983.
63. Thompson RE, Mandel R, Kaplan AP: Studies of binding of prekallikrein and factor XI to high molecular weight kininogen and its light chain. J Clin Invest 60:1376, 1977.
64. Verdon TA, Forrester RH, Crosby WH: Hemolytic anemia after open heart repair of ostium primum defects. N Engl J Med 269:444, 1963.
65. Waldman JD, Czapek EE, Paul MH, et al: Shortened platelet survival in cyanotic heart disease. J Pediatr 87:77-79, 1975.
66. Ward A, Brogden R, Heel R, et al: Amrinone: A preliminary review of its pharmacological properties and therapeutic use. Drugs 26:468, 1983.
67. Wedemeyer AL, Edson R, Krivit W: Coagulation in cyanotic congenital heart disease. Am J Dis Child 124:656-660, 1972.
68. Westaby S, Turner MW, Stark J: Complement activation and anaphylactoid response to protamine in a child after cardiopulmonary bypass. Br Heart J 53:574-576, 1985.
69. Young JA, Kisker T, Doty DB: Adequate anticoagulation during cardiopulmonary bypass determined by activated clotting time and appearance of fibrin monomer. Ann Thorac Surg 26:231-240, 1978.
70. Zilliacus H, Ottenhin AM, Mattsson T: Blood clotting and fibrinolysis in human fetuses. Biol Neonate 10:108-112, 1966.

16. DeLeon SY, Ilbawi MN, Tubeszewski K, et al: Resternotomy in patients with valved conduits adherent to the sternum. Ann Thorac Surg 52:569-571, 1991.
17. DeLeon SY, Ilbawi MN, Wilson WR, et al: Surgical options in subaortic stenosis associated with endocardial cushion defects. Ann Thorac Surg 52:1076-1083, 1991.
18. DeLeon SY, LoCicero J, Ilbawi MN, Idriss FS: Repeat median sternotomy in pediatrics: Experience in 164 consecutive cases. Ann Thorac Surg 41:184-188, 1986.
19. DeLeon SY, Freeman JE, Ow EP, et al: Obligatory Glenn shunt in fenestrated Fontan. Ann Thorac Surg, in press.
20. Doty DB, Knott HW, Hoyt JL, Koepke JA: Heparin dose for accurate anticoagulation in cardiac surgery. J Cardiovasc Surg 20:597-604, 1979.
21. Ekelund H, Funnsstrom O: Fibrinolysis in pre-term infants small for gestational age. Acta Paediatr Scand 61:185-196, 1972.
22. Ekert H, Gilchrist GS, Stanton R, Hammond D: Hemostasis in cyanotic congenital heart disease. J Pediatr 76:221-230, 1970.
23. Feusner JH: Normal and abnormal bleeding times in neonates and young children utilizing a full standardized template technic. Am J Clin Pathol 74:73, 1980.
24. Gill JC, Wilson AD, Endres-Brooks J, Montgomery RR: Loss of the largest von Willebrand factor multimers from the plasma of patients with congenital cardiac defects. Blood 67:758-781, 1986.
25. Gross SJ, Stuart MJ: Hemostases in the premature infant. Clin Perinatalol 4:259-304, 1977.
26. Haneda K, Sato S, Ishizawa E, Horiuchi T: The importance of colloid osmotic pressure during open heart surgery in infants. Tohoku J Exp Med 147:65-71, 1985.
27. Hathaway WE: The bleeding newborn. Semin Hematol 12:175-188, 1975.
28. Henriksson P, Varendh G, Lundstrom NR: Haemostatic defects in cyanotic congenital heart disease. Br Heart J 41:23-27, 1979.
29. Horkay F, Martin P, Rajah SM, Walker DR: Response to heparinization in adults and children undergoing cardiac operations. Ann Thorac Surg 53:822-826, 1992.
30. Ilbawi MN, Quinn K, Idriss FS, et al: The surgical management of left ventricular outflow tract obstruction due to tricuspid valve pouch in complete transposition of the great arteries. J Thorac Cardiovasc Surg 87:66-73, 1984.
31. Iolster NJ: Blood coagulation in children with cyanotic congenital heart disease. Acta Paediatr Scand 59:551-557, 1970.
32. Jumean HG, Sudah F: Monitoring of anticoagulant therapy during open-heart surgery in children with congenital heart disease. Acta Haematol 70:392-395, 1983.
33. Kane WH, Davie EW: Blood coagulations factor V and VIII: Structural and functional similarities and their relationship to hemorrhagic and thrombotic disorders. Blood 71:539-555, 1988.
34. von Kaulla KN, Paton BC, Rosenkrantz JG, et al: Preoperative correction of coagulation in tetralogy of fallot. Arch Surg 94:107-111, 1967.
35. Kawaguchi A, Bergsland J, Subramanian S: Total bloodless open heart surgery in the pediatric age group. Circulation 70:I-30-I-37, 1984.
36. Kawamura M, Minamikawa O, Yokochi H, et al: Safe limit of hemodilution in cardiopulmonary bypass—comparative analysis between cyanotic and acyanotic congenital heart disease. Jpn J Surg 10:206-211, 1980.
37. Kern FH, Morana NJ, Sears JJ, Hickey PR: Coagulation defects in neonates during cardiopulmonary bypass. Ann Thorac Surg 54:541-546, 1992.
38. Komp DM, Sparrow AW: Polycythemia in cyanotic heart disease—a study of altered coagulation. J Pediatr 76:231-236, 1970.
39. Kontras SB, Sirak HD, Newton WA Jr: Hematologic abnormalities in children with congenital heart disease. JAMA 195:99-103, 1966.
40. Lavee J, Martinowitz U, Mohr R, et al: The effect of transfusion of fresh whole blood versus platelet concentrates after cardiac operations. J Thorac Cardiovasc Surg 97:204-212, 1989.
41. Lawless S, Burckart G, Diven W, et al: Amrinone in neonates and infants after cardiac surgery. Crit Care Med 17:751-754, 1989.
42. Lopes AAB, Maeda NY, Ebaid M, Chamone DAF: Aggregation of platelets in whole blood from children with pulmonary hypertension. Int J Cardiol 28:173-178, 1990.
43. Manno CS, Hedberg KW, Kim HC, et al: Comparison of the hemostatic effects of fresh whole blood, stored whole blood, and components after open heart surgery in children. Blood 77:930-936, 1991.
44. Martin P, Horkay F, Rajah SM, Walker DR: Monitoring of coagulation status using thrombelastography during paediatric open heart surgery. Int J Clin Monit Comput 8:183-187, 1991.

CONCLUSION

Anticoagulation and hemostasis in children undergoing CPB have different perioperative considerations compared with adults. The coagulation system in children, which is not fully developed until 6 months of age, can be affected by cyanosis, turbulent flows in certain congenital heart diseases, and severe illness that may affect liver function.

The prime volume, which is proportionally larger in children than in adults, causes greater hemodilution and significant changes in the coagulation factors. Such changes are more pronounced in neonates. Children also require more heparin because the biologic half-life during bypass is shorter. Use of the heparin dose/response curve and/or circulating free heparin levels after CPB has led to more accurate doses of protamine compared with conventional protocols.

The use of the hemofilter and cell-saver systems has led to minimal blood usage. Warm fresh whole blood offers better platelet function, but because of logistic problems with procurement and completion of necessary screening tests, blood-component therapy with platelets, cryoprecipitate, and fresh frozen plasma may offer a viable and practical alternative.

REFERENCES

1. Aballi AJ, Puapondh Y, Desposito F: Platelet counts in thriving premature infants. Pediatrics 42:685-689, 1968.
2. Abbott TR: Changes in serum calcium fractions and citrate concentrations during massive blood transfusions and cardiopulmonary bypass. Br J Anaesth 55:753-760, 1983.
3. Akl BF, Vargas GM, Neal J, et al: Clinical experience with the activated clotting time for the control of heparin and protamine therapy during cardiopulmonary bypass. J Thorac Cardiovasc Surg 79:97-102, 1980.
4. Ambrus CM, Ambrus JL, Choi TS, et al: The fibrinolytic system and its relationship to disease in the newborn. Am J Pediatr Hematol/Oncol 1:251, 1979.
5. Andrew M, Paes B, Miner R, et al: Development of the human coagulation system in the full term infant. Blood 70:165-172, 1987.
6. Andrew M, Castle V, Saigal S, et al: Clinical impact of neonatal thrombocytopenia. J Pediatr 110:457-464, 1987.
7. Babacan MK, Tasdemir O, Yakut C, et al: Heparin need of the patients with cyanotic congenital heart disease during cardiopulmonary bypass. J Cardiovasc Surg 30:348-350, 1989.
8. Bleyer WA, Hakami N, Shepard T: The development of hemostasis in the human fetus and newborn infant. J Pediatr 79:838-853, 1971.
9. Breyer RH, Engelman RM, Rousou JA, Lemeshow SA: A comparison of cell saver versus ultrafilter during coronary artery bypass operations. J Thorac Cardiovasc Surg 90:736-740, 1985.
10. Bull BS, Korpman RA, Huse WM, Briggs BD: Heparin therapy during extracorporeal circulation. J Thorac Cardiovasc Surg 69:674-684, 1975.
11. Campbell FW, Jobes DR, Ellison N: Coagulation management during and after cardiopulmonary bypass. In Hensley FA, Martin DE (eds): The Practice of Cardiac Anesthesia. Boston, Little, Brown, 1990, pp 546, 579.
12. Cardoso PFG, Yamazaki F, Keshavjee S, et al: A reevaluation of heparin requirements for cardiopulmonary bypass. J Thorac Cardiovasc Surg 101:153-160, 1991.
13. Cromme-Dijkhuis AH, Henken CMA, Bijleveld CMA, et al: Coagulation factor abnormalities as possible thrombotic risk factors after Fontan operations. Lancet 336:1087-1090, 1990.
14. DeLeon SY, Ilbawi M, Arcilla R, et al: Choreoathetosis after deep hypothermia without circulatory arrest. Ann Thorac Surg 50:714-719, 1990.
15. DeLeon SY, Ilbawi MN, Roberson DA, et al: Conal enlargement for diffuse subaortic stenosis. J Thorac Cardiovasc Surg 102:814-820, 1991.

procedures. Other postoperative coagulation studies, however, could not explain the increased loss in patients receiving reconstituted blood; it was suggested that improvement in platelet functions may eliminate the difference. With attention to technical details[16,18,37,43] and compensation with more platelet transfusion, blood-component therapy may produce surgical results comparable with those of fresh whole blood. One of our last 100 patients needed exploration for postoperative bleeding after blood-component therapy.

In neonates, hemodilution has produced profound reduction in platelets and coagulation factors. In 30 neonates undergoing deep hypothermic CPB, Kern and colleagues[37] reported 70% reduction in platelet count and 50% reduction in coagulation factors (fibrinogen, factor II, VII, IX, and X) during CPB. They found that neither deep hypothermia nor prolonged exposure to extracorporeal surfaces has further effect on the coagulation factors. After weaning from CPB, they used fresh whole blood ($\leq$48 hours old); after administration of protamine, blood-component therapy was used. No exploration for bleeding was needed in any of the patients. Based on these data, they feel that platelet concentration and cryoprecipitate may be effective alternatives to fresh whole blood.

With transfusion of either whole blood or components, it is important to provide adequate calcium supplementation.[2,47] Calcium is depleted by use of citrate-phosphate-dextrose blood and by binding to albumin and other plasma proteins. Calcium is vitally important not only for adequate cardiac function but also for the binding of the various factors in the clotting cascade and for platelet adhesion and function. Our policy is to administer 100 mg of calcium gluconate for each 50 cc of blood, blood product, or albumin.

Postoperative Considerations

The postoperative period in regard to anticoagulation and hemostasis after CPB in children can be divided into early (first 24 hours) and late (after 24 hours).

Early Postoperative Period. Problems in the first 24 hours postoperatively are extensions of intraoperative events. Postoperative bleeding can occur or continue because of inadequate neutralization of heparin, incomplete correction of coagulation factor deficits, or technical problems associated with surgery. Heparin rebound can also occur 2–3 hours after CPB in children.[37,55] Management requires administration of protamine and either fresh whole blood or blood components, such as platelets, cryoprecipitate, and fresh frozen plasma.

Late Postoperative Period. After the first 24 hours postoperatively, the problems are different. Drugs such as nitroprusside and amrinone,[41,66] which are frequently used in children, especially in those with reactive pulmonary vascular bed, can cause thrombocytopenia. Patients receiving such drugs should have daily platelet counts. In the presence of thrombocytopenia, an alternative drug such as nitroglycerin can be used. We do not transfuse platelets unless the count is <50,000/cc. Residual defects after open-heart surgery are not uncommon in children. Residual left ventricular outflow tract obstruction, mitral insufficiency after canal repair, and use of cardiac prostheses such as valve conduits or homografts can cause platelet activation and hemolysis.[30,50,54,64] Such problems with coagulation, however, are usually self-limiting.

ACTs ≥250 seconds and ≥450 seconds. Experience with extracorporeal membrane oxygenator support has shown that ACT ≥200 seconds is safe.

Protamine can be administered in several ways to neutralize heparin after CPB. The conventional method has been to give 1.2-1.5 mg of protamine for every mg/heparin. This empirical method clearly gives more protamine than necessary, because the half-life of heparin and the effects of hypothermia and hemodilution are not taken into consideration. A more accurate method of giving protamine is to use the heparin dose/response curve. From the graph of ACT in response to heparin doses, the remaining heparin at the end of CPB can be calculated.[10] More recently, the circulating free heparin has been determined with the Hepcon; protamine is then given accordingly.[29]

Because of known reactions to protamine, we combine calcium chloride (10-20 mg/kg) with the protamine infusion, which is given slowly.[68]

Hemofilter and Cell-saver Systems

Before terminating CPB, we use the hemofilter (Cobe Cardiovascular, Inc., Arvada, CO) to remove plasma, water, and dissolved solutes from the blood, thus increasing the hematocrit. The volume removed depends on the circulating volume needed to maintain adequate CPB flow just before bypass is terminated. After CPB we process most of the remaining blood and solution in the extracorporeal circuit through the cell-saver and use the blood for transfusion. With the use of hemofilter and cell-saver systems[9,48] infants and young children generally require 1-2 units of blood, unless bleeding is excessive.

Fresh Whole Blood vs. Components in Infants

Infants and small children undergoing CPB are subjected to significant hemodilution with major alterations in the blood's oxygen-carrying capacity, in coagulation factors, and in other blood components. These changes are more pronounced in infants <6 months of age, who have underdeveloped coagulation systems.[37]

Most pediatric cardiac surgeons believe that the use of warm fresh whole blood (≤6 hours old) at the end of CPB minimizes the effect of hemodilution in infants and small children, as well as gives excellent coagulation factors and therefore the best surgical result.[43] Because of logistic problems in procuring a steady supply of warm fresh whole blood that has passed the necessary screening test and because of the ready availability of blood components believed to have hemostatic characteristics similar to fresh blood, blood banks encourage the use of blood components.[37,40,43]

In a study of 161 children undergoing open-heart surgery, Manno and colleagues[43] found that warm fresh whole blood (≤6 hours old) and whole blood that is relatively fresh (≤48 hours old) are quite similar in terms of postoperative bleeding and platelet functions. Relatively fresh whole blood allows completion of all necessary tests before usage. In patients who received reconstituted blood (packed red blood cells, fresh frozen plasma, platelets), the postoperative blood loss was significant, and the PTT and fibrinogen levels were more abnormal compared with patients receiving the other two types of fresh blood. The difference in postoperative loss was more significant in children who are less than 2 years of age and/or undergoing more complex rates) in 2.4% of patients (range: 0-6.8%), with fatal bleeding in 1.7% (range: 0-4.1%).[41,55] Expressed in more directly comparable terms, major bleeding occurred at a rate varying between 0.8-4.1 episodes per 100 patient-years (median: 1.7 bleeds per 100 patient-years). Fatal bleeding occurred at a rate between 0.2-2.3 fatalities per 100 patient-years (median: 0.8 per 100 patient-years). The overall occurrence rates for bleeding varied between 1.8-14.0 events per 100 patient-years (median: 5.7). Thus, estimated average risk ratings for overall, major, and fatal hemorrhagic complications per 100 patient-years, are approximately 6.0, 2.0, and 0.8, respectively.[40]

The generally accepted indices of serious bleeding are any hemorrhagic event necessitating hospitalization, transfusion, reversal of anticoagulant therapy, or surgery to control or correct the bleeding. A thromboembolic event has been defined as a transient or permanent neurologic deficit not explained by a coexisting disease process (e.g., endocarditis) and includes any systemic arterial embolization as well. Clearly interpretive leeway is exercised; not all studies that report incidence rates use similarly precise definitions or criteria by which direct comparisons may be made. Furthermore, patient characteristics may play an important role in determining risk or likelihood of bleeding.[40]

CLARIFYING THE CONFUSION

Herein lies the conundrum: What constitutes adequate anticoagulation? What is excessive? What is the best method to determine, maintain, and monitor these levels of intensity? Fortunately, as more solidly based answers and clarifying information continue to emerge from a previously muddled data pool, conclusions can be drawn and recommendations made. Much of the information is collated and disseminated by authorities in the field of hemostasis and representatives of relevant clinical disciplines, working as consensus panels. The first group met in Leuven in 1984. The second, under the auspices of the British Society for Haematology, also met in 1984, and its recommendations were slightly revised and published in 1990.[8]

The third such panel of experts, appointed as a special working group by the American College of Chest Physicians (ACCP) in conjunction with the National Heart, Lung and Blood Institute (NHLBI), was convened under the cochairmanship of Drs. James E. Dalen and Jack Hirsh. This group, which first met in 1984, set about to reach agreement on criteria for evaluating the burgeoning issues and increasingly large number of publications addressing antithrombotic therapy in cardiovascular disease. Eight task forces were established to examine the use of antithrombotic therapy in the following interrelated categories: cardiovascular disease; valvular heart disease; prosthetic heart valves; coronary artery bypass graft surgery; atrial fibrillation; venous thrombosis and pulmonary embolism; pulmonary vascular disease; and cerebrovascular disease. Recommendations, published in 1986,[3] were based on the consensus reached by each task force and approved after final review and revision by the entire group.

Meticulous and critical reconsideration of increasing data and relevant points of information has been instrumental in updating conclusions and making new or modified graded recommendations (from A, the most strongly supported, to C, the least supported). These recommendations are based upon

TABLE 1. Criteria for Recommendations on the Use of Antithrombotic Agents

Grades of Recommendations	Levels of Evidence
A: Supported by at least 1 (and preferably >1) level I trial.	I. Randomized trials with low alpha (false positive) and low beta (false negative) errors (high power).
B: Supported by at least 1 level II randomized trial.	II. Randomized trials with high alpha and/or beta errors (low power).
C: Supported only by level III, IV, or V evidence.	III. Nonrandomized concurrent cohort comparisons between contemporaneous patients who did not receive antithrombotic agents.
	IV. Nonrandomized historical cohort comparisons between current patients who received antithrombotic agents and former patients (from the same institution or from the literature) who did not.
	V. Case series without controls.

various levels of evidence (from level I, randomized study with low alpha and beta errors, to level V, case-series only, with no controls) (Table 1).[53,54]

The panels, whose membership consisted of cardiologists, pulmonologists, hematologists, neurologists, vascular surgeons, thoracic surgeons, and epidemiologists, meet jointly every three years, with timely publication of the proceedings of each conference as a special supplement in the journal *Chest*. The second such meeting was held in June 1988, with publication in February 1989.[2] The proceedings of the third conference were published in October 1992.[1]

Guided by the results of a number of recently concluded interim and continuing studies, several insightful therapeutic modifications have been advanced.[19,27,29,49,58] One of the more significant changes is the recommended use of lower doses of warfarin in patients with prosthetic heart valves. The therapeutic ranges of anticoagulation recommended in the Second ACCP Conference were limited to 2 levels of intensity: less intense (INR: 2.0-3.0; prothrombin time ratio [PTR]: approximately 1.3-1.5) and more intense (INR: 3.0-4.5; PTR: approximately 1.5-1.8). These levels were clearly defined and the terms used with consistency.[35,59] In the larger sense, the terms "low, lower, or less," "mild, moderate, or intermediate," and "more or high" intensity have little or no intrinsic meaning; they have been used with different and sometimes overlapping connotations, even in supposedly explicit articles. Stated in terms of the commonly used PTR, recommendations remain significantly inconsistent and variable, rendering such usage inherently flawed, often to the extent of contributing to possibly harmful mistakes in the use of oral anticoagulants.[10,24,28,30,31]

Therefore, when any such term is used hereafter, it is uniformly qualified; i.e., anticoagulation intensity is described in specifically fixed terms of the INR, a standard measure of intensity of anticoagulation that is corrected for the sensitivity of the local thromboplastin (TPL) reagent used in determining the prothrombin time (PT). The prothrombin time ratio (PTR) is simply expressed as follows:

$$\frac{\text{PT observed (patient) (seconds)}}{\text{PT control (seconds)}} = \text{prothrombin time ratio (PTR)}$$

Otherwise expressed, the PTR represents the multiplication factor by which a patient's PT exceeds the control value.

The widespread practice of using the PTR alone as the guide for anticoagulant therapy, with no adjustment for the responsiveness of the TPL reagent, has led to errors in reporting the level of intensity of anticoagulation.[10,24,28,30,31] In turn, these discrepancies can lead to errors in the interpretation of study data and serious mistakes in day-to-day clinical practice.[10,24,28-31,42,49] The pressing need to adopt and apply the INR as a standard measure for monitoring warfarin anticoagulation cannot be overemphasized, as Hirsh has cogently explained in editorial comment and correspondence,[29-31,33] expanding upon extensive background information and supporting data.[6,10,24,28,50]

Responsiveness to warfarin anticoagulation varies markedly among various TPL preparations used in performing the one-step PT test. This determination, introduced in 1935 by Quick,[51] remains the basis of testing most often used to monitor anticoagulant therapy. However, because of variability in responsiveness, neither the PT alone (time expressed in seconds) nor the PTR (the commonly used ratio of the observed [patient] PT to control PT) accurately measures the degree of reduction of the vitamin K-dependent procoagulants, which determines the actual intensity of anticoagulation. Levels of anticoagulation intensity can be meaningfully expressed and compared only by taking into account the TPL responsiveness. This issue has been addressed by expanding the PTR to the INR.[28-32,50]

Commercial preparations of rabbit brain TPL used in North America since the 1970s are not only less responsive to warfarin anticoagulation but also vary much more in their responsiveness than previously suspected.[6,10,24] Responsiveness may vary even from batch to batch supplied by a given manufacturer.[10] These discrepancies in TPL responsiveness may distort anticoagulation monitoring and result in uncertainty about outcomes and complication rates. The unannounced change in source and nature of the TPL preparations available in North America involved a switch from a responsive TPL in the 1940s-1960s to relatively less responsive commercial TPL preparations in the 1970s and 1980s. This change resulted in significant overanticoagulation and consequent hemorrhagic complications when using the PTR of 2.0-2.5 (PT 2.0-2.5 times control) originally recommended in 1948 by the American Heart Association.[66] This PTR range corresponds to an INR well over 4.5-5.0, the threshold for greatly enhanced risk of bleeding.[29,42,64]

The INR, which is easily used, can simplify further study and improve anticoagulation therapy. This measure requires that each manufacturer/vendor of the TPL reagents (there are three principal suppliers in North America) provide the verified International Sensitivity Index (ISI), which has been established as a standardized measure of responsiveness, for each batch of TPL reagent supplied. The ISI, designated by convention as superscript C, is a numerical representation of the responsiveness of a given TPL as calibrated against a standard or reference TPL preparation (Fig. 1). Any clinical laboratory assessing PTs simply applies this number, ISI = superscript C, in the following equation:

$$\left[\frac{PT\ (observed)}{PT\ (control)}\right]^C \text{ or PTR raised to the power of } C = (PTR)^C = INR$$

The INR is based on a standard reference TPL preparation developed in 1977 under the auspices of the World Health Organization (WHO). After further refinement, this standardized usage was adopted in 1982 and is

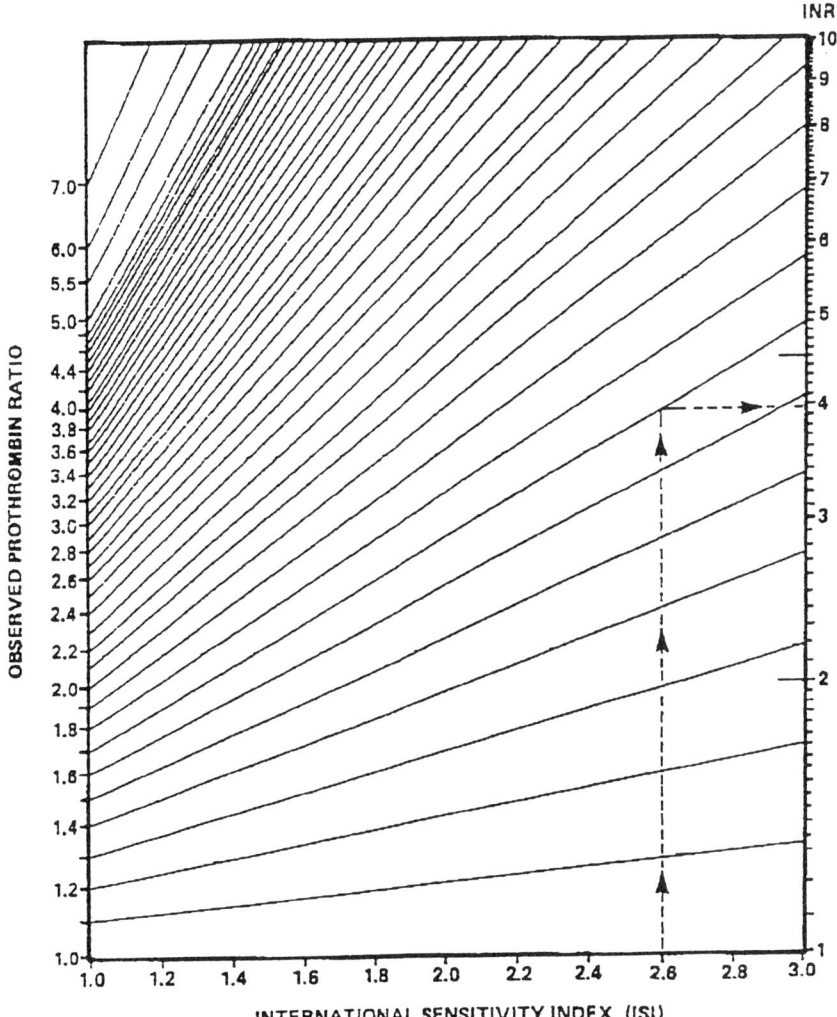

FIGURE 1. Nomogram devised for conversion of PTR to INR (or vice versa) over a range of ISI values from 1.0–3.0.[50] Use of this graph allows quick derivation of the INR from a given PTR, when the ISI value of the TPL reagent is known. Arrows indicate an example in which the observed ratio of 1.7 is measured using thromboplastin with an ISI of 2.6 and an INR of 3.97. (From Poller L: A simple nomogram for the derivation of international normalized ratios for the standardization of prothrombin times. Thromb Haemost 60:18–20, 1988, with permission.)

becoming increasingly accepted, although still falling far short of the pressing goal of universal use. Even with certain imperfections, the INR provides the best standard gauge of the intensity of anticoagulation. Practitioners as well as laboratory supervisors must understand and apply this concept and its operative principals.[6,10,24,29–31,36]

For quite some time the TPL preparations now in use in North America were believed to fall within a relatively narrow range of responsiveness,

TABLE 2. Effect of the International Sensitivity Index on the International Normalized Ratio

	INR		
	PTR: 1.3	PTR: 1.5	PTR: 2.0
ISI 1.4	1.4*	1.8	3.6
ISI 2.8	2.1	3.1	7.0†

* Represents undercoagulation by current recommendations; INR ≤1.8 reflects an increased risk for thromboembolism for mechanical valves.[58]
† This is well into the range of sharply increased risk of bleeding (INR >4.5-5) and indicates overanticoagulation in most instances.

comprising ISIs of 2.2–2.6.[35] Recent studies, however, have shown that the preparations vary in sensitivity over a much wider range (ISI of 1.4–2.8) and in an unpredictable fashion.[6,10,24] A small difference in the ISI, or TPL responsiveness, has a large effect on the resultant INR, which represents the standard and consistent measure of the functional intensity of anticoagulation (Table 2).

Another comparative tabulation shows the variation in PTR, depending on TPL responsiveness, for currently recommended therapeutic target INR ranges (Table 3).

The foundation of these concepts, including the need and method for standardizing anticoagulation testing, is instructive in its basic scientific underpinnings and historically spans almost three decades. Interested readers may find the details elsewhere.[8,28,30-32,35,50]

Although less intense oral anticoagulation regimens were increasingly studied in the past decade and have been gaining favor as recommended therapy for patients prone to thromboembolic events (e.g., patients with deep vein thrombosis, pulmonary embolism, and atrial fibrillation[9,15,22,48,61] as well as those with prosthetic heart valves [see below]), differences of opinion and confusion still exist.[27,36,42,49,58] Although the trend for lower warfarin dosage reflects the prevailing opinion in the western hemisphere and the United Kingdom, a countervailing view labelled the Dutch Policy has been strongly voiced by Loeliger and associates in the Netherlands.[42,45]

ANTICOAGULATION IN PATIENTS WITH PROSTHETIC HEART VALVES

Tissue Valves

In the Second ACCP/NHLBI Conference, the less intense range of warfarin anticoagulation (INR 2.0–3.0, corresponding roughly to PTR of

TABLE 3. Effect of Variations in Prothrombin Time Ratio on the International Normalized Ratio

INR	PTR		
	ISI: 1.8	ISI: 2.3	ISI: 2.8
2.0–3.0	1.5–1.8	1.4–1.6	1.3–1.5
2.5–3.5	1.7–2.0	1.5–1.7	1.4–1.6

1.3-1.5, using a "typical" North American TPL reagent [see above]), was recommended for patients with tissue heart valve replacement.[43] This grade A recommendation (based on one level I study) advised such treatment for the first 3 months after bioprosthetic valve insertion in the mitral position, with warfarin anticoagulation optional for patients in sinus rhythm with a tissue valve in the aortic position. It was further recommended (grade C, based on a single unconfirmed level IV study) that all patients with bioprosthetic valves who are in sinus rhythm "be optionally treated, long-term" with aspirin (325 mg/day). These recommendations remain the same through the Third ACCP Conference in 1992.[27,58] However, the recommendations have been changed for patients with bioprosthetic valves who (1) have a history of prior systemic embolization; (2) have a left atrial thrombus; or (3) are in atrial fibrillation. The earlier statement in 1989[59] advocated that such patients be treated with the more intense regimen of warfarin therapy (INR: 3.0-4.5; PTR: approximately 1.5-2.0) for the first 3 months, after which the intensity may be decreased (INR: 2.0-3.0; PTR: approximately 1.3-1.5). This grade C recommendation was based on a level IV study: duration of long-term therapy as well as the appropriate intensity of warfarin therapy were acknowledged to be "uncertain."[59]

Current recommendations call for patients in these categories to have long-term treatment with warfarin (target INR: 2.0-3.0; PTR: 1.3-1.5). The duration of such therapy is again "uncertain" for patients with evidence of a left atrial thrombus at surgery; 3-12 months for patients with a history of systemic embolism; and *permanently* (authors' emphasis) for those in atrial fibrillation (grade C, level I).[58]

Turpie and associates,[63] in a randomized study of 210 patients with tissue heart valve replacements, found a lower intensity of warfarin therapy (INR: 2.0-2.25; PTR: 1.3-1.4) in 108 patients to be as effective as the higher intensity (INR: 2.5-4.0; PTR: 1.5-1.8) in 102 patients, but with significantly less bleeding: 5.9% (6 patients, none with major bleeding) vs. 13.9% (15 patients, 5 with major bleeding). This study has been widely referenced, but it included only 3 months of postoperative anticoagulant treatment, although warfarin was continued in patients considered at high risk for thromboembolism. In spite of evidence that the first 3 postoperative months are the time span with the highest reported incidence of thromboembolic events, a retrospective study found that thromboembolic events occur in a linear manner.[43] This linearity, which has also been found in patients with nonvalvular atrial fibrillation, is an important factor arguing for long-term, lower-dose anticoagulant therapy in such patients.[29] The study by Turpie and associates has been criticized and its interpretations and determinations challenged[42,45]; but the conclusions have also been strongly defended,[33] and the debate continues.

Mechanical Valves

In 1986 and 1989 the recommendation (grade C, based on level III evidence) of the consensus committees for patients with mechanical prosthetic heart valves was a more intensive range of anticoagulation (INR: 3.0-4.5; PTR: approximately 1.5-2.0) to be maintained life-long.[2,3,59] Dipyridamole (400 mg/day) was recommended as optional therapy with a grade A rating, based on 1 level I and 3 level II studies.[59] The present recommendation (strongly reiterated, despite remaining grade C) is for permanent therapy with warfarin at a target INR of 2.5–3.5 (PTR: approximately 1.5–1.7; levels II and V).[58]

Dipyridamole (400 mg/day) in addition to warfarin, as outlined above, remains an optional recommendation because studies differ in attributing any additional therapeutic benefits (varying from favorable to favorable trend to no benefit).[58] Drawbacks include added cost, compliance, and possible side effects of another drug; however, no persuasive evidence suggests that dipyridamole causes or promotes more bleeding.[13,21] Aspirin (160 mg/day, as extrapolated from a level I study[62]) may offer added protection without undue risk, but larger doses (i.e., 500 mg/day or more) combined with warfarin have been found to increase bleeding and should be avoided.[58]

In the presence of systemic embolization despite warfarin therapy, the addition of dipyridamole (400 mg/day) was recommended in 1989 as standard therapy—again rated grade A, based on the same 4 studies as optional use.[59] An alternative optional recommendation (grade A) for this group of patients is that aspirin (160 mg/day) be added to the warfarin regimen instead of dipyridamole.[19,58] Although this option was extrapolated from the same level I study cited above,[62] the patients in that study group did not have emboli.

The level II study by Altman et al.[4] is credited with providing the basis for the final modification recommended for patients considered to be at high risk for bleeding. Thus, if full-dose warfarin, currently defined as the amount required for an INR target range of 2.5–3.5, is contraindicated, the dose may be lowered to achieve anticoagulation at a target INR of 2.0–3.0, and used in combination with dipyridamole (75 mg twice daily) and aspirin (330 mg twice daily). This recommendation contrasts with that of 1989 (grade C), which called for the addition of dipyridamole (400 mg/day) combined with warfarin to a target INR of 2.0–3.0 for such patients.[59] Whether aspirin (160 mg/day) without dipyridamole, added to warfarin at the targeted INR of 2.0–3.0 or perhaps 2.5–3.5, would be as effective and safe remains speculative.[58] Specifically designed, controlled trials seem appropriate to answer this question; judgment of extrapolative interpretations, such as those derived from the study in question,[62] is best reserved. Ongoing studies, such as that of Turpie and associates,[62] may provide more definitive information.

Isolated studies have advocated the use of antiplatelet agents alone in selected situations—e.g., St. Jude valves in the aortic position.[26] However, results were inconsistent, and antiplatelet agents alone have not been shown to confer sufficient protection from thromboembolism to warrant their usage as primary therapy in patients with mechanical prosthetic heart valves.[18,46,47,58] Furthermore, some question remains as to the efficacy of dipyridamole as an in-vivo antithrombotic agent.[7,21,23] There is, however, increasing interest in trials of aspirin and other antiplatelet agents in conjunction with reduced dosage of anticoagulants such as warfarin.[19,27,29,49,58,62] Such therapy, as reflected in the Third ACCP Conference recommendations,[1] advocated by Altman et al.,[4] studied by Turpie et al.,[62] and considered by Hirsh,[29] shows promise for acceptance as frontline therapy. As new antiplatelet agents are approved for clinical trials,[14] they need to be tested in conjunction with warfarin therapy.

Several recent trials[4,10,37,55,65] have provided strong evidence that the lower ranges of intensity of anticoagulation (INR as low as 2.0–3.0[55,65]) can be used in patients with mechanical prosthetic heart valves without loss of efficacy in preventing thromboembolic events, yet with greater safety by virtue of a marked reduction in minor and major bleeding episodes.

Wilson and associates[65] retrospectively studied 101 patients with 123 prosthetic valves, covering a period of 17 years from 1972-1988. They found that low intensity anticoagulation (PTR:1.3-1.5) proved to be equally effective as higher intensity (PTR: 1.6-2.0) in preventing thromboembolism (2.5 and 2.2 events per 100 patient-years, respectively) and resulted in fewer bleeding complications (3.8 and 5.5 events per 100 patient-years, respectively). These data support the use of the lower range warfarin therapy in patients with mechanical heart valve prostheses. Patients whose PTR was <1.3 experienced 2.9 thromboembolic events per 100 patient-years; in patients with PTR >2.1, hemorrhagic events occurred at a rate of 12.2 per 100 patient-years.

Another recent blinded study[4] randomized 99 patients with mechanical prosthetic heart valves between less intense anticoagulation (INR: 2.0-3.0) (group A) and a more intense regimen (INR: 3.0-4.5) (group B). The investigators concluded that the less intense level of anticoagulation was equivalent to the more intense regimen in preventing thromboembolic events, with a statistically significant reduction ($p < 0.02$) of bleeding complications (3.8 per 100 patient-years for group A, compared with 24.7 per 100 patient-years in group B). All patients in both groups in this trial were also treated with antiplatelet agents, receiving aspirin (330 mg twice daily) and dipyridamole (75 mg twice daily, compared with the usual 400 mg/day). The oral anticoagulant was acenocoumarol, a coumarin congener of warfarin. The authors are strong advocates for the use of antiplatelet agents in combination with low-dose anticoagulation and suggest, but do not substantiate, that this regimen not only allows a lower, hence safer, dosage of the anticoagulant for therapeutic equivalency but may also reduce the severity as well as the incidence of thromboembolic events. They also suggest that hemorrhagic complications may be less severe, although perhaps of higher incidence, than with similarly effective anticoagulant monotherapy, at least compared with the trial reported by Kopf.[37] A brief critique and responsive defense of this study, published in conjunction with the original article, offer insight into the complexities as well as the central points at issue.[57]

It is prudent to note the many variables involved in attempting to reconcile the various studies. Such variables include type and number of prosthetic valves; their position; status of the patient; length and stringency of follow-up; method of monitoring; and differences in definitions. These and other factors, such as drug-drug interactions[5,32,52,64] or extreme (fad) diets affecting vitamin K intake, may enhance or retard the effectiveness of warfarin and thus make it difficult and potentially misleading to attempt point-by-point comparisons or to draw precise and specific conclusions from analysis of diversely designed and disparate studies. Thrombogenicity of prosthetic heart valves and consequent thromboembolic events follow these general trends (from greater to less risk): mechanical > tissue; porcine > bovine valves; older > newer mechanical valves; mitral > aortic position; and multiple > single valves.

Another variable, running as a thread through the central theme, centers on the consistency of long-term maintenance of target anticoagulant intensity. In a general sense, this may be likened to the tightness of glycemic control in diabetes and depends on patient compliance, accurate monitoring, and appropriate therapeutic adjustments, with obvious bearing on outcome and complication rates.[20] Loeliger[42] emphasizes a more stringently structured system of monitoring antithrombotic therapy with currently accepted methods of measurement, along with higher warfarin doses, and individual adjustments as indicated. This may be more practical in a small, closely-linked country, such as Holland, with a relatively homogeneous, well-educated, compliant patient population.

Completion of current and proposed studies will allow a more precise estimation of the incidence of complications of antithrombotic therapy, subtending the extremes of too little (leading to more thromboembolism) and too much (leading to increased bleeding) as well as more definitive recommendations for optimal dosage and combination(s) of agents suitably tailored for a given patient within a selected subset. Application of meta-analytic techniques may serve to convert "multiple small level II trials into a single level I overview," as posited by Sackett[53]; however, if INR is not used, even meta-analysis becomes suspect.

DISCUSSION

Predicated on preliminary data from clinical trials, combined with extrapolations from historical and interrelated studies,[20,29,56,62] it seems reasonable to speculate that further reduction in thromboembolic events may be achieved with a combined regimen (e.g., lower intensity warfarin and low-dose aspirin). Such a combination may also confer added benefits in preventing or lessening artery-to-artery systemic embolization (e.g., carotid to cerebral), hence decreasing the incidence of stroke as well as helping to reduce secondary (and possibly primary) coronary events arising from thrombosis with critical occlusion. If this presumption proves to be correct, such combined therapeutic regimen could be expected to fulfill the promise of significantly reducing overall cardiovascular morbidity and mortality.[29,62] (also personal communication with authors).

Preliminary evidence that added benefits can be achieved by the use of low-dose combination regimens stems from the initial findings of a study in progress of some 370 patients wiith prosthetic heart valves (mostly mechanical but some patients considered to be at high risk for thromboembolism received tissue valves). The achieved INRs were mostly in the low 3.0s, although the targeted INR range was 3.0-4.5[29,62] (also personal communication with the authors). Results indicate that this level of warfarin-induced anticoagulation, combined with aspirin (100 mg/day), was more effective in reducing major thromboembolic events and was virtually as safe in terms of major hemorrhage as the same dose of warfarin plus placebo (same INR range). Furthermore, the combined regimen resulted in a striking reduction in overall mortality (9 of 186 patients or 4.8% of those receiving warfarin plus aspirin, compared with 22 of 184 patients or 11.9% of those receiving warfarin plus placebo; p <0.011).[62] This reduction in mortality was ascribed entirely to a decrease in cardiovascular deaths due to coronary events (e.g., myocardial infarction).[29] This benefit was found not only in patients with associated coronary artery disease, many of whom had undergone coronary artery bypass grafting, but also in patients without known coronary artery disease.[29]

Multicenter primary intervention studies of healthy adults are currently underway in the United Kingdom with an even lower dose of warfarin (target

INR: 1.6). Subjects were chosen for this trial because they had high levels of fibrinogen or factor VII coagulant activity, both of which are considered to be major risk factors for ischemic heart disease.[44] A recent study,[38] which found several rheologic abnormalities, including an increase in fibrinogen, after heart valve replacement, further supports the use of long-term oral anticoagulant therapy for patients with substitute heart valves.

Another potential benefit of warfarin in patients with bioprosthetic valves may be slowing or reducing the calcification that occurs in spontaneously degenerating tissue valves. This effect of warfarin may be mediated by its inhibition of the synthesis of gammacarboxyglutamic acid, a vitamin K-dependent enzymatic process. The reduction of this calcium-binding amino acid has been postulated as the means by which calcification of porcine valves is reduced.[60] This effect could add to the longevity of such valves as well as to a decrease in thromboembolic events.[59]

Whether even lower (true mini-dose) regimens of warfarin may be effective in selective patients with prosthetic heart valves and for other indications is under study. At present, however, such regimens cannot be routinely recommended.[29]

Despite all the variables, uncertainties, and expressed disagreements, fundamental understanding of the complex, important, and broadly encompassing field of antithrombotic therapy continues to advance, and basic differences in approach and recommendations may be more narrow than deep. Thus, within the relatively close INR ranges recommended, appropriate targets of anticoagulant intensity may be selected—i.e., lower INR for patients judged to be at high risk of bleeding and higher INR for those judged to be at higher risk for thromboembolic events.[39] Furthermore, the promise of more efficacious combination(s) of drugs presently in use for antithrombotic therapy and the development of newer antithrombotic agents[14] portend further progress—from basic research through clinical trials to routine use—in the evolution of broadly applicable strategies.

SUMMARY

Intensity of anticoagulation lower than and/or otherwise modified from the levels recommended by the Second ACCP/NHLBI Conference[59] is now advised by the Third ACCP Conference panelists and others,[49,58] although this approach has not been undisputed.[42,45] The formal revisions have been outlined above; additional implied and inferred points of revision, outlined below, are aimed at achieving a useful working overview of current knowledge, trends, and recommendations for therapy in patients with prosthetic heart valves, whether mechanical or tissue.

For patients with mechanical prosthetic heart valves, permanent therapy with warfarin (INR: 2.5–3.5; PTR: approximately 1.5–1.7) is strongly recommended (grade C)[19,58] with a small daily dose of aspirin (perhaps 80–160 mg),[29] even without a history of systemic embolism. The target INR range of 2.5–3.5 is supported by level II and V studies.[28]

For patients with tissue valves who are in sinus rhythm, the Third ACCP consensus recommendations (grade A, level I) remain the same as in 1989—i.e., 3 months of therapy with warfarin (INR: 2.0–3.0) for patients with bioprosthetic mitral valve replacement. This regimen is optional for patients with a tissue valve in the aortic position. Also reiterated as optional for all patients with bioprosthetic valves is long-term therapy with aspirin (325 mg/day), based on one level IV study.[58]

For patients at higher risk for thromboembolism, longer-term warfarin therapy is recommended (targeted INR: 2.0-3.0) (grade C, level IV). Such patients include those with atrial fibrillation, a history of systemic embolization, or evidence of left atrial thrombus at surgery.[58]

The optimal dosage of aspirin and the possibility of lowering anticoagulant intensity even further are currently under study. The objective, as always, is to achieve increased efficacy (decreased incidence and possibly decreased severity of thromboembolic events) combined with increased safety (decreased incidence and possibly decreased severity of hemorrhagic events).

REFERENCES

1. ACCP/NHLBI: Third ACCP Consensus Conference on Antithrombotic Therapy. Chest 104:303S-549S, 1992.
2. ACCP/NHLBI: Second ACCP Conference on Antithrombotic Therapy. Chest 95:1S-162S, 1989.
3. ACCP/NHLBI: National Conference on Antithrombotic Therapy. Chest 89(Suppl):1S-106S, 1986.
4. Altman R, Rouvier J, Gurfinkel E, et al: Comparison of two levels of anticoagulant therapy in patients with substitute heart valves. J Thorac Cardiovasc Surg 101:427-431, 1991.
5. American Hospital Formulary Service Drug Information-1992: Coumarin and Indandione Derivatives. General Statement. 771-776 warfarin sodium: 777-778.
6. Ansell JE: Oral anticoagulant drugs. N Engl J Med 326:368, 1992.
7. Antiplatelet Trialists' Collaboration: Secondary prevention of vascular disease by prolonged antiplatelet treatment. BMJ 296:320-331, 1988.
8. British Society for Haematology: Guidelines on oral anticoagulation, 2nd ed. J Clin Pathol 43:177-183, 1990.
9. Boston Area Anticoagulant Trial for Atrial Fibrillation Investigators (BAATAF): The effect of low-dose warfarin on the risk of stroke with nonrheumatic atrial fibrillation. N Engl J Med 323:1506-1511, 1990.
10. Bussey HI, Force RW, Bianco TM, et al: Reliance on prothrombin time ratios causes significant errors in anticoagulation therapy. Arch Intern Med 152:278-282, 1992.
11. Butchart EG, Lewis PA, Grumkmeier GL, et al: Low risk of thrombosis and serious embolic events despite low-intensity anticoagulation. Circulation 78(Suppl):166-176, 1988.
12. Chesebro JH, Ezekowitz M, Badiman L: Intracardiac thrombi and systemic thromboembolism: Detection, incidence, and treatment. Annu Rev Med 36:579-605, 1985.
13. Chesebro JH, Fuster V, Elveback LR, et al: Trial of combined warfarin plus dipyridamole or aspirin therapy in prosthetic heart valve replacement: Danger of aspirin compared with dipyridamole. Am J Cardiol 51:1537-1541, 1983.
14. Coller BS: Antiplatelet agents in the prevention and therapy of thrombosis. Annu Rev Med 43:171-180, 1992.
15. Connolly SJ, Laupacis A, Gent M, et al: Canadian atrial fibrillation anticoagulation (CAFA) study. J Am Coll Cardiol 18:349-355, 1991.
16. Cortina JM, Martinell J, Artiz V, et al: Comparative clinical results with Omniscience (STM1), Medtronic-Hall, and Bjork-Shiley convexo-concave (70 degrees) prostheses in mitral valve replacement. J Thorac Cardiovasc Surg 91:174-183, 1986.
17. Czer LSC, Matloff JM, Chaux A, et al: Comparative clinical experience with porcine bioprosthetic and St. Jude valve replacement. Chest 91:503-514, 1987.
18. Czer LSC, Matloff JM, Stewart AE, et al: The St. Jude valve analysis of thromboembolism in warfarin related hemorrhage and survival. Curr Cardiol Am Heart J 114:389-397, 1987.
19. Dalen JE, Hirsh J: Third ACCP Consensus Conference on Antithrombotic Therapy. Chest 104:303S-304S, 1992.

20. Dalen JE: An apple a day or an aspirin a day? Arch Intern Med 151:1066-1069, 1991.
21. Edmunds LH: Thrombotic and bleeding complications of prosthetic heart valves (collective review). Ann Thorac Surg 44:430-445, 1987.
22. Ezckowitz MD, Bridges SL, James KE, et al: Interim analysis of VA cooperative study: Stroke prevention in nonrheumatic atrial fibrillation (SPINAF). Am Heart Assoc Abstr Nov:11-14, 1991.
23. FitzGerald GA: Dipyridamole. N Engl J Med 316:1247-1257, 317:1734-1736, 1987.
24. Force R, Roush M, Bussey HI: Comment: Warfarin and the international normalized ratio. Ann Pharm Ther 26:430-431, 1992.
25. Friedli B, Aerichide N, Grondin P, et al: Thromboembolic complications of heart valve prostheses. Am Heart J 81:702-708, 1971.
26. Hartz RS, LoCicero J III, Kucich V, et al: Comparative study of warfarin versus antiplatelet therapy in patients with a St. Jude valve in the aortic position. J Thorac Cardiovasc Surg 92:684-690, 1986.
27. Hirsh J: Oral anticoagulants: Mechanism of action, clinical effectiveness and optimal therapeutic range. Chest 102:312S-326S, 1992.
28. Hirsh J: Oral anticoagulant therapy: Urgent need for standardization. Circulation 86:1332-1335, 1992 [editorial].
29. Hirsh J: New approaches to antithrombotic therapy, heparin and warfarin: Their limitations and what's new Program #TELE U4009. Presented as a Med Grand Rnds Med Coll of WI and Dept of VA Affairs, Milwaukee, WI. Sponsored by DuPont, August 5, 1992.
30. Hirsh J: Inadequate monitoring of warfarin dosage. Blood 80:562-563, 1992 [editorial].
31. Hirsh J: Substandard monitoring of warfarin in North America: Time for change. Arch Intern Med 152:257-258, 1992 [editorial].
32. Hirsh J: Oral anticoagulant drugs. N Engl J Med 324:1865-1875, 1991.
33. Hirsh J: Replies to vdMeer FJM and Answell J. N Engl J Med 326:68-69, 1992.
34. Hirsh J: Influence of low-intensity warfarin treatment on patients' perceptions of quality of life. Arch Intern Med 151:1921-1922, 1991 [editorial].
35. Hirsh J, Poller L, Deykin D, et al: Optimal therapeutic range for oral anticoagulants. Chest 95:5S-11S, 1989.
36. Hoskison T, Boomer WM: Anticoagulation and prothrombin time ratios. Arch Intern Med 152:1720, 1992 [letter with reply by Hirsh J].
37. Kopf GS, Hammond GL, Geha AS, et al: Long-term performance of the St. Jude medical valve: Low incidence of thromboembolism and hemorrhagic complications with modest doses. Circulation 76(Suppl III):132-136, 1987.
38. Koppensteiner R, Meritz A, Schlick W, et al: Blood rheology after cardiac valve replacement with mechanical prostheses or bioprostheses. Am J Cardiol 67:79-83, 1991.
39. Lechner K: Oral anticoagulant treatment: Is mild beautiful? Ann Hematol 64:51, 1992.
40. Levine MN, Hirsh J, Landefeld S, et al: Hemorrhagic complications of anticoagulant treatment. Chest 104:352S-363S, 1991.
41. Levine MN, Rashob G, Hirsh J: Hemorrhagic complications of long-term anticoagulant therapy. Chest 95:26S-36S, 1989.
42. Loeliger EA: Therapeutic target values in oral anti-coagulation: Justification of Dutch policy and a warning against the so-called moderate-intensity regimens. Ann Hematol 64:60-65, 1992.
43. Magillian DJ Jr, Lewis JW Jr, Tilley B, et al: The porcine bioprosthetic valve—twelve years later. J Thorac Cardiovasc Surg 89:499-507, 1985.
44. Meade TW, Wilkes HC, Stirlina Y, et al: Randomized controlled trial of low dose warfarin in the primary prevention of ischemic heart disease in men at high risk: Design and pilot study. Eur Heart J 4:836-843, 1988.
45. vdMeer FJM, Rosendaal RR, Cannegieter SC, et al: Oral anticoagulant drugs (with reply by Hirsh J). N Engl J Med 326:68-69, 1992.
46. Mok CK, Boey J, Wang R, et al: Warfarin versus dipyridamole-aspirin and pentoxifylline-aspirin for the prevention of prosthetic heart valve thromboembolism: A prospective randomized clinical trial. Circulation 72:1059-1063, 1985.
47. Myers ML, Lawrie GM, Crawford ES, et al: The St. Jude valve prosthesis: Analysis of the clinical results in 815 implants and the need for systemic anticoagulation. J Am Coll Cardiol 13:57-62, 1989.
48. Petersen P, Boysen G, Godtfredsen E, et al: Placebo-controlled randomized trial of warfarin and aspirin for prevention of thromboembolic complications in atrial fibrillation: The Copenhagen AFASAK study. Lancet 1:175-178, 1989.

49. Poller L: Therapeutic ranges for oral anticoagulation in different thromboembolic disorders. Ann Hematol 64:52-59, 1992.
50. Poller L: A simple nomogram for the derivation of international normalized ratios for the standardization of prothrombin times. Thromb Haemost 60:18-20, 1988.
51. Quick AJ: The prothrombin time in hemophilia and obstructive jaundice. J Biol Chem 109:73-74, 1935.
52. Roush MK, Bussey HL, Bianco IM: Fluoroquinolones alter the effects of warfarin therapy? Arch Intern Med 152:1534-1535, 1992 (letter with reply by Jolson et al.].
53. Sackett DL: Rules of evidence and clinical recommendations on the use of antithrombotic agents. Chest 95:2S-4S, 1989.
54. Sackett DL: Rules of evidence and clinical recommendations on the use of antithrombotic agents. Chest 89:2S-4S, 1986.
55. Saour JN, Sieck JO, Mamo LRM, et al: Trial of different intensities of anticoagulation in patients with prosthetic heart valves. N Engl J Med 322:428-432, 1990.
56. Smith P, Arnesen H, Holme I: The effect of warfarin on mortality and reinfarction after myocardial infarction (WARIS). N Engl J Med 323:147-152, 1990.
57. Stein B, Fuster V: Invited letter concerning: Anticoagulant plus platelet inhibitor therapy in patients with mechanical valve prostheses. J Thorac Cardiovasc Surg 101:557-558, 1991 [with reply by Altman R, et al. 559].
58. Stein PD, Alpert JS, Copeland J, et al: Antithrombotic therapy in patients with mechanical and biological prosthetic heart valves. Chest 104:445S-455S, 1992.
59. Stein PD, Kantrowitz A: Antithrombotic therapy in mechanical and biological prosthetic heart valves and saphenous vein bypass grafts. Chest 95:107S-117S, 1989.
60. Stein PD, Riddle JM, Kemp SR, et al: Effect of warfarin on calcification of spontaneously degenerated porcine bioprosthetic valves. J Thorac Cardiovasc Surg 90:119-125, 1985.
61. Stroke Prevention in Atrial Fibrillation (SPAF) study group investigators: Preliminary report. N Engl J Med 322:863-868, 1990.
62. Turpie AGG, Gent M, Laupacis A, et al: Reduction in mortality by adding aspirin (100 mg) to oral anticoagulants in patients with heart valve replacement. J Am Coll Cardiol 19:103A, 1992 [abstract 738-1].
63. Turpie AGG, Alexander GG, Gunstensen J, et al: Randomized comparison of two intensities of oral anticoagulant therapy after tissue heart valve replacement. Lancet 1:1242-1245, 1988.
64. Wessler S, Gitel SN: Warfarin—from bedside to bench. N Engl J Med 311:645-652, 1984.
65. Wilson DB, Dunn MJ, Hassanein K: Low-intensity anticoagulation in mechanic cardiac prosthetic valves. Chest 100:1553-1557, 1991.
66. Wright IS, Marple CD, Beck DF: Report of the committee for the evaluation of anticoagulants in the treatment of coronary thrombosis with myocardial infarction. Am Heart J 36:801-815, 1948.

Chapter 22

Perioperative Antiplatelet Therapy and Management in Cardiovascular Surgery: Assessment of Bleeding Risk

Thomas P. Lecompte, M.D., Pierre L. Julia, M.D., Simone Massonnet-Castel, M.D., and Michel Meyer Samama, M.D.

Cardiovascular surgery typifies the surgical challenge of bleeding vs. thrombosis. This chapter focuses mainly on cardiac surgery with cardiopulmonary bypass (CPB) and the effects of perioperative administration of an antiplatelet agent (APA), which have been the subject of numerous studies. The patient receiving an APA raises special concerns about bleeding. Changes in hemostasis, particularly in platelet number and function, have been well documented after CPB[9,14,27] and may accentuate the otherwise minimally significant effect of preoperative ingestion of an APA. Early reoperation for bleeding is associated with a substantial increase in morbidity and mortality. On the other hand, the thrombotic risk may be so high that treatment with an APA seems necessary even in a patient scheduled for surgery; for example, a patient with unstable and refractory angina awaiting coronary artery bypass grafting (CABG). It was also thought that preoperative administration of an APA could help to prevent acute thrombosis and late occlusion of the graft. For such reasons particular attention has been paid to the effects of APA on perioperative hemostasis in the context of CABG surgery, which requires CPB.

PHARMACOLOGY OF ANTIPLATELET AGENTS

None of the currently available molecules aimed at depressing platelet behavior to prevent arterial thrombosis are direct inhibitors of aggregation per se; that is, of the binding of fibrinogen with activated glycoproteins IIb-IIIa.

True inhibitors of aggregation, including monoclonal antibodies directed at glycoproteins IIb-IIIa and proteins from snake venoms (such as disintegrins) will become available for clinical use in the near future. Although these agents may have greater antithrombotic potency, they may also result in a higher risk of bleeding compared with the currently used APAs (Table 1).

Aspirin, ticlopidine, and prostacyclin and its analogues impair the process of platelet activation.[15] Aspirin inhibits synthesis of thromboxane, whereas ticlopidine selectively inhibits the platelet-activating effect of adenosine diphosphate (ADP) from injured cells or previously activated platelets (through the release reaction). Both agents inhibit only amplification pathways of platelet activation, which are important but not essential. By contrast, prostacyclin, which increases intraplatelet levels of cyclic adenosine monophosphate (c-AMP), is able, at least in vitro, to decrease dramatically (and even abolish) platelet responses to all agonists. However, its powerful vasodilating effects preclude clinical use of high dosages.

Both aspirin and ticlopidine have a long-lasting effect because of irreversible inhibition of circulating platelets, in contrast with prostacyclin and its currently available chemically stable analogs.[15] Thus total recovery of platelet function requires the complete turnover of the peripheral pool of platelets (i.e., 10 days). Because improvement is gradual, normalization of the bleeding risk after administration of an APA is probably achieved within a shorter time, although this point has not yet been proved (see below). Rapid absorption aspirin, at a starting dose of 160 mg, results in immediate, almost total suppression of thromboxane synthesis. The maximal effect of ticlopidine (currently recommended dosage: 250 mg twice daily) is achieved after several days (about 5) of administration.

Finally, aspirin on average induces a mild (prolongation factor: × 1.5 to 2) increase in the Ivy bleeding time (BT). But some subjects appear to be exquisitely sensitive to aspirin[7] for as yet unknown reasons (almost complete inhibition of thromboxane synthesis is achieved). The prolongation of the BT with ticlopidine therapy is generally greater than that observed with aspirin; in contrast with aspirin, the prolongation with ticlopidine is dose-dependent. Sensitivity to ticlopidine varies markedly among individuals, in terms of both BT and ex vivo platelet aggregation.

Dipyridamole, which can be safely administered alone before surgery,[25] is not specifically considered in this chapter.

ASSESSMENT OF THE BLEEDING RISK

Aspirin and Cardiac Surgery

The magnitude of the problem is underscored by the fact that nearly one-half of patients with ischemic heart disease awaiting surgery take aspirin. The Transfusion Medicine Academic Award Group[12] recently audited 540 patients undergoing elective primary CABG at 18 institutions (tertiary-care hospitals associated with schools of medicine) for the purpose of describing the variability in transfusions and the determining factors. The study reported 220 instances of aspirin ingestion within 7 days before surgery. In the study of Bashein et al.[1] a pilot chart review at one institution revealed the proportion of

TABLE 1. Antiplatelet Agents Most Extensively Studied in Clinical Settings

Name	Mechanism of Action	Duration of Effect
Aspirin	Inhibition of thromboxane	Platelet life-span
Flurbiprofen	Same	Reversible (<24 hours)
Ticlopidine	Inhibition of adenosine diphosphate	Platelet life-span
Prostacyclin and analogs	Increase in cyclic adenosine monophosphate	Short-lasting (minutes)
n-3 fatty acids	Changes in membrane and eicosanoids	Long-lasting

patients using aspirin within 7 days of surgery to be 41% (95% confidence interval: 38-44%). On the other hand, approximately 5% of CABG patients are believed to require reoperation to control hemorrhage or to relieve pericardial tamponade caused by hemorrhage.[27]

Most studies suggest that patients taking aspirin before CPB have excessive and prolonged mediastinal bleeding and are at higher risk for reoperation.[27] For example, in a recent prospective, randomized, double-blind trial[11] increased bleeding complications were seen with preoperative aspirin therapy compared with aspirin started 6 hours postoperatively. Either 325 mg aspirin or placebo was administered the night before surgery; after surgery all patients received 325 mg aspirin daily, with the first dose administered through the nasogastric tube 6 hours postoperatively. The reoperation rate for bleeding was 6.3% in the group receiving preoperative aspirin compared with 2.4% in the placebo group. More transfusions were also required (median: 900 vs. 725 ml). Median chest-tube drainage within the first 6 hours was significantly, but only slightly, increased: 500 vs. 448 ml.

This effect of preoperative aspirin was suggested by the results of an earlier trial conducted by the same group of investigators,[10] in which preoperative aspirin (325 mg 12 hr before surgery) was compared with placebo given throughout the study period. Patients receiving aspirin showed an increase in mediastinal bleeding, transfusion, and reoperation rate (4-9%).

The assessment of the extent of post-CPB bleeding, however, seems to vary widely among studies and institutions[24]; the assessment of the effects of aspirin is no exception. In multicenter studies the involvement of several surgeons and different CPB techniques results in wide variations in bleeding volumes. Thus, although most authors strongly advise against use of preoperative aspirin, especially because early postoperative administration seems to provide the same protective effect for CABG patency,[8,11] others still advocate that the increase in bleeding risk related to aspirin is marginal and almost always clinically irrelevant.[25]

The clinical trials devoted to the study of the effects of APAs on CABG provide an objective assessment of the aspirin-related bleeding risk, but only under the particular circumstances of each study and with postoperative continuation of aspirin. Thus they are not relevant to the management of patients who receive only preoperative aspirin—a group that is common in clinical practice. Three studies with different designs attempt to address the question from a more practical point of view. Torosian et al.[26] studied 100 consecutive patients operated by the same surgeon. The only surgical procedure was CABG, and the surgical technique remained constant throughout the 5-month study period. The CPB technique is also well described.

Thirteen patients received preoperative aspirin, with administration terminated from 2-7 days before surgery. For the second through fourth hours, hourly chest-tube drainage was significantly increased in these patients compared with 64 patients who received no treatment impairing hemostasis (<100 ml/hr). Mean mediastinal loss was about 900 ml vs. about 400 ml and mean chest-tube duration 34 ± 6 vs. 20 ± 1 hours (mean $\pm$ SEM) in the aspirin group and in the control group, respectively. Only 3 patients (including 1 who received aspirin) were returned to the operating room for reexploration related to excessive postoperative bleeding; each had a surgically correctable lesion.

Ferraris et al.[7] carried out a small, non-blinded study of 40 patients scheduled for urgent or elective CABG. The patients were randomized to receive either 1 aspirin tablet (325 mg) or no aspirin the day before operation. Three staff surgeons performed or supervised the procedures. Patients in the aspirin group had a template BT determination between 2 and 10 hours after ingestion of aspirin. Because six patients were excluded because of excessively prolonged preoperative BT (according to the authors' criterion), 16 aspirin-treated patients were compared with 18 controls. Aspirin-treated patients showed an increase in chest-tube drainage 12 hours after surgery ($1,513 \pm 977$ vs. 916 ± 482 ml, respectively) and a statistically significant increase in transfusion requirements (packed red blood cells, platelets, fresh-frozen plasma). Moreover, 6 patients, all in the aspirin group, had postoperative bleeding that required intervention in the form of hemostatic drugs (4 patients), such as 1-deamino-8-D-arginine vasopressin (DDAVP) (see below) or epsilon-aminocaproic acid, or reoperation (2 patients).

Bashein et al.[1] carried out a case-control study of 2,355 patients who underwent CABG only operations at one institution during a 4-year period. Ninety analyzable cases with reoperation for bleeding before discharge were matched with 180 controls. The proportions of patients who received aspirin within 7 days before surgery were 34.4% (reoperative patients) and 22.2% (controls), with an estimated odds ratio for reoperation after aspirin ingestion of 1.82 (95% confidence interval: 1.23-3.32). The differences in preoperative template (Simplate) BT were statistically significant but said to be clinically unimportant: 5.5 ± 2.2 compared with 4.9 ± 1.1 (mean $\pm$ SD) in reoperative patients and controls, respectively.

Aspirin and Vascular Surgery

Data regarding aspirin and peripheral vascular surgery are, to our knowledge, more scarce. In McCollum's double-blind study,[23] 549 patients undergoing femoropopliteal vein bypasses were randomized to receive either the combination of aspirin (300 mg) plus dipyridamole, starting 2 days before surgery, or placebo. No significant differences in operative complications were reported between the 2 groups: 18 vs. 9 reoperations for bleeding and 12 vs. 14 hematomas for APA treatment and placebo, respectively.

Data have also been collected in the particular context of heparin-induced thrombocytopenia (HIT) with thrombosis requiring surgery. Gruel et al.[13] recently reported 2 patients with arterial thrombosis. First heparin was stopped, and aspirin and dipyridamole were administered. Then surgical revascularization was successfully attempted with intraoperative unfractionated heparin

(UFH) and IV infusion of the prostacyclin analogue, iloprost. This short reexposure led to neither bleeding nor recurrent thrombosis. We analyzed 14 consecutive patients with HIT,[6] who were prospectively managed with UFH withdrawal and use of the low-molecular-weight heparin, enoxaparin (75 IU/kg twice daily subcutaneously) combined with aspirin (300 mg intravenously, once daily). Thrombectomy had to be performed in 5 patients; no severe hemorrhage occurred.

Ticlopidine

Six small prospective studies,[4] involving a total of >100 patients, were designed to improve CABG patency with preoperative administration of ticlopidine. Ticlopidine was administered 3-5 days before surgery; thus the maximal antiplatelet effect was presumably not achieved. A trend for increased bleeding was noticed, but the rate of reoperation was not significantly higher. Two studies with ticlopidine (250 mg twice daily, beginning 48 hours after surgery), are cited by Stein et al.[25] No increase in bleeding risk was reported, and graft patency was found to be improved.[2,20] The authors thus conclude that postoperative ticlopidine may be considered as a safe alternative for aspirin-allergic patients, at least in terms of perioperative bleeding.

In addition, the data collected through the 2 large-scale trials (CATS and TASS) of ticlopidine as a means of decreasing cardiovascular events in patients with cerebrovascular disease do not seem to indicate a dramatic risk of operative bleeding.[4] Protocols recommended discontinuation of the drug 10 days before elective surgery. A substantial variety of surgical procedures (precise nature unfortunately unknown) were performed on this therapy, with only one reported case of abnormal intraoperative bleeding.

Prostacyclin and Iloprost

Chemically synthetized prostacyclin, known as epoprostenol, has been studied in 4 controlled trials,[18] with dosages up to 50 ng $\times$ kg^{-1} $\times$ min^{-1}. With the higher dosage, some platelet preservation was reported, as well as a trend toward decreased blood loss and blood transfusion. These results illustrate the apparent paradox that preservation of platelets from consumption and from alterations due to CPB by intraoperative administration of an APA may in fact improve postoperative hemostasis.

Iloprost, a chemically stable analog of prostacyclin, was infused to 11 patients with HIT and thrombosis who required cardiac or vascular surgery and thus were reexposed to unfractionated heparin.[17] The infusion was started after induction of anesthesia and before CBP. The maximal dose for each patient, which varied from 10-48 ng $\times$ kg^{-1} $\times$ min^{-1}, was reportedly sufficient to prevent further platelet activation in vivo in the presence of heparin. Blood pressure had to be controlled with phenylephrine, but no perioperative complications occurred. Iloprost was also studied by one of us[22] in a double-blind, randomized, placebo-controlled, pilot study involving 30 patients undergoing CABG, with a mean CPB duration of about 90 minutes. Iloprost was infused in incremental doses, up to 12 ng $\times$ kg^{-1} $\times$ min^{-1}. The infusion was begun before CPB and stopped at the time of protamine injection. No significant difference in post-bypass bleeding was observed between the iloprost and the placebo groups. Iloprost appeared to preserve platelet function. Two patients in the iloprost group experienced severe hypotension, and the infusion had to be stopped prematurely.

Some data suggest that both prostacyclin and iloprost can potentiate the effects of unfractionated heparin on coagulation tests.[5,22]

Polyunsaturated, n-3 Fatty Acids

Dietary n-3 fatty acids from marine oils have many biologic effects, including some degree of inhibition of platelet aggregation. One study focuses on preoperative administration of fish oil to patients scheduled for CABG. Despite an ex-vivo documented decrease in platelet aggregation and thromboxane generation during whole blood clotting and a prolongation of bleeding time, no excessive bleeding was reported.[3]

No careful clinical assessment of the combination of n-3 fatty acids with aspirin therapy is available; however, the combination carries, at least theoretically, an enhanced bleeding risk.

MANAGEMENT

Because of the evidence—small though it be— for an increased bleeding risk due to preoperative administration of aspirin, we strongly recommend its avoidance whenever possible. Although fewer data are available, the same holds true for ticlopidine, particularly because it induces in most of the cases a striking impairment of ADP-induced aggregation (far beyond the effect of aspirin) and a marked prolongation of bleeding time. For both of these APAs the maximal safety interval is 10 days.

The up-dated recommendations of the Third North American (ACCP) Consensus Conference[25] state that (1) aspirin, started 6 hours after CABG at 325 mg/day, is safer than aspirin of the same dosage started before operation and results in a similar rate of occlusion; (2) if postoperative bleeding prevents the administration of aspirin at 6 hours after surgery, then starting as soon as possible thereafter is advised; and (3) dipyridamole may be started safely before surgery.

The following discussion and suggestions thus apply only to patients with inadvertent aspirin use in whom it is not possible to defer the operation until the effect has worn off, or to patients scheduled for surgery and thought to require permanent antiplatelet theapy because of high risk of arterial thrombosis.

As discussed above, patients vary in their response to aspirin (in terms of BT) and to ticlopidine (in terms of both BT and platelet aggregation). Taking also into account the at least rough relationship between prolongation of BT and type and degree of an inherited platelet or von Willebrand's factor defect, it is tempting to speculate that BT would help in identifying patients on APA therapy at highest risk for bleeding.[7] Unfortunately, the clinical value of BT is controversial, as is the method of measurement, although the Ivy technique, with an horizontal incision, is by far the most studied. Moreover, despite progress in standardization with the availability of automatic devices, the observer's skill still remains of crucial importance. Thus the predictive value of

TABLE 2. Methods to Prevent or to Stop Excessive Bleeding on Antiplatelet Therapy

Agent	Mechanism of Action (Likely or Alleged)
Steroids	Unknown (vessel wall?)
DDAVP	Increase in plasma levels of von Willebrand's (desmopressin) factor (endothelial release)
Aprotinin	Inhibitor of plasmin, the key enzyme of the fibrinolytic system; relationship with the effects on primary hemostasis not yet fully elucidated
Platelet transfusion	Replacement therapy

BT for surgical bleeding risk is at best not yet established.[21] This point, combined with the assumption that the overall increase in bleeding risk due to preoperative administration of an APA is low, suggests that no systematic attempt to improve hemostasis is warranted.

In contrast, obsessional attention must be paid to other correctable factors, including surgical technique, quality of intraoperative hemostasis, hematocrit (threshold for prolongation of the BT due to low hematocrit: 30%), and use of other drugs, such as nitrates or beta-lactam antibiotics, that definitely, or even possibly, impair hemostasis. If despite all these precautionary measures, serious bleeding occurs intraoperatively, then platelet transfusion should be quickly effective.

Several nontransfusional therapies to improve defects in primary hemostasis due to antiplatelet therapy have been proposed (Table 2): a 20-mg bolus injection of methylprednisolone, which may shorten the BT in platelet defects; infusion of DDAVP (also known as desmopressin acetate), which dramatically increases plasma levels of von Willebrand's factor in most subjects[9]; and aprotinin, a powerful inhibitor of plasmin, the crucial enzyme of the fibrinolytic system, in which interest has been renewed, especially in the setting of CPB.[24] In a recent double-blind, randomized, placebo-controlled, cross-over study of 10 healthy volunteers after aspirin ingestion, desmopressin (0.3 $\mu g/kg$) produced a transient decrease in template BT.[19] Unfortunately, a clinical study in the setting of CPB did not demonstrate a beneficial effect of such an infusion following protamine in 39 patients who received aspirin within 7 days before operation.[16] In this study, however, an increase in bleeding due to aspirin therapy could not be evidenced. We agree entirely with the authors' conclusions: routine administration of desmopressin to aspirin-taking patients undergoing CPB is not recommended; however, aspirin-treated patients who bleed excessively after operation may benefit from desmopressin.

High-dose aprotinin therapy is strongly recommended by Royston[24] as a safe treatment to prevent diffuse bleeding in patients receiving aspirin and undergoing cardiac surgery with CPB. An alternative approach of interest is to deliver aprotinin after completion of CPB in patients with excessive bleeding; this approach, in our opinion, deserves to be studied.

If preoperative therapy to prevent arterial thrombosis is absolutely required, one may either assume the bleeding risk of aspirin or ticlopidine or switch the antithrombotic therapy to more convenient drugs with a short-term effect: either unfractionated heparin (a dosage aimed at reaching a twofold prolongation of APTT) or a reversible cyclooxygenase inhibitor such as flurbiprofen.

ACKNOWLEDGMENT

We thank Dr. K. Phuong Phan (Heart Institute, Ho Chi Minh City, Viet-Nam) for her helpful comments, and Dr. J.C. Arcan (Sanofi-Winthrop, Gentilly, France) for providing us with data from Sanofi and Syntex files.

REFERENCES

1. Bashein G, Nessly ML, Rice AL, et al: Preoperative aspirin therapy and reoperation for bleeding after coronary artery bypass surgery. Arch Intern Med 151:89-93, 1991.
2. Chevigné M, David JL, Rigo P, Limet R: Effect of ticlopidine on saphenous vein bypass patency rates: A double-blind study. Ann Thorac Surg 37:371-378, 1984.
3. DeCaterina R, Giannessi D, Mazzone A, et al: Vascular prostacyclin is increased in patients ingesting omega-3 polyunsaturated fatty acids before coronary artery bypass graft surgery. Circulation 82:428-438, 1990.
4. Ellis DJ: Summary of surgical experience in ticlopidine treated patients. Personal communication, 1991.
5. Fabiani JN, O'Grady J, Terrier E, et al Etude clinique des effets de la prostacycline lors des circulations extra-corporelles en chirurgie cardiaque à coeur ouvert. Coeur 12:149-151, 1981.
6. Farkas JC, Lecompte T, Luo SK, et al: Heparin induced thrombocytopenia: Treatment with a combination of aspirin and low molecular weight heparin. Thromb Haemost 65:1283, 1991 [abstract 2129].
7. Ferraris VA, Ferraris SP, Lough FC, Berry WR: Preoperative aspirin ingestion increases operative blood loss after coronary artery bypass grafting. Ann Thorac Surg 45:71-74, 1988.
8. Gavaghan TP, Gebski V, Baron DW: Immediate postoperative aspirin improves vein graft patency early and late after coronary artery bypass graft surgery: A placebo-controlled, randomized study. Circulation 83:1526-1533, 1991.
9. George JN, Shattil SJ: The clinical importance of acquired abnormalities of platelet function (review article). N Engl J Med 324:27-39, 1991.
10. Goldman S, Copeland J, Moritz T, et al: Improvement in early saphenous vein graft patency after coronary artery bypass surgery with antiplatelet therapy. Circulation 77:1324-1332, 1988.
11. Goldman S, Copeland J, Moritz T, et al: Starting aspirin therapy after operation: Effects on early graft patency. Circulation 84:520-526, 1991.
12. Goodnough LT, Johnston MFM, Toy PTCY, and the Transfusion Medicine Academic Award Group: The variability of transfusion practice in coronary artery bypass surgery. JAMA 265:86-90, 1991.
13. Gruel Y, Lermusiaux P, Lang M, et al: Usefulness of antiplatelet drugs in the management of heparin-associated thrombocytopenia and thrombosis. Ann Vasc Surg 5:552-555, 1991.
14. Harker LA, Malpass TW, Branson HE, et al: Mechanisms of abnormal bleeding in patients undergoing cardiopulmonary bypass: Acquired transient platelet dysfunction associated with selective alpha granule release. Blood 56:824-833, 1980.
15. Hirsh J, Dalen JE, Fuster V, et al: Aspirin and other platelet-active drugs: The relationship between dose, effectiveness, and side effects. Chest 102:327S-336S, 1992.
16. Horrow J, van Riper D, Parmet J, Osborne BS: Desmopressin does not decrease bleeding after aspirin. Anesthesiology 75:A985, 1991.
17. Kappa JR, Fisher CA, Todd B, et al: Intraoperative management of patients with heparin-induced thrombocytopenia. Ann Thorac Surg 49:714-723, 1990.
18. Kerins DM, Murray R, FitzGerald GA: Prostacyclin and prostaglandin E1: Molecular mechanisms and therapeutic utility. Prog Hemost Thromb 10:307-337, 1991.
19. Lethagen S, Rugarn P: The effect of DDAVP and placebo on platelet function and prolonged bleeding time induced by oral acetylsalicylic acid intake in healthy volunteers. Thromb Haemost 67:185-186, 1992.
20. Limet R, David JL, Magotteaux P, et al: Prevention of aorta-coronary bypass graft occlusion: Beneficial effect of ticlopidine on early and late patency rates of venous coronary bypass grafts: A double-blind study. J Thorac Cardiovasc Surg 94:773-783, 1987.
21. Lind SE: The bleeding time does not predict surgical bleeding (review article). Blood 77:2547-2552, 1991.
22. Massonnet-Castel S, Farge D, Tournay D, et al: Utilisation d'une prostacycline de synthèse en circulation extracorporelle. Presse Méd 21:113-118, 1992.

23. McCollum C, Alexander C, Kenchington G, et al: Antiplatelet drugs in femoropopliteal vein bypasses: A multicenter trial. J Vasc Surg 13:150-162, 1991.
24. Royston D: High-dose aprotinin therapy: A review of the first five years' experience (review article). J Cardiothorac Vasc Anesth 6:76-100, 1992.
25. Stein PD, Dalen JE, Goldman S, et al: Antithrombotic therapy in patients with saphenous vein and internal mammary artery bypass grafts and following percutaneous transluminal coronary angioplasty. Chest 102:508S-515S, 1992.
26. Torosian M, Michelson EL, Morganroth J, MacVaugh H: Aspirin and coumadin-related bleeding after coronary-artery bypass graft surgery. Ann Intern Med 89:325-328, 1978.
27. Woodman RC, Harker LA: Bleeding complications associated with cardiopulmonary bypass (review article). Blood 76:1680-1697, 1990.

Chapter 23

Anticoagulants for Peripheral Vascular Disease

Hans Klaus Breddin, M.D., Piotr Radziwon, M.D., and Barbara Boczkowska-Radziwon, M.D.

The term anticoagulants is used for heparins and heparinlike drugs, for vitamin K antagonists, and for thrombin inhibitors such as hirudin. Acetylsalicylic acid (aspirin), used as an antithrombotic agent mainly in arterial disease, is discussed in this chapter only in comparison with anticoagulants in peripheral arterial diseases. In general, anticoagulants are used to prevent thrombotic vascular occlusions. An exception is the treatment of deep venous thrombosis with heparin, which may enhance the regression of thromboses.

Primary or prophylactic treatment with anticoagulants involves the identification of patients at risk of thromboembolism and the application of anticoagulants to prevent thromboembolic complications before they occur. Secondary treatment involves therapy for patients with existing thromboembolic disease in whom anticoagulants are used mainly to prevent the extension or recurrence of thromboses or their complications.

Warfarin and other vitamin K antagonists, which require several days to achieve their full effect, are used mainly for long-term outpatient treatment, most often after initial administration of heparin. Dose levels depend on the underlying thromboembolic risk. In special circumstances vitamin K antagonists are also administered for primary prophylaxis in hospitalized patients in place of low-dose heparin or low-molecular-weight heparins.

Heparin, vitamin K antagonists, and aspirin have been used in short-term trials to prevent new arterial occlusions in patients with peripheral occlusive arterial disease (POAD) and new thrombotic occlusions after successful revascularization. Which of these drugs should be used to prevent thromboses or rethromboses in a specified clinical setting remains open to debate.

Oral anticoagulants and aspirin have been compared in long-term studies for prevention of thrombotic reocclusions in patients with symptoms of POAD or after previous revascularization. In contrast with studies of coronary disease, these studies are small and inconclusive. The need for further investigations is obvious.

EARLY PREVENTION OF THROMBOSES WITH HEPARIN AFTER ACUTE ARTERIAL OCCLUSIONS OR ACUTE INTERVENTION

Heparin or low-molecular-weight heparins provide instant anticoagulation and must be administered parenterally; they are mainly used for short-term anticoagulation in hospitalized patients or in outpatients for a limited time.

Different dose regimens are used. Frequently 5000 IU of unfractionated heparin (UFH) are administered intravenously, followed by continuous infusion of 15–20 IU/kg/hr. In general, high-dose intravenous heparin is monitored by activated partial thromboplastin time (APTT) or thrombin time with the aim of achieving a prolongation 2–3 times the baseline values.[72] In principle, low-molecular-weight heparins can be administered subcutaneously for the same indications, but prospective trials in patients with POAD have not yet been published.

Heparin is frequently used after successful revascularization or after catheter dilatation to prevent thrombotic reocclusions. Heparin is also administered intravenously after embolectomy. Many reports but few clinical trials have proved the effectiveness of this form of heparin prophylaxis.

Prevention of Complications of Arterial Catheterization

Heparin has been used with and without protamine sulfate neutralization for the prevention of iatrogenic thromboembolic complications during and after catheter procedures in peripheral, carotid, and coronary arteries. Walker et al.[93] described the effective and safe prevention of thromboembolic complications by intravenous application of 3000–7000 IU of heparin during percutaneous coronary arteriography.

In a prospective study of 400 patients with transfemoral angiography, Antonovic et al.[5] observed two femoral arterial occlusions in the control group and no occlusions in the group treated with heparin. Major bleeding and minor hematoma were evenly divided between the two groups. Delayed bleeding occurred more frequently in the heparin group. The authors concluded that systemic heparinization confers benefit in transfemoral angiography.

Debrun et al.[25] investigated the effect of an infusion that contained heparin (250 IU/hr) and aspirin (250 mg/hr) in 57 consecutive patients undergoing diagnostic and interventional neuroradiology. They concluded that the combination was superior to a continuous heparin infusion for the prevention of thromboembolic complications. Similar results with heparin were reported by Girod et al.[34] Aspirin alone was not effective in a similar trial.[30]

Thus heparin may be used to prevent acute thromboses during angiography in patients at high risk of thrombolic complications because of either local or general thrombosis-promoting factors.

Surgical Management of Severe Lower-Extremity Ischemia

Lower-extremity ischemia can be caused by trauma, by embolism (mainly from a cardiac source), and by local thrombus formation at atherosclerotic plaques or after vascular surgery. Data on the frequency of embolization vary from 8%-85%.[28] The need for acute interventions depends on the cause of occlusion and even more on the condition of the extremity. A previously existing stenosis may have induced collateral formation, which may keep the limb viable even after total occlusion of the stenosis.

Many surgeons administer heparin to patients with acute critical ischemia to prevent thrombus propagation from the occlusion site. Retrospective data suggest that heparin followed by oral anticoagulation prevents recurrence after embolectomy.[28,50] Huber[51] recommended anticoagulation after operative desobliteration in patients with acute mesentery artery occlusions. Blaisdell et al.[8] advised high-dose heparin in addition to embolectomy, revascularization, or amputation in patients with acute lower-extremity arterial ischemia. Yeager et al.[96] operated on 74 patients with lower-extremity ischemia, of whom 7 were amputated, 42 received inflow reconstructions, 20 received outflow reconstructions, and 9 were treated by embolectomy. Of these patients, 86% received conventional doses of heparin with no bleeding and only minor reperfusion complications.

High-dose heparin treatment, in addition to early surgical repair, seems to be the treatment of choice in patients with acute lower-extremity arterial ischemia due to embolism and thrombosis. Close monitoring reduces bleeding complications.[21] The benefits of postoperative anticoagulation, however, have not been established in a prospective, randomized trial. Early preoperative heparinization probably reduces mortality in such patients.[8] Whether it increases the risks of bleeding or white-clot syndrome[19,50] should be established in future trials.

Dissection of the Internal Carotid Artery

Dissections of internal carotid arteries are not frequent. Such patients have a high rate of thromboembolic complications, and several authors have reported good results with heparin followed by a vitamin K antagonist for at least several months.[64,69,83] The patients received intravenous heparin for several days, followed by phenprocoumon and in some patients by aspirin.

Thus patients with internal carotid artery dissections diagnosed by angiography, computerized tomography, magnetic resonance imaging, and extracranial or transcranial Doppler sonography should be treated initially with intravenous heparin; some should also receive subsequent vitamin K-antagonist treatment for a maximum of 6 months.

Acute Arterial Occlusion

In patients with acute arterial occlusions thrombolytic treatment and/or surgical revascularization are the methods of choice. Heparin may be administered before and after surgical repair as well as before and after thrombolysis. After an initial bolus of 5000 IU/kg, intravenous infusion should be maintained at 15-20 IU/kg/hr with dosage adjustment according to APTT values.

Vitamin K antagonists play no major role in the prevention of acute reocclusions after successful reopening procedures. Aspirin also has been tried to prevent arterial reocclusions in such patients. Intraoperative anticoagulation with heparin is frequently used, but its benefit needs to be proved by controlled studies. A rational regimen may consist of a bolus of 5000 IU, followed initially by continuous infusion during the first days of treatment and subsequently by either oral anticoagulation or aspirin in patients with a high risk of reocclusion (e.g., after bypasses with prosthetic material, long bypasses to small arteries [infrapopliteal], complex reconstructions, and poor distal runoff).

Prevention of Acute Thrombotic Complications after Peripheral Percutaneous Transluminal Angioplasty

In one study of a large and probably representative patient population, the primary success rate of percutaneous transluminal angioplasty (PTA) was 82% in the iliac region and 74% in the ileofemoral region.[98] Most authors heparinize patients during femoropopliteal PTA, then institute prophylaxis with Coumadin or aspirin for 6–12 months. Heparinization may not be necessary in PTA of iliac arteries, but it is probably beneficial during and after PTA of the femoropopliteal region.[33,55,62,80,85,97]

Our patients with PTA of the femoropopliteal region receive heparin during the procedure and, if the procedure is successful, thereafter for 2–3 days as a continuous infusion of 10–15 IU/kg/hr. Prospective trials should clarify which treatment prevents early reocclusions in patients with different risks after successful PTA.

LONG-TERM PREVENTION OF THROMBOSES AND VASCULAR OCCLUSIONS

Heparin

Shulman et al.[78] presented animal and clinical evidence for the role of long-term, low-dose heparin in prevention of atherosclerosis but stressed the need for larger clinical trials. Mannarino et al.[63] recruited 44 patients with intermittent claudication for a randomized, double-blind, controlled study. Twenty-two patients were treated for 6 months with a single daily subcutaneous dose of 15,000 anti-Xa units of a low-molecular-weight heparin, and 22 received placebo. After 6 months low-molecular-weight heparin had improved walking capacity; however, this small study provided no proof of a direct reduction of vascular occlusions in the treatment group.

New trials are at present underway in patients after myocardial infarction or coronary angioplasty. The long-term prevention of new peripheral occlusions in patients with POAD by heparins and other glycosaminoglycans is also a worthwhile aim for future clinical trials.

Oral Anticoagulants: Vitamin K Antagonists, Aspirin, and Dipyridamole

In Patients with Peripheral Occlusive Arterial Disease

Whether treatment with vitamin K antagonists (usually warfarin or Coumadin) inhibits the progression of atherosclerotic lesions remains an open question because only a few small controlled clinical trials exist. Hess[45] showed that well-controlled, long-term anticoagulation significantly reduced vascular occlusions in patients with POAD. Burkhalter et al.[16] demonstrated that progression of vascular disease was minimally influenced, but during continuous anticoagulation with a vitamin K antagonist the number of new occlusions was reduced. A few relatively small trials[13,16,47] have demonstrated the effects of long-term treatment with vitamin K antagonists in patients with POAD, but further studies are necessary.

After Vascular Reconstructive Surgery

Several investigators have studied whether the reocclusion rate can be reduced by vitamin K antagonists after vascular surgery. Saggau[76] observed a reduced rate of reocclusions (19%) in a small group of patients compared with an untreated control group (27%). In this investigation the quality of anticoagulation seemed to have no effect on the outcome of treatment. After venous bypass operation Brunner et al.[14] and Waibel[91,92] reported a slightly superior patency rate (1-5 years postoperatively) with vitamin K antagonists in comparison with the combination of aspirin and dipyridamole.

Buda et al.[15] reported a slightly higher patency rate in patients with venous bypass or Dacron prostheses treated with oral anticoagulants 3 years postoperatively in comparison with an untreated cohort (52% vs. 47%). Holm and Schersten[50] observed reduced rates of amputation and mortality in patients who were treated at least 3 months with oral anticoagulants. In a recent randomized prospective trial with reversed saphenous vein femoropopliteal bypasses a significant reduction in bypass occlusions (18% in the treated group vs. 37% in the control group) was observed after a follow-up of 30 months.[56] These results are promising, but the beneficial effect on patency and survival should be confirmed by other trials before long-term oral anticoagulation can be generally recommended for patients undergoing femoropopliteal bypass surgery or other peripheral vascular operations. The risk-benefit ratio of oral anticoagulants compared with aspirin also has to be studied in further trials.

Some experimental studies suggest that antiplatelet treatment reduces neointimal hyperplasia.[41,65,66] This finding was corroborated by Bomberger et al.[10] The progressive narrowing of saphenous vein coronary grafts due to neointimal hyperplasia was not reduced by treatment with aspirin plus dipyridamole.[32]

The long-term studies on the effect of platelet function inhibitors and anticoagulants in patients undergoing vascular surgery are summarized in Table 1. Bollinger et al.[9] studied the rate of reocclusions after endarterectomy of the femoropopliteal segment in a prospective randomized study of 90 patients. A significant reduction in reocclusions was observed during the first 3 months with aspirin alone or together with dipyridamole. Patients in the control group received vitamin K antagonists.

Aspirin and dipyridamole reduce platelet adherence to polytetrafluoroethylene (PTFE) grafts[70] and to thrombendarterectomy sites[27] or atherosclerotic lesions.[79] Goldman[35] described a reduced platelet deposition on prosthetic femoropopliteal grafts in patients with venous grafts receiving aspirin alone or in combination with dipyridamole. In a double-blind, controlled trial with 428 patients, Ehresmann et al.[26] observed 11.2% postoperative occlusions in the aspirin-treated group compared with 20.2% in the placebo group 1 year after thrombarterectomy. This study strongly supports the benefit of aspirin after

TABLE 1. Clinical Trials of the Effect of Aspirin or Anticoagulation in Peripheral Occlusive Disease

Authors	Year	Drug	Dose (mg/d)	Control Group	Endpoint	No. on ASA	Patency Rate (%)	No. of Controls	Patency Rate (%)	Duration	p
Linke[60]	1975	ASA	1500	Placebo	New occlusion	50	68	50	44	3 yr	—
Zekert et al.[99]	1976	ASA	1500	Placebo	Reocclusion after vascular surgery	149	88	150	81	Wks	NS
Ehresmann et al.[26]	1977	ASA	1500	Placebo	Reocclusion rate after vascular surgery	215	53	213	47	1 yr	<0.03
Hess et al.[47]	1978	ASA	1500	Placebo	New occlusion	134	94	124	13.7	2 yr	<0.05
Brunner et al.[14]	1979	ASA + dipyridamole	1000 225	VKA	Reocclusion rate after bypass surgery	61	73	30	66	3 mo–2 yr	NS
Bollinger et al.[9]	1981	ASA + dipyridamole	1000 225	VKA	Reocclusion rate after thrombectomy	81	80	39	58	3 mo–2 yr	<0.02
Green et al.[36]	1982	ASA + dipyridamole ASA	975 225 975	Placebo	PTFE grafts above knee	9 10	100 100	9	50	1 yr	0.05
		ASA + dipyridamole ASA	975 225 975	Placebo	PTFE grafts below knee	9 6	19 65	8	21	1 yr	NS
Broomé et al.[11]	1982	ASA + dipyridamole	1000	Placebo	Thrombectomy	83	85	64	65	2 yr	<0.001
Albert et al.[1]	1982	ASA	1500	VKA	Patency rate after thrombendarteriectomy	37	86	28	93	2 yr	NS
Kohler et al.[54]	1984	ASA ASA + dipyridamole	1500 975 225	VKA Placebo	Patency rate after bypass surgery Patency rate	11 44	55 43	10 44	90 33	2 yr 2 yr	<0.05 NS
Hess et al.[46]	1985	ASA ASA + dipyridamole	990 990 225	Placebo	Score-system angiography	67 63	95.6 97.8	69	93.8	2 yr	<0.01
Clyne et al.[20]	1987	ASA + dipyridamole ASA + dipyridamole	300* 400 300 400	Placebo Placebo	Patency rate venous bypass Patency rate prosthetic bypass	49 29	83 85	44 26	72 53	1 yr 1 yr	NS 0.005
Kretschmer et al.[56]	1988	VKA	Controlled	No treatment	Cumulative survival after femoropopliteal vein bypass	60**	75.2	59	57	5 yr	<0.05

* Treatment period of 6 wk. ** Phenprocoumon.

ASA = aspirin; NS = not significant; VKA = vitamin K antagonist.

suboptimal reconstruction. Zekert et al.[99] came to a similar conclusion in 300 patients who were treated with aspirin or placebo after vascular surgery.

A small prospective trial in patients treated with dipyridamole and aspirin revealed a significant reduction of reocclusions after vascular reconstruction, whereas the reduction in patients treated with dipyridamole or aspirin alone was insignificant.[43] In a randomized, double-blind trial of patency rates of expanded PTFE grafts in the infrainguinal position, Green et al.[36] observed a significantly higher rate in the above-knee grafts of patients treated with aspirin or aspirin plus dipyridamole compared with placebo. The difference in patients with below-knee grafts was statistically insignificant, but even in these patients the patency rate was higher with aspirin or aspirin plus dipyridamole.

The conclusions reached in the reports on venous coronary bypass grafts cannot be directly extrapolated to bypass grafts in the peripheral arterial circulation. Five studies have shown a statistically significant reduction in vein bypass occlusion in treated patients.[82] However, other large, well-designed, randomized prospective trials have shown no benefit of antithrombotic treatment in maintaining early patency of venous aortofemoral bypass grafts. The main difference in the studies showing no benefit was that antithrombotic treatment was started 2-5 days after the operation. Thus early initiation of treatment may be an important factor. Lorenz et al.[61] showed a significant improvement in patency with aspirin alone. Brown et al.[12] found no difference in occlusion rates between groups treated with aspirin alone or aspirin plus dipyridamole. Although recently lower doses (100-300 mg/day) have been used, no optimal dose of aspirin has yet been established.

It is likely that aspirin treatment should begin as soon as possible after operation; unless contraindicated, it should even be started preoperatively.

Clinical Studies with Platelet Function Inhibitors in Peripheral Occlusive Arterial Disease

The mechanism by which aspirin is an antithrombotic agent is still not fully understood. Dipyridamole in the usually applied dosage of 3×75 mg/day inhibits platelet aggregation only for a short time and not in all patients. The antithrombotic effect of this agent, which has been demonstrated in animal models, may be explained by its inhibitory effect on platelet adhesion and platelet stimulation. Ticlopidine, a progressive inhibitor of platelet aggregation, probably inhibits the adenosine diphosphate (ADP) receptor for fibrinogen on the platelet surface.

Linke[60] reported the effect of aspirin in 100 diabetics with POAD who were observed for 3 years. Vascular occlusions were reduced from 20% in the placebo group to 7% in the aspirin-treated group. Hess[48] reported 258 patients who were observed for 2 years and randomized to receive either aspirin (1.5 g/day) or placebo. New peripheral arterial occlusions occurred with significantly less frequency in the treatment group (6%) than in the control group (13.7%).

In a controlled, double-blind trial Schoop[77] investigated 300 men with POAD who had occlusions of the femoral arteries. One hundred patients each received 3×330 mg of aspirin, 3×330 mg of aspirin plus 3×75 mg of dipyridamole, or placebo. After an observation period of 5 years with angiographic control after 2 years in the two treatment groups, new arterial occlusions occurred with significantly greater frequency in the group receiving placebo. Broomé et al.[11] reported that in patients with arterial reconstructions aspirin and dipyridamole, given for the first 6 postoperative months, significantly reduced the rates of thrombectomies; however, this was not a prospective, randomized trial.

In a small double-blind trial comparing ticlopidine and placebo in patients with POAD, Stiegler et al.,[84] using a new angiographic score system, observed a significant reduction of new vascular lesions in the treatment group. In a similar but larger trial Balsano et al.[6] described an improvement in walking distance in the ticlopidine-treated group. It is likely that ticlopidine reduced the thrombotic progression of atherosclerotic lesions. Larger trials in the area of POAD, however, are still needed.

Prevention of Reocclusions After Percutaneous Transluminal Angioplasty

Cunningham et al.[22] and Minar et al.[67] observed the inhibition of platelet deposits on angioplasty sites during the first days after angioplasty with aspirin treatment. When the primary success rate is taken as 100%, the 5-year results of PTA in femoropopliteal arteries show patency rates around 60%.[33,55,85] Krepel et al.[55] treated patients with either Coumadin or aspirin (80 mg/day) plus dipyridamole (3 × 75 mg/day) for 1 year after the procedure. Stokes et al.[85] used 81 mg of aspirin once daily for 6 months–1 year. Gallino[33] used phenprocoumon for 1 year in patients with femoral PTA and aspirin for 1 year in patients with iliac PTA. Freimann et al.[31] reported a 2-year patency rate of 75% after PTA of femoral arteries without anticoagulation.

In several studies the effect of aspirin was compared with either placebo or other anticoagulants after angioplasty (Table 2). The results of long-term aspirin prophylaxis in patients with POAD and in patients with vascular operations strongly suggest that aspirin improves the patency rate after femoropopliteal angioplasty. In a controlled trial of the early prevention of reocclusions by aspirin or vitamin K antagonists,[97] patients were observed for 10 days after PTA. After dilatation of the femoral artery patients received either aspirin (3 × 0.5 g) with vitamin K antagonists or vitamin K antagonists alone. The 10-day reocclusion rate was 16% in the aspirin-treated group, 21% in the group treated with aspirin and vitamin K antagonist, and 30% in the group treated with vitamin K antagonists alone.

In a similar small study[46] a higher patency rate was observed in patients receiving aspirin (900 mg) plus dipyridamole (225 mg) compared with patients who were treated with aspirin alone (Table 2). In a prospective double-blind trial Heiss et al.[44] observed a significant retardation of the progression of atherosclerotic lesions on repeat angiography 6 months after successful angioplasty in a group of patients receiving aspirin (990 mg/day) plus dipyridamole (225 mg/day) compared with placebo. The lower-dose regimen (300 mg aspirin plus 225 mg dipyridamole) was less effective (Table 2).

Recently different doses of aspirin have been compared in patients after angioplasty. Ranke et al.[73] found no difference in reocclusions between daily doses of 100 and 900 mg in a study of 359 patients after successful angioplasty. In a similar trial Weichert et al.[94] observed no difference in reocclusion rate in patients receiving either 300 or 1200 mg/day of aspirin after angioplasty.

TABLE 2. Clinical Trials of the Effect of Aspirin on the Reocclusion Rate After Peripheral Percutaneous Transluminal Angioplasty

Authors	Year	ASA Dose (mg/day)	No. on ASA	Occlusion Rate (%)	Control Group	No. of Controls	Occlusion Rate (%)	Duration	p
Zeitler[97]	1973	1500	87	4.6	VKA	19	21	10 days	<0.05
					VKA + ASA	90	6.7	10 days	—
Hess et al.[47]	1978	990	50	30	ASA 990 mg + 225 mg dipyridamole	50	16	14 days	<0.1
Heiss et al.[44]	1990	990 + 225 dipyridamole	66	51	Placebo	67	63	6 months	0.0
		300 + 225 dipyridamole	66	39					
Ranke et al.[73]	1992	900	175	15.1	ASA 50 mg/day	184	16.2	1 year	NS
Weichert et al.[94]	1993	1000	111	18	300	112	16	1 year	NS

ASA = aspirin; NS = not significant; VKA = vitamin K antagonist.

The rate of side effects did not differ between the two dosage groups in either trial (Table 2).

Cardiogenic Embolism

Cardiogenic embolism, which accounts for more than 150,000 strokes/year in the United States, is a major public health problem. The main causes of cardiogenic embolism are nonvalvular atrial fibrillation (45%), ischemic heart disease (25%), chronic valvular disease (10%), and prosthetic valve replacement (10%).[42,72]

In patients at risk for cardiogenic embolism, prophylaxis mostly involves long-term Coumadin treatment. The exceptions are patients with acute myocardial infarction, prosthetic valve(s), or fresh intracardial thrombi. Patients with large myocardial infarctions and significant left ventricular dysfunction and rhythmic abnormalities should be treated with a short course of either intravenous[74,81,87] or high-dose (12,500 IU twice daily) subcutaneous[86,89] heparin. All patients with mechanical valves, as well as patients with bioprosthetic and mitral valve replacements,[18,24,81] are treated initially with intravenous heparin, followed by long-term treatment with a vitamin K antagonist. A slightly less intensive anticoagulation (INR: 2.0-2.25) was as effective as more intensive treatment (INR: 2.5-4.0).[88] Treatment with intravenous heparin is optional in patients after bioprosthetic valve replacements but should be considered if additional risk factors are present (e.g., an associated mitral disease).[18,81] This approach has been reviewed by Harrington and Ansell.[42]

A combination of oral anticoagulation with aspirin was first successfully used by Dale et al.[23] in a prospective trial. In another trial the combination of Coumadin and aspirin (500 mg/day) increased the frequency of excessive bleeding; a trend toward reduced thromboembolism favored a combination of warfarin and dipyridamole (400 mg/day).[17] In comparison with platelet function inhibitor combinations warfarin was clearly superior in preventing thromboembolic episodes in similar patients.[68]

SIDE EFFECTS OF ANTICOAGULANTS AND ASPIRIN

Heparins

Hemorrhage

Spontaneous hemorrhage is rare if the APTT is within the therapeutic range. The hemorrhagic risk increases with excessive prolongation of the APTT, but the risk of bleeding is also modified by other factors such as recent surgery, presence of gastrointestinal ulcers, malignancy, advanced age, underlying defects in platelet function or coagulation, and other drug therapy (e.g., aspirin).

Heparin-induced Thrombocytopenia

Heparin-induced thrombocytopenia (HIT) was observed as early as 1948.[29] Its increasingly frequent combination with thromboses was described in 1973,[75] and during the last 10 years many case reports and reviews have been published on this complication. In a prospective study 1 of 54 patients treated with bovine and 2 of 50 patients treated with porcine heparin developed HIT type I.[4] HIT is probably the most frequent drug-induced thrombocytopenia.[3,7,52,53,57,59,71] The risk of HIT seems to increase with the duration of heparin administration.

HIT has been seen with standard heparins, low-molecular-weight heparins, and heparinlike molecules after intravenous or subcutaneous administration. The occurrence is not dose-dependent; HIT has been observed even after administration of very low heparin concentrations to prevent occlusions of intravenous catheters and with heparin-coated catheters.[58]

HIT Type I. In HIT type I the platelet count is reduced early after the onset of treatment (1-3 days). The platelet count rarely decreases to values lower than $100,000/\mu l$. Thromboembolic complications do not occur, and the platelet count normalizes even if heparin is continued.

HIT Type II (White Clot Syndrome). HIT type II is seen usually 7-20 days or even later after the start of heparin treatment. In patients with previous exposure to heparin it may occur a few hours after reexposure. Platelet counts drop to values below $100,000/\mu l$ but rarely below $10,000/\mu l$. They normalize only if heparin administration is discontinued. Bleeding complications are rare, but the patients are at a high risk for new venous and arterial occlusions even if platelet counts are low. The incidence rate of HIT type I probably lies between 3-30% and for HIT type II between 0.1-5%. These estimates may be too high.

The grade of sulfation of different oligosaccharides seems to be correlated with cross-reactivity in serum of patients with HIT type II.[37] Thus HIT type II apparently is not caused by a heparin-specific antibody. HIT type II may be associated with the formation of antibodies that bind to a neoantigen on the platelet surface or to a platelet membrane-heparin complex. Newer trials strongly suggest that a heparin-antiheparin IgG complex activates platelets via a receptor for IgG that leads to their destruction. Amiral et al.[2] recently reported that the platelet component reacting with the antibody is platelet factor 4. A heparin-specific antibody or specific antigen on the platelet surface has not yet been detected. Several methods have been described to detect the antibodies; the most frequently used are platelet aggregation tests with higher diluted plasma.[38,59,95] The tests used to detect antibodies may become negative within weeks.[57]

If HIT type II is suspected, heparin treatment should be discontinued, and if antibodies can be detected, treatment with other heparins or low-molecular-weight heparins should be considered only if no cross-reaction[90] is seen with in vitro testing. Good results have been described if patients are treated with the heparan-dermatan preparation, Organon 10172. Cross-reactions with this agent seem to be rare.[39] The risk of HIT type II can be reduced if, in all patients treated with heparin, platelets are counted preferably twice weekly, but at least once per week.

Hypersensitivity

Hypersensitivity reactions are rare, but skin reactions, such as urticaria, and local allergic reactions with skin necroses have been reported.

Osteoporosis

Clinically significant osteoporosis is a rare complication of long-term heparinization (>6 months).

Vitamin K Antagonists

Bleeding, a frequent side effect of treatment with vitamin K antagonists, is directly connected to their pharmacologic effects. The risk of bleeding increases with increasing intensity of treatment. Common bleeding locations include the urinary tract, the gastrointestinal tract, and, less frequently, the central nervous system.

Coumarin derivatives should not be administered to pregnant women because of the high risk of a fetal warfarin syndrome. Multiple interactions with other drugs are described elsewhere.[40,49]

Gastrointestinal complaints are relatively rare. A severe complication is the cutaneous necrosis that occurs in about 0.1% of patients treated with coumarins. Coumarin necroses have been associated with defects in protein C. This complication, however, occurs in only a portion of affected patients. Several of our patients developed skin necrosis when receiving antibiotics with vitamin K antagonists, without an additional protein C deficiency. A reduced starting dose of vitamin K antagonists is likely to reduce the risk of skin necrosis.

CONCLUSION

Anticoagulants and platelet function inhibitors are frequently used to prevent both local vascular occlusions at an already affected vascular area and peripheral thromboembolism. For some indications, such as prosthetic heart valves, the advantage of continuous oral anticoagulation is clear. For others, such as prevention of new occlusions in patients with POAD and reocclusions after vascular surgery or successful PTA, anticoagulants and platelet function inhibitors have been found to be of some value. New studies, however, are urgently needed to define which agents are optimal for a specific indication. The hypothesis that heparin and heparinlike structures reduce atherosclerosis will be studied in the future. At present clinical trials provide no validation for this treatment. New antithrombotic agents, such as hirudin and other thrombin inhibitors as well as inhibitors of platelet glycoproteins, may prove in the near future to be better drugs for prevention of vascular occlusions.

REFERENCES

1. Albert JP, Regensburger D, Rudolf I, et al: Rezidivprophylaxe operativ korrigierter Arterienverschlüsse der unteren Extremitäten. Med Welt 33:1829-1831, 1982.
2. Amiral J, Bridey F, Dreyfus M, et al: Platelet factor 4 complexed to heparin is the target for antibodies generated in heparin-induced thrombocytopenia. Thromb Haemost 68:95-96, 1992.
3. Ansell JE, Deykin D: Heparin-induced thrombocytopenia and recurrent thromboembolism. Am J Hematol 8:325-332, 1980.
4. Ansell JE, Price JM, Shah S, Beckner RR: Heparin-induced thrombocytopenia: What is its real frequency? Chest 88:878-883, 1985.
5. Antonovic R, Rösch J, Dotter CT: The value of systemic arterial heparinization in transfemoral angiography: A prospective study. Am J Roentgenol 127:223-225, 1976.
6. Balsano F, Coccheri S, Libretti A, et al: Ticlopidine in the treatment of intermittent claudication: A 21-month double-blind trial. J Lab Clin Med 114:84-91, 1989.
7. Bell WR: Heparin-associated thrombocytopenia and thrombosis. J Lab Clin Med 111:600-605, 1988.
8. Blaisdell FW, Steele M, Allen RE: Management of acute lower extremity arterial ischemia due to embolism and thrombosis. Surgery 84:822-834, 1978.
9. Bollinger A, Schneider E, Pouliadis G, et al: Thrombozytenfunktionshemmer und Antikoagulantien nach gefäßrekonstruktiven Eingriffen im femoro-poplitealen Bereich. In Breddin K (ed): Thrombose und Atherogenese. Pathophysiologie und Therapie der arteriellen Verschlußkrankheit; Bein-Beckenvenen-Thrombose. Baden-Baden, Witzstrock, 1981, pp 276-279.
10. Bomberger RA, DePalma RJ, Ambrose TA, Manalo P: Aspirin and dipyridamole inhibit endothelial healing. Arch Surg 117:1459-1464, 1982.
11. Broomé A, Davidsson T, Eklöf B, Hansson L: Effect of platelet aggregation inhibitors on the rate of thrombectomy following arterial reconstructions with Gore-Tex prostheses: A retrospective study. Vasa 11:210-212, 1982.
12. Brown BG, Cukingnan RA, DeRouen T, et al: Improved graft patency in patients treated with platelet inhibiting therapy after coronary bypass surgery. Circulation 90:373-377, 1985.
13. Bruhn HD, Jipp P, Schellmann J, et al: Zur Antikoagulantienprophylaxe bei chirurgischer und konservativer Therapie chronischer Becken-Bein-Arterienverschlüsse. Med Klinik 67:1514-1519, 1972.
14. Brunner U, Bollinger A, Schneider E, Witschi B: Endarteriektomie und autologer Venenbypass: Rezidivprophylaxe mit Aggregationshemmern und Antikoagulantien. In Wagener O, Kubina VK (eds): Der Rezidivverschluß nach Gefäßkonstruktionen an der unteren Extremität. Wien, Egermann, 1979, pp 99-107.
15. Buda JA, Weber CJ, McAllister EF, Voorhees AB: Factors influencing patency of femoropopliteal artery bypass grafts. Am J Surg :8-12, 1970.
16. Burkhalter A, Widmer LK, Glans L: Chronischer Gliedmaßenverschluß und Langzeitantikoagulation. Vasa 3:185-189, 1974.
17. Chesebro JH, Fuster V, Elveback CR, et al: Trial of combined warfarin plus dipyridamole or aspirin therapy in prosthetic heart valve replacement. Danger of aspirin compared with dipyridamole. Am J Cardiol 51:1537-1541, 1983.
18. Chesebro JH, Adams PC, Fuster V: Antithrombotic therapy in patients with valvular heart disease and prosthetic heart valves. J Am Coll Cardiol 8:41B-56B, 1986.
19. Clagett GP, Genton E, Salzman EW: Antithrombotic therapy in peripheral vascular disease. Chest 95:128S-139S, 1989.

20. Clyne CAC, Archer TJ, Atuhaire LK, et al: Random control trial of a short course of aspirin and dipyridamole (Persantine) for femorodistal grafts. Br J Surg 74:246-248, 1987.
21. Collins GJ, Rich NM, Clagett GP, et al: Heparin: Efficacy and safety after arterial operations. Arch Surg 116:1077, 1981.
22. Cunningham DA, Kumar B, Siegel BA, et al: Aspirin inhibition of platelet deposition of angioplasty sites: Demonstration by platelet scintigraphy. Radiology 151:487-490, 1984.
23. Dale J, Myhre E, Storstein O, et al: Prevention of arterial thromboembolism with acetylsalicylic acid. Am Heart J 94:101-111, 1977.
24. Dalen JE: Valvular heart disease, infected valves and prosthetic heart valves. Am J Cardiol 65:29C-31C, 1990.
25. Debrun GM, Vinuela FV, Fox AJ: Aspirin and systemic heparinization in diagnostic and interventional neuroradiology. AJNR 3:337-340, 1982.
26. Ehresmann U, Alemany J, Loew D: Prophylaxe von Rezidivverschlüssen nach Revaskularisationseingriffen mit Acetylsalicylsäure. Med Welt 28:1157-1162, 1977.
27. Ehringer H, Marosi L, Schöfl R: Reduction of thrombotic layers on the new inner vessel wall following thrombendarterectomy (TEA) of the carotid artery by means of ASA (1.0 g/day) treatment. In Maurer CP, Becker HM, Heidrich H, et al (eds): What is New in Angiology? Trends and Controversies. München, W. Zuckschwerdt Verlag, 1986, pp 298-300.
28. Elliott JP, Hageman JH, Szilagyi E: Arterial embolization: Problems of source, multiplicity, recurrence and delayed treatments. Surgery 88:833, 1980.
29. Fidlar E, Jaques LB: The effect of commercial heparin on the platelet count. J Lab Clin Med 33:1410-1414, 1948.
30. Freed MD, Rosenthal A, Fyler D: Attempts to reduce arterial thrombosis after cardiac catheterization in children: Use of percutaneous technique and aspirin. Am Heart J 87:283-286, 1974.
31. Freimann DB, Spence R, Gatenby R, et al: Transluminal angioplasty of the iliac and femoral arteries: Results without anticoagulation. Radiology 141:437-450, 1981.
32. Fuster V, Chesebro JH: Role of platelets and platelet inhibitors in aortocoronary vein graft disease. Circulation 73:227-232, 1986.
33. Gallino A, Mahler F, Probst P, Nachbur B: Percutaneous transluminal angioplasty of the arteries of the lower limbs. A 5-year follow-up. Circulation 70:619-623, 1984.
34. Girod DA, Horwitz RA, Caldwell RL: Heparinization for prevention of thromboses following pediatric percutaneous arterial catheterization. Pediatr Cardiol 3:175-179, 1982.
35. Goldman MD, Simpson D, Hawker RJ, et al: Aspirin and dipyridamole reduce platelet deposition on prosthetic femoro-popliteal grafts in man. Ann Surg 198:713-716, 1983.
36. Green RM, Roedersheimer RL, DeWeese JA: Effects of aspirin and dipyridamole on expanded polytetrafluorethylene graft patency. Surgery 92:1016-1026, 1982.
37. Greinacher A, Michels I, Müller-Eckhardt C: Heparin-associated thrombocytopenia: The antibody is not heparin specific. Thromb Haemost 67:545-549, 1992.
38. Greinacher A, Müller-Eckhardt C: Diagnostik der Heparin-assoziierten Thrombozytopenie. Dtsch Med Wschr 116:1479-1482, 1991.
39. Greinacher A, Müller-Eckhardt C: Therapie der Heparin-assoziierten Thrombozytopenie. Dtsch Med Wschr 116:1483-1484, 1991.
40. Griffin JP, Darcy PF, Speirs CJ: A Manual of Adverse Drug Interactions. London, Wright, 1988, pp 139-158.
41. Hagen PO, Wang ZG, Mikat EM, Hackel B: Antiplatelet therapy reduces aortic intimal hyperplasia distal to small diameter vascular prostheses (PTFE) in non-human primates. Ann Surg 195:328-343, 1982.
42. Harrington R, Ansell J: Risk-benefit assessment of anticoagulant therapy. Drug Saf 6:54-69, 1991.
43. Harjola PT, Meurala H, Frick MH: Prevention of early reocclusion by dipyridamole and ASA in arterial reconstructive surgery. Cardiovasc Surg 22:141-144, 1981.
44. Heiss HW, Just H, Middleton D, Deichsel G: Reocclusion prophylaxis with dipyridamole combined with acetylsalicylic acid following PTA. Angiology 41:263-269, 1990.
45. Hess H: Die Antikoagulantien- und Fibrinolysebehandlung bei arteriellen Gefäß verschlüssen. Therapiewoche 17:1617-1619, 1967.
46. Hess H, Mietaschk A, Deichsel G: Drug-induced inhibition of platelet function delays progression of peripheral occlusive arterial disease. Lancet 1:415-419, 1985.
47. Hess H, Müller-Fassbender H, Ingrisch H, Mietaschk A: Verhütung von Wiederverschlüssen nach Rekanalisation obliterativer Arterien mit der Kathetermethode. Dtsch Med Wschr 103:1994-1997, 1978.

48. Hess H, Keil-Kuri E: Theoretische Grundlagen der Prophylaxe obliterierender Arteriopathien mit Aggregationshemmer und Ergebnisse einer Langzeitstudie mit ASS (Colfarit). In Marx R, Breddin HK (eds): Colfarit-Symposium III. Köln, Bayer, 1975, pp 80-87.
49. Hirsh J: Oral anticoagulant drugs. N Engl J Med 324:1865-1873, 1990.
50. Holm J, Schersten T: Anticoagulant treatment during and after embolectomy. Acta Chir Scand 138:68, 1972.
51. Huber FB: Zur Therapie des akuten Mesenterialarterienverschlusses. Thoraxchirurgie-Vaskuläre Chirurgie 18:137-145, 1970.
52. Kelton JG: Heparin-induced thrombocytopenia. Hemostasis 16:173-186, 1986.
53. Kirchmaier CM, Bender N: Heparin-induzierte Thrombopenie mit arterieller und venöser Thrombose. Inn Med 15:174-178, 1988.
54. Kohler TR, Kaufmann IL, Kacoyanis G, et al: Effect of aspirin and dipyridamole on the patency of lower extremity bypass grafts. Surgery 96:462-466, 1984.
55. Krepel VM, van Andel GJ, van Erp WFM, Breslau PJ: Percutaneous transluminal angioplasty of the femoropopliteal artery: Initial and long term results. Radiology 156:325-328, 1985.
56. Kretschmer G, Schemper M, Ehringer H, et al: Influence of postoperative anticoagulant treatment on patient survival after femoro-popliteal vein bypass surgery. Lancet 1:797-799, 1988.
57. Laster J, Cikrit D, Walker N, Silver D: The heparin-induced thrombocytopenia syndrome: An update. Surgery 102:763-770, 1987.
58. Laster J, Nichols K, Silver D: Thrombocytopenia associated with heparin-coated catheters in patients with heparin-associated antiplatelet antibodies. Arch Intern Med 149:2285-2287, 1989.
59. Linde N, Tsakiris A, Vogt A, Marbet GA: Heparin-induzierte Thrombozytopenie. Perspektiven in einem therapeutischen Dilemma. Vasa 20:157-163, 1991.
60. Linke H: Langzeitprophylaxe mit ASS (Colfarit) bei arteriellen Angiopathien, insbesondere bei der Angiopathia diabetica. In Marx R, Breddin HK (eds): Colfarit Symposium III. Köln, Bayer, 1975, pp 88-103.
61. Lorenz RL, Schacky CV, Weber M, et al: Improved aortocoronary bypass patency by low dose aspirin effects on platelet aggregation and thromboxane formation. Lancet 1:1261-1264, 1984.
62. Mahler F, Nachbur B, Probst P: Die perkutane Katheterbehandlung arterieller Stenosen und Verschlüsse der unteren Extremitäten. Schweiz Rundschau für Medizin (Praxis) 68:1250-1253, 1979.
63. Mannarino E, Pasqualini L, Innocente S, et al: Efficacy of low-molecular-weight heparin in the management of intermittent claudication. Angiology 42:1-7, 1991.
64. Marx A, Messing B, Storch B, Busse O: Spontane Dissektionen hirnversorgender Arterien. Nervenarzt 58:8-18, 1987.
65. McCann RL, Hagen PO, Fuchs JCA: Aspirin and dipyridamole decrease intimal hyperplasia in experimental vein grafts. Ann Surg 191:238-243, 1980.
66. Metke MP, Lie JT, Fuster V, Kaye JM: Reduction of intimal thickening in canine coronary bypass vein grafts with dipyridamole and aspirin. Am J Cardiol 43:1144-1148, 1979.
67. Minar E, Ehringer H, Ahmadi R, et al: Platelet deposition at angioplasty sites and platelet survival time after PTA in iliac and femoral arteries: Investigations with indium-111-oxine labelled platelets in patients with ASA (1.0 g/day)-therapy. Thromb Haemost 58:718-723, 1987.
68. Mok CK, Bocy BS, Wang R, et al: Warfarin versus dipyridamole-aspirin and pentoxifylline-aspirin for the prevention of prosthetic heart valve thromboembolism: A prospective randomized clinical trial. Circulation 72:1059-1063, 1985.
69. Müllges W, Ringelstein EB, Weiller C, et al: Dissektionen der A. carotis interna—neue diagnostische und pathogenetische Aspekte. Fortschr Neurol Psychiat 59:12-24, 1991.
70. Oblath RW, Buckley FO, Green RM, et al: Prevention of platelet aggregation and adherence to prosthetic vascular grafts by aspirin and dipyridamole. Surgery 84:37-44, 1978.
71. Ockelford P: Heparin 1986: Indications and effective use. Drugs 31:81-92, 1986.
72. Petersen TR: Thromboembolic complications of atrial fibrillation and their prevention: A review. Am J Cardiol 65:246-280, 1990.
73. Ranke C, Creutzig A, Luska G, et al: Controlled trial of high versus low dose aspirin treatment after percutaneous transluminal angioplasty in patients with peripheral vascular disease. Lancet 1993 (in press).
74. Resnekov L, Chediak J, Hirsh J, Lewis D: Antithrombotic agents in coronary artery disease. Chest 95:52S-72S, 1989.
75. Rhodes GR, Dixon RH, Silver D: Heparin-induced thrombocytopenia with thrombotic and hemorrhagic manifestations. Surg Gynecol Obstet 136:409-416, 1973.

76. Saggau W: Antikoagulantientherapie in der Gefäßchirurgie. In Marx R, Thies HL (eds): Klinische und ambulante Anwendung klassischer Antikoagulantien. Stuttgart, Schattauer, 1977, pp 171-176.
77. Schoop W: Prognose und Prophylaxe der peripheren arteriellen Verschlußkrankheit. In Trübestein C (ed): Arterielle Verschlußkrankheit und tiefe Beinvenenthrombose. Stuttgart, G. Thieme Verlag, 1984, pp 172-176.
78. Shulman AG: Heparin and atherosclerosis: An investigative report on the treatment of atherosclerosis. Biomed Parhamcother 44:303-306, 1990.
79. Sinzinger H, O'Grady J, Fitscha P: Platelet deposition on human atherosclerotic lesions is decreased by low-dose aspirin in combination with dipyridamole. J Int Med Res 16:39-43, 1988.
80. Spencer K, Freiman DB, Gotenby R, et al: Long term results of transluminal angioplasty of the iliac and femoral arteries. Arch Surg 116:1377-1386, 1981.
81. Stein B, Fuster V: Antithrombotic therapy in acute myocardial infarction: Prevention of venous, left ventricular and coronary artery thromboembolism. Am J Cardiol 64:33B-40B, 1989.
82. Stein PD, Kantrowitz A: Antithrombotic therapy in mechanical and biological prosthetic heart valves and saphenous vein bypass grafts. Chest 95:107S-117S, 1989.
83. Steinke W, Aulich A, Hennerici M: Diagnose und Verlauf von Carotisdissektionen. Dtsch Med Wschr 114:1869-1875, 1989.
84. Stiegler H, Hess H, Mietasch K, et al: Einfluß von Ticlopidin auf die periphere obliterierende Arteriopathie. Dtsch Med Wschr 109:1240-1243, 1984.
85. Stokes KR, Strunk HM, Campbell DR, et al: Five year results of iliac and femoropopliteal angioplasty in diabetic persons. Radiology 174:977-982, 1990.
86. Tarazzi L: Heparin in acute myocardial infarction. Hemostasis 20:122-128, 1990.
87. Turpie AGG: Anticoagulant therapy after acute myocardial infarction. Am J Cardiol 65:20C-23C, 1990.
88. Turpie AGG, Gunstensen J, Hirsh H, et al: Randomised comparison of two intensities of oral anticoagulant therapy after tissue heart valve replacement. Lancet 1:1242-1245, 1988.
89. Turpie AGG, Robinson JG, Doyle DJ, et al: Comparison of high-dose with low-dose subcutaneous heparin to prevent left ventricular mural thrombosis in patients with acute transmural anterior myocardial infarction. N Engl J Med 320:352-357, 1989.
90. Vitoux JF, Matieu JF, Roncato M, et al: Heparin-associated thrombocytopenia treatment with low molecular weight heparin. Thromb Haemost 55:37-39, 1985.
91. Waibel P: The value of anticoagulation in arterial reconstruction. Vasa 8:121, 1979.
92. Waibel P, Geering P: Spätresultate bei Rekonstruktionen wegen Verschlußkrankheit der unteren Extremität. Vasa 10:308-309, 1981.
93. Walker JW, Mundall SL, Broderick HG, et al: Systemic heparinization for femoral percutaneous coronary arteriography. N Engl J Med 288:826-830, 1973.
94. Weichert W, Meentz H, Abt K, et al: Acetylsalicylic acid: Reocclusion-prophylaxis after angioplasty (ARPA-study). A randomized controlled trial of different dosages of ASA in patients with peripheral occlusive arterial disease. Vasa 1993 (in press).
95. Wolf II, Nowack H, Wick G: Detection of antibodies interacting with glycosaminoglycan polysulfate in patients treated with heparin or other polysulfated glycosaminoglycans. Int Arch Allerg Appl Immunol 70:157-163, 1983.
96. Yeager RA, Moneta GL, Taylor LM, et al: Surgical management of severe acute lower extremity ischemia. J Vasc Surg 15:385-393, 1992.
97. Zeitler E, Reichold J, Schoop W, Loew D: Einfluß von Acetylsalicylsäure auf das Frühergebnis nach perkutaner Rekanalisation arterieller Obliterationen nach Dotter. Dtsch Med Wschr 98:1285-1288, 1973.
98. Zeitler E, Richter E, Roth FJ, Schoop W: Results of percutaneous transluminal angioplasty. Radiology 146:57-60, 1983.
99. Zekert F, Kohn P, Vormittag E, Piza F, Thien W: Zur Acetylsalicylsäure prophylaxe von sofort verschluessen nach gefaesschirurgischen Eingriffen. In Marx R, Breddin (eds): Colfarit Symposium III. Bayer, 1975, pp 109-119.

Chapter 24

Potential Use of New Thrombin Inhibitors and Low-molecular-weight Heparins as Anticoagulants in Cardiopulmonary Bypass Surgery

Jeanine M. Walenga, Ph.D., Michael J. Koza, B.S., MT(ASCP), and Roque Pifarré, M.D.

Cardiopulmonary bypass (CPB) surgery requires a high level of anticoagulation to keep the extracorporeal circuit free of blood clots. Although heparin has been the only anticoagulant of choice for this indication, disadvantages of its use include lot-to-lot variations in potency as well as variations in patient response. Heparin may also cause thrombocytopenia, arterial thrombosis, platelet dysfunction, and severe bleeding.[8,16] In other patients a deficiency of antithrombin III may render heparin ineffective, or heparin rebound may occur, causing postoperative bleeding.[17] Furthermore, the use of protamine to neutralize heparin after CPB can also be associated with side effects such as hypotension, anaphylaxis, respiratory compromise, and shock.[12] Thus an alternative anticoagulant would be useful.

The low-molecular-weight (LMW) heparins, which are derived from a depolymerization of standard heparin, retain the activities of heparin but in varying proportions. The advantages of LMW heparins include a better defined structure,[3] varying biological/chemical properties[6] that may lead to decreased bleeding potential and fewer platelet interactions, and a decreased probability of heparin-induced thrombocytopenia. Studies are needed to confirm these assumptions. LMW heparins have proved antithrombotic effects in animal models and in humans when used prophylactically to reduce postoperative thrombosis.[6,10,20] Previous studies, however, have produced conflicting results in evaluating LMW heparin and a heparinoid as anticoagulants in CPB surgery.[1,7,9,14,16,18,19]

Peptide inhibitors of serine proteases for coagulation proteins have been under development for many years.[4,5] The primary enzyme of the coagulation system in terms of kinetics is thrombin. Thrombin is also the final product of the activated coagulation cascade, which directly converts fibrinogen to fibrin (clot). It is, therefore, reasonable to consider specific thrombin inhibitors as anticoagulants. Different types of thrombin inhibitors, such as hirudin (derived from the leech) and oligopeptides, have been shown to be potent antithrombotic agents.[2,11,13,15] Thrombin inhibitors have four advantages over heparin: (1) they are a pure material of one chemical structure; (2) they have a single mechanism of action (thrombin inhibition), as opposed to multiple sites of activity (coagulation enzymes, platelets, fibrinolysis) for heparin; (3) they are independent of antithrombin III for expression of activity; and (4) their short half-life may negate the need to neutralize anticoagulant activity.

We have evaluated two synthetic peptide inhibitors of thrombin (a recombinant hirudin and a boroarginine peptide) as well as a LMW heparin for use in CPB surgery. In vitro and in vivo evaluation of thrombosis in animal models have shown all three to be active antithrombotic agents. This chapter describes our results from a canine model of CPB surgery in which each of the three agents was used as an anticoagulant.

MATERIALS AND METHODS

Cardiopulmonary Bypass Model

Male mongrel dogs (average weight: 28 kg) were anesthetized intravenously with pentobarbital (30 mg/kg), intubated, and ventilated to 3 cm peak end-expiratory pressure (PEEP). Vascular access lines and a drip injection of lactated Ringer's solution were established. After midsternal thoracotomy CPB was immediately initiated with cannulation through the right atrial appendage and ascending aorta (70 ml/kg flow; 55-70 mmHg mean arterial pressure [MAP]) by means of a Travenol pump (Travenol Labs, Ann Arbor, MI) and a variable prime Cobe membrane lung blood oxygenator (Cobe, Lakewood, CO) with surgical grade Tygon S-50-HL tubing and EC-3840 Pall blood filters. CPB was continued for exactly 60 minutes and followed by an observation period of 120 minutes.

Blood pressure, heart rate, hemodynamics, and blood gases were monitored. Measurements included hematocrit value (manual method); platelet count (manual); level of fibrinogen (Clauss method, Dade, Miami, FL); celite activated clotting time (ACT) (International Technidyne, Edison, NJ); an in-house kinetic rate assay of chromogenic substrate anti-factor IIa (thrombin) specific for measuring the inhibition of thrombin (performed on both plasma and urine); the bleeding time test (Simplate, Organon Teknika, Durham, NC), performed on the gingiva; complete blood counts; and leukocyte differentials.

For assessment of efficacy of anticoagulation, pumpline filters were collected, washed with saline (1.0 L) and dried by forced air. Deposits (clots) were measured by the Folin-Ciocalteu assay for fibrinogen and protein. Tissue samples of liver, lung, heart, spleen, adrenal gland, and kidney were preserved in formalin and examined for microthrombi. For assessment of safety, blood loss was measured by weight of aspirated blood collected from the chest cavity during the postoperative observation period. The amount of blood oozing from tissues and cut surfaces intra- and postoperatively was also recorded.

The studies were conducted in the Animal Research Facilities of Hines Veterans Affairs Hospital (Hines, IL), which is accredited by the American Association for the Accreditation of Laboratory Animal Care (AALAC).

Anticoagulants

Four separate protocols were used for anticoagulation:

1. Heparin was administered as a single bolus into the right atrial space at 2.5 mg/kg (250 U/kg). During the pump run approximately 0.15 mg/kg was injected to maintain the ACT at 350 seconds (the bolus heparin ACT response). Protamine sulfate was administered at 2.5 mg/kg at the end of the pump run.

2. r-Hirudin, obtained from Transgene-Sanofi (Paris, France) (lot no. RHE15) and Knoll AG (Ludwigshafen, Germany) (lot no. 00300), is a recombinant derived peptide which specifically inhibits thrombin. The original hirudin was isolated from the leech *Hirudo medicinalis*. r-Hirudin was administered as a bolus (1.5 mg/kg) plus an infusion into the femoral artery (1.5 mg/kg/hr) during the pump run. No antagonist was used to reverse the anticoagulant effect after the pump run.

3. DuP 714 (lot no. 21), a boroarginine peptide obtained from duPont-Merck (Wilmington, DE), is a specific inhibitor of thrombin with slight factor Xa and kallikrein inhibitory activity.[11] This agent was administered as a bolus (0.25 mg/kg) plus an infusion via the femoral artery (0.50 mg/kg/hr) during the pump run. No antagonist was used to reverse the anticoagulant effect after the pump run.

4. The low-molecular-weight heparin (lot no. 341169) obtained from Sandoz AG (Nürnberg, Germany), is a fraction of standard heparin produced by a chemical depolymerization using isoamyl nitrate in an acidic medium that cleaves the larger-molecular-weight components into smaller ones (mean molecular weight: 6,000 daltons). The anti-Xa activity is approximately 95 U/mg; the anti-IIa activity is approximately 50 U/mg. Therefore, the anti-Xa:anti-IIa ratio is 2:1, whereas heparin has a ratio of 1:1. The LMW heparin was administered as a bolus at 3.0 mg/kg and supplemented with injections (0.15 mg/kg) to maintain the ACT at 200 seconds (the ACT response of bolus LMW heparin) during the pump run. Protamine sulfate (3.0 mg/kg) was given at the end of the pump run.

RESULTS

The LMW heparin, r-hirudin and DuP 714 groups show no difference in efficacy of anticoagulation, as measured by the deposits in the pumpline filter (Fig. 1). A trend toward slightly more deposits with the new anticoagulants was not significant in comparison with heparin.

The safety of anticoagulation as measured by postoperative blood loss revealed no difference between the three new agents and heparin (Fig. 2). Blood oozing from the cut surfaces (sternum and muscles at the femoral cutdown sites for catheter insertion), however, was much more pronounced and longer-lasting with the LMW heparin than with heparin, whereas the surgical fields were dry with r-hirudin and DuP 714.

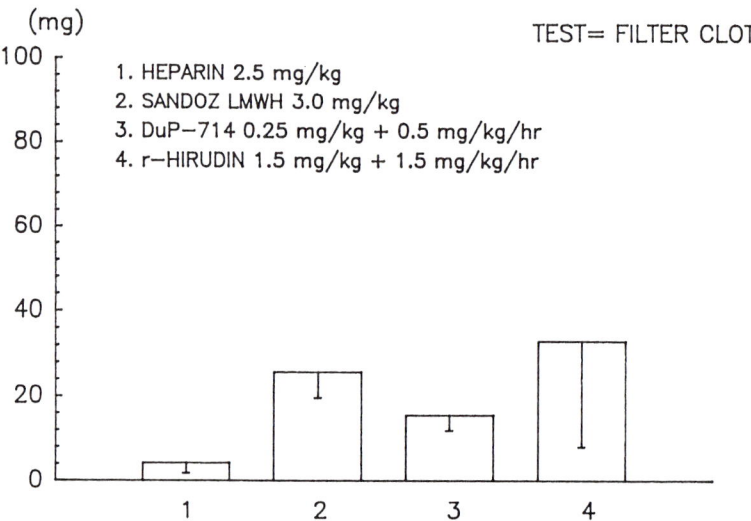

FIGURE 1. Comparison of the efficacy of various anticoagulants in a canine model of cardiopulmonary bypass surgery. Protein deposits in the arterial line filter were quantitated after a 60-minute pump run. (Mean ± 1 SEM; n = 8–12/group)

The ACT typically used to monitor heparin dosing during CPB surgery was used in this study to determine whether the new anticoagulants could be monitored by the same test system. Heparin gave an expected response of 350 seconds (Fig. 3). The LMW heparin, however, gave only a 200-second response, even though the actual dose was higher than the dose of heparin and the

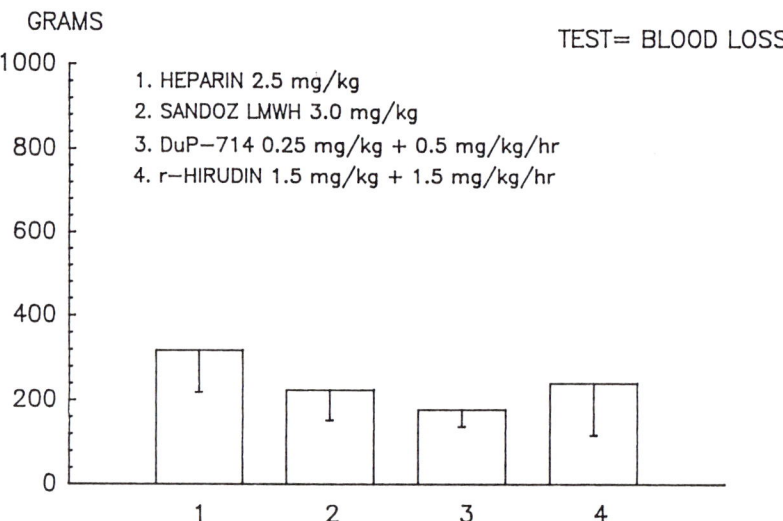

FIGURE 2. Comparison of the safety of various anticoagulants in a canine model of cardiopulmonary bypass surgery. Blood loss was measured as aspirated blood collected from the chest cavity during the first two postoperative hours. (Mean ± 1 SEM; n = 8–12/ group)

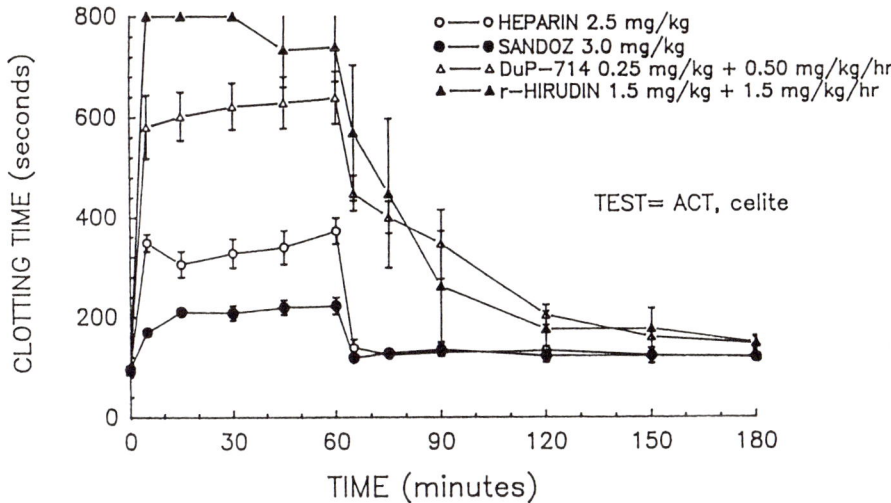

FIGURE 3. Monitoring the effect of various anticoagulants in a canine model of cardiopulmonary bypass surgery. The ACT was performed at various times before, during, and after the 60-minute pump run. (Mean ± 1 SEM; n = 8–12/group)

anticoagulant efficacy of the two drugs was equivalent. Both anticoagulants were reversed by protamine sulfate, as demonstrated by the ACT.

The ACT response of DuP 714 was about 600 seconds, of r-hirudin about 800 seconds, as compared with 350 seconds for heparin. Both DuP 714 and r-hirudin, however, were equivalent to heparin in anticoagulant efficacy (Fig. 3). Neither was reversed with a neutralizing agent but cleared the body through natural renal elimination. By 1 hour after CPB ACT values had returned to baseline.

The chromogenic anti-IIa (anti-thrombin) assay was used as a more sensitive monitor of blood level. Even though equivalent anticoagulation was obtained, the inhibition of thrombin was highest with r-hirudin (Fig. 4). The anti-IIa assay showed natural elimination of r-hirudin and DuP 714 immediately after coming off pump. However, some residual activity was observed up to 1½–2 hours after CPB, particularly for r-hirudin. The LMW heparin showed less anti-IIa activity than DuP 714 but significantly higher activity than heparin (Fig. 4). After reversal by protamine sulfate, the LMW heparin showed a significant rebound effect, and anti-IIa activity was detected up to 2 hours after CPB. This effect was not observed for heparin. The advantage of the anti-IIa assay over the ACT was the readable endpoints for the high activity levels of r-hirudin and the more sensitive detection of low activity levels for the LMW heparin.

Platelet count was not effected by the LMW heparin, DuP 714, or r-hirudin during the pump run (Fig. 5). An initial decrease due to hemodilution was observed but no further change in count. Both thrombin inhibitors, however, showed a trend toward increase to baseline values within 2 hours after the pump run. This trend was not observed with either heparin or LMW heparin.

As a measure of the overall coagulation status, the bleeding time test was performed on the gingiva of the animals. LMW heparin and heparin gave

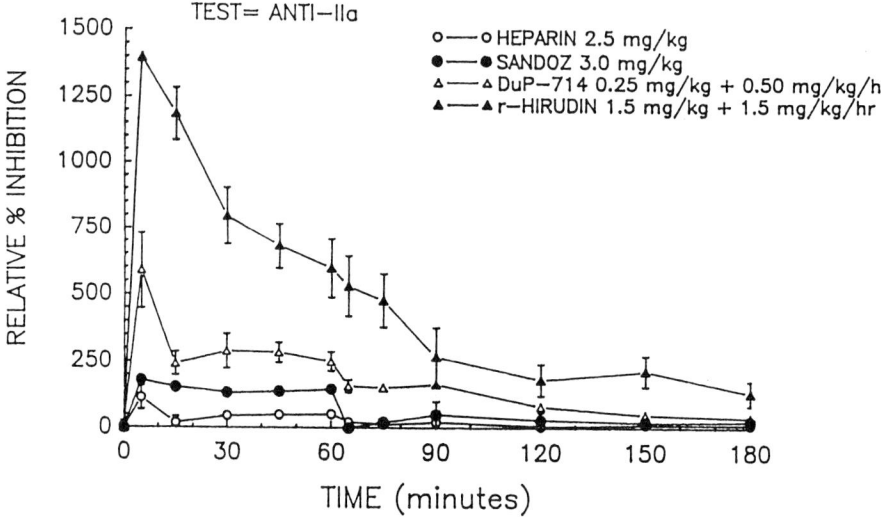

FIGURE 4. Monitoring the effect of various anticoagulants in a canine model of cardiopulmonary bypass surgery. The chromogenic antithrombin assay was performed at various times before, during, and after the 60-minute pump run. (Mean ± 1 SEM; n = 8–12/group)

nearly identical data (>15 minutes bleeding time on pump), whereas DuP 714 did not prolong the bleeding time as much (12 minutes bleeding time on pump). Both agents, like heparin, showed a decrease to near normal within 30 minutes of coming off pump (Fig. 6). r-Hirudin had a minimal effect on prolonging the bleeding time, even on pump.

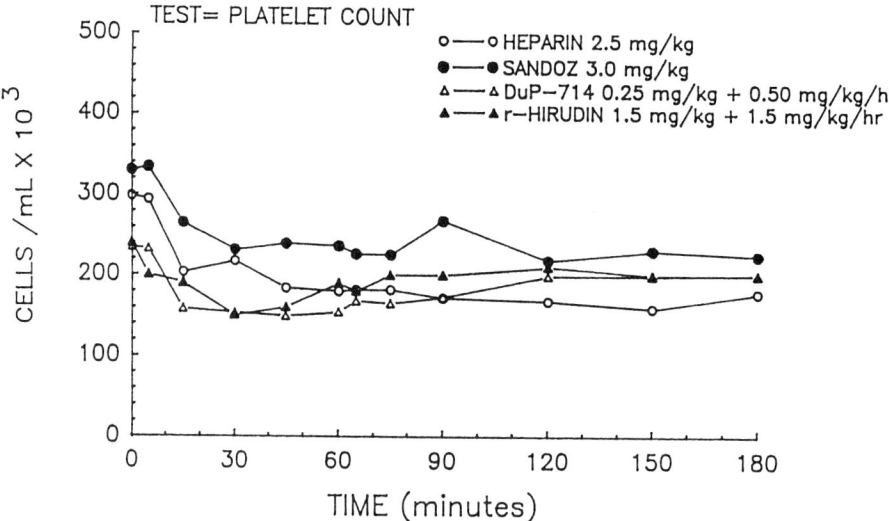

FIGURE 5. Comparison of the effect of various anticoagulants in a canine model of cardiopulmonary bypass surgery. Platelet counts were made at various times before, during, and after the 60-minute pump run. (Mean ± 1 SEM; n = 8–12/group)

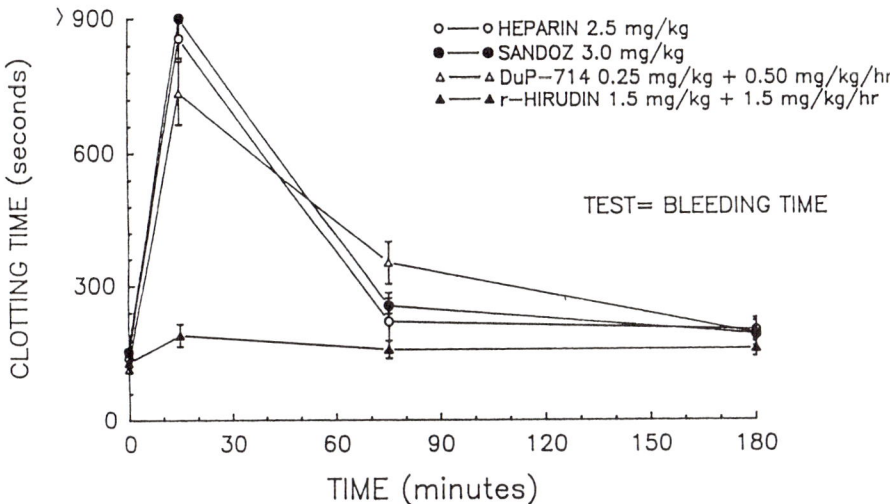

FIGURE 6. Comparison of the effect of various anticoagulants in a canine model of cardiopulmonary bypass surgery. The bleeding time test was performed at various times before, during, and after the 60-minute pump run (Mean ± 1 SEM; n = 8–12/group)

DISCUSSION

The purpose of this study was to determine if the new antithrombotic agents can be used with efficacy and safety as anticoagulants in CPB surgery. It is clinically important to know whether alternatives to heparin are available for patients who have developed heparin-induced thrombocytopenia, who are allergic to protamine sulfate, or who have low levels of antithrombin III. In addition, patients with platelet dysfunction or patients who bleed excessively from heparin may better tolerate another anticoagulant, and heparin rebound may be reduced.

The two thrombin inhibitors tested act by directly binding to, and thereby inactivating, thrombin. r-Hirudin specifically inhibits thrombin, whereas DuP 714 inhibits to a small degree both factor Xa and kallikrein, in addition to inhibiting thrombin. The LMW heparin acts, like heparin, via binding to antithrombin III and subsequent inactivation of factor Xa and thrombin.

The doses of the three new anticoagulants evaluated in this study were chosen on the basis of data from studies in the same model in which a dose/response for each agent was established.[21,22] Administration by infusion was incorporated because of the short half-life of both r-hirudin and DuP 714. A bolus only regimen resulted in significant clotting during the pump run because of incomplete anticoagulant protection.

In terms of anticoagulant efficacy, as determined by filter protein deposits (clots), r-hirudin, DuP 714, and the LMW heparin were equal to heparin. The individual dosing of each agent differed from a total dose of 0.75 mg/kg/hr for DuP 714 to 3.0 mg/kg for the LMW heparin. The thrombin inhibitors showed a much stronger potency than either of the heparins, and DuP 714 was more potent than r-hirudin. The LMW heparin was less potent than heparin.

In terms of safety, the postoperative blood loss associated with the three new anticoagulants was similar to that caused by heparin. Heparin and LMW heparin were reversed with protamine sulfate, but no neutralizing agent was used for DuP 714 or r-hirudin. DuP 714, however, showed a trend toward less blood loss attributed to anticoagulation than heparin. The safety index (bleeding) appears to be rather large for DuP 714; higher doses prolonged the time to clot of all laboratory assays studied but did not lead to additional blood loss.

With DuP 714 and r-hirudin, no intraoperative oozing of blood, as is commonly observed with heparin used in humans and in the canine model, occurred from the cut muscles, the catheter insertion sites, or the sternum. On the other hand, LMW heparin had significantly more intra- and postoperative oozing than heparin, even after the administration of protamine.

None of the agents produced unexpected hemodynamic effects. The hematocrit and fibrinogen changes during CPB were the same as for heparin. r-Hirudin, DuP 714, and LMW heparin had no effect on the complete blood count (CBC) different from heparin. There were no differences in survival rates among the groups.

In general, for all parameters considered, the two thrombin inhibitors produced reproducible responses in the canine model, whereas individual variation was observed in the anticoagulation response to heparin and LMW heparin.

The return to baseline value of the platelet count after CPB appeared to be better with DuP 714 and r-hirudin 2 hours post-CPB than with heparin or LMW heparin. This could be a major advantage of the thrombin inhibitors over heparin.

The bleeding time test, which was markedly prolonged for heparin, was similarly prolonged for LMW heparin. The lesser effect by DuP 714 and the relative lack of effect by r-hirudin were likely due to their different mechanisms of action. Thrombin inhibitors are not associated with the platelet effects and the inhibition of coagulation enzymes induced by heparin. Perhaps these actions are related to bleeding. The elevated bleeding time test (and elevated activated partial thromboplastin time) of LMW heparin and heparin may be an indicator of the higher degree of oozing blood from cut surfaces.

The ACT whole-blood clotting assay (celite activated) is routinely used to monitor heparinization during CPB. This same assay can be used for DuP 714 and LMW heparin. However, whereas adequate heparin anticoagulation is achieved at an ACT of 350–450 seconds, an adequate anticoagulation response with DuP 714 is achieved at an ACT of 600–700 seconds and with LMW heparin at an ACT value of 200–250 seconds. Thus no one ACT value that relates to appropriate anticoagulation or to bleeding is optimal. The ACT value is a function of the mechanism of action of the drug; thus its response as related to bleeding or thrombosis must be judged on the basis of the individual drug monitored.

No pharmacologic agent appears to be necessary to neutralize the anticoagulant effect of the thrombin inhibitors after CPB, provided that the dosing is regulated through the ACT or other blood assay. The blood loss was equal to or less than that of heparin and the surgical field was drier both intra- and postoperatively with DuP 714 and r-hirudin. These drugs have short half-lives and are cleared rapidly from the blood, appearing in the urine, whereas heparin has a much longer half-life and is not filtered through the kidneys. On the other hand, LMW heparin has a longer half-life than heparin, the efficacy of protamine reversal of the anticoagulant effect of LMW heparin is not optimal, and the oozing of blood into the surgical field intra- and postoperatively needs to be addressed further.

SUMMARY

The three agents evaluated as potential alternatives to heparin anticoagulation during CPB—r-hirudin, a boroarginine peptide (a thrombin inhibitor, DuP 714) and a LMW heparin—were shown to be effective in a canine model. None of the three agents altered the hemodynamics, hematologic parameters, or survival rates in a manner different from heparin. Due to differing mechanisms of action, the bleeding time test and the platelet count were less effected by DuP 714 and r-hirudin than by LMW heparin or heparin.

DuP 714 produced less bleeding than heparin, and r-hirudin showed a bleeding effect equivalent to that of heparin. Both agents produced less intra- and postoperative oozing of blood from cut surfaces. For monitoring the level of anticoagulation, the ACT can be used for the boroarginine peptide (at a level of 600–700 seconds, compared with 350–400 seconds for heparin) and for r-hirudin (approximately 800 seconds). No antagonist should be needed to reverse the anticoagulant effect of either DuP 714 or r-hirudin because of their short half-life.

The LMW heparin, although effective at preventing clotting without significant blood loss immediately after surgery, showed signs of blood oozing from cut surfaces that were not observed with the two other agents and were more pronounced than those observed with heparin. An ACT of 200–250 seconds corresponded with adequate anticoagulation. Protamine sulfate did not reverse all effects of the LMW heparin.

These studies revealed several new agents as possible alternative anticoagulants to heparin for CPB surgery. Based on the data presented here, further studies are warranted to validate their safety for use in humans.

REFERENCES

1. Aiach M, Dreyfus G, Michaud A, et al: Low molecular weight heparin derivatives in experimental extracorporeal circulation. Haemostasis 14:325–332, 1984.
2. Bajusz S, Barabas E, Tolnay P, et al: Inhibition of thrombin and trypsin by tripeptide aldehyde. Int J Peptide Protein Res 12:217–221, 1978.
3. Casu B: Structure of heparins and their fragments. Nouv Rev Fr Hematol 26:211–219, 1984.
4. Coggins JR, Kray W, Shaw E: Affinity labelling of proteinases with tryptic specificity by peptides with C-terminal lysine chloromethyl ketone. Biochem J 137:579–585, 1974.
5. Fareed J, Messmore HL, Kindel G, Balis JU: Inhibition of serine proteases by low molecular weight peptides and their derivatives. NY Acad Sci 370:765–784, 1981.
6. Fareed J, Walenga JM, Hoppensteadt D, et al: Chemical and biological heterogeneity in low molecular weight heparins: Implications for clinical use and standardization. Semin Thromb Hemost 15:440–463, 1989.
7. Gouault-Heillmann M, Huft Y, Contant G, et al: Cardiopulmonary bypass with low molecular weight heparin fraction. Lancet 11:1374, 1983.
8. Green D: Heparin-induced thrombocytopenia. Med J Aust 44:HS37-HS39, 1986.
9. Henny CP, Ten Cate H, Ten Cate JW, et al: A randomized blind study comparing standard heparin and a new low molecular weight heparinoid in cardiopulmonary bypass surgery in dogs. J Lab Clin Med 106:187–196, 1985.

10. Hirsh J: From unfractionated heparins to low molecular weight heparins. Acta Chir Scand 55(Suppl):42-50, 1990.
11. Kettner C, Mersinger L, Knabb R: The selective inhibition of thrombin by peptides of boroarginine. J Biol Chem 265:18289-18297, 1990.
12. Levy JH, Zaidan JR, Faraj B: Prospective evaluation of risk of protamine reactions in patients with NPH insulin-dependent diabetes. Anesth Analg 65:739-742, 1986.
13. Markwardt F, Fink G, Kaiser B, et al: Pharmacological survey of recombinant hirudin. Pharmazie 43:202-207, 1988.
14. Massonet-Castel S, Pelissier E, Dreyfus G, et al: Low-molecular-weight heparin in extracorporeal circulation. Lancet 1(8387):1182-1183, 1984.
15. Okamoto S, Hijikata A, Ikezawa K, et al: A new series of synthetic thrombin inhibitors (OM-inhibitors) having extremely potent and selective action. Thromb Res 8(Suppl II):77-82, 1976.
16. Olinger GN, Hussey CV, Olive JA, Malik MI: Cardiopulmonary bypass for patients with previously documented heparin induced platelet aggregation. J Thorac Cardiovasc Surg 87:673-677, 1984.
17. Pifarre R, Babka R, Sullivan HJ, et al: Management of postoperative heparin rebound following cardiopulmonary bypass. J Thorac Cardiovasc Surg 81:378-381, 1981.
18. Reber G, Schweizer A, De Moerloose PH, et al: Comparison between a low molecular weight and standard heparin for anticoagulation during extracorporeal CO_2 removal in the dog. Thromb Res 49:157-168, 1988.
19. Roussi JH, Houbouyen LL, Goguel AF: Use of low molecular weight heparin in heparin-induced thrombocytopenia with thrombotic complications. Lancet 1:1183, 1984.
20. Thomas DP: Prevention of post-operative thrombosis by low molecular weight heparin in patients undergoing hip replacement. Thromb Haemost 67:491-493, 1992.
21. Walenga JM, Bakhos M, Messmore HL, et al: Potential use of recombinant hirudin as an anticoagulant in a cardiopulmonary bypass model. Ann Thorac Surg 51:271-277, 1991.
22. Walenga JM, Chomiak PN, Koza MJ, Pifarre R: Investigation of a thrombin inhibitor peptide as an alternative to heparin in cardiopulmonary bypass surgery. Submitted for publication.

Chapter 25

Antithrombotic Biomaterials for Cardiovascular Surgery

Julian Breillatt, Ph.D., and Li-Chien Hsu, Ph.D.

The development of antithrombotic materials began in the 1960s in response to the explosive progress in cardiovascular surgery during that decade.[14,15,17] They were perceived as a way to avoid coagulation and to minimize formation of mural thrombi on implanted devices and the associated risk of thromboemboli.[14] By contrast, antithrombotic surfaces are now perceived as a means to retain near-normal coagulation properties in blood during cardiopulmonary bypass (CPB) surgery. The key to success has been shown to be the low systemic heparinization made possible by antithrombotic extracorporeal circuits.[63] Lower heparin levels result in reduced blood loss, with attendant lower transfusion requirements and diminished return of activated blood from cardiotomy suction. The heparinized surface, coupled with lower protamine dosage, reduces the stimuli to complement activation and inflammatory response.[7,52]

STRATEGIES FOR ANTITHROMBOTIC MATERIALS

The endothelial lining of the mammalian vascular system is uniquely able to hold blood in its native state, because it participates with blood to maintain hemostatic balance and to minimize blood loss when the vascular wall is breached. Exposure of blood to a foreign surface, such as an extracorporeal circuit, or simple exposure of extracellular matrix by abrasion of a vessel initiates a cascade of reactants designed to seal the breach and to stimulate the vascular wall and its endothelial lining to repair themselves. However, when the reactants are directed toward a device containing a nonparticipating, surrogate vascular wall, they produce thrombotic and embolic events that can both defeat the function of the device and compromise the patient.[45] In the search for hemocompatible materials and surfaces that do not initiate such events, researchers in biomaterials have developed many synthetic surfaces, ranging from passively nonthrombogenic to actively antithrombotic, that have been incorporated into a wide variety of blood-contacting devices with varying degrees of success. Passive properties, such as surface texture, surface morphology, electrocharge, free energy, and wettability, have been found to affect blood compatibility. However, none of these properties or any combination thereof has consistently produced thromboresistance.[14,45] Thus, full systemic anticoagulation with heparin, followed by neutralization with protamine, is still the standard method of supporting the multimaterial, high-surface-area devices used in cardiac surgery. The undesirable sequelae of this method include intra- and postoperative bleeding, reinfusion of activated blood from cardiotomy suction, requirements of exogenous transfusion with risk of viral infection, and reactions related to heparin-protamine complexes.

The irony is that although **soluble** heparin blocks the fluid-phase reactions of the coagulation cascade, thereby preventing the propagation of clotting, it is a poor regulator of surface-induced activation of the contact system,[39] of complement,[24] and of the inflammatory response; it can also initiate platelet activation.[45] However, **surface-immobilized** heparin effectively limits activation of the complement system[24,32] and may limit contact activation[13] in a manner analogous to the heparan sulfate proteoglycan that coats the luminal surface of the endothelium.[33,34] In practice, antithrombotic coatings that contain immobilized heparin with functional antithrombin III (AT III) binding sites have consistently provided hemocompatible surfaces for cardiopulmonary devices.[66]

Kazatchkine and Fearon demonstrated that immobilized heparin blocks complement activation by promoting enhanced surface binding of factor H, an inhibitor of the alternate pathway C3 convertase.[24] Immobilized heparin has also been shown to limit inflammatory reactions, as measured by release of myeloperoxidase and lactoferrin from activated leukocytes.[51]

Until recently the antithrombotic activity of surface-bound heparin has been attributed to its anti-Xa and antithrombin activity; the argument is made that in flowing blood the esterases of the coagulation cascade are convectively transported to the luminal wall and there inactivated.[1,29] However, Olsson recently reported that the formation of factor XIIa from factor XII was markedly inhibited on immobilized heparin surfaces that contained AT III binding sites; thus the antithrombotic properties of heparinized surfaces may proceed in part from ab initio inhibition of contact activation.[13] This indication of an early role for surface-bound heparin is supported by our observation that whereas blood drawn without anticoagulant demonstrates only limited activation during hours of flow in a Chandler loop lined with covalently attached heparin, it will quickly clot in an identical loop with hirudin covalently attached to the luminal wall. However, an equal quantity of hirudin immobilized on micron-sized Latex beads dispersed in the blood prevents both clotting and formation of fibrinopeptide A.[8]

Similarly, Lindon has shown that immobilized heparin surfaces containing bound AT III tend neither to activate nor to adhere platelets.[31] Moreover, low-molecular-weight heparin fractions can be designed to possess markedly reduced platelet-binding activity while retaining appreciable anti-Xa activity.[46] This suggests why antithrombotic immobilized heparin surfaces prepared from low-molecular-weight heparin exhibit reduced platelet adhesion.[29]

Thus the device surfaces that promise marked reduction in requirements for systemic anticoagulation during cardiovascular surgery seek to mimic the native endothelial surface by placing heparin or heparinlike molecules with AT III binding sites at the interface between blood and the vascular wall.

Three currently realizable approaches use (1) heparin coatings of the device and tubing surfaces comprising the extracorporeal blood flow path,[20,21,29] (2) synthetic materials containing heparin or heparin analogs,[16,35] and (3) endogenous endothelial cells growing on the surface of synthetic implants.[23,44] Currently available systems and components for clinical use in cardiovascular surgery are mostly based on heparin coatings, although some devices are made from heparin-containing materials. Endothelialized synthetic grafts have been used clinically for peripheral revascularization but are still in the research phase.

HEPARIN SURFACE COATINGS

Resistance to Thrombus Formation and Embolization

Heparin-coated surfaces retrieved from perfusion circuits are remarkably free of thrombus, whether at the visual or scanning electron microscope level,[20,38,53,66] except in areas of blood stagnation.[1,3,59] Clinical studies,[6,26,43,61-63] ranging from several hours to many days, have confirmed the results of animal experiments.[27,48,54,55,57-60,64,66]

Retrieval of clean surfaces usually indicates either nonthrombogenic surfaces or surfaces that shed emboli efficiently.[28] Three experimental studies in animal models suggest that thromboembolization from heparinized surfaces is significantly less than from uncoated controls:

1. Thrombus formation and subsequent embolization from heparin-coated arterial filters were greatly reduced in in-vitro baboon blood, as demonstrated by transfilter pressure drop and microaggregate sizing and counting by laser scattering.[41]

2. Two animal studies showed that heparin-coated ventricular assist devices (VADs) can function for 1-6 hours in the absence of systemic heparin with reduced clotting and no sign of generalized embolization; however, renal microemboli were found in both studies.[9,64]

3. The kinetics of thrombus formation and embolization during cardiopulmonary bypass (CPB) in a pig model, using indium 111-labeled platelets and full systemic heparinization, showed that the arterial filter was the principal source of emboli. When a heparin-coated circuit was substituted for the uncoated one, the quantity of thrombus and rate of embolization were significantly reduced.[11,12]

These studies, although indicating efficacy, cannot predict the extent of embolization from heparinized surfaces during CPB in humans. A newly developed light-scattering system that can continuously monitor the number and size of emboli in the arterial line of a bypass circuit during surgery is expected to provide a definitive answer.[36]

Reduced Blood Loss During Cardiopulmonary Bypass

Perfusion of a CPB circuit moves blood from the vascular compartment (Fig. 1), where it maintains hemostasis, into the CPB compartment, which presents a full spectrum of surface stimuli to the thrombotic and hemostatic system. Hydrophilic anionic surfaces promote activation of factor XII and

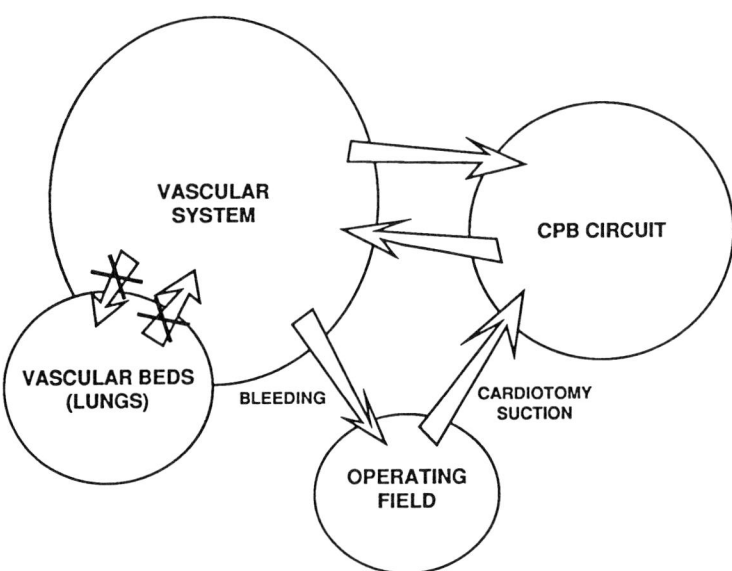

FIGURE 1. The four compartments perfused by blood during cardiopulmonary bypass. Each compartment has a unique potential to activate the host defense systems present in the blood.

kallikrein, which progresses to coagulation, fibrinolysis, and inflammatory responses. Complement activation proceeds primarily via the alternate pathway with concomitant leukocyte activation. Hydrophobic surfaces adsorb fibrinogen, among other proteins, which in turn binds platelets via their GPIIb/IIIa receptors. The most significant clinical effect on platelets is a decrease in the surface receptors, GPIb and GPIIb/IIIa. A 50% loss of GPIb receptors occurs during the first 5 minutes of CPB.[42,49,50] This loss of GPIb receptors, which selectively bind von Willebrand's factor, compromises the platelet's ability to recognize and attach to collagen exposed in breaches of the vascular wall, a primary mechanism by which vessel incisions are plugged and healed. The decrease in GPIIb/IIIa, the fibrinogen receptor, reduces the ability of the platelets to aggregate and to consolidate into a clot by attachment to fibrin strands. The net result of combining this compromised platelet population with the systemic levels of heparin required to limit the coagulation cascade by minimizing formation of fibrin and to maintain patency of the CPB compartment is a hemostatic system that cannot plug leaks. Therefore, bleeding occurs into a third compartment, the extravascular operating field (Fig. 1). Here, in contact with cut tissue, the host defense systems in the blood become more fully activated. Return of that blood via cardiotomy suction to the CPB and vascular compartments consumes the reserve capacity of the natural inhibitors and further decreases the ability of the hemostatic system to seal suture lines. These phenomena are responsible for the transfusion requirements commonly associated with CPB.

Currently, two approaches attempt to reverse this blood loss. The first maintains partial activity of the coagulation cascade. Von Segesser[63] demonstrated that when the entire CPB circuit is coated with heparin, the amount of systemic heparin needed to maintain patency is reduced. Thus the coagulation cascade can generate sufficient thrombin to form a platelet plug held together by the interaction of GPIIb/IIIa receptors with fibrin. The second approach maintains platelet function by using aprotinin to block contact activation and its immediate sequelae and to prevent the loss of platelet GPIb and GPIIb/IIIa receptors.[49]

The efficacy of the first approach has been confirmed by numerous studies, systematically pursued over several years, that use two principal heparin-coating methods, Bentley's Duraflo II[47] and the Carmeda Bioactive Surface.[29] Experiments in animal models have evaluated heparin-coated perfusion systems, including left-heart bypass,[60,67] CPB,[55,57,58,65] extracorporeal membrane oxygenation/extracorporeal carbon dioxide removal (ECMO/ECCO$_2$R),[5,27,48] and left VADs[54,59] with normal, reduced, and no systemic heparin. These experiments concluded that heparin-coated circuits can be safely used for cardiovascular surgery with reduced systemic heparinization.[66]

Clinical studies with heparinized systems have confirmed the safety of these procedures and demonstrated significant reduction in blood loss and transfusion requirements during CPB.[61] In a randomized prospective study of full vs. low systemic heparin during coronary revascularization, von Segesser[63] demonstrated that in both instances heparin-coated CPB circuits decrease blood loss and transfused red blood cells by 3- and 9-fold, respectively (Table 1).

Von Segesser also used heparin-coated perfusion equipment with low systemic heparin for partial CPB during resection of thoracic aortic aneurysms to achieve significant reductions in mortality compared with historical controls using simple aortic cross-clamping.[62,63] Although the bleeding propensities of this group of patients was overcome by low heparin levels, total heparinless bypass was necessary to rewarm a patient in deep hypothermia with severe cranial trauma[53] and in another case to provide ECMO to a patient with intractable bleeding and postoperative cardiopulmonary failure.[30]

Use of low heparin levels to control bleeding in compromised patients during bypass requires special attention to blood flow rates in the extracorporeal circuits. A shunt is recommended to allow recirculation between the arterial and venous lines to avoid stagnation of blood within the lines.[53,56,63] A slow rate of flow leading to stagnation of blood can result in surface thrombus formation at normal heparin levels in any device, whether or not it is coated with heparin,

TABLE 1. Effect of Heparin Level on Blood Loss During Cardiopulmonary Bypass for Coronary Artery Revascularization*

	Low Systemic Heparin (n = 12)	Full Systemic Heparin (n = 10)
Activated clotting time (sec)	>180	>480
Heparin (IU)	8041 ± 1270	52,500 ± 17,000
Blood loss (ml)	831 ± 373	2345 ± 1815
Transfused red blood cells (ml)	281 ± 415	2731 ± 2258
Patients transfused	5/12	10/10
Postoperative hematocrit (%)	35.0 ± 2.0	24.7 ± 2.7
Protamine (IU)	7875 ± 1918	31,400 ± 14,000

* Adapted from von Segesser LK, Weiss BM, Garcia E, et al: Reduction and elimination of systemic heparinization during cardiopulmonary bypass. J Thorac Cardiovasc Surg 103:790–799, 1992.

or even in undamaged endothelial-lined surfaces.[1,29] Stagnation of blood in cardiotomy reservoirs is of particular concern, and although coated reservoirs are now available,[56] continuous blood flow must be maintained and monitored to avoid prolonged accumulation. In settings other than acute trauma and intractable bleeding, maintenance of a low level of systemic heparin is recommended, particularly to neutralize the increased thrombin that appears in the circulation after release of the aortic cross-clamp.[19]

Inflammatory Response

The activation of complement via the alternate pathway during CPB by the components of the circuit, followed by a protamine-dependent activation via the classical pathway, is well documented.[10,25] The relationship of complement activation to the appearance of inflammatory mediators in the circulation after release of the aortic cross-clamp and reperfusion of the lungs has also been the object of continued research in an attempt to understand the postperfusion organ dysfunction syndrome and to reduce its frequency and morbidity.[68]

Heparin-coated circuits exhibited lower concentrations of complement and leukocyte activation markers during and after CPB in experimental[37,40,51] and clinical[7,18,52] studies. Reduced activation of humoral factors was demonstrated in a controlled clinical study during which C3a and the terminal complement complex (C5a-C9) were activated to a lesser degree in coated CPB circuits.[52] In both circuits the activated complement components began appearing in the circulation at the start of CPB, accelerated after release of the cross-clamp, then gradually disappeared over a 6-hour period after termination of the procedure.

Both humoral and cellular indices were measured in a clinical study that tested the ability of coated CPB circuits to reduce the inflammatory response as measured by C3a, tumor necrosis factor (TNF), and leukocyte elastase.[18] The group of patients using coated circuits did not exhibit the marked increase in C3a and TNF that occurred after protamine administration in the group that used uncoated circuits. Whereas the increase in C3a may reflect protamine neutralization of heparin, the increase in TNF probably reflects an earlier activation step, given the time delay inherent in its synthesis and release from macrophages.[2,22] Both groups demonstrated increased leukocyte degranulation after cross-clamp release, as measured by elastase concentration, with the patients on coated systems reflecting a lesser cell activation. However, the finding of equal concentrations of elastase in the left and right atria of the patients of the coated circuit group 5 minutes after clamp release indicated that leukocytes were not further activated in the lungs during reperfusion; in contrast, the left atrial blood contained twice the elastase concentration as the right atrium in the uncoated group.[18]

A controlled clinical trial exploring the effect of heparin-coated circuits on cellular responses during CPB demonstrated that although leukocyte degranulation occurred continuously during the procedure, it was markedly lower in the coated circuits.[7] The release in heparin-coated circuits of myeloperoxidase and lactoferrin, two oxidative enzymes that can mediate tissue destruction, was suppressed to 37% and 46% of uncoated control levels by the end of the procedure.

Heparin-coated CPB circuits obviously reduce the inflammatory response of the patient. The lesser activation of complement during CPB by heparin-coated devices was anticipated from the basic work of Kazatchkine.[24] Heparin-coated circuits can also reduce the cellular inflammatory response during CPB. However, the effect of such coatings on the leukocyte response is more difficult to explain, because the response characteristically follows release of the aortic cross-clamp and reperfusion of the lung microvasculature. Because other vascular beds are also fully reperfused at that time, additional variables are introduced, such as introduction of endotoxins from the splanchnic capillary bed.[22] A description of the mechanism by which this process occurs must await more data than are available from the limited series of trials.

SUMMARY

Full systemic heparin does not prevent surface thrombus formation and subsequent embolic events. Heparin-surfaced blood conduits, however, block build-up of surface thrombus except in areas of blood stagnation. Heparinized surfaces appear to reduce significantly the number and size of thromboemboli during CPB, but the actual extent of this phenomenon in the clinical setting has yet to be adequately quantified.

When heparin-coated devices are used in conjunction with reduced systemic heparin dosage, intra- and postoperative bleeding is markedly reduced, with an attendant reduction in transfusion requirements. Heparin-coated CPB circuits activate complement to a lesser extent than controls and appear to protect leukocytes from inflammatory stimuli, especially after aortic cross-clamp release.

REFERENCES

1. Arnander C, Olsson P, Larm O: Influence of blood flow and the effect of protamine on the thromboresistant properties of a covalently bonded heparin surface. J Biomed Mater Res 22:859–868, 1988.
2. Beutler B, Milsark IW, Cerami A: Cachectin/tumor necrosis factor: Production, distribution, and metabolic fate in vivo. J Immunol 135:3972–3977, 1985.
3. Bianchi JJ, Swartz MT, Raithel SC, et al: Initial clinical experience with centrifugal pumps coated with the Carmeda process. ASAIO Trans 38:143–146, 1992.
4. Bindslev L, Bohm C, Jolin A, et al: Extracorporeal carbon dioxide removal performed with surface heparinized equipment in patients with ARDS. Acta Anaesthesiol Scand 35:125–131, 1991.
5. Bindslev L, Gouda I, Inacio J, et al: Extracorporeal elimination of carbon dioxide using a surface-heparinized veno-venous bypass system. ASAIO Trans 32:530–533, 1986.
6. Borowiec J, Thelin S, Bagge L, et al: Heparin-coated cardiopulmonary bypass circuits and 25-percent reduction of heparin dose in coronary artery surgery—a clinical study. Ups J Med Sci 97:55–66, 1992.
7. Borowiec J, Thelin S, Bagge L, et al: Heparin-coated circuits reduce activation of granulocytes during cardiopulmonary bypass. J Thorac Cardiovasc Surg 104:642–647, 1992.
8. Breillatt J, Johnson RJ, Ku C, et al: Recombinant hirudin analog designed for attachment to polymers. FASEB J 6:A1320, 1992.
9. Campanella C, Cameron E, Sinclair C, et al: Preliminary results of left heart bypass in pigs using a heparin-coated centrifugal pump. Ann Thorac Surg 52:245–249, 1991.
10. Chenoweth DE, Cooper SW, Hugli TE, et al: Complement activation during cardiopulmonary bypass. N Engl J Med 304:497–503, 1981.

11. Dewanjee MK, Palitianos GM, Kapadvanjwala M, et al: Quantification of embolus with Indium-111 labeled platelets in hollow-fiber oxygenator and arterial filter during cardiopulmonary bypass (CPB) in a pig model. Proc Cardiovasc Sci Technol Conf: AAMI/NHLBI, Bethesda, MD, December 2-4, 1991, p 148.
12. Dewanjee MK, Palitianos GM, Kapadvanjwala M, et al: Rate constants of embolization and quantification of emboli from the hollow-fiber oxygenator and arterial filter during cardiopulmonary bypass. ASAIO Trans 38:317-321, 1992.
13. Elque G, Sanchez J, Egberg N, et al: Novel antithrombin independent properties of surface bound heparin. Thromb Haemost 65:864, 1991.
14. Gott VL, Furuse A: Anithrombogenic surfaces, classification and in vivo evaluation. Fed Proc 30:1679-1685, 1971.
15. Gott VL, Whiffen JD, Dutton RC: Heparin bonding colloidal graphite surfaces. Science 142:1297-1298, 1963.
16. Grainger DW, Knutson K, Kim SW, et al: Poly(dimethylsiloxane)-poly(ethyleneoxide)-heparin block copolymers. II: Surface characterization and in vitro assessments. J Biomed Mater Res 24:403-431, 1990.
17. Grode GA, Anderson SJ, Grotta HM, et al: Nonthrombogenic material via a simple coating process. ASAIO Trans 15:1-5, 1969.
18. Gu YJ, Van Oerveren W, Akkerman C, et al: Reduction of inflammatory response during cardiopulmonary bypass by the use of heparin-coated extracorporeal circuit. Ann Thorac Surg (in press).
19. Gu YJ, van Oeveren W, van der Kamp KWHJ, et al: Heparin-coating of extracorporeal circuits reduces thrombin formation in patients undergoing cardiopulmonary bypass. Perfusion 6:221-225, 1991.
20. Hsu LC: Principles of heparin-coating techniques. Perfusion 6:209-219, 1991.
21. Hsu LC, Loar ME, Tong SD: Thromboresistant properties of surface-modified arterial blood filter materials. Trans Soc Biomater 14:112, 1991.
22. Jansen NJG, van Oeveren W, Gu YJ, et al: Endotoxin release and tumor necrosis factor formation during cardiopulmonary bypass. Ann Thorac Surg 54:744-748, 1992.
23. Jarrell BE, Williams SK, Stokes G, et al: Use of freshly isolated capillary endothelial cells for the immediate establishment of a monolayer on a vascular graft at surgery. Surgery 100:392-399, 1986.
24. Kazatchkine MD, Fearon DT, Silbert JE, et al: Surface-associated heparin inhibits zymosan-induced activation of the human alternative complement pathway by augmenting the regulatory action of the control proteins on particle-bound C3b. J Exp Med 150:1202-1215, 1979.
25. Kirklin JK, Chenoweth DE, Naftel DC, et al: Effects of protamine administration after cardiopulmonary bypass on complement, blood elements, and the hemodynamic state. Ann Thorac Surg 41:193-199, 1986.
26. Knoch M, Kollen B, Dietrich G, et al: Progress in venovenous long-term bypass techniques for the treatment of ARDS—Controlled clinical trial with the heparin coated bypass circuit. Int J Artif Organs 15:103-108, 1992.
27. Koul B, Vesterqvist O, Egberg N, et al: Twenty-four-hour heparin-free veno-right ventricular ECMO: An experimental study. Ann Thorac Surg 53:1046-1051, 1992.
28. Kusserow D, Larrow R, Nichols J: Observations concerning prosthesis-induced thromboembolic phenomena with an in vivo embolus test system. ASAIO Trans 16:58-62, 1970.
29. Larm O, Larsson R, Olsson P: A new non-thrombogenic surface prepared by selective covalent binding of heparin via a modified reduced terminal residue. Biomater Med Devices Artif Organs 11:161-173, 1983.
30. Laub GW, Muralidharan S, Clancy R, et al: Use of ECMO for intractable postoperative cardiopulmonary failure. Circulatory Support Meeting, San Francisco, November 1991 [abstract].
31. Lindon JN, Salzman EW, Merrill EW, et al: Catalytic activity and platelet reactivity of heparin covalently bonded to surfaces. J Lab Clin Med 105:219-226, 1985.
32. Maillet F, Petitou M, Choay J, et al: Structure-function relationships in the inhibitory effect of heparin on complement activation: Independency of the anti-coagulant and anti-complementary sites on the heparin molecule. Mol Immunol 25:917-923, 1988.
33. Marcum JA, McKenney JB, Rosenberg RD: Acceleration of thrombin-antithrombin complex formation in rat hind quarters via heparin-like molecules bound to the endothelium. J Clin Invest 74:341-350, 1984.
34. Marcum JA, Rosenberg RD: The biochemistry, cell biology, and pathophysiology of anticoagulantly active heparin-like molecules of the vessel wall. Biochem Biophys Res Commun 126:365-372, 1985.

35. Migonney V, Fougnot C, Jozefowicz M: Heparin-like tubings. Biomaterials 9:145-149, 1988.
36. Mohammad SF, Solen KA, Olsen DB, et al: Thrombogenesis in blood pumping devices. Proc Cardiovasc Sci Technol Conf: AAMI/NHLBI, Bethesda, MD, December 12-14, 1992, p 11.
37. Nilsson L, Storm KE, Thelin S, et al: Heparin-coated equipment reduces complement activation during cardiopulmonary bypass in the pig. Artif Organs 15:90-95, 1991.
38. Peters J, Redermacher P, Kuntz ME, et al: Extracorporeal CO_2 removal with a heparin coated artificial lung. Intens Care Med 14:578-584, 1988.
39. Pixley RA, Shapira M, Colman RW: Effect of heparin on the inactivation rate of human activated factor XII by antithrombin III. Blood 66:198-203, 1985.
40. Plotz FB, van Oeveren W, Hultquist KA, et al: A heparin-coated circuit reduces complement activation and the release of leukocyte inflammatory mediators during extracorporeal circulation in a rabbit. Artif Organs 16:366-370, 1992.
41. Reynolds L, Clarke R, Drumm G: In vitro efficacy tests for arterial filter materials. Trans Soc Biomater 11:115, 1985.
42. Rinder CS, Mathew JP, Rinder HM, et al: Modulation of platelet surface adhesion receptors during cardiopulmonary bypass. Anesthesiology 75:563-570, 1991.
43. Rossaint R, Slama K, Lewandowski K, et al: Extracorporeal lung assist with heparin-coated systems. Int J Artif Organs 15:29-34, 1992.
44. Rupnick MA, Hubbard FA, Pratt K, et al: Endothelialization of vascular prosthetic surfaces after seeding or sodding with human microvascular endothelial cells. J Vasc Surg 9:788-795, 1989.
45. Salzman EW, Merrill EW: Interaction of blood with artificial surfaces. In Colman RW, Hirsh J, Marder VI, Salzman EW (eds): Hemostasis and Thrombosis. Philadelphia, J.B. Lippincott, 1987, pp 1335-1347.
46. Sobel M, Suda Y, Kermode JC, et al: Heparin binding to platelets: Dissociation of platelet binding and anticoagulant properties of heparin, based on structural specificities of the glycosaminoglycan. Proc Cardiovasc Sci Technol Conf: AAMI/NHLBI, Bethesda, MD, December 2-4, 1991, p 132.
47. Tong SD, Rolfs MR, Hsu LC: Evaluation of Duraflo II heparin immobilized cardiopulmonary bypass circuits. ASAIO Trans 36:654-656, 1990.
48. Toomasian JM, Hsu LC, Hirschl RB, et al: Evaluation of Duraflo II heparin coating in prolonged extracorporeal membrane oxygenation. ASAIO Trans 34:410-414, 1988.
49. van Oeveren W, Eijsman L, Roozendaal KJ, et al: Platelet preservation by aprotinin during cardiopulmonary bypass. Lancet 2:644, 1988.
50. van Oeveren W, Harder MP, Roozendaal KJ, et al: Aprotinin protects platelets against the initial effect of cardiopulmonary bypass. J Thorac Cardiovasc Surg 99:788-797, 1990.
51. Videm V, Nilsson L, Venge P, et al: Reduced granulocyte activation with a heparin coated device in an in vitro model of cardiopulmonary bypass. Artif Organs 15:90-95, 1991.
52. Videm V, Svennevig JL, Fosse E, et al: Reduced complement activation with heparin-coated oxygenator and tubings in coronary bypass operations. J Thorac Cardiovasc Surg 103:806-813, 1992.
53. von Segesser LK, Garcia E, Turina M: Perfusion without systemic heparinization for rewarming in accidental hypothermia. Ann Thorac Surg 52:560-561, 1991.
54. von Segesser LK, Lachat M, Gallino A, et al: Performance characteristics of centrifugal pumps with heparin surface coating. Thorac Cardiovasc Surg 34:224-228, 1990.
55. von Segesser LK, Lachat M, Leskosek B, et al: Cardiopulmonary bypass with low systemic heparinization: An experimental study. Perfusion 5:267-276, 1990.
56. von Segesser LK, Pasic M, Leskosek B, et al: Heparin-coated cardiotomy reservoirs with improved thromboresistance. Cah CECEC 36:9-16, 1991.
57. von Segesser LK, Turina M: Cardiopulmonary bypass without systemic heparinization. Performance of heparin-coated oxygenators in comparison with classic membrane and bubble oxygenators. J Thorac Cardiovasc Surg 98:386-396, 1989.
58. von Segesser LK, Turina M: Long term cardiopulmonary bypass without systemic heparinization. Int J Artif Organs 13:687-691, 1990.
59. von Segesser LK, Weiss BM, Bisang B, et al: Ventricular assist with heparin surface coated devices. ASAIO Trans 37:278-279, 1991.
60. von Segesser LK, Weiss BM, Gallino A, et al: Superior hemodynamics in left heart bypass without systemic heparinization. Eur J Cardiothorac Surg 4:384-389, 1990.
61. von Segesser LK, Weiss BM, Garcia E, et al: Reduced blood loss and transfusion requirements with low systemic heparinization: Preliminary clinical results in coronary artery revascularization. Eur J Cardiothorac Surg 4:639-643, 1990.

62. von Segesser LK, Weiss BM, Garcia E, et al: Perfusion with low systemic heparinization during resection of descending thoracic aortic aneurysms. Eur J Cardiothorac Surg 6:246-250, 1992.
63. von Segesser LK, Weiss BM, Garcia E, et al: Reduction and elimination of systemic heparinization during cardiopulmonary bypass. J Thorac Cardiovasc Surg 103:790-799, 1992.
64. von Segesser LK, Weiss BM, Hanseler E, et al: Improved biocompatibility of heparin surface-coated ventricular assist devices. Int J Artif Organs 15:301-306, 1992.
65. von Segesser LK, Weiss BM, Pasic M, et al: Experimental evaluation of heparin-coated cardiopulmonary bypass equipment with low systemic heparinization and high-dose aprotinin. Thorac Cardiovasc Surg 39:251-256, 1991.
66. von Segesser LK, Weiss BM, Turina MI: Perfusion with heparin-coated equipment: Potential for clinical use. Semin Thorac Cardiovasc Surg 2:373-380, 1990.
67. Weiss BM, von Segesser LK, Vetter W, et al: Heparin-coated left heart bypass: Renal function and hormonal reponse. Int J Artif Organs 14:792-799, 1991.
68. Westaby S: Organ dysfunction after cardiopulmonary bypass: A systemic inflammatory reaction initiated by the extracorporeal circuit. Intens Care Med 13:89-95, 1987.

Chapter 26

Medicolegal Aspects of Blood Transfusions

Joy V. Cunningham, J.D., and Jill M. Rappis, J.D.

Today's surgeon practices in an atmosphere that is legally as well as technologically and medically different from the era of his predecessors. The legal climate in which the surgeon currently practices was not contemplated fifty years ago or even more recently than that. As a result, most physicians have been faced with the concept of practicing defensive medicine. For some physicians this means ordering extra tests and performing procedures that may have been omitted if not for concern about later suits. The physician who is well informed with respect to legal trends as they affect the practice of medicine is in a better position to defend himself should the occasion arise. This knowledge is far more important than attempting to second-guess whether to order additional tests and procedures that the patient may not need—just in case.

This chapter addresses the legal risks facing the surgeon with respect to blood transfusions and the administration of blood products as well as other relevant legal issues.

Unless one has been asleep for the last ten years, it comes as no surprise that medical malpractice and personal injury litigation has steadily increased. One area that has seen considerable activity over the last five years is litigation arising from blood transfusions. According to the Centers for Disease Control, approximately 6,000 Americans, both adults and children, have contracted Acquired Immune Deficiency Syndrome (AIDS) as a result of receiving tainted blood or blood products in the course of a transfusion. The figure has no doubt increased since these statistics were obtained. Attorneys representing the patients are earnestly seeking ways to recover large judgments or settlements on behalf of their injured clients.

The media attention given to these AIDS-related stories has raised the level of public awareness regarding transfusions and related issues. AIDS may become the most litigated disease in the history of American jurisprudence.

Traditionally, plaintiffs have not fared well in litigation against blood banks and suppliers of blood products. They have, however, scored a number of victories against hospitals and physicians. Rather than pursue the blood bank and suppliers who, for the most part, are protected by blood shield statutes, lawyers representing injured patients are seeking ways to hold physicians and hospitals accountable. This trend is likely to continue since it has yielded the most success.

THEORIES OF LIABILITY

It is not sufficient that the plaintiff merely allege an injury after medical treatment. Any lawsuit brought against a physician or hospital requires the plaintiff to set forth a theory of liability—that is, a legal basis on which to state a cause of action. The most common are negligence, breach of contract, and strict liability.

Negligence

In order to bring a suit for medical malpractice based on negligence, the plaintiff must show that the physician was required to exercise a certain degree of care in his treatment of the plaintiff, that the physician's treatment fell below the acceptable standard of care, and that injury to the plaintiff resulted. The plaintiff must also claim that he is entitled to damages as a result of the injury. Once the plaintiff has stated these facts, he has reached the necessary threshold to maintain a lawsuit against the physician based on negligence.

Breach of Contract

Some innovative attorneys have sued physicians on the basis of breach of contract. In such a situation, the plaintiff asserts that he and the physician entered into a contract, and that, in return for the plaintiff's paying or agreeing to pay the physician's fee, the physician agreed to perform certain procedures and render treatment in accordance with the contract. Such a complaint alleges that the physician breached the contract by not performing in the manner agreed upon.

Strict Liability

The theory of strict liability is usually advanced against sellers of products when personal injury has resulted from use of the product. It is generally limited to the sale of a product rather than the performance of a service. In fact, courts are reluctant to allow a case to proceed under a strict liability theory when the service is deemed to be a professional service such as medicine or surgery.

In a California case, a patient sued under the theory of strict liability (in addition to others), based on the implantation of an allegedly defective pacemaker.[1] The court found that a strict liability theory was inappropriate despite the patient's argument that the hospital and surgeon were sellers of a product rather than providers of a service. The court emphasized that strict liability is imposed to ensure that the cost of injuries resulting from defective products is borne by the manufacturers who place the products on the market. The implanting of a pacemaker was held to be a medical/surgical service rather than the sale of a product; thus, because hospitals and physicians are not primarily engaged in the selling of products or equipment used in the course of surgery, strict liability was inappropriate.

In Illinois, on the other hand, a woman brought suit against a hospital under a strict liability theory when she contracted hepatitis after a blood transfusion. The court stated that under the concept of strict liability, an entity that distributes a defective product for human consumption should bear the legal consequences of injury caused by the product. Accordingly, the Illinois Supreme Court permitted the plaintiff to proceed against the hospital under a theory of strict liability.[2]

Under a strict liability theory, all that needs to be shown is that the product or thing that caused the injury was unreasonably dangerous when it was placed in the stream of commerce. Fault is not a prerequisite for a finding of liability under this theory.

Some courts have found certain contaminated blood products to be "unreasonably dangerous." In those instances, usually the seller of the product rather than the provider of the service, is held liable. However, the plaintiff may still proceed against the health-care provider under a theory based on negligence or fault.

WHAT THEORY WILL A PLAINTIFF CHOOSE?

Although one cannot predict which theory an attorney for the plaintiff will advance in any given case, the theory most often advanced against a surgeon is based on negligence or fault. Although strict liability and breach of contract may be legitimate grounds on which to sue, it is difficult to maintain an action under these theories. Most experienced attorneys recognize that courts are reluctant to hold hospitals and surgeons strictly liable for injuries sustained after blood transfusion when there has been no demonstrable negligence on the part of the surgeon or hospital. Under a contract theory, moreover, the amount of money that may be recovered is limited. Plaintiffs' attorneys find it more attractive to sue under the theory of negligence because recovery can be virtually limitless. In an action for negligence, the plaintiff alleges that the surgeon was in some way at fault for the plaintiff's injuries. The physician failed to do something that could and should have been done to prevent the injuries.

The assessment of liability under a negligence or fault theory can also extend to harm caused to third parties. In Illinois a young woman brought suit against the hospital and a surgeon as a result of a transfusion that she had received ten years earlier when she was 13 years old. The suit was brought on behalf of both the woman and her child, who had not yet been conceived at the time of the transfusion.

The suit charged that ten years earlier the surgeon and the hospital negligently transfused the 13-year-old girl during the course of surgery. She was Rh-negative and received Rh-positive blood. When the suit was filed many years after the occurrence, the woman stated that she first discovered that she had been improperly sensitized by the Rh-positive transfusion during routine blood work in the course of prenatal care.

The Illinois court held for the first time that a plaintiff could maintain a suit for wrongful conduct that occurred prior to the child's conception. The court found that the physician and the hospital had a duty to the woman to perform the transfusion in a manner that conformed to an acceptable standard of care. They further found that it was foreseeable that the transfusion of a young Rh-negative female with Rh-positive blood could result in difficulties if she later became pregnant.[3]

The court pointed out that the concept of the defendant's duty to act reasonably within the accepted standard of care was not a static one and that an expansion of that duty may be appropriate under certain circumstances. This case imposed on the physician not only a duty to the transfused patient but also, by implication, to her child, who had not been conceived at the time of the allegedly negligent act. The case also demonstrates the willingness of the courts to move beyond established boundaries in extending theories under which plaintiffs may bring suit for transfusion-related injuries.

LIKELY TARGETS IN A TRANSFUSION-RELATED LAWSUIT

Most medical malpractice actions that result from the administration of blood or blood products include not only the surgeon, but the hospital, the anesthesiologist, other caregivers, and often the blood bank, the blood supplier, or the manufacturer of the blood product. Most plaintiffs' attorneys initially include as many parties and theories of liability as possible. Thus, in a transfusion-related lawsuit, the surgeon is likely to find himself in the company of many of his colleagues as well as the hospital. However, the theories of liability against each defendant may be significantly different.

Vicarious Liability

The theory of vicarious liability essentially makes one person liable for the acts of another if the liable person directs and supervises the activity of the other and exercises control over him. Theoretically, this concept could make surgeons liable for the actions of residents or surgical assistants performing under their direction and control. By the same theory, a hospital is held liable for the actions of a nurse who is found negligent during the course of nursing duties.

Creative attorneys have increasingly fashioned theories of liability against the surgeon, although the injury may have occurred as a result of the negligence of another person. A surgeon may be found vicariously liable for the actions of others even if they are not the surgeon's employees or directly under the surgeon's control. In such situations, the plaintiff is likely to assert that he had no choice regarding the caregiver in question and submitted to care and treatment by that person on the basis of the surgeon's recommendations. The secondary caregiver could be an anesthesiologist, nurse anesthetist, resident, surgical assistant, or a specifically requested nurse who works only with that surgeon.

This theory may also apply to a surgeon who recommends a particular hospital for surgery. Many surgeons have admitting privileges at more than one hospital. If it can be shown that the hospital to which the surgeon sent the patient experienced several prior transfusion-related incidents and that the surgeon either knew or should have known about such a history, the plaintiff may be able to fashion a theory of vicarious liability against the surgeon.

Because the hospital is usually considered the "deep pocket" in medical malpractice litigation, most attorneys try to find some way to keep the hospital in the lawsuit. The hospital is responsible for the actions of its nurses, its technicians, in-house blood bank personnel, and possibly physicians. A recent case in Illinois suggests that the hospital can even be held vicariously liable for the negligent acts of physicians who are independent contractors.[4]

Illinois is not the only jurisdiction that has suggested extension of vicarious liability to hospitals. By legislative fiat, New York hospitals may also be found vicariously liable for the negligence of the blood bank or blood service.[5] That liability has been described by a New York court as nondelegable.[6] This theory is designed to allow plaintiffs expanded access to redress for injuries suffered as a result of receiving contaminated blood. Hospitals, blood banks, and surgeons who are sued under this theory have a unique commonality of interest in terms of assessed liability.

Some jurisdictions recognize the "captain of the ship" doctrine, which makes the surgeon responsible for most events occurring in the operating room. Fortunately, this doctrine has been rejected in most jurisdictions and is severely limited even in the jurisdictions where it remains.

With regard to transfusion of blood and blood products, the surgeon is held to the same standard of care that is applicable to other aspects of treatment. In order to be held vicariously liable, the surgeon must be shown to have some level of control, direction, supervisory authority, and responsibility for the actions of those through whom a plaintiff seeks to attach liability.

THE MOST COMMON CAUSES OF TRANSFUSION-RELATED LAWSUITS

During the course of a surgical procedure involving blood transfusion, various occurrences may give rise to a lawsuit. However, most transfusion-related lawsuits have their genesis in a limited number of occurrences.

Attorneys representing plaintiffs in transfusion-related lawsuits are well aware of the pitfalls in presenting their case, and ultimately prevailing, if the suit is predicated purely on a transfusion-related theory. The goal is to recover damages for the client. In order to do so, the attorney employs as many theories as are appropriate and available. The most commonly used theories are discussed below.

Administration of Contaminated Blood

The administration of contaminated blood is probably the cause of the majority of transfusion-related lawsuits. This type of suit has grown in notoriety in recent years because of the spread of human immunodeficiency virus (HIV) and growing public awareness. Lawsuits related to other blood-borne pathogens are also worthy of discussion because the potential liability for the surgeon is the same, no matter what the contaminant. In fact, in some instances, a contaminant other than HIV may present greater liability for the surgeon.

As mentioned above, it is difficult to sue blood banks, suppliers, manufacturers of blood products, and others under a strict liability theory. Almost all states have blood-shield statutes that limit the circumstances under which a plaintiff can bring an action against these entities. A majority of the case law has also rejected the use of a strict liability theory for the administration of contaminated blood. Thus, a plaintiff usually proceeds under a theory of negligence—that is, he must show that the blood bank, supplier, or manufacturer knew that the particular disease could be transmitted through blood and failed to test for the contaminant or to prevent the circulation and use of tainted blood and that, as a result, the plaintiff suffered injury. In such situations, industry-wide standards are used as a gauge to measure acceptable practice. For example, if no blood bank in the country was performing a particular screening test, it probably would not be sufficient to show that the test was known to researchers and probably could have been used by making special arrangements.

Most of the cases involving HIV-tainted blood arise from transfusions administered before March 1985, when a reliable means of testing for the virus in blood became commercially available. Plaintiffs have tried to circumvent the argument that HIV could not have been detected because adequate screening was not available at the time in question, as the following case from Texas demonstrates.

The parents of a four-year-old child who died of AIDS contracted during a 1982 blood transfusion shortly after birth brought suit against the hospital and the blood supplier based on negligence. As a result of that transfusion, the child tested positive for cytomegalovirus (CMV) and HIV.

Testimony established that at the time of the transfusion the transmission of HIV was not well understood and that the test for the antibody was not mandated for use by blood banks until sometime between March and July of 1985. Nevertheless, the plaintiffs were able to avoid dismissal of their case by showing that the hospital's failure to test for CMV was negligent. The plaintiffs' expert testified that a test for CMV was available and in use at the time of the child's transfusion and that groups at significantly increased risk for CMV were the same groups at risk for HIV. The court found that the expert testimony sufficiently raised the question of whether proper screening of the blood for infectious agents other than HIV would have shown contamination by CMV, thereby preventing transfusion of blood that turned out to be also infected with HIV.[7] This case is unusual because the blood contained two separate and distinct contaminants. The basic principle could also be applied to the transmission of hepatitis, as testimony established that the same groups of donors would be at risk for infection with hepatitis.

In a New York case, a 46-year-old woman who contracted HIV after a two-unit blood transfusion during surgery in 1981 sued the hospital, the blood supplier, the surgeons, and other physicians.[8] She advanced several theories in pursuing her case.

One theory argued that the hospital did not have proper procedures in place to protect her against the transmission of blood-borne diseases other than HIV, which were well known in 1981. She contended that if the hospital had employed screening procedures for blood-borne diseases such as hepatitis, those procedures would have been effective in screening for HIV-infected blood. The court looked to industry standards for screening and testing procedures in use at the time the plaintiff received the blood. No one was employing the procedures that the plaintiff claimed would have prevented her infection. Although the plaintiff's clever argument did not prevail, it is nonetheless noteworthy because the same or similar arguments have been used in other cases and in all likelihood will continue to be used.

Litigation arising from the administration of contaminated blood or blood products is definitely on the rise, but it is by no means the only risk of liability regarding the use of blood or blood products during surgery.

Mismatched Transfusions

In addition to contaminated blood, mismatched transfusions present the kind of facts which make it easier for the plaintiff to prove his or her case. A hypothetical case involves a young married woman of child-bearing age with a serious congenital heart defect that requires surgical correction. The operation is a technical success, but the patient receives blood containing an incompatible Rh factor. The patient is later told of the error and her recovery is uneventful. Does she have a cause of action against the surgeon, the hospital, and others? The answer is yes.

The transfusion issue is only one of several that could be raised by the patient. In addition to injury from the mismatched blood, a likely claim would be the fear of childbearing because of Rh sensitivity caused by transfusing Rh-incompatible blood. It can reasonably be argued that a woman with a serious congenital heart defect should avoid pregnancy. However, the patient's truthfulness about childbearing aspirations could never be proved and could not effectively be used as a defense.

Failure To Transfuse Appropriately

In the event blood transfusion is necessary, the physician must determine which blood product should be administered. However, the determination must be made with diligence and care. When more than one alternative is available, the physician should make a reasoned choice within the scope of his or her medical knowledge. A physician is not liable if, after careful thought and exercise of reasonable medical judgment, he makes a choice that later turns out to have been wrong. However, the physician must be able to show that the choice was reasonable and may have been made by other well-qualified physicians under similar circumstances.

Such cases are never clear cut. The plaintiff who believes that the physician made a wrong choice that resulted in injury will certainly seek and, in all likelihood, find medical expert testimony to support the contention that a well-qualified physician under similar circumstances would not have made that choice.

Administration of Insufficient Blood

Administration of an insufficient amount of blood or blood products may also be the basis for liability. The administration of blood or blood products is always a carefully considered decision. Most physicians agree that blood or blood products should be ordered only if absolutely necessary and only in amounts that, in the physician's medical judgment, are necessary under the circumstances. With the benefit of hindsight, the plaintiff who believes that the physician ordered an insufficient amount of blood or blood products will challenge the reasonableness of the physician's judgment.

Failure To Recognize the Need for Transfusion

The physician's failure to recognize the necessity for transfusion may also be the basis for liability. In one case a surgeon was sued after the death of a patient who did not receive a blood transfusion. The plaintiff's expert testified that if a blood transfusion had been given, the patient in all probability would have survived. Predictably, the defendant's expert disagreed. In his judgment, the condition from which the patient suffered had a 25% mortality rate under all treatment regimens, including blood transfusion. Thus, it was his opinion that no one could say with certainty that transfusion would have saved the patient's life.[9] It was the jury's role to weigh the testimony of the experts and to determine whether malpractice had been committed.

Improper Technique or Equipment

The surgical technique is one of the most obvious and often used vehicles for charges of malpractice on the part of the surgeon. The surgeon may be faulted for using a technique that, in the plaintiff's argument, resulted in an abnormal blood loss, thereby necessitating transfusion. The plaintiff may also assert that the surgeon's lack of skill prolonged the surgery or that the surgery was performed in an unusual or inappropriate manner that created a need for transfusion that would not have occurred with the proper technique.

A plaintiff may also attempt to show that the equipment used by the surgeon was substandard or that it was used in an improper manner. If, for example, the patient develops an infection at the site of a line through which the blood is transfused, he may assert that the technique used in placing the line was the cause of the infection. Thus, although the transfusion itself is not the issue, the plaintiff asserts that poor technique resulted in injury. In such a situation, even though surgery and recovery may have been successful, the plaintiff may bring suit for the infection. The success of the surgery and recovery is not considered in determining whether a surgeon is liable for the injury suffered as a result of the alleged improper technique.

An obviously related issue is the extent of a plaintiff's injury. In one case the defendants argued that the gift of life outweighed the injury sustained by the plaintiff. Therefore, because the plaintiff sustained no injury greater than the benefit conferred upon her, the defendants sought dismissal of the lawsuit. The court acknowledged some merit to the defendants' argument but rejected it nevertheless. Although agreeing that life is preferable to death, the court stated that the issue could not be viewed as broadly as the defendants proposed.[10] The court added that a reasonable standard of care must be exercised by physicians even when saving a life. In all situations, a physician has a duty to act in a way that minimizes injury to the patient. Any breach that results in unnecessary injury to the patient is negligence and constitutes a valid cause of action for medical malpractice.

Failure To Recognize an Adverse Transfusion Reaction

Although the surgeon may decide whether to administer blood to the patient and how much blood should be administered, it is usually not the surgeon's responsibility to carry out the procedural checks prior to transfusion or to administer the transfusion itself. Other members of the team are responsible for cross-checking the blood with the patient's identification to ensure that the correct blood or blood product is administered to the correct patient. Even in the best of institutions, the system can sometimes break down, and a transfusion error may result. Although someone else may have created the problem and will probably be held accountable, the surgeon may also be faced with liability for failure to recognize a hemolytic reaction. Once a transfusion error has been committed, if the surgeon fails to recognize signs of an adverse reaction in a timely manner, the surgeon may be held accountable.

The question of whether the signs were obvious or occult is a question of fact that will not prevent the surgeon from being sued. Expert testimony will assert that a reasonably well-qualified surgeon under similar circumstances would have identified the hemolytic reaction in a timely manner and responded appropriately. In such situations, the surgeon is likely to be part of a larger defendant dragnet that involves the hospital, anesthesiologist, residents, nurses, and perhaps the blood bank.

SHIFTING THE FOCUS TO RELATED ISSUES SURROUNDING TRANSFUSIONS

As discussed above, proceeding under theories of strict liability against the manufacturer of blood products, the supplier, the hospital, or the surgeon is usually not the easiest route for a plaintiff to pursue. Plaintiffs bring lawsuits because they want compensation for an injury; therefore, they pursue the theories that are more likely to net recovery.

This goal can sometimes be achieved by shifting the focus of the lawsuit. For example, a plaintiff may assert that if the physician had diagnosed a particular problem earlier and treated it appropriately, the transfusion may not have been necessary. Therefore, the sufficiency of the transfusion or the transfusion itself would not be an issue if it had not been for the physician's negligence in related care and treatment.

Furthermore, if the plaintiff claims that the surgery was unnecessary, then clearly the transfusion exposed the plaintiff to an unnecessary risk. Similarly, the plaintiff may claim that the transfusion was unnecessary and thus resulted in unnecessary exposure to contaminated blood.

The same argument of unnecessary exposure may be used if a patient loses 500 cc or less of blood during surgery. The plaintiff in a New York case argued that the physician was negligent in ordering a transfusion because her blood loss was not large enough to warrant transfusion.[11] Her theory was that because the blood loss was minimal, the physician, exercising reasonable medical judgment, should have employed other measures to replace her blood volume. Further, she argued that the risk of an untoward reaction from receiving a single unit of blood was greater than the risk if no blood had been administered. Although the plaintiff did not prevail for reasons unrelated to her factual arguments, under other circumstances this theory could well be accepted as a basis on which to impose liability.

When looking at any of the theories of liability most frequently used by plaintiffs in transfusion-related lawsuits, one should be mindful that a physician is not negligent simply because he makes a mistake or error in judgment, as long as he exercises reasonable medical skill under the circumstances.

INFORMED CONSENT

The evolving doctrine of informed consent, which is a relatively recent judicial creation, is often cited as a major contributor to the increasing number of malpractice claims and constitutes a great source of discomfort for many physicians. The claim of lack of informed consent essentially means that a patient was not reasonably apprised of potential adverse consequences of surgery or other treatment and would not have consented if the risk that materialized had been disclosed. Underlying the concept of informed consent is the acknowledgment of each person's right to autonomy in medical treatment. Health-care providers often discover a fine line between adequately advising patients of possible risks associated with a particular course of treatment and providing them with hope and reassurance at a time when they are anxious and fearful.

The subject of blood transfusion has recently become a candidate for the requirement of informed consent, primarily because of the advent of transfusion-associated diseases such as AIDS and the resultant rise in public awareness. Lack of informed consent in blood transfusion cases has been advanced against physicians because they are generally detached from the process of blood collection and transfusion; therefore, it provides a viable theory under which to establish the physician's liability.

Although earlier case law characterized the failure to obtain adequately informed consent as battery on the part of the physician,[12] in the great majority of jurisdictions informed consent is now essentially a negligence theory. The concept is predicated on the duty to disclose information to a patient about his or her medical condition and the duty to obtain the patient's consent before rendering treatment. With respect to this second duty, the law also requires that the consent be informed—that is, the patient must have been given enough information to make a knowledgeable decision.

An informed choice discussion should be a mutual exchange of information. The physician discusses the possible risks and benefits of a procedure, conveys to the patient that the practice of medicine has no guarantees, and that alternatives are available. The patient expresses concerns, asks questions, gains an understanding of the proposed treatment, and makes an informed choice.

As a side benefit, this discussion can enhance the physician–patient rapport that is essential in reducing malpractice litigation. A significant number of malpractice claims can be traced to a patient's psychological dissatisfaction with the medical treatment. An open line of communication between physician and patient reduces the risk of a lawsuit if the outcome is less than optimal.

A question that logically follows in considering disclosure of risks to a patient is "how much is enough information?" The seminal case that sets the standard for disclosure arose in the District of Columbia. In that case[13] the court applied a patient-oriented standard that requires disclosure of risks that would be "material" to a patient's decision whether or not to undergo a treatment or procedure. This approach has been adopted in the majority of jurisdictions. In assessing whether the standard for full disclosure of material information has been met, most courts rely on what a reasonably prudent medical practitioner would disclose under the same or similar circumstances.

Discussion of Risks Associated with Transfusion

As stated above, blood transfusion has quickly evolved as a topic in most consent-for-treatment discussions. Although transfusion is usually incidental to another procedure, it should nonetheless be incorporated into the discussion.

The risks of blood transfusion that must be disclosed to the patient are determined by what the reasonable physician would communicate under the same circumstances. Although the case law makes clear that not all risks need to be disclosed, particularly those which are obvious or that stand a statistically insignificant chance of materializing, the risk of AIDS transmission should be mentioned, even though it is extremely low. The reason is simple: the subject of AIDS is emotionally charged. Public awareness has been enhanced, and many patients are fearful of the threat of AIDS. This discussion can be an opportunity for the physician to educate his patient about the blood screening techniques that are in place and help to reduce substantially the risk of transfusion-transmitted disease.

Case law clearly suggests that because the severity of the harm posed by AIDS is great, the fully informed patient might possibly refuse to accept blood transfusion from an anonymous donor and may even refuse to undergo surgery, particularly if it is elective.[14] Thus it is too risky for the physician to withhold a discussion about HIV-contaminated blood. In the current legal climate a jury could impose liability on a physician for failure to do so.

Exceptions to Requirement for Consent

The exceptions to the requirement for informed consent are limited. The first is an emergency, which is defined differently from state to state. In general, however, an emergency is a situation in which the loss of life or limb is threatened. The law assumes that a reasonable person would want medical care in an emergency and that the patient, if conscious and able to give consent, would do so. In the case of surgery during which blood transfusion becomes medically necessary, however, the physician cannot hide behind the emergency exception if the likelihood of transfusion was reasonably contemplated beforehand.

The second exception is patient waiver. The reasonable physician should be wary of the patient who does not "want to know all the gory details" and just wants the doctor to "do what you think is best." The physician should make every effort to inform the patient fully about the contemplated course of treatment, despite the patient's protests.

Another exception is therapeutic privilege, which permits the physician to withhold information from a patient whom the physician believes is not capable of coping with the knowledge. This exception, which tends to be one of the most overused by medical practitioners, is not an automatic bar to liability. If the surgeon chooses to invoke this exception, several precautions should be taken. First, the decision should be discussed in detail with the spouse or a family member of the patient. Second, the surgeon should consult with the patient's family physician or psychiatrist. Third, the medical record should carefully reflect why the information was withheld from the patient and identify the persons consulted, including the patient's spouse or other relatives as well as other physicians.

Disclosure of Alternatives

The informed consent discussion of blood transfusion should also provide the patient with a list of available alternatives, including blood conservation, preoperative autologous donation, and directed donations by family and friends. The crucial point is to hold the discussion well in advance of the contemplated surgery to allow the patient time to exercise these options. This goal is easily accomplished with elective or non-emergent surgery.

Other Issues Relating to Consent

The belief that inadequate disclosure automatically results in liability for patient injury is a source of anxiety for many surgeons. But claims based on lack of informed consent are often defeated in the absence of proof of malpractice because of the common knowledge that surgery involves risks. Thus, if it is shown that treatment was medically justified and properly performed, it may be quite difficult for a plaintiff to argue persuasively that the treatment would have been refused with knowledge of risks. The claim of lack of informed consent has more obvious validity in cases of elective surgery.

A surgeon's discussion with the patient about risks of transfusion should be complemented with documentation in the chart to justify the need for transfusion. Most lawyers whose clients contract a disease from a tainted transfusion, for example, spend a great deal of time poring over the medical record to determine whether the blood was actually necessary. If no indications are documented in the record, the physician has an uphill battle relieving himself of liability.

Informed Refusal

Another twist to the issue of informed consent is the doctrine of informed refusal, which was introduced in a California case.[15] The decision suggests that physicians need to tell patients that refusal to consent to a particular procedure might place their health or life in jeopardy. In the California case, the physician recommended to a patient that she undergo a Papanicolaou smear. The patient refused. The physician failed to advise her of the risks associated with refusing the test. After the patient died from cervical cancer, her estate filed a lawsuit for wrongful death against the physician, claiming that he had an obligation to inform his patient of the importance of the test. The California Supreme Court upheld the cause of action.

This decision makes quite clear that physicians must tell patients not only that treatment of disease poses certain risks, but also that failure to treat specific conditions also poses certain risks.

Disclosure of HIV Status

An issue that is currently heavily debated in both the medical and legal environments is whether a physician has a duty to inform the patient if the physician's HIV or hepatitis status is positive. Few courts have been asked to decide this question. Many medical associations, however, as well as the Centers for Disease Control (CDC), advocate that HIV infected health professionals should stop performing exposure-prone procedures unless they obtain the informed consent of the patient beforehand. Many physicians have opposed both the CDC guidelines and proposed legislation that calls for mandatory testing of health-care workers and patient notification in the event of positive findings. The argument is that the risk of transmission to patients is insignificant; therefore, the potential loss of hospital privileges and the possibility of lawsuits do not warrant disclosure. Furthermore, many physicians are reluctant to disclose matters of such a private nature.

Courts have not yet entered the debate over mandatory testing of health-care workers, and very few cases have addressed the need to inform patients that a health-care worker is HIV positive. As a result, the CDC guidelines may set the standard for disclosure in claims by infected patients or by noninfected patients who experience serious emotional distress after learning of their physician's health status. The guidelines are persuasive and may influence a court's determination of what constitutes proper disclosure on the part of a medical practitioner.

In one of the few cases to discuss this issue at length, the New Jersey Supreme Court imposed the duty of disclosing the risk of transmission of HIV on a surgeon diagnosed with AIDS.[16] The court found that although the risk of transmission was low, the risk of a surgical accident (such as a needlestick or scalpel cut) existed. These two risks created a reasonable probability of substantial harm which a reasonable patient would consider in determining whether to consent to the proposed procedure.

The court also considered the nature of the specific procedure in an effort to quantify the risk. In this case, the physician specialized in ear and mouth surgery, which was particularly susceptible to transmission of HIV if a surgical accident should occur because of contact with mucous membranes. The court, recognizing its strong commitment to the concept of a fully informed patient, rejected the physician's argument that patient reaction was more likely to be based on public hysteria than on a studied assessment of the actual risk involved. The court stated that it was the physician's responsibility to allay those fears and that the difficulties created by the public reaction to AIDS should not deprive the patient of making the ultimate decision about medical treatment with full knowledge of the potential risk.

This case is significant because it recognized that requiring a physician to reveal HIV infection in a discussion of informed consent would amount to a *de facto* termination of surgical privileges. Nonetheless, the court gave priority to the patient's right to know over the physician's right to perform surgery as a practice of his profession. The case also suggests that failure to discuss a key element that may be integral to the patient's decision is actionable.

Many health-care workers argue that required HIV disclosure is outweighed by the loss of privacy, possible discrimination, low risk of transmission, and loss of certain hospital privileges. The debate is still relatively new, but the issue has already resulted in litigation. And more lawsuits are likely to follow. Attorneys will continue to advance creative theories to hold physicians liable for transmission of HIV or for emotional distress resulting from the failure to disclose HIV positivity. The only assurance that a physician's duty has been discharged is full disclosure of HIV-positive status to the patient about to undergo an invasive procedure. This discussion also affords the physician an opportunity to provide accurate information to the patient and to dispel many of the myths that have been perpetuated as a result of public AIDS hysteria.

Refusal of Consent and Forced Transfusion

Competent adults can refuse to give consent for medical treatment, even if it is life-sustaining, and in particular they can refuse blood transfusion. The vast majority of cases in this area concern refusal on the basis of religious beliefs, but as AIDS awareness increases and the risk of transmission through blood transfusion becomes more of a concern for patients, problems related to patient refusal may also increase.

Because the decision to accept blood can be one of life or death, on occasion, courts have chosen to intervene to protect the sanctity of life. They have addressed this issue in a variety of contexts, dealing with children, pregnant women, and adults.

Children. In the case of a child, the parents generally have the right to make decisions about medical treatment. However, many states have a statutory basis for the court to intervene and order that the needed medical treatment be provided for the child, even if it includes blood transfusion. This power is particularly enforced when the child's life is threatened. The case law is quite uniform that under such circumstances, the interest in preserving the child's life outweighs even religious beliefs.

Pregnant Women. The special cases posed by pregnant women are similar to those involving children. Most courts generally find that they have a duty to preserve human life. If fetal well-being is at risk and blood transfusion is necessary to preserve the fetus, courts will intervene and order the treatment.

Adults. The competent adult presents a much more difficult situation. Earlier cases justified compulsory transfusion, but many courts have shown a growing trend to affirm the rights of Jehovah's Witnesses to decline transfusion because of a patient's right to self-determination. Many physicians find these opinions troublesome, arguing that in essence the courts are forcing physicians to provide less than optimal care when they are prohibited from transfusing a patient in need of blood.

One response to this concern can be found in an opinion of the Michigan Appellate Court, which ruled that a physician would not be held liable for ordering life-saving blood for a Jehovah's Witness patient who had previously refused to receive blood.[17] In that case, the plaintiff was admitted to the hospital for delivery of twins. While preregistering approximately two months before admission, she signed a Refusal To Permit Blood Transfusion.

After delivery, the plaintiff bled profusely from her uterus. She was taken to surgery, during which the bleeding could not be controlled, and her blood pressure dropped significantly. The doctor ordered a blood transfusion, in spite of knowing that the patient was a Jehovah's Witness and had previously documented her refusal to be transfused.

The trial court found that the patient's refusal of blood some two months earlier was based on the expectation of routine elective surgery with no threat to life. Therefore, it could not be said that she made the decision to refuse a blood transfusion in a competent state with full awareness that death would result from refusal. The medical record reflected the unexpected development of a medical emergency that required transfusion to prevent death. On this basis, the court found that the patient did not have an action against the physician for ordering the transfusion. The appellate court affirmed the decision, stating that in an emergency calling for an immediate decision, nothing less than a fully conscious contemporaneous decision by the patient is sufficient to override the implied consent that the law recognizes for treatment necessary to preserve a patient's life.

The fact that an emergency exception exists should not be viewed as an absolute entitlement to proceed with treatment without patient consent. Courts will continue to scrutinize the use of this exception because many of them believe that an adult has the right to refuse medical treatment. Each situation will be evaluated by the court on a case-by-case basis and the facts, as they are borne out in the medical record, will determine whether a physician is held liable.

In a related case, the patient made it clear to the surgeon before surgery that under no circumstances should a transfusion be administered because of her religious beliefs. The patient was borderline anemic. During the course of the surgery, an inadvertent laceration caused a massive hemorrhage. The surgeon made an heroic attempt to bring the bleeding under control. When it became clear that he was losing the battle, the hospital's attorney was contacted for legal authorization to proceed with a blood transfusion. Within fifteen minutes, the authorization had been received and the transfusion started. Unfortunately, by that time, the patient had lost too much blood and later expired. The patient's husband sued. He asserted that the surgeon should have begun the blood transfusion immediately after the patient began to hemorrhage. The husband also claimed that after the surgeon received the authorization to perform the transfusion, he did so negligently. The court noted that before surgery the surgeon had specifically informed the patient that a blood transfusion may be necessary to save her life. Neither the plaintiff nor the defendant disputed that the patient was unequivocal in withholding her consent to transfusion, even in the face of death. Nevertheless, the jury found for the plaintiff (the husband).

The appellate court reversed the verdict. The court said no physician should be forced to stand by helplessly while a patient dies, even if the patient instructs the surgeon to do just that. By the time the surgeon was allowed to use all available methods, including transfusion, to save the patient, it was too late. Such a situation involved no liability.[18] Although this case was eventually resolved in the surgeon's favor, many lessons can be learned.

Most situations involving refusal of treatment do not contemplate negligence on the part of the physician, which will undoubtedly alter the outcome in the event a lawsuit is filed. An example is a wrongful death action brought by the widow of a patient who died after surgery. The patient was advised by his surgeon that he needed a blood transfusion, but the patient refused on religious grounds. The surgeon testified that he advised the patient and his wife that a blood transfusion was imperative as the only remaining treatment available to alleviate the patient's internal bleeding. The surgeon also advised the patient and his wife that without a blood transfusion the patient could die. Both the patient and his wife refused the transfusion.

The patient and his wife were asked to sign a release document that stated in substance that the patient understood that his refusal to accept the blood transfusion would "seriously imperil [his] life." The release also stated that all of the attendant risks of the refusal had been explained to the patient and his wife and that the hospital, its nurses, employees, and the surgeon were released from any liability whatsoever for following the patient's wishes and direction. The patient died, and his wife later sued for malpractice.

The trial court granted summary judgment in favor of the surgeon, reasoning that the patient's refusal of the blood transfusion barred any recovery for wrongful death. The wife appealed. The appellate court reversed the trial court and reinstituted the lawsuit. The appellate court held that the release signed by the patient and his wife did not bar recovery against the surgeon because the release did not contemplate the surgeon's alleged negligent treatment of the patient, which was unrelated or only indirectly related to the transfusion issue.[19]

CONCLUSION

The courts have seen a drastic increase in the number of transfusion-related lawsuits as a result of heightened public concern over adverse consequences of transfusion. Traditional theories of liability have focused on the anesthesiologist, hospital, and blood bank. However, plaintiffs' attorneys have also sought to include in the list of defendants the surgeon and other caregivers, basing liability on various creative theories.

The best defense for the surgeon is to be aware of the legal risks that confront him in the course of treating a patient and to minimize those risks by adequately educating the patient, maintaining good documentation, and practicing in a manner that is consistent with the care provided by other reasonably well-qualified surgeons in his area of specialty.

GLOSSARY

Actionable: furnishing legal ground for an action or lawsuit.
Appellate court: a court having jurisdiction of appeal and review, which is the power to examine a trial court's actions in an earlier proceeding.
Battery: any unlawful touching of a person without his or her consent.
Blood shield statutes: statutes that prohibit claimants from bringing a legal action against a blood bank, blood supplier, or manufacturer of blood products without some evidence of negligence on the part of that entity.
Breach: the violation of a duty, either by commission or omission.
Case law: an aggregate collection of reported cases which form a body of law and upon which many courts rely when ruling on matters before them.
Complaint: the initial document filed in court at the commencement of a lawsuit which sets forth the claim being made and the recovery being sought.
Damage: loss, injury, or deterioration caused by the negligence of another; money or compensation for loss.

Defendant: the party against whom relief is sought in a legal action.
Duty: an obligation to which the law will give recognition and effect to conform to a particular standard of conduct toward another.
Liability: an imposed responsibility for a loss.
Negligence: the failure to use such care as a reasonably prudent and careful person would use under similar circumstances; the doing of some act which a person of ordinary prudence would not have done under similar circumstances; or the failure to do what a person of ordinary prudence would have done under similar circumstances.
Material: having influence or effect.
Plaintiff: the party who complains or sues in a legal action and seeks remedial relief for an injury.
Pleadings: the formal allegations by the parties, in written form, that are filed in court.
Proximate cause: any cause which, in natural or probable sequence, produced the injury complained of; it need not be the only cause, nor the last or nearest cause.
Release: the relinquishment of a right, claim, or privilege by the person who has a right to it, to the person against whom it might have been enforced.
Strict liability: liability without fault. A legal doctrine that holds sellers and manufacturers responsible for products that are in a defective condition and are unreasonably dangerous at the time they reach the consumer.
Summary judgment: a procedure which allows a resolution of a lawsuit on the basis of written pleadings, without a trial. The party seeking summary judgment must show that there is no material issue of fact and that as a matter of law, the court must rule in his favor. The court's ruling has the same effect as if the matter had been fully tried.
Wrongful death action: a type of lawsuit brought on behalf of a decedent's beneficiaries, alleging that his death was attributable to the negligence of another.

REFERENCES

1. *Hector v. Cedars Sinai Medical Center*, 180 Cal. App. 3d 493, 225 Cal. Rptr. 595 (1986).
2. *Cunningham v. MacNeal Memorial Hospital*, 47 Ill. 2d 443, 226 N.E.2d 897 (1970).
3. *Renslow v. Mennonite Hospital*, 67 Ill. 2d 348, 367 N.E. 2d 1250 (1977).
4. *Uhr v. Lutheran General Hospital*, 226 Ill. App. 3d 236, 589 N.E.2d 723 (1992). This opinion was vacated by the Illinois Supreme Court on March 9, 1993 on procedural grounds, but there is no reason to expect that the appellate court, if presented with similar facts, would reach a different conclusion.
5. 10 N.Y.C.R.R. 400.4(a); 405.2(a), 405.2(h).
6. *Mondello v. New York Blood Center, et al.*, 175 A.D.2d 718, 573 N.Y.S. 2d 665 (1991).
7. *Longoria v. McAllen Methodist Hospital*, 771 S.W.2d 663 (Tex. Ct. App. 1989).
8. *Hoemke v. New York Blood Center, et al.*, 720 F. Supp. 45 (N.Y. Cir. 1989).
9. *Corlett v. Caserta*, 204 Ill. App. 3d 403, 562 N.E.2d 257 (1990).
10. *Scott v. Brooklyn Hospital*, 125 Misc. 2d 765, 480 N.Y.S.2d 270 (1984).
11. *Hoemke v. New York Blood Center, et al.*, 720 F. Supp. 45 (N.Y. Cir. 1989).
12. *Schloendorff v. Society of N.Y. Hosps.*, 211 N.Y. 125, 105 N.E. 92 (1914).
13. *Canterbury v. Spence*, 464 F.2d 772 (D.C. Cir. 1972).
14. See, e.g., *Valdiviez v. U.S.*, 884 F.2d 196 (5th Cir. 1989).
15. *Truman v. Thomas*, 165 Cal. Rptr. 308, 611 P.2d 902 (1980).
16. *Estate of Behringer v. Princeton Medical Center*, 249 N.J. Super. 597, 592 A.2d 1251 (1991).
17. *Werth v. Taylor*, 190 Mich. App. 141, 475 N.W.2d 426 (1991).
18. *Randolph v. The City of New York*, 501 N.Y.S.2d 837, 117 A.D.2d 44 (1986).
19. *Corlett v. Caserta*, 204 Ill. App. 3d 403, 562 N.E.2d 257 (1990).

RECOMMENDED READING LIST

Berry CL: AIDS and hospital liability. In For the Defense. Chicago, Defense Research Institute, 1990.
Brenner, Gerken: Informed consent: Myths and risk management alternatives. Risk Management and Quality Assurance: Issues and Interactions. Chicago, Joint Commission on Accreditation of Hospitals, 1986.
Clark GM (ed): Medicolegal Aspects of Blood Collection and Transfusion. Arlington, VA, American Association of Blood Banks, 1983.
Clark GM (ed): Legal Issues in Transfusion Medicine: Managing Risk in a Changing Environment. Arlington, VA, American Association of Blood Banks, 1986.
Closen ML, et al: Supplement to AIDS, Cases and Materials. Houston, TX, John Marshall Publishing, 1990.
Curran WJ, et al: Health Care Law, Forensic Science, and Public Policy, 4th ed. Boston, Little, Brown, 1990.
Eckert RD, Wallace EL: Securing a Safer Blood Supply: Two Views. Washington, DC: American Enterprise Institute for Public Policy Research, 1985.
Evans GF Jr: Medicolegal aspects of blood transfusions. State Art Rev 5:133–141, 1991.
Fiscina SF, et al: A Source Book for Research in Law and Medicine. Owing Mills, MD, National Health Publishing Company, 1985.
Gerber S, et al (eds): The Heart: A Law Medicine Problem. Cleveland, Institute of Law–Medicine, 1958.
Greenlaw PS: HIV antibody testing: Legal considerations and sound hospital policy. J Health Hosp Law 25(3):80-85, 1992.
Hayt E: Law of Hospital, Physician and Patient, 3rd ed. Berwyn, IL, Physicians' Record Company, 1972.
N.Y. Pub. Health Law, sec. 2805(d) (McKinney 1988).
Official Compilation of Codes, Rules and Regulations of the State of New York, secs. 400.4(a)(4), 405.2(a), 405.2(h) (1992).
Richards EP III, Rathburn KC: Medical Risk Management: Preventive Legal Strategies for Health Care Providers. Rockville, MD, Aspen Systems Corporation, 1983.
Rosenblum JB, Curry CL: Medical Malpractice: Handling Cardiology and Cardiovascular Surgery Cases. Colorado Springs, CO, Shepard's/McGraw-Hill, 1991.
Widmann FK (ed): Informed Consent for Blood Transfusion: Transcribed Proceedings of a National Conference and Issues Forum. Arlington, VA, American Association of Blood Banks, 1989.

INDEX

Acenocoumarol, 310
Acquired immune deficiency syndrome (AIDS), blood transfusion-related, 215, 363
Activated clotting time (ACT)
  in acute myocardial infarction, 180
  of aprotinin, 141–142, 157–163, 182
  during cardiopulmonary bypass, 68–69, 71, 72
    in children, 294–295
  of heparin, 57, 58, 61, 78–79, 80, 81, 112
  measurement of, 160–163
Activated partial thromboplastin time (APTT), 11
  during cardiopulmonary bypass, 69, 71, 72
  heparin-related prolongation of, 113, 328, 336
  preoperative evaluation of, 31, 78
    in acute myocardial infarction patients, 180
  thermoelastography comparison with, 71
  of total artificial heart patients, 239–240
  transfusion thresholds of, 217
Acyl-plasminogen-streptokinase activator complex, 29–30
Adenosine-3′,5′-cyclic monophosphate (cAMP)
  in platelet aggregation inhibition, 100
  in platelet degranulation, 247–248
  prostacyclin interaction with, 131, 318
Adenosine diphosphate (ADP)
  in platelet activation, 96, 98, 99
  in platelet adhesion, 2
  in platelet aggregation, 27, 274
  as platelet release reaction inducer, 24–25
  in primary hemostasis, 289
  in salvaged blood syndrome, 91
  ticlopidine-related inhibition of, 318, 319
Adenylate cyclase
  inhibitors of, 26
  stimulators of, 26
Adrenocorticotropic hormone (ACTH), plasmin-induced degradation of, 29
Albumin, as plasmapheresis replacement colloid, 226
Allergic reactions
  to aprotinin, 139
  to heparin, 58
Alpha-2-antiplasmin, as fibrinolytic system inhibitor, 30
Alpha-2-macroglobulin, as fibrinolytic system inhibitor, 30
Aminocaproic acid
  concomitant desmopressin use with, 37

Aminocaproic acid *(cont.)*
  epsilon (EACA)
    adverse effects of, 39, 44
    as antifibrinolytic therapy contraindication, 181
    for perioperative hemorrhage control, 39, 44, 131, 279, 280
    as streptokinase inhibitor, 277
    as fibrinolytic system inhibitor, 30
Amrinone, pediatric use of, 296
Anaphylaxis, protamine-related, 62–63
Ancrod, 67, 193, 195
Anemia, autoimmune hemolytic, 230
Angina pectoris
  peptide conjugate anticoagulant therapy for, 116–117
  unstable
    antithrombotic therapy for, 101–102
    pathophysiology of, 100, 101
Angioplasty
  percutaneous transluminal coronary, 116–117
    mechanical revascularization and, 177–178
    thrombosis prevention in, 103–104, 334–335
  transfemoral, 328
Anisoylated plasminogen-streptokinase activator complex, 178–179, 276, 277–278
Antibodies
  heparin-dependent, 187–189, 222
  plasmapheresis-related decrease of, 228
Anticoagulants, **111–128**
  comparison with antithrombotics, 111–116
  for coronary artery bypass patients, 179
  definition of, 327
  endothelial effects of, 119
  intensity measures of
    INR measure, 304, 305–306, 307, 308–310, 311–313
    prothrombin time ratio, 304–305, 306, 307–308, 309, 310, 312
    TPL measure, 304, 305–308
  natural, 6, 8–9
  new, 111, 116–120
  oral, 15–18
    side effects of, 123
  pediatric use of, 292
  as peripheral vascular disease prophylactics, **327–341**
    for early prophylaxis, 327, 328–330
    for long-term prophylaxis, 327, 330–336
  pharmacology of, 1–21

381

Anticoagulants *(cont.)*
  for postsurgical thromboembolism
    prophylactics, 111, 120-125
  for prosthetic heart valve patients, 45-46
  synergistic interactions of, 118
  systemic monitoring of, **65-76**
Antiplatelet therapy
  during coronary artery bypass surgery, 179,
    317-325
    hemorrhage management of, 322-323
    hemorrhage risk assessment for, 318-322
  pediatric use of, 292, 293
  pharmacology of, 317-318
Antithrombinic potential index, 240, 244
Antithrombin III (AT III)
  activation of, 8, 9
  aprotinin-related decrease of, 140-141
  as disseminated intravascular coagulation
    indicator, 38
  heparin binding of, 6, 8, 58, 122, 123, 354
  neonatal levels of, 288
  plasmapheresis-related decrease of, 228
  as procoagulant system inhibitor, 30
  serum content determination of, 252
  thrombin inhibiting action of, 6, 8, 251
  of total artificial heart patients, 240, 244
Antithrombin III deficiency, 115
  heparin resistance and, 62
Antithrombin peptides, synthetic, 116,
  117-118
Antithrombin potential index, 252-253
Antithrombotics, **95-110**
  for acute coronary syndromes, 100-103
  in coronary artery bypass graft surgery,
    104-105
  emergency cardiac surgery following use of,
    177-184
    coagulation restoration for, 181-182
    preoperative evaluation for, 179-180
  as hemorrhage cause, 138, 178-179, 276-278
  monitoring assays of, 121
  as myocardial infarction therapy, 177-181
  new selective thrombin inhibitors, 105-106
  in percutaneous transluminal coronary
    angioplasty, 103-104
  in prosthetic heart valve surgery, 105
Aorta, as heparin-induced thrombocytopenia
  site, 191, 193, 194
Aortocoronary bypass graft
  hemorrhage risk evaluation for, 209-210
  thromboembolic complications of, 210-212
Apheresis, in cardiac surgery, **225-235**
  cellular apheresis, 231-234
  centrifugation techniques for, 225
  complications of, 226
  erythrocyte exchange, 234
  preoperative, 233-234
  therapeutic plasma exchange, 227-231
  volume replacement during, 225-226
Aprosulfate, 116, 124

Aprotinin, 67, **147-166**
  activated clotting time prolongation effect
    of, 141-142, 157-163, 182
  for acute myocardial infarction, 181
  cell-saver-related loss of, 151-152
  chemistry of, 149-150
  as contact activating system inhibitor, 149
  efficacy criteria of, 152-156
  hemostatic restoration mechanism of, 119
  heparin interaction of, 119, 158-163
  high-dosage, 150-157
    adverse effects of, 212
    as aspirin-related hemorrhage
      prophylaxis, 323
    for children, 151
    modifications of, 151-157
  kallikrein inactivation units of, 149-150
  as perioperative blood-conserving therapy,
    129-145, 279, 280
    during coronary artery surgery, 133
    dosage regimen for, 133
    during infective endocarditis, 134
    multicenter studies of, 134-137
    during reoperative surgery, 133-134,
      135-136
    risk/benefit considerations in, 140-143
    safety of, 138-140
  timing of administration, 156-157
  trypsin inhibitory units of, 149
Aquamephyton, 181
Arachidonic acid
  conversion of, 25-26
  in platelet activation, 100
  in salvaged blood syndrome, 91
Argatroban, 105-106
Arteparon, 126
Arterial occlusion, thrombosis management
  following, 328-330
Arteriography, percutaneous coronary,
  thromboembolism prevention during,
  328
Arvin time, 180
Aspirin
  antiplatelet activity of, 248-249, 318
  as antithrombotic agent, 112, 123, 193
    for cardiogenic embolism prophylaxis,
      335
    for coronary artery bypass graft patients,
      104-105, 179, 322
    for femoral artery occlusion prophylaxis,
      333-334
    for internal carotid artery dissection
      patients, 329
    for myocardial infarction patients, 179
    for percutaneous transluminal angio-
      plasty patients, 103-104, 334-335
    for prosthetic heart valve patients, 45, 46,
      105
    for total artificial heart patients,
      248-250

INDEX 383

Aspirin *(cont.)*
   as antithrombotic agent *(cont.)*
      for unstable angina pectoris patients, 101-102
      for vascular reocclusion prophylaxis, 331, 332, 333
   bleeding time prolongation effect of, 179, 180, 181
   concomitant heparin therapy, 14
   concomitant warfarin therapy, 17, 309, 310, 311, 312-313
   as cyclooxygenase inhibitor, 26
   as postoperative hemorrhage cause, 14, 137-138, 209-210, 276
      desmopressin therapy for, 323
      reoperation for, 319, 320
   preoperative use of, 78, 82, 272-273, 276
      incidence of, 318-319
   side effects of, 123
Atherogenesis, process of, 95-96
Atherosclerosis, heparin prophylaxis of, 330
Atherosclerotic plaques
   formation of, 95, 97, 98
   as heparin-induced thrombi site, 191
   rupture of, 98, 100
      in acute ischemic coronary syndromes, 100-101
      angioplasty balloon-related, 103

Basement membrane, as platelet release reaction inducer, 24
B-beta 15-42-related peptides, 43, 44
Bernard-Soulier syndrome, 189, 289
Beta-lactam antibiotics, 323
Bioavailability, 9
Biomaterials, antithrombotic, for cardiovascular surgery, **353-358**
   heparin surface coatings of, 353, 354, 355-358
   thromboelastographic testing of, 69-71
BioMedicus extracorporeal centrifugal pump, 265, 268
Biotransformation, 10
Bleeding time
   antiplatelet agent-related prolongation of, 318, 322-323
   aspirin-related prolongation of, 179, 180, 181
   during cardiopulmonary bypass, 69
   following cardiopulmonary bypass, 274-275
   in congenital heart disease, 291, 292
   for heparin monitoring, 69
   preoperative evaluation of, 78
Blood banks
   blood-shield statutes for, 363-364, 368
   processing costs of, 77
Blood components
   allogenic, hematocrit indicator for, 217
   autologous, 219-221

Blood components *(cont.)*
   autologous *(cont.)*
      preoperative donation of, 219, 220
      salvage technique for, 219, 220
   pediatric use of, 295-296
   transfusion thresholds of, 216, 217
Blood conservation, intraoperative, **77-83**
   blood transfusion risks and, 129-130
   cell saver device for, 79-80, 82
   cell salvage process of, 86-89
   by postoperative drainage reinfusion, 82
   salvaged blood syndrome and, **85-93**
Blood sampling techniques, 71-72
Blood shield statutes, 363-364, 368, 378
Blood transfusions
   in acute myocardial infarction, 182
   adverse reactions to
      incidence of, 215
      physician's failure to recognize, 371-372
      during plasmapheresis, 226
   allogenic, risks of, 215
   aprotinin and, 133, 134, 135, 136, 137
   autologous, 232-233
      during cardiopulmonary bypass, 78-79
   blood-shield statutes regarding, 363-364, 368, 378
   of contaminated blood, 232, 367-369
   following failed thrombolytic therapy, 182
   medicolegal aspects of, **363-380**
      informed consent and, 372-378
      lawsuits, 367-370
      liability theories of, 364-366
   during open-heart surgery, 171, 172
   refusal of consent for, 376-378
   risks of, 129-130, 215
Blood viscosity, anticoagulant-related reduction of, 118, 119
Blood volume
   anticoagulant-related reduction of, 118, 119
   of children, 292, 293
Bradykinin, 148, 203-204
Breach of contract, 364

Calcium
   in hemostasis, 289, 290
   in thrombin formation, 250, 251
γ-Carboxylated glutamic acid, 15-16
   in coagulation localization, 4
   warfarin-related inhibition of, 312
Cardiac surgery. *See also* specific types of cardiac surgery
   blood transfusion requirements during, 129-130
   hemostasis during, 129-131
Cardiopulmonary bypass
   blood conservation during, **77-83**
   blood perfusion during, 355-356
   blood transfusions during, 215
   in children, **287-299**

Cardiopulmonary bypass *(cont.)*
  in children *(cont.)*
    anticoagulation and hemostasis techniques for, 292-297
    intraoperative techniques for, 292-296
    preoperative conditions affecting, 291-292
  hemostasis during, 31-41, 65, 66, 130-131, 167-168
  heparin anticoagulation protocol during, **57-64**
    inadequate, 61
  of heparin-induced thrombocytopenia patients, 193-195
  platelet count during, 32, 33, 195, 274
  as platelet function defect cause, 33-37, 195, 202-203, 274
  postoperative hemorrhage of, 274-276
    mediastinal reexploration for, 66, 216
    ventricular assist devices and, 266
  salvaged blood syndrome and, **85-93**
    platelet pathophysiology during, 89-91
    refractory platelets and, 91-92
  systemic anticoagulation monitoring during, **65-76**
Cardiotomy, platelet damage by, 274
Cardiotomy reservoir, blood stagnation in, 358
Carotid artery, internal dissection of, 329
Catecholamines, as platelet release reaction inducer, 24-25
Catheterization, arterial, prevention of complications of, 328
Cell-saver device, 79-80, 82
  as blood loss cause, 276
  pediatric use of, 295
Cell separators, 231-232
Centrifugal pump, 265, 268
Cerebrovascular disease patients, ticlopidine therapy for, 321
Chest-tube drainage, as reexploration indicator, 278
Children
  aprotinin dosage for, 151
  cardiopulmonary bypass in
    anticoagulation and hemostasis techniques for, 292-297
    intraoperative techniques for, 292-296
    preoperative factors affecting, 291-292
  compulsory blood transfusions for, 376
  congenital heart disease of, 207, 291, 292
  hemodilution in, 207, 292-294, 295-296
  hemostatic system development in, 287-288
  heparin resistance in, 162, 294
  normal hemostasis in, 289-291
Cholinesterase, plasmapheresis-related decrease of, 228
Circulating antigen-antibody complex, 24-25
Coagulation
  cascade of, 5, 6-7

Coagulation, cascade of *(cont.)*
  extrinsic pathway of, 3-4, 5, 99, 100, 289, 290
  intrinsic pathway of, 3, 5, 99, 100, 289, 290
  contact activation system of, 130, 131, 132, 147-149, 203-204
  initiation of, 5, 100
  injury-site localization of, 4-5
  serine protease inhibition during, 158
  in total artificial heart patients, 250-256
Coagulation factors, 27-29. *See also* specific coagulation factors
  in hemostasis, 26
  neonatal, 288
  synonyms of, 27
  warfarin-related inhibition of, 15-16
COBE Spectra system, 225, 234
Cold agglutinin disease, 230-231
Collagen
  in platelet activation, 24, 96, 98, 100
  in platelet adhesion, 2
  in platelet aggregation, 100, 274
Collagen-chamber test, 205
Communication, patient-physician, malpractice inplications of, 372
Complement
  aprotinin-related inhibition of, 132
  cardiopulmonary bypass-related activation of, 130, 358, 359
  in disseminated intravascular coagulation, 27
  extracorporeal circulation-related alterations of, 208
  in hemostasis, 26-27, 30
  heparin-related inhibition of, 354
  plasmapheresis-related activation of, 226
  protamine-related activation of, 67
  in salvaged blood syndrome, 220
Complement C3a degradation products, 275
Complement CSB-9, extracorporeal circulation-related increase of, 203
Congenital heart disease
  acyanotic, 291, 292, 293
  cyanotic, 40, 207, 272, 291, 293
Contact activating system, of coagulation, 130, 131, 132, 147-149, 203-204
Coronary artery bypass graft, occlusion of, 95-96, 98
Coronary artery bypass graft surgery
  for acute myocardial infarction, 178, 179
  antiplatelet therapy for, 104-105, **317-325**
  mechanical revascularization and, 177-178
  postoperative hemorrhage of
    aspirin-related, 209-210, 318-319
    incidence of, 271, 272
    management of, 169-172, 322-323
    risk assessment of, 318-322

Coronary artery surgery, aprotinin blood-conserving therapy during, 133
Coronary vein graft, aprotinin-related occlusion of, 139-140
Coumadin
  as cardiogenic embolism prophylactic, 335-336
  contraindications to
    in children, 292
    during pregnancy, 337
  as hemorrhage risk factor, 216
  as heparin alternative, 192
  preoperative use of, 78
  by heart transplant patients, 272
Cryoglobulin screening, preoperative, 273
Cryoprecipitates, for postoperative hemorrhage control, 218
CY 222, 14, 123
Cyanotic congenital heart disease
  in children, 207, 291, 293
  extracorporeal circulation-related platelet count decrease in, 207
  hemostatic disorders of, 291
  perioperative hemorrhage risk of, 40, 272
Cyclooxygenase, 100
  inhibition of, 26
Cytomegalovirus infection, blood transfusion-related, 232, 368

Dalen, James E., 303
D-dimer, 42, 43, 44
Defibrotide, 126
Dermatan sulfates, as venous thrombosis prophylactics, 124
Desmopressin
  as aspirin-related hemorrhage therapy, 323
  for cardiopulmonary bypass-related hemorrhage control, 36-37, 131, **165-175**, 182, 195, 279-280
Dextran, 15, 112, 123, 193
Dicoumarol, 15
Dipyridamole
  action mechanism of, 247-248, 333
  as adenosine-3'-5'-monophosphate inhibitor, 247-248
  as antithrombotic agent, 333
  in coronary artery bypass graft surgery, 104-105
  for femoral artery occlusion prophylaxis, 333-334
  as myocardial infarction prophylaxis, 103
  in percutaneous transluminal coronary angioplasty, 103-104
  for prosthetic heart valve patients, 45, 46, 105, 308-309, 310
  for total heart patients, 249-250
  for vascular reocclusion prophylaxis, 331, 332, 333
  preoperative administration of, 248, 272, 273, 322

Disintegrin, 318
Disseminated intravascular coagulation (DIC), 41
  as antifibrinolytic therapy contraindication, 181
  antithrombin III as indicator of, 38
  cardiopulmonary bypass-related, 38-39, 41, 266, 275
  complement in, 27
  as heart transplantation contraindication, 242-243
  as heparin complication, 58, 186
  hypotension and, 30, 216
  hypothermia and, 120
  kinin in, 27
  pathophysiology of, 5
  pinching phenomenon and, 241, 242, 244, 245-246
  salvaged blood syndrome and, 220
  shock in, 30
  thrombocytopenia and, 32
  in total artificial heart patients, 241-246, 259
D-Me-Phe-Pro-Arginal, 116
D-Phenyl-L-prolyl-L-arginyl-chloromethyl ketone, 106
DuP 714, 345-351

Ecchymoses, vascular permeability-related, 24
Edema, pulmonary, with left ventricular dysfunction, 182
Eicosanoids, antithrombin action of, 112
Embolectomy, heparin administration following, 328, 329
Embolism
  cardiogenic
    anticoagulant prophylaxis of, 335-336
    perfusion circuit-related, 355
    as prosthetic heart valve complication, 45-46
    ventricular assist device-related, 266-267
  pulmonary
    non-heparin therapy for, 193
    prophylaxis of, 120-125
Endarterectomy, reocclusion prevention following, 331, 332
Endocarditis, infective, 134
Endothelial plasminogen activator, 29
Endothelium, vascular
  cellular interactions of, 24
  function of, 353
  surgery-related injury of, 96
Endotoxin, as platelet release reaction inducer, 24-25
Enoxaparin, 14
Epidermal growth factor, in atherosclerosis, 98
Epinephrine, in primary hemostasis, 289
Epoprostenol, 321
Erythrocyte damage, during extracorporeal circulation, 208

Erythrocyte deformability, cardiopulmonary
  bypass-related decrease of, 275–276
Erythrocyte exchange, 234
Erythropoietin, 222–223
Euglobulin lysis time, 39
Extracorporeal circulation. *See also*
  Cardiopulmonary bypass
  hemostatic activation during, 201–204
  heparin-coated circuits of, **353–362**
  platelet monitoring during, 204–209

Factor II
  anticoagulant-related inhibition of, 252
  cardiopulmonary bypass-related inhibition
    of, 38, 275
  neonatal levels of, 288
  prothrombin time of, 216
Factor IIa
  heparin-antithrombin III complex-related
    inhibition of, 158, 160
  in thrombin formation, 251
Factor III, in thrombin formation, 250–251
Factor V
  activation of, 6, 30
  cardiopulmonary bypass-related inhibition
    of, 38, 275
  heparin-related inhibition of, 252
  neonatal levels of, 288
  plasmin-induced degradation of, 29
  in thrombin formation, 251
Factor Va
  protein C-related inactivation of, 8, 9
  in secondary hemostasis, 290
  in thrombin formation, 250–251
Factor VII
  anticoagulant-related inhibition of, 252
  as hypercoagulability marker, 142
  neonatal levels of, 288
  phospholipid membrane attachment by, 4
  prothrombin time measurement of, 216
  tissue factor binding by, 5
  warfarin-related inhibition of, 15, 16
Factor VIIa, in thrombin formation, 250, 251
Factor VII:C, cardiopulmonary bypass-related
  inhibition of, 38
Factor VIII
  activation of, 6
  hemodilution-related release of, 120
  neonatal levels of, 288
  plasmapheresis-related inhibition of, 228
  plasmin-related degradation of, 29
  in secondary hemostasis, 290
  in thrombin formation, 250
Factor VIIIa
  protein C-related inactivation of, 8, 9
  in thrombin formation, 251
Factor VIII:C, activation of, 30
Factor IX
  activation of, 5, 6–7
  anticoagulant-related inhibition of, 252

Factor IX *(cont.)*
  in fibrin clot formation, 27–28
  phospholipid membrane attachment by, 4
  plasmin-related degradation of, 29
  prothrombin time measurement of, 216
  warfarin-related inhibition of, 15, 16
Factor IXa
  activation of, 5
  antithrombin-related inhibition of, 8, 30
  in fibrin clot formation, 27–28
  heparin-antithrombin III complex-related
    inhibition of, 12, 158
  in secondary hemostasis, 290
  in thrombin formation, 250, 251
Factor X
  activation of, 4, 5, 6–7
    in total artificial heart patients, 240
  anticoagulant-related inhibition of, 252
  cardiopulmonary bypass-related inhibition
    of, 275
  neonatal levels of, 288
  phospholipid membrane attachment by, 4
  prothrombin time measurement of, 216
  warfarin-related inhibition of, 15, 16
Factor Xa
  activation of, 5, 6–7
  factor Va association of, 6–7
  formation of, 5, 28, 29
  hypercoagulability effect of, 254
  inhibition of
    by antithrombin, 8, 9, 30
    by heparin, 14, 113
    by heparin-antithrombin III complex,
      12, 158
    by recombinant tick anticoagulant
      peptide, 106
  in secondary hemostasis, 290
  serum level measurement of, 254
  in thrombin formation, 250–251
Factor XI
  activation of, 5, 6–7
  cardiopulmonary bypass-related inhibition
    of, 275
  neonatal levels of, 288
  plasmin-induced degradation of, 29
  in secondary hemostasis, 289
Factor XIa
  antithrombin-related inhibition of, 8
  in fibrin clot formation, 27–28
  heparin-antithrombin III complex-related
    inhibition of, 12, 158
  in secondary hemostasis, 290
Factor XII
  activation of, 5, 203
    during cardiopulmonary bypass, 39, 40,
      41, 130–131, 132, 148, 355–356
  deficiency of, 4
  in fibrin clot formation, 27
  neonatal levels of, 288
  in secondary hemostasis, 289–290

INDEX 387

Factor XIIa
  antithrombin-related inhibition of, 8, 30
  heparin-antithrombin III complex-related inhibition of, 12, 158
  immobilized heparin-related inhibition of, 354
  as inflammatory mediator, 148
  in secondary hemostasis, 289–290
Factor XIIb, as fibrinolysis stimulator, 148
Factor XIII
  activation of, 29
  in complement activation, 30
  in fibrinolytic system activation, 29
  neonatal levels of, 288
Factor XIIIa
  activation of, 29
  in secondary hemostasis, 290
Femoral artery occlusion, prevention of, 328, 333–334
Femoropopliteal vein bypass patients
  preoperative aspirin use by, 320
  reocclusion prevention for, 331, 332
Fetal warfarin syndrome, 337
Fetus, hemostatic system of, 287, 288
Fibrin
  binding site exposure for, 100
  formation of, 29
Fibrin clot. *See* Hemostatic clot
Fibrin degradation products, 291
  of cardiopulmonary bypass patients, 34, 275
  in cardiopulmonary bypass-related hemorrhage, 42, 43
  as platelet release reaction inducers, 24–25
  protamine-related increase of, 38
Fibrin glue, 43–44, 280
Fibrin monomer
  formation of, 6, 29
  as platelet release reaction inducer, 24–25
Fibrinogen
  cryoprecipitate-induced increase of, 181
  neonatal levels of, 288
  plasmapheresis-related decrease of, 228
  in platelet adhesion, 2
  in platelet aggregation, 2
  preoperative evaluation of, 272
    in acute myocardial infarction patients, 180
  transfusion thresholds of, 217
Fibrinolysis, 290–291
  aprotinin-related inhibition of, 132
  during cardiopulmonary bypass, 37–38, 39–40, 41, 43, 118, 130, 131, 266, 275, 280
  definition of, 105
  in neonates, 288
  management of, 44
  in total artificial heart patients, 241–246
Fibrinolytic system
  activation pathways of, 29–30

Fibrinolytic system *(cont.)*
  in hemostasis, 26
  inhibition of, 30
  of total artificial heart patients, 240
Fibrinopeptide, in congenital heart disease-related hemostasis, 291
Fibrinopeptide A
  in primary fibrinolysis, 43, 44
  in total artificial heart patients, 240
Fibrin polymers, as clot stabilizers, 6
Fibronectin, in platelet adhesion, 2
Fistula, ascending aortic, 280
Fitzgerald factor, 27. *See also* Williams factor
Flaujac factor, 27
Fletcher factor, 27. *See also* Prekallikrein
Flurbiprofen, 319, 323
Fontan operations, in children, 292
Fragment X, as platelet release reaction inducer, 24–25
Fragmin, 14
Free fatty acids, as platelet release reaction inducers, 24–25
Free radicals, 148, 149
Fresh frozen plasma, 218
  for heparin resistance reversal, 62
  for presurgical coagulation restoration, 181–182
Fujiwara factor, 27. *See also* Kininogen, high-molecular-weight

Gammaglobulin-coated surfaces, as platelet release reaction inducers, 24–25
Ghost particles, 202
Glue, for perioperative hemorrhage control, 43–44, 280
Glycoprotein(s), extracorporeal circulation-related changes of, 202–203
Glycoprotein Ib, 203
  cardiopulmonary bypass-related decrease of, 356, 357
  deficiency of, 289
  as platelet binding mediator, 2, 3
  platelet complex of, 189
  as von Willebrand's factor binding site, 96
Glycoprotein IIb/IIIa, 203
  cardiopulmonary bypass-related decrease of, 356, 357
  as von Willebrand's factor binding site, 96
Glycoprotein IV, 203
Glycosaminoglycan(s), as thromboembolism prophylactics, 124–125
Glycosaminoglycan-derived agents, anticoagulant activity of, 116, 117
Granulocyte-colony stimulating factor, 222–223

Hageman factor. *See* Factor XIII
HeartMate left ventricular assist device, 265, 267, 268–269

Heart transplantation
  contraindications to
    disseminated intravascular coagulation, 242-243
    pinching phenomenon, 244-245
    incidence of, 272
    ventricular assist devices and, 265, 266
Hematocrit
  during cardiopulmonary bypass, 275
  as hemodilution indicator, 206-207
  postoperative decrease of, 279
  of total artificial heart patients, 239
  transfusion thresholds of, 217
Hemoclar, 126
Hemodialysis, heparin substitutes for use during, 195
Hemodilution
  acute normovolemia, 219
  in children, 292-294, 295-296
  effect on anticoagulant responses, 120
  as hemorrhage risk factor, 216
  platelet count effects of, 206-207
  preoperative, 207
Hemofilter, pediatric use of, 295
Hemoglobin, transfusion thresholds of, 217
Hemolysis, effect on platelet function, 208
Hemophilia, desmopressin therapy for, 279, 280
Hemophilia A, 168
Hemorrhage, perioperative, **271-285**
  in acute myocardial infarction patients, 182
  antiplatelet agent-related, 317, 318-323
    management of, 322-323
    risk assessment of, 318-322
  aprotinin therapy for. *See* Aprotinin
  aspirin-related, 14, 137-138, 209-210
    desmopressin therapy for, 323
    reoperation for, 319, 320
  aspirin/warfarin concomitant therapy-related, 17
  causes of, 273-278
  complications of, 271
  desmopressin therapy for. *See* Desmopressin
  diagnosis of, 41-43
  fibrinolysis activation-related, 118
  heparin-related, 14, 58, 66, 335, 336, 343
  incidence of, 271-272
  intracranial, as thrombolytic therapy contraindication, 179
  management of, 43-44, 279-281, 322-323
  mechanisms of, 167-168, 355-356
  patterns of, 278-279
  plasmapheresis-related, 228
  predisposing factors for, 41
  preoperative hemostasis screening for, 31-32
  preoperative patient evaluation for, 272-273
  prevention of, 31-32, 168-172

Hemorrhage *(cont.)*
  reexploratory surgery for, 66, 133-134, 135-136, 278-279, 319, 320
  thrombolytic drug-related, 178-179
  in total artificial heart patients, 243
  types of, 42
  ventricular assist device-related, 266
  vitamin K antagonist-related, 337
  warfarin-related, 17-18
Hemostasis
  during cardiac surgery, 129-131
    anticoagulant interactions and, 118-119
  during cardiopulmonary bypass, 31-41, 65, 66, 167-168
    pathology of, 32-40
  initiation of, 3-4
  normal, 1-9
  patient variability in, 142
  physiology of, 23-31
  preoperative screening of, 31-32
  primary, 1, 2, 23-24, 289
  secondary, 1-2, 3-6, 289
Hemostatic clot, formation of, 2, 23-24, 255
Hemostatic system, development of, 287-288
HemoTec Heparin Management System, 160-162
Hemotrauma, during extracorporeal circulation, 207
Heparin, **57-64**, 255-256
  action mechanisms of, 12, 13, 58, 111, 113
  activated clotting time of, 57, 58, 61
    in autologous transfusions, 78-79
    dosing regimen application of, 80, 81
  in acute conditions, 329-330
  administration protocol of, 58-60
  alternatives to, 67, 111, 116-120, 192-195
  antithrombin binding by, 12
  antithrombin III binding by, 6, 8, 58, 122, 123, 158, 159-160, 354
  aprotinin interaction of, 119
  as cardiogenic embolism prophylactic, 335
  in chronic conditions, 330
  complications of, 58, 66
  concomitant aprotinin administration, 141-142, 158-163
  concomitant aspirin administration, 328
  disadvantages of, 343
  endogenous cofactors of, 120
  factor Xa interaction of, 254
  half-life of, 14
    in children, 294
  hemodilution and, 120
  immune reactions of, 188-192, 194-195, 222
  inadequate dosage of, 40
  intravenous administration of, 328
  low-dose, use during cardiopulmonary bypass, 256
  low-molecular-weight, 112-116
    action mechanisms of, 14
    advantages of, 343

Heparin *(cont.)*
  low-molecular-weight *(cont.)*
    anticoagulant efficacy of, 345, 346–347, 349
    bleeding time effects of, 347–348, 349, 350, 351
    as deep venous thrombosis prophylactic, 120–123
    hemodynamic effects of, 347, 350
    inability to inhibit thrombin, 12
    as low-dose heparin substitute, 122
    new applications of, 114–115
    safety of, 345, 350–351
  monitoring of, 57, 58–60, 61
  as myocardial infarction therapy, 179
  neutralization of, 12, 14. *See also* Protamine
  nitroglycerin interaction of, 14
  pediatric use of, 294–295
  as perioperative hemorrhage risk factor, 14, 58, 66, 335, 336, 343
    evaluation assay for, 42, 43
  pharmacology of, 11–14
  platelet count effects of, 205
  platelet retention effects of, 206
  as polycomponent drug, 112, 113
  preoperative administration of, 67, 78, 272
    heparin resistance and, 162
  as prosthetic materials coating, 353, 354, 355–358
  side effects of, 115, 118. *See also* Thrombocytopenia, heparin-induced
  structure of, 11–12
  synthetic analogues of, 116
  systemic, monitoring of, 66–72
  thrombin binding by, 12, 13
  as thrombin inhibitor, 252
  titration of, 80, 81, 82
  for total artificial heart patients, 257–258
  unfractionated
    intraoperative use of, 320–321
    potentiation of, 322
    preoperative use of, 323
  as unstable angina pectoris therapy, 101–102
  as ventricular assist device coating, 267
Heparin-antithrombin III complex, activated clotting time
  prolongation effects of, 159–160
Heparin cofactor II, 122, 240, 251
Heparin concentration test, 69
Heparin dose/activated clotting time response, 162
Heparin dose curve/response, 294
Heparin dose/response technique, 294, 295
Heparin-induced platelet antibodies, 187–188, 222
Heparin rebound, 60–61, 343
  as cardiopulmonary bypass-related hemorrhage cause, 40, 275
  in children, 296

Heparin rebound *(cont.)*
  management of, 44
  prevention of, 81, 82
Heparin resistance, 61–62, 115
  in children, 162, 294
  heparin preoperative administration and, 67
Heparin sulfates, as venous thrombosis prophylactics, 124
Hirsh, Jack, 303
Hirudin, 116–117, 119
  antithrombotic activity of, 18, 105, 106, 112
  as heparin alternative, 67
  recombinant, 106, 117–118
    comparison with heparin, 345–351
    in heparin-induced thrombocytopenia patients, 195
  as thrombosis prophylactic, 126
  as surgical anticoagulant, 117–118
Hirulog, antithrombotic efficacy of, 18
Histamine, protamine-induced release of, 62–63
Hospitals, vicarious liability of, 366–367
Human immune deficiency virus (HIV) infection
  blood transfusion-related, 367–369, 372, 373
  of physicians, disclosure of, 375–376
Human immune deficiency virus (HIV) testing, of blood, 368
Hydroxyethyl starch, as plasmapheresis replacement colloid, 226
Hypercoagulability
  factor VII marker of, 142
  of total artificial heart patients, 242, 243–244, 246
Hyperplasia, neointimal, 331
Hypersensitivity, heparin-related, 337
Hyperviscosity syndrome, plasmapheresis for, 229
Hypocoagulability, thrombodynamic potential index of, 253–254
Hypofibrinogenemia, during cardiopulmonary bypass, 37, 38
Hypotension
  of autologous blood donors, 220
  hypoxemia-related, 216
  mediastinal blood transfusion-related, 220–221
Hypothermia
  for children, 294
  as cold agglutinin disease cause, 230–231
  effect on anticoagulant action, 119–120
  as hemorrhage risk factor, 40, 216
  for neonates, 296
  preoperative tests for, 31–32

Iloprost, 193, 321–322
Immune responses, endothelial-cellular interactions in, 24

Immune system, extracorporeal circulation response of, 208
Immunocompromised patients, plasmapheresis in, 228
Immunoglobulin G
  in heparin-induced thrombocytopenia, 186, 187, 188
  plama exchange removal of, 227
Immunoglobulin M, plasma exchange removal of, 227, 228, 231
Infants
  fresh whole blood vs. blood component transfusions for, 295–296
  hypothermia for, 296
  platelet counts of, 287
Inflammatory mediators, endothelial-cellular interactions in, 24
Inflammatory response. *See also* Coagulation, cascade of
  cardiopulmonary bypass-related, 130, 131, 355–356
  contact activation system-mediated, 147–149
  heparin-coated circuits and, 358–359
Informed consent
  for blood transfusions, 372–378
  legal exceptions to, 373–374
Informed refusal, 374
Internal mammary artery bypass, perioperative hemorrhage risk of, 272, 273, 278
International Sensitivity Index, of coagulation, 306–307
Intraaortic balloon counterpulsation
  in heparin-induced thrombocytopenia patients, 195
  heparin resistance and, 162
Ischemia, lower-extremity, 328–329
Ischemic coronary syndromes, pathophysiology of, 100–101
Ivy bleeding time
  antiplatelet agent-related increase of, 318
  preoperative, 273
  in total artificial heart patients, 240

Jehovah's Witnesses, blood transfusion refusal by, 376–377

Kallikrein
  activation of, during cardiopulmonary bypass, 130, 355–356
    blockage of, 132, 133
  antithrombin-related inhibition of, 8, 30
  as fibrinolysis stimulator, 148
  formation of, 203–204
  heparin-antithrombin III complex-related inhibition of, 158
  as inflammatory mediator, 148
  in secondary hemostasis, 289–290

Kallikrein inactivation units, 149–150
Kinin
  in disseminated intravascular coagulation, 27
  in hemostasis, 26
  in thrombohemorrhage, 30
Kininogen
  conversion to bradykinin, 203
  high-molecular-weight, 27
    deficiency of, 4
    neonatal levels of, 288
    prekallikrein complex, 5, 6–7
  high-molecular-weight *(cont.)*
    in secondary hemostasis, 289

Lactobionic acid amide, 124
Left ventricular dysfunction, in acute myocardial infarction, 178, 182
Liability
  in blood transfusion-related lawsuits, 364–367
  definition of, 379
Lipoprotein-associated coagulation inhibitor, 251
Liver disease, prothrombin time prolongation in, 180, 181–182
Lomoparan, 125–126, 193, 194–195
Loyola University Medical Center, blood preservation protocol of, **77–83**

Macrophage, in primary hemostasis, 24
Malpractice lawsuits
  blood transfusion-related, **363–380**
    informed consent and, 372–378
    liability theories of, 364–366
    legal terminology of, 378–379
Mediastinal blood, autologous transfusion of, 220–221
Methylprednisolone, 323
Myeloproliferative disorders, platelet dysfunction in, 34
Myocardial infarction
  aprotinin-related, 139, 140
  aspirin prophylaxis for, 102, 103
  aspirin therapy for, 102–103
  cardiogenic shock following, 265
  following failed thrombolysis, **177–184**
    coagulation restoration in, 180–182
    presurgical evaluation of, 179–180
  heparin prophylaxis for, 102
  pathophysiology of, 100, 102
  reinfarction prevention in, 102, 103
  streptokinase therapy for, 102

Negligence
  blood transfusion-related, 364, 366–367, 371–372
  definition of, 379
  vicarious liability for, 366–367

Neutrophil
  in primary hemostasis, 24
  in salvaged blood syndrome, 90–91
Neutrophil-activating peptide-2, 91
Nitrates, hemostatic system impairment by, 323
Nitroglycerin, interaction with heparin, 14
Nitroprusside, pediatric use of, 296
Novacor pulsatile device, 265, 268

Oncotic pressure maintenance, in children, 293–294
Open-heart surgery. *See also* Cardiopulmonary bypass
  hemorrhage control during, 169–172
ORG 10172, 14, 67
Osteoporosis, heparin-related, 337
Oxygenation
  bubble, 274, 275
  effect on contact activation system, 147
  as hemotrauma cause, 208
  membrane, 357
    activated clotting time during, 160
    comparison with bubble oxygenation, 275
    pediatric use of, 293
    steroid administration with, 275
    platelet aggregation effects of, 36
  as thrombocytopenia cause, 33

Pacemaker, defective, legal liability for, 364–365
Partial thromboplastin time (PTT)
  in cyanotic congenital heart disease, 291
  preoperative, 273
Pentasaccharide, with antithrombin III affinity, 123–124
Peptide conjugates, anticoagulant activity of, 116–117, 119
Peripheral vascular disease, anticoagulants for, **327–341**
  for early thrombosis prevention, 327, 328–330
  for long-term thrombosis prevention, 327, 330–336
Peripheral vascular surgery patients, preoperative aspirin use by, 320
Petechiae, vascular permeability-related, 24
Pharmacodynamics, 2, 11
Pharmacokinetics, 1, 2, 9–11
Pharmacology
  of anticoagulation, **1–21**
    normal hemostasis and, 1–9
    of specific anticoagulants, 11–18
  clinical, 1, 2
Phenprocoumon, 15
Phospholipase A_2
  activation of, 25
  serin-related inhibition of, 157–158

Physical examination, preoperative, 273
Physicians, disclosure of HIV status by, 375–376
Pinching phenomenon, 240, 241, 242, 244, 245–246, 253–254
Plasma half-life, 10
Plasmapheresis
  in heparin-induced thrombocytopenia patients, 195
  indications for, 229–231
  plasma volume exchange during, 227–228
  volume replacement colloid for, 226
Plasma products, autologous transfusion of, 232–234
Plasma protein, in hemostasis, 26–27
Plasma saver, 215
Plasmin
  antithrombin-related inhibition of, 8
  as complement activator, 30
  formation of, 29
  heparin-antithrombin III complex-related inhibition of, 158
  proteolytic activity of, 29, 291
Plasminogen
  conversion to plasmin, 29, 30
  neonatal levels of, 288
  synthetic substrate level evaluation of, 42
  in total artificial heart patients, 240
Plasminogen activation pathway, 290–291
Plasminogen activator inhibitors, 30
Platelet
  fetal development of, 287
  pseudopod formation by, 25
  zones of, 24
Platelet activation, 25
  adenosine diphosphate-related, 96, 98, 99
  during cardiopulmonary bypass, 168, 202–203
  during extracorporeal circulation, 202–203
  heparin-induced thrombocytopenia-dependent, 189–190, 192
  prostacyclin related inhibition of, 131–132
  prostaglandin-related, 98, 99, 100
  serotonin-related, 98
  in unstable angina pectoris, 101
Platelet adhesion, 25, 26
  aprotinin-related inhibition of, 157–158
  cardiopulmonary bypass-related inhibition of, 34
  mechanisms of, 2, 3
  in thrombosis, 96, 98
  ticlopidine-related inhibition of, 249
Platelet aggregation
  aprotinin-related inhibition of, 157
  during cardiopulmonary bypass, 35–36, 167–168, 202, 203
  extracorporeal circulation-related, 202, 203
  in heparin-induced thrombocytopenia, 186, 187

Platelet aggregation *cont.*)
 inducing agents of, 98, 100
 inhibitors of, 157, 317-318
 mechanisms of, 2-3
 neonatal, 287
 in oxygenator reservoir, 202, 203
 secondary wave of, 25
 in thrombosis, 96, 98-100
 in total artificial heart patients, 239, 246-250
Platelet-associated immunoglobulin, in total artificial heart patients, 240
Platelet cohesion, 25, 26
Platelet concentrate, for hemorrhage control, 218-219
Platelet count
 cardiopulmonary bypass-related changes of, 32, 33, 167-168, 202, 205, 274-275
 for cardiopulmonary bypass-related hemorrhage evaluation, 42
 hemodilution effects on, 206-207
 heparin-related decrease of, 66, 185
 neonatal, 287
 preoperative evaluation of, 31, 78, 273
 in acute myocardial infarction, 180
 of total artificial heart patients, 239
 transfusion thresholds of, 217
Platelet degranulation
 during cardiopulmonary bypass, 35, 202
 in total artificial heart patients, 247-248, 249-250
Platelet-derived growth factor, in atherosclerosis, 98
Platelet dysfunction
 aspirin-related, 272-273
 cardiopulmonary bypass-related, 33-37, 41, 43, 44, 130
 drug-related, 119
 heparin-related, 67
Platelet factor 3, 25
Platelet factor 4
 cardiopulmonary bypass-related increase of, 35-36
 in congenital heart disease-related hemostasis, 291
 extracorporeal circulation-related release of, 202
 hemodilution-related release of, 120
 in heparin-induced thrombocytopenia, 336-337
 platelet adhesion-related release of, 4
 recombinant, as heparin antagonist, 14
 in total artificial heart patients, 239, 246, 247, 248, 249
Platelet function, 24-26, 289. *See also* Hemostasis
 factors affecting, 24, 25, 34-36
 monitoring of, **201-213**
  with platelet reactivity test, 209-212

Platelet function inhibitors. *See also* Antiplatelet therapy
 in peripheral occlusive arterial disease, 333-334
Platelet reactivity index, 209-210, 211
Platelet reactivity test, 209-212
Platelet release reaction. *See also* Platelet activation
 induction of, 24-25
Platelet retention test, 205, 206, 207
Platelet-rich plasma, preoperative autologous, 221-222
Polycythemia, in cyanotic congenital heart disease, 291
Polytetrafluoroethylene graft, platelet deposition on, 331, 332, 333
Positive end-expiratory pressure (PEEP), 281
Postperfusion organ dysfunction syndrome, 358
Pregnancy
 compulsory blood transfusions during, 376
 coumadin contraindication during, 337
Prekallikrein, 27
 conversion to kallikrein, 203-204
 neonatal levels of, 288
 in secondary hemostasis, 289
Prekallikrein-high-molecular-weight kininogen complex, 5, 6-7
Procoagulant fraction, neonatal levels of, 288
Procoagulant system
 thrombin inhibition equilibrium of, 252
 of total artificial heart patients, 239-240
Procoagulation reactions, 27-29. *See also* Coagulation
Prostacyclin
 adenosine-3'-5'-cyclic adenosine interaction of, 131, 318
 for cardiopulmonary bypass hemorrhage control, 131-132, 168, 321
 chemically-synthesized, 321
 as platelet activation inhibitor, 319
 therapeutic use of, 26
Prostaglandin(s), as platelet activators, 98, 99, 100
Prostaglandin G_2, 25-26, 100
Prostaglandin H_2, 25-26, 100
Prostaglandin I_2, 100
Prosthetic heart valve patients
 antithrombotic therapy for, 105, **301-315**
 dosage recommendations for, 304-307
 mechanical valve patients, 308-311, 312
 tissue valve patients, 307-308, 312-313
 thromboembolism incidence in, 302
Prosthetic heart valves
 complications of, 45
 hemostasis and, 44-46
Prosthetic materials
 as extacorporeal circulation circuit coating, **353-362**
 as intrinsic coagulation initiators, 5

Protamine, 57, 60–61
　administration protocol for, 67
　adverse reactions to, 62–63, 66, 67, 343
　dosage calculations for, 58–60
　dosage requirements of, 67
　as fibrinogen degradation product stimulator, 38
　as hemorrhage cause, 40–41, 66
　heparin dosage relationship of, 209
　heparin interaction of, 67
　Hepcon titration of, 80–81, 82
　pediatric use of, 295
　platelet membrane effects of, 274
　split injections of, 81, 82
　timing of administration, 209
Protein C
　activation of, 8, 9, 118
　anticoagulant-related inhibition of, 252
　neonatal levels of, 288
　phospholipid membrane attachment by, 4
　as procoagulant system inhibitor, 30
　as thrombin inhibitor, 251
　in total artificial heart patients, 240
　warfarin-related inhibition of, 15, 16
Protein kinase C, cAMP-related inhibition of, 247
Protein S, 8, 9
　anticoagulant-related inhibition of, 252
　phospholipid membrane attachment by, 4
　as procoagulant system inhibitor, 30
　as thrombin inhibitor, 251
　in total artificial heart patients, 240
　warfarin-related inhibition of, 15
Proteins induced by vitamin K absence (PIVKAs), 29
Prothrombin
　normal form of, 28
　plasma abnormal form of, 28
　warfarin-related inhibition of, 15, 16
Prothrombinase, in thrombin formation, 250
Prothrombin time (PT), 11
　in cardiopulmonary bypass-related hemorrhage, 42, 216
　in cyanotic congenital heart disease, 291
　decrease of, 254
　definition of, 216
　liver disease-related prolongation of, 180, 181–182
　normal, in hemorrhage, 216
　for oral anticoagulant monitoring, 253
　preoperative evaluation of, 31, 78, 273
　　in acute myocardial infarction patients, 180
　prolongation factors of, 180
　in total artificial heart patients, 239–240
　transfusion thresholds of, 217
　warfarin-related prolongation of, 17, 179
Prothrombin time ratio, of warfarin therapy, 304–305, 306, 307–308, 309, 310, 312

Prothrombosis, aprotinin-related, 139–140, 142
Pulmonary artery catheterization, for left ventricular dysfunction, 182
Pulmonary artery shunt, in children, 292
Purpura, vascular permeability-related, 24

Raby's K test, 240
Raby's transfer test, 240, 255, 256
Red factor, 27
Refusal of consent, for blood transfusions, 376–378
Reoperative cardiac surgery, for hemorrhage control, 66, 278–279, 319, 320
　aprotinin blood-conserving therapy during, 133–134, 135–136
Reptilase time
　in acute myocardial infarction patients, 180
　for cardiopulmonary bypass-related hemorrhage evaluation, 42, 43
　in total artificial heart patients, 240
Respiratory distress
　aprotinin therapy for, 132
　salvaged blood syndrome-related, 85, 92
Revascularization
　of heparin-induced thrombocytopenia patients, 320–321
　mechanical, following thrombolytic therapy, 177–178
　myocardial, aprotinin therapy for, 152, 153, 154, 155
　reoperative, 272
Rheumatic valve disease, 45
Rh sensitization, blood transfusion-related, 365–366, 369

Salvaged blood syndrome, **85–93**, 220
Saphenous vein graft, occlusion of, 104
Serine proteases, 147–148
　inhibitors of, 149, 343–344
Serotinin
　as platelet activator, 98
　in primary hemostasis, 289
Serotonin release test, 186, 187
Shock, postcardiotomy cardiogenic, 265
Sickle-cell hemoglobinopathy, preoperative erythrocyte exchange in, 234
SMA 12/60 biomedical screening survey, 31
Sternal closure, delayed, 280–281
Streptokinase
　fibrinogen depleting effect of, 178–179
　as fibrinolytic system activator, 29–30
　as hemorrhage risk factor, 276, 277
　as plasminogen activator stimulator, 277
　as surgical revascularization adjunct, 178
　systemic, 277
Strict liability, 364–365
Stroke, hemorrhagic, aspirin-related, 102

Sudden ischemic death, 100, 101
Suleparoide, 124-125
Sulfinpyrazone
  as angina therapy, 101
  as cyclooxygenase inhibitor, 26
  as prosthetic heart valve-related thromboembolism prophylactic, 45

Tamponade, controlled, 281
Template bleeding time, 31
Therapeutic privilege, 373-374
Thoratec pulsatile assist device, 265
Thrombin
  formation of, 4, 6-7, 28, 29, 100, 250-251, 289
  functions of, 6-7, 29
  phospholipid membrane attachment by, 4
  as platelet aggregation promoter, 100
  in platelet-mediated arterial thrombosis, 105
  as platelet release reaction inducer, 24-25
  as protein C activator, 118
  in secondary hemostasis, 289, 290
Thrombin inhibitors, 30, 251-252. *See also* Antithrombotics
  as heparin alternative, 344
  new, 343-352
  selective, 18, 105-106
Thrombin time
  for cardiopulmonary bypass-related hemorrhage evaluation, 42, 43
  in myocardial infarction therapy, 180
Thrombocytopenia. *See also* Platelet count
  activated clotting time in, 69
  in acute myocardial infarction, 181
  cardiopulmonary bypass-related, 32-33, 205
    in children, 296
  cardiopulmonary bypass hemorrhage and, 41, 44, 266, 273, 274
  in congenital heart disease, 291, 292
  extracorporeal circulation-related decrease of, 205
  heparin-induced, 58, **185-199**, 336-337
    aspirin therapy for, 320
    diagnosis of, 186-187
    incidence of, 14
    management of, 192-195
    as morbidity cause, 66-67
    as mortality cause, 66-67
    pathophysiology of, 187-192
    plasmapheresis for, 229-230
    prevention of, 195-196
    revascularization for, 320-321
    with thrombosis, 14, 320-321. *See also* Thrombosis, heparin-induced
  neonatal, 287
  types of, 274-275
Thrombodynamic potential index, 240, 244, 253-254

Thromboelastography, 69-71
  clot formation time measurement by, 69-70
  as postoperative hemorrhage indicator, 157
  of total artificial heart patients, 240, 243-244
Thromboembolism. *See also* Embolism; Thrombosis
  prosthetic heart valve-related, 45-46
  ventricular assist device-related, 265, 266-267
β-Thromboglobulin
  in congenital heart disease-related hemostasis, 291
  extracorporeal circulation-related release of, 202
  in total artificial heart patients, 239, 247, 248, 249
Thrombolytic therapy. *See* Antithrombotics
Thrombomodulin, 8, 9
Thrombosis
  anticoagulant prophylaxis of, **327-341**
    in acute conditions, 328-330
    in chronic conditions, 330-336
    side effects of, 336-337
  in aortocoronary bypass graft patients, 210-212
  deep-vein
    non-heparin therapy for, 193
    heparin therapy for, 327
    prophylaxis of, 114-115, 120-125
  heparin-induced, 14, 58, 185-186, 320-321
    as amputation cause, 190-191
    arterial, 190, 191, 192, 193
    plasmapheresis for, 229
  in ischemic coronary syndromes, 100, 101, 102
  mechanisms of, 96-100
Thrombospondin, in platelet adhesion, 2
Thromboxane, 63, 318, 319
Thromboxane A_2
  formation of, 26
  in platelet activation, 100
  in platelet aggregation, 2
  in primary hemostasis, 289
Thromboxane B_2
  aprotinin-related inhibition of, 157-158
  aspirin-related inhibition of, 272, 273
  in congenital heart disease-related hemostasis, 291
  extracorporeal circulation-related increase of, 202
Tick anticoagulant peptide, recombinant, 106
Ticlopidine
  antithrombotic activity of, 333, 334
  as aspirin alternative, 321
  as platelet activation inhibitor, 318
  as platelet adhesion inhibitor, 249
  as postoperative hemorrhage risk factor, 322
  pre-coronary artery bypass graft administration of, 321

Tissue factor
  as coagulation initiator, 5
  factor VII complex of, 290
Tissue factor pathway inhibitor, 5, 8, 9, 112
Tissue plasminogen activator
  desmopressin-related release of, 37
  endothelial release of, 148
  as fibrinolytic system activator, 29-30
  as hemorrhage risk factor, 276, 277
  inhibitors of, 30
  recombinant, 178-179, 240
  in total artificial heart patients, 240
Total artificial heart, long-term use of, 256-258
Total artificial heart patients, hemostasis control and treatment in, **237-264**
  assessment tests for, 239-241
  therapeutic objectives in, 241-256
Tranexamic acid
  dosage of, 44
  as fibrinolytic system inhibitor, 30
  for perioperative hemorrhage control, 131, 279, 280
  for presurgical coagulation restoration, 181
Transforming growth factor-beta, in atherosclerosis, 98
Transfusion medicine specialist, 215, 216, 222-223
Transfusion thresholds, 216, 217
Trypsin inhibitory units, 149
Tumor necrosis factor, 358

Urokinase
  fibrinogen depleting effects of, 178-179
  as fibrinolytic system activator, 29-30
  as hemorrhage risk factor, 276, 277

Valve replacement. *See also* Prosthetic heart valve patients
  in children, 292
  incidence of, 272
Vascular injury, types of, 95
Vascular occlusion, long-term prevention of, 330-336
Vascular reconstructive surgery, reocclusion prevention following, 331-333
Vasculature, in hemostasis, 23-24
Vasoactive substances, extracorporeal circulation-related increase of, 203, 208
Venous bypass, reocclusion prevention following, 331, 332, 333
Venous bypass graft disease, phases of, 95-96
Venous occlusion test, in total artificial heart patients, 240

Ventricular devices, **265-270**
  anticoagulation protocols for, 267-269
  complications of, 265, 266-267
  heparin-coated, 355
Viruses, as platelet release reaction inducers, 24-25
Vitamin K
  in fibrin clot formation, 28-29
  in internal carotid artery dissection, 329
Vitamin K antagonists, 15-18, 252, 253
  long-term use of, 327
  for percutaneous transluminal angioplasty patients, 334
  for vascular occlusion prevention, 330-331
  side effects of, 337
Vitamin K deficiency, 181
Vitamin K-dependent coagulation factors, 28
  abnormal, 29
  neonatal levels of, 288
Vitronectin, in platelet adhesion, 2
von Willebrand's disease, 289
  desmopressin therapy for, 168, 279, 280
  platelet dysfunction in, 34
von Willebrand's factor
  in acyanotic congenital heart disease, 292
  deficiency of, 289
  desmopressin interaction of, 131
  neonatal levels of, 288
  as platelet binding mediator, 2, 3
  in primary hemostasis, 289

Warfarin
  action mechanism of, 15-16
  antagonists of, 17
  contraindication during pregnancy, 18
  as deep-vein thrombosis therapy, 193
  drug interactions of, 17
  fetal syndrome of, 337
  as hemorrhage cause, 17-18, 40
  long-term use of, 327
  as myocardial infarction therapy, 179
  pharmacology of, 16-17
  for prosthetic heart valve patients, 45, 46, **301-315**
    dosage recommendations for, 304-307
  prothrombin time effect of, 182
  as skin necrosis cause, 18
White clot, 185-186
  of aorta, 194
White-clot syndrome, 329, 336-337
Williams factor, 27
Wrongful death action
  blood transfusion-related, 377-378
  definition of, 379
Wu-Hoak coefficient, 249
Wu-Hoak test, 240